CANCER
MANAGEMENT
in Small Animal Practice

CANCER MANAGEMENT
in Small Animal Practice

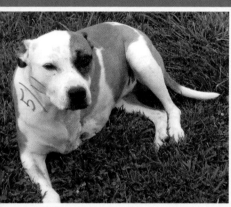 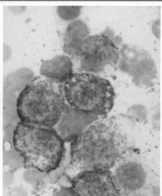 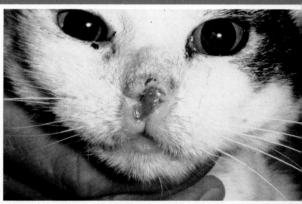

Carolyn J. Henry, DVM, MS, DACVIM (Oncology)
Professor of Oncology
Department of Veterinary Medicine and Surgery
College of Veterinary Medicine, and
Division of Hematology/Oncology
School of Medicine;
Director
Tom and Betty Scott Endowed Program in Veterinary Oncology
University of Missouri
Columbia, Missouri

Mary Lynn Higginbotham, DVM, MS, DACVIM (Oncology)
Assistant Professor of Oncology
Department of Clinical Sciences
College of Veterinary Medicine
Kansas State University
Manhattan, Kansas

SAUNDERS

ELSEVIER

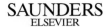

3251 Riverport Lane
Maryland Heights, Missouri 63043

CANCER MANAGEMENT IN SMALL ANIMAL PRACTICE
Copyright © 2010 Saunders, an imprint of Elsevier, Inc.

ISBN: 978-1-4160-3183-3

Notice

Knowledge and best practice in this field are constantly changing. As new research and experience broaden our knowledge, changes in practice, treatment and drug therapy may become necessary or appropriate. Readers are advised to check the most current information provided (i) on procedures featured or (ii) by the manufacturer of each product to be administered, to verify the recommended dose or formula, the method and duration of administration, and contraindications. It is the responsibility of the practitioner, relying on their own experience and knowledge of the patient, to make diagnoses, to determine dosages and the best treatment for each individual patient, and to take all appropriate safety precautions. To the fullest extent of the law, neither the Publisher nor the Authors assume any liability for any injury and/or damage to persons or property arising out of or related to any use of the material contained in this book.

The Publisher

Library of Congress Cataloging in Publication Data
Cancer management in small animal practice / [edited by] Carolyn J. Henry, Mary Lynn Higginbotham.
    p. ; cm.
    Includes bibliographical references and index.
    ISBN 978-1-4160-3183-3 (pbk. : alk. paper) 1. Veterinary oncology. I. Henry, Carolyn J. II. Higginbotham, Mary Lynn.
    [DNLM: 1. Cat Diseases–therapy. 2. Neoplasms–veterinary. 3. Dog Diseases–therapy. SF 986.C33 C215 2010]
    SF910.T8C36 2010
    636.089'6994–dc22

2009042648

Vice President and Publisher: Linda Duncan
Senior Acquisitions Editor: Anthony Winkel
Developmental Editor: Maureen Slaten
Publishing Services Manager: Patricia Tannian
Senior Project Manager: John Casey
Design Direction: Margaret Reid

Printed in Canada

Last digit is the print number: 9   8   7   6   5   4   3   2   1

Contributors

Gregory T. Almond, DVM, DACVR
Clinical Assistant Professor
Department of Radiation Oncology
College of Veterinary Medicine
Auburn University
Auburn, Alabama
Radiation Therapy: Management of Radiation Toxicity and Complications

Kathryn J. Atkinson, DVM, MS, DACVIM (Cardiology)
Cardiologist
Cardiology Northwest
Portland, Oregon
Tumors of the Thoracic Cavity: Cardiac and Heart-Based Tumors

Linda M. Berent, DVM, PhD, DACVP
Clinical Assistant Professor
Department of Veterinary Pathobiology
College of Veterinary Medicine
University of Missouri
Columbia, Missouri
The Cytology of Neoplasia

Philip J. Bergman, DVM, MS, PhD, DACVIM (Oncology)
Chief Medical Officer
BrightHeart Veterinary Centers
Armonk, New York
Immunotherapy

David A. Bommarito, DVM, DACVR (Radiation Oncology)
Resident, Medical Oncology
Department of Veterinary Medicine and Surgery
College of Veterinary Medicine
University of Missouri
Columbia, Missouri
Radiation Therapy: External Beam Radiation Therapy (Teletherapy) and Brachytherapy

William R. Brawner, DVM, DACVR
Professor
Department of Clinical Sciences
College of Veterinary Medicine
Auburn University
Auburn, Alabama
Radiation Therapy: Management of Radiation Toxicity and Complications

Matthew Breen, PhD, C.Biol, M.I.Biol
Professor
Department of Molecular Biomedical Sciences
College of Veterinary Medicine
North Carolina State University
Raleigh, North Carolina
Genetic Basis of Cancer

William G. Brewer, Jr., DVM, DACVIM (Oncology and Internal Medicine)
Staff Oncologist and Internist
Affiliated Animal Care
Chesapeake, Virginia
Imaging Methods in Cancer Diagnosis: Endoscopy

Bonnie Brugmann, DVM
Resident
Department of Clinical Sciences
College of Veterinary Medicine
Auburn University
Auburn, Alabama
Tumors of the Abdominal Cavity: Liver, Gall Bladder, and Non-Endocrine Pancreatic Tumors

Jeffrey N. Bryan, DVM, MS, PhD, DACVIM (Oncology)
Assistant Professor
College of Veterinary Medicine
Washington State University
Pullman, Washington
Radiation Therapy: Radioisotopes in Cancer Therapy
Photodynamic Therapy
Tumors of the Abdominal Cavity: Renal Tumors
Tumors of the Abdominal Cavity: Prostate Tumors
Tumors of the Hematopoietic System: Lymphoma
Tumors of the Hematopoietic System: Leukemia
Tumors of the Hematopoietic System: Multiple Myeloma
Tumors of the Endocrine System: Adrenal and Pituitary Tumors
Tumors of the Endocrine System: Thyroid Tumors
Tumors of the Endocrine System: Parathyroid Tumors
Tumors of the Endocrine System: Pancreatic Tumors

Ruthanne Chun, DVM, DACVIM (Oncology)
Clinical Associate Professor
Department of Medical Sciences
School of Veterinary Medicine
University of Wisconsin
Madison, Wisconsin
Paraneoplastic Syndromes

Craig A. Clifford, DVM, MS, DACVIM (Oncology)
Director of Clinical Research
Red Bank Veterinary Hospital
Tinton Falls, New Jersey
Advanced Imaging Modalities: Computed Tomography (CT) and Magnetic Resonance Imaging (MRI)
Tumors of the Skin, Subcutis, and Other Soft Tissues: Histiocytic Diseases

Joan R. Coates, DVM, MS, DACVIM (Neurology)
Associate Professor
Neurology/Neurosurgery Service Leader
Department of Veterinary Medicine and Surgery
College of Veterinary Medicine
University of Missouri
Columbia, Missouri
Nervous System Neoplasia

Cristi R. Cook, DVM, MS, DACVR
Clinical Assistant Professor, Radiology
Head of Imaging, Comparative Orthopaedic Laboratory
Department of Veterinary Medicine and Surgery
College of Veterinary Medicine
University of Missouri
Columbia, Missouri
Advanced Imaging Modalities: Nuclear Scintigraphy

Deborah J. Davenport, DVM, MS, DACVIM
Adjunct Professor
Department of Clinical Sciences
College of Veterinary Medicine
Kansas State University
Manhattan, Kansas;
Executive Director
Mark Morris Institute
Topeka, Kansas
Supportive Care of the Cancer Patient: Nutritional Management of the Cancer Patient

Amy E. DeClue, DVM, MS, DACVIM (Internal Medicine)
Assistant Professor
Department of Veterinary Medicine and Surgery
College of Veterinary Medicine
University of Missouri
Columbia, Missouri
Tumors of the Endocrine System: Adrenal and Pituitary Tumors
Tumors of the Endocrine System: Thyroid Tumors
Tumors of the Endocrine System: Parathyroid Tumors
Tumors of the Endocrine System: Pancreatic Tumors

Louis-Philippe de Lorimier, DVM, DACVIM (Oncology)
Staff Medical Oncologist
Hôpital Vétérinaire Rive-Sud
Brossard (Québec)
Canada
Supportive Care of the Cancer Patient: Assessment and Management of Pain in the Cancer Patient

Nikolaos G. Dervisis, DVM, DACVIM (Oncology)
Assistant Professor
Center for Comparative Oncology
College of Veterinary Medicine
Michigan State University
East Lansing, Michigan
Pathophysiology and Tumor Cell Growth

Ravinder S. Dhaliwal, DVM, MS, DACVIM (Oncology), DABVP
Consultant in Medical Oncology
Department of Oncology
All Care Animal Referral Center
Fountain Valley, California;
Pet Care Veterinary Hospital
Santa Rosa, California
Managing Oncologic Emergencies: Tumor- and Treatment-Related Complications

Stephanie C. Essman, DVM, MS, DACVR
Assistant Professor, Radiology
Department of Veterinary Medicine and Surgery
College of Veterinary Medicine
University of Missouri
Columbia, Missouri
Imaging Methods in Cancer Diagnosis: Ultrasound

Timothy M. Fan, DVM, PhD, DACVIM (Internal Medicine and Oncology)
Assistant Professor
Department of Veterinary Clinical Medicine
College of Veterinary Medicine
University of Illinois
Urbana, Illinois
Supportive Care of the Cancer Patient: Assessment and Management of Pain in the Cancer Patient

Deborah M. Fine, DVM, MS, DACVIM (Cardiology)
Assistant Professor
Department of Veterinary Medicine and Surgery
College of Veterinary Medicine
University of Missouri
Columbia, Missouri
Tumors of the Thoracic Cavity: Cardiac and Heart-Based Tumors

Anthony J. Fischetti, DVM, MS, DACVR
Department Head of Diagnostic Imaging
The Animal Medical Center
New York, New York
Advanced Imaging Modalities: Computed Tomography (CT) and Magnetic Resonance Imaging (MRI)

S. Dru Forrester, DVM, MS, DACVIM
Scientific Affairs
Hill's Pet Nutrition, Inc.
Topeka, Kansas;
Adjunct Faculty
Department of Clinical Sciences
College of Veterinary Medicine
Kansas State University
Manhattan, Kansas
Supportive Care of the Cancer Patient: Nutritional Management of the Cancer Patient

Leslie E. Fox, DVM, MS, DACVIM (Internal Medicine)
Associate Professor
Department of Veterinary Clinical Sciences
College of Veterinary Medicine
Iowa State University
Ames, Iowa
Tumors of the Thoracic Cavity: Primary Respiratory Tumors
Tumors of the Thoracic Cavity: Rib and Pleural Tumors
Tumors of the Abdominal Cavity: Stomach Tumors

Tracy Gieger, DVM, DACVIM (Internal Medicine and Oncology), DACVR (Radiation Oncology)
Assistant Professor of Veterinary Medical and Radiation Oncology
Department of Veterinary Clinical Sciences
School of Veterinary Medicine
Louisiana State University
Baton Rouge, Louisiana
Tumors of the Skin, Subcutis, and Other Soft Tissues: Skin Tumors

Helen P. Gill, BS
Director of Small Animal Pharmacy
Department of Clinical Sciences
College of Veterinary Medicine
Auburn University
Auburn, Alabama
Chemotherapy: Chemotherapy Preparation

Elizabeth A. Giuliano, DVM, MS, DACVO
Assistant Professor
Department of Veterinary Medicine and Surgery
College of Veterinary Medicine
University of Missouri
Columbia, Missouri
Tumors of the Head and Neck: Ocular and Periocular Tumors

Justin M. Goggin, DVM, DACVR (Radiology)
Metropolitan Veterinary Radiology, Ltd.
Montclair, New Jersey
*Advanced Imaging Modalities: Computed Tomography
(CT) and Magnetic Resonance Imaging (MRI)*

Carolyn J. Henry, DVM, MS, DACVIM (Oncology)
Professor of Oncology
Department of Veterinary Medicine and Surgery
College of Veterinary Medicine, and
Division of Hematology/Oncology
School of Medicine;
Director Tom and Betty Scott Endowed Program
  in Veterinary Oncology
University of Missouri
Columbia, Missouri
*Veterinary Cancer Etiology: Environmental, Chemical,
  and Physical Carcinogens*
*Veterinary Cancer Etiology: Hormonal Impact on
  Carcinogenesis*
*Methods of Tumor Diagnosis: Fine-Needle Aspiration and
  Biopsy Techniques*
Chemotherapy: Chemotherapy Drug Interactions
*Chemotherapy: Formulary and Sources of
  Chemotherapeutic Agents*
*Tumors of the Head and Neck: Oral and Salivary Gland
  Tumors*
Tumors of the Head and Neck: Nasal Tumors
Tumors of the Head and Neck: Skull Tumors
Tumors of the Abdominal Cavity: Mammary Tumors
*Tumors of the Abdominal Cavity: Bladder and Urethral
  Tumors*

**A. Elizabeth Hershey, DVM, DACVIM
  (Oncology), CVA**
Integrative Veterinary Oncology, PC
Phoenix, Arizona
*Tumors of the Thoracic Cavity: Metastatic Respiratory
  Tumors*

**Mary Lynn Higginbotham, DVM, MS, DACVIM
  (Oncology)**
Assistant Professor, Oncology
Department of Clinical Sciences
College of Veterinary Medicine
Kansas State University
Manhattan, Kansas
*Chemotherapy: Formulary and Sources of
  Chemotherapeutic Agents*
*Supportive Care of the Cancer Patient: Prevention and
  Management of Nausea and Vomiting*
*Tumors of the Head and Neck: Oral and Salivary Gland
  Tumors*
Tumors of the Head and Neck: Nasal Tumors
Tumors of the Head and Neck: Aural Tumors
Tumors of the Head and Neck: Esophageal Tumors
*Tumors of the Abdominal Cavity: Liver, Gall Bladder,
  and Non-Endocrine Pancreatic Tumors*
*Tumors of the Skin, Subcutis, and Other Soft Tissues:
  Perianal and Anal Sac Tumors*

**Ann E. Hohenhaus, DVM, DACVIM (Internal
  Medicine and Oncology)**
Staff Veterinarian
The Animal Medical Center
New York, New York
*Managing Oncologic Emergencies: Transfusion
  Considerations*

**Gayle C. Johnson, DVM, MPVM, MS, PhD,
  DACVP**
Professor
Department of Veterinary Pathobiology
College of Veterinary Medicine
University of Missouri
Columbia, Missouri
Nervous System Neoplasia

Kim D. Johnson, DVM, DACVIM (Oncology)
Assistant Professor
Department of Clinical Sciences
College of Veterinary Medicine
Mississippi State University
Mississippi State, Mississippi
Tumors of the Abdominal Cavity: Splenic Tumors
*Tumors of the Skin, Subcutis, and Other Soft Tissues:
  Nail Bed Tumors*
*Tumors of the Skin, Subcutis, and Other Soft Tissues:
  Foot Pad Tumors*

Chand Khanna, DVM, PhD, DACVIM (Oncology)
Head, Tumor and Metastasis Biology Section
Pediatric Oncology Branch
Director, Comparative Oncology Program
Center for Cancer Research
National Cancer Institute
Bethesda, Maryland
Clinical Trial Design and Access to Clinical Research
  Studies

Barbara E. Kitchell, DVM, PhD, DACVIM
  (Internal Medicine and Oncology)
Professor and Director
Center for Comparative Oncology
Department of Small Animal Clinical Sciences
College of Veterinary Medicine
Michigan State University
East Lansing, Michigan
Pathophysiology and Tumor Cell Growth

Jimmy C. Lattimer, DVM, MS, DACVR
  (Radiology and Radiation Oncology)
Associate Professor
Veterinary Medicine and Surgery
Veterinary Medical Teaching Hospital
University of Missouri
Columbia Missouri
Imaging Methods in Cancer Diagnosis: Radiography
Radiation Therapy: External Beam Radiation Therapy
  (Teletherapy) and Brachytherapy
Radiation Therapy: Radioisotopes in Cancer Therapy

Amy K. LeBlanc, DVM, DACVIM (Oncology)
Assistant Professor of Oncology
Department of Small Animal Clinical Sciences
College of Veterinary Medicine
University of Tennessee
Knoxville, Tennessee
Advanced Imaging Modalities: Positron Emission
  Tomography (PET)

Dennis W. Macy, DVM, MS, DACVIM
Professor Emeritus
Department of Clinical Sciences
College of Veterinary Medicine
Colorado State University
Fort Collins, Colorado;
Chief
Department of Medical Oncology
Desert Veterinary Specialist
Palm Desert, California;
Owner and Chief of Staff
Cancer Care Specialist
West Flamingo Animal Hospital
Las Vegas, Nevada
Veterinary Cancer Etiology: Viral Carcinogenesis

Dudley L. McCaw, DVM, DACVIM
  (Internal Medicine and Oncology)
Professor
Department of Clinical Sciences
College of Veterinary Medicine
Kansas State University
Manhattan, Kansas
Photodynamic Therapy
Tumors of the Skin, Subcutis, and Other Soft Tissues:
  Mast Cell Tumors

Jaime F. Modiano, VMD, PhD
Perlman Professor of Oncology
Department of Comparative Medicine
College of Veterinary Medicine
Masonic Cancer Center
University of Minnesota
Minneapolis, Minnesota
Genetic Basis of Cancer

Nicole Northrup, DVM, DACVIM (Oncology)
Associate Professor
Department of Small Animal Medicine and Surgery
College of Veterinary Medicine
University of Georgia
Athens, Georgia
Tumors of the Skin, Subcutis, and Other Soft Tissues:
  Skin Tumors

Melissa C. Paoloni, DVM, DACVIM (Oncology)
Comparative Oncology Program
National Institutes of Health
National Cancer Institute
Bethesda, Maryland
Clinical Trial Design and Access to Clinical Research Studies

Eric R. Pope, DVM, MS, DACVS
Professor of Surgery
School of Veterinary Medicine
Ross University
Basseterre, St. Kitts, West Indies
*Methods of Tumor Diagnosis: Fine-Needle Aspiration and
    Biopsy Techniques*
Surgical Interventions in Cancer

E. Scott Pretorius, MD
Director of MRI, USTeleradiology
Palm Springs, California
*Advanced Imaging Modalities: Computed Tomography
    (CT) and Magnetic Resonance Imaging (MRI)*

**Wendi Velando Rankin, DVM, MS, DACVIM
    (Oncology)**
Associate Medical Oncologist
Veterinary Medical Specialists
Dublin, California
Chemotherapy: Chemotherapy Drug Interactions

Kimberly B. Reeds, DVM
Medical Oncology Resident
Department of Clinical Sciences
College of Veterinary Medicine
Kansas State University
Manhattan, Kansas
Veterinary Cancer Etiology: Viral Carcinogenesis

Kerry C. Rissetto, DVM
Medical Oncology Resident
Department of Veterinary Medicine and Surgery
College of Veterinary Medicine
University of Missouri
Columbia, Missouri
*Tumors of the Thoracic Cavity: Primary Respiratory
    Tumors*
Tumors of the Abdominal Cavity: Intestinal Tumors

**Carlos O. Rodriguez, Jr., DVM, PhD, DACVIM
    (Oncology)**
Continuing Lecturer
Veterinary Medical Teaching Hospital
University of California
Davis, California;
Staff Oncologist
San Francisco Veterinary Specialists
San Francisco, California
Chemotherapy: Basic Chemotherapy Principles
*Chemotherapy: Formulary and Sources of
    Chemotherapeutic Agents*

Philip Roudebush, DVM, DACVIM
Director
Scientific Affairs
Hill's Pet Nutrition, Inc
Topeka, Kansas
*Supportive Care of the Cancer Patient: Nutritional
    Management of the Cancer Patient*

Natalie S. Royer, LVT
Department of Oncology
Small Animal Teaching Hospital
Auburn University
Auburn, Alabama
Chemotherapy: Safe Handling of Chemotherapy Drugs

**David Ruslander, DVM, DACVIM (Oncology),
    DACVR (Radiation Oncology)**
Veterinary Specialty Hospital of the Carolinas
Cary, North Carolina
Tumors of the Musculoskeletal System

Kim A. Selting, DVM, MS, DACVIM (Oncology)
Assistant Teaching Professor
Department of Veterinary Medicine and Surgery
College of Veterinary Medicine
University of Missouri
Columbia, Missouri
Tumors of the Abdominal Cavity: Intestinal Tumors
*Tumors of the Skin, Subcutis, and Other Soft Tissues:
    Soft-Tissue Sarcomas*

Eric R. Simonson, RLAT
Co-Clinical Instructor
Department of Medical Oncology
Veterinary Medical Teaching Hospital
School of Veterinary Medicine
University of California
Davis, California
Management of Oncologic Emergencies:
   Treatment of Chemotherapy Extravasations

Katherine A. Skorupski, DVM, DACVIM (Oncology)
Assistant Professor of Clinical Medical Oncology
Department of Surgical and Radiological Sciences
College of Veterinary Medicine
University of California
Davis, California
Tumors of the Skin, Subcutis, and Other Soft Tissues:
   Histiocytic Diseases

Annette N. Smith, DVM, MS, DACVIM (Oncology and Internal Medicine)
Associate Professor
Department of Clinical Sciences
College of Veterinary Medicine
Auburn University
Auburn, Alabama
Tumors of the Thoracic Cavity: Mediastinal Tumors

Jamie D. Steffy-Morgan, BS, CVT
Faculty Instructor
Veterinary Technology Program
Southern Illinois Collegiate Common Market
Herrin, Illinois
Chemotherapy: Chemotherapy Administration

Kathryn H. Taylor, DVM, MS, DACVIM (Oncology)
Veterinary Oncologist
Veterinary Specialty Care, LLC
Mount Pleasant, South Carolina
Tumors of the Abdominal Cavity: Female Reproductive
   Tumors
Tumors of the Abdominal Cavity: Male Reproductive Tumors

Chelsea Tripp, DVM
Medical Oncology Resident
Department of Veterinary Clinical Sciences
Veterinary Teaching Hospital
Washington State University
Pullman, Washington
Tumors of the Hematopoietic System: Multiple Myeloma

†**Jeff W. Tyler, DVM, MPVM, PhD, DACVIM**
Professor
Director of Strategic Program Initiatives
Director of Clinical Research
Department of Veterinary Medicine and Surgery
College of Veterinary Medicine
University of Missouri
Columbia, Missouri
Cancer Epidemiology and Statistics

Jarrod M. Vancil, DVM
Resident, Medical Oncology
Veterinary Cancer Group
Tustin, California
Tumors of the Head and Neck: Skull Tumors

Jose Armando Villamil, DVM, MS
Oncology Resident and PhD Candidate
Department of Small Animal Medicine and Surgery
   (Oncology)
College of Veterinary Medicine
University of Missouri
Columbia, Missouri
Cancer Epidemiology and Statistics

Elizabeth M. Whitley, DVM, MS, PhD, DACVP
Associate Professor
Department of Veterinary Pathology
College of Veterinary Medicine
Iowa State University
Ames, Iowa
Histopathology, Immunohistochemistry, and Tumor
   Grading

Marlyn S. Whitney, DVM, PhD, DACVP
Clinical Associate Professor
Department of Veterinary Pathobiology
Veterinary Medical Diagnostic Lab
College of Veterinary Medicine
University of Missouri
Columbia, Missouri
The Cytology of Neoplasia

†Deceased.

Valerie J. Wiebe, Pharm D, FSVHP, DICVP
Assistant Clinical Professor
Clinical Pharmacy Coordinator
Department of Medicine and Epidemiology
Veterinary Medical Teaching Hospital
University of California
Davis, California
Managing Oncologic Emergencies: Treatment of
*   Chemotherapy Extravasations*

Jennifer E. Winter, DVM, DACVIM
Medical Oncologist
Southeast Veterinary Oncology
Orange Park, Florida
Tumors of the Head and Neck: Laryngeal and Tracheal
*   Tumors*

J. Paul Woods, DVM, MS, DACVIM (Oncology
**   and Internal Medicine)**
Professor
Department of Clinical Studies;
Co-Director
Institute for Comparative Cancer Investigation
College of Veterinary Medicine
University of Guelph
Guelph, Ontario, Canada
Supportive Care of the Cancer Patient: Palliative Care for
*   the Cancer Patient*

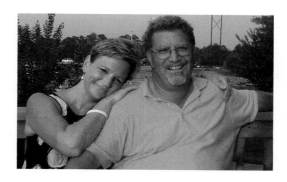

We dedicate this book to

Jeff W. Tyler
May 31, 1957 – May 17, 2009

A dedicated scientist, clinician, educator, mentor, and "number cruncher";
a beloved husband, father, son, brother, uncle, colleague, and friend;
a tireless advocate for children and underdogs worldwide;
and a quiet soul whose mate was found and blessed from that day forward.

———◆———

To the world you may be one person,
But to one person you may be the world
~Anonymous

Preface

What began several years ago as a simple suggestion to expand a continuing education lecture on a topic I coined the "onco-logical" approach to small animal cancer diagnosis and treatment into a pocket-sized oncology handbook for practicing veterinarians has grown into a larger, more comprehensive text than originally envisioned. During the past year of development, my co-editor, Mary Lynn Higginbotham, and I were told that this could no longer be called a "handbook" because that would falsely imply it would fit in one hand. Indeed, the final product is larger in both actual size and in depth of discussion than first planned, with contributions from leading experts in all aspects of veterinary oncology.

What became apparent during the writing of this text was that key pieces of information relevant to the day-to-day practice of oncology were difficult for practitioners to find. Examples include a readily available resource on how to handle cytotoxic drug overdoses and extravasations, worksheets for outlining supplemental nutrition plans, a listing of sites offering various forms of radiation therapy, and easy-reference charts useful for selecting drugs for anti-emetic therapy, pain management, and antimicrobial therapy. We have included these items in the text or on the accompanying website (www.smallanimaloncology.com) so that the information will be at the practitioner's fingertips. In keeping with the original goal envisioned for this book, we provide a logical approach to diagnosis and case management in small animal oncology with an emphasis on the practical issues facing veterinarians in general practice.

One overarching criterion for all sections of the text is that they be well-referenced, so as not to include anecdotal information. Accordingly, we have limited references to the peer-reviewed literature whenever possible. When information can be found only in textbooks or abstracts, it is referenced as such, and these citations are meant to provide the reader with a clear indication of the body of evidence for the topic at hand and to serve as a starting point for readers wanting to determine if a study or finding has since been published in the peer-reviewed literature. Our emphatic advice to the reader is to use an evidence-based approach to make case management decisions and to avoid applying findings from non-peer-reviewed literature. An annotated list of selected references appears at the end of each section, and a complete reference list is included on the accompanying website, including links to the original and related articles where available.

We envision this practice guide to be a countertop resource that will be referenced regularly by practitioners and students. This book is divided into five parts. **Part I** covers **cancer principles and concepts,** providing the background information necessary to understand why cancer occurs and how it progresses. **Part II** addresses **evidence-based approaches to cancer in companion animals.** The topics of cancer epidemiology, statistics, and clinical trial research are made relevant to the general practitioner who wants to understand concepts and terminology related to reading and assessing journal articles in veterinary oncology, as well as participating in and referring cases for oncology clinical trials. **Part III** covers **cancer diagnosis and staging,** discussing and illustrating techniques in tumor diagnosis and imaging, as well as describing the paraneoplastic syndromes that may accompany underlying cancer. **Part IV** covers the **management of cancer,** discussing the different therapeutic modalities, as well as offering guidelines for supportive care (including nutrition, pain management, and palliative care of patients for whom owners opt out of definitive therapy), diagnosis and treatment of life-threatening problems that can arise during the course of cancer and its treatment, and safe handling and administration of chemotherapeutic agents. **Part V** addresses **specific tumors** using a unique **head-to-tail approach,** with diagnoses covered as one would encounter them in a physical exam, beginning with those occurring in the CNS and head and neck, followed by the thoracic cavity, abdominal cavity, skin, subcutis, and other soft tissues, and the musculoskeletal system. This head-to-tail approach concludes with the systemic tumors affecting the hematopoietic system and endocrine neoplasia. As such, the practitioner finding an abnormality during a physical examination can refer to the relevant section of the book by body location and gain information regarding an appropriate diagnostic plan, differential diagnoses, and associated prognosis and treatment options. This enables a logical approach to case management from the time of first identification of a lesion, rather than initiating this approach only after a final diagnosis is established.

Numerous boxes, tables, and appendices provide valuable and practical information including step-by-step instructions for diagnostic techniques, dosing recommendations, summaries of findings from clinical studies, forms for tumor staging and monitoring therapy, OSHA recommendations for prevention of employee exposure to hazardous drugs, and more. Printable handouts for medical records and client information serve as useful resources for veterinarians practicing oncology. High-quality figures and illustrations aid in recognition of specific cancers and related abnormalities, as well as provide a resource to facilitate discussions with clients regarding planned procedures and potential complications.

The editors and contributing authors of this practice guide have made every effort to provide the most up-to-date and comprehensive information in a format that is useful and relevant to veterinarians caring for small animal oncology patients. This is a text by clinicians for clinicians and is designed to provide veterinarians who are practicing oncology in their clinics with easy-to-access, clinically relevant details for complete care of the small animal cancer patient, while considering the needs, concerns, and capabilities of the client/caregiver. It is also intended to facilitate the establishment of a stronger, cooperative team approach between client and clinical staff and with oncology specialists, who also may be involved in patient care. For those who are new to the practice of veterinary oncology, consultation with a board-certified oncologist is recommended before administering any new therapy with which one is unfamiliar. The practice of oncology is often a rewarding aspect of veterinary medicine and is an area of unprecedented growth in terms of both case load and body of knowledge. It is our hope that this textbook will serve as a useful resource in your practice of high-quality medicine and compassionate cancer care.

Carolyn Henry and Mary Lynn Higginbotham

Acknowledgments

I begin these acknowledgements by recognizing the significant contributions made by my co-editor, Mary Lynn Higginbotham. Mary Lynn, your amazing efforts and willingness to step in when I most needed your help made all the difference in seeing this project to completion. Thank you for going above and beyond for me. The contributing authors of this textbook are some of the finest individuals with whom one could ever work. It is only through their individual expertise, commitment to quality, and unending patience with me that this book has made it to print and will serve as a valuable resource for veterinarians. I am proud to call them colleagues and am indebted to them for their contributions to this book. From its inception, Dr. Tony Winkel was the driving force behind this book and is solely to blame for my original interest in taking on this project. Thank you for your friendship and for your tenacity and vision, Tony. The field of veterinary publications lost a tremendous resource as you moved on from your post at Elsevier, but I wish you well in your future endeavors in the field of nutrition. To Maureen Slaten at Elsevier, I offer my most sincere gratitude for navigating the peaks and valleys of this project through the past few years. You have offered the organizational skills and consistency needed to help us create a product of which we can be proud. And to Penny Rudolph and John Casey at Elsevier—thank you for attending to the final details of editing and production so that we could see this long-awaited text become a reality. Through the course of writing this book, content and context have been altered in part due to comments, questions, and suggestions of countless veterinary students, technicians, house officers, clinicians, referring veterinarians, clients, and continuing education seminar attendees. It has been through the unique perspective of each of these individuals that we have been able to create a text that is most relevant to a broad audience. Thank you to all of you who have read through rough drafts, edited, and commented on content until we got it right. My original in-house copy editor, Ginny Dodam, is surely eligible for some form of sainthood for her tireless attention to detail in editing and for her more recent assistance in making my schedule more manageable. The oncology service staff, faculty, and house officers at the University of Missouri, along with making it possible for me to have time to edit this book, have made significant contributions to its content and quality. The same can be said for their contributions to my life. You are all part of my extended family and will forever hold a special place in my heart. To my immediate family, I am indebted to you for your encouragement, patience, and understanding when time spent working on this book meant time not spent with you. Thank you, Mom, for teaching me perseverance at an early age through your example. Thank you Barb and Kat for leading my cheering section, and Morgan, Cody, and Trevor for lifting me up with your own personal strength and love. To Reggie, Tarnue, Sydney, Praise, and Quinn, you are my greatest inspirations and sources of pride. Thank you for always believing in me and for reminding me what is most important in life. And finally, to my late husband, Jeff Tyler, you are the reason I had the confidence to pursue my dreams. You made me a better scientist, clinician, teacher, and colleague, all through your example and unyielding commitment to excellence. The sacrifices you made to allow me to write this book are magnified by the fact that you did not live to see it published. As expected, your contribution (Chapter 4) was finished ahead of schedule, in no need of editing, and reflects your combination of innate intelligence and common sense approach to difficult subjects. Veterinary medicine lost a great one this year. Thank you for 20 wonderful years and for all the reasons you have given me to continue to put one foot in front of the other.

Carolyn Henry

First, and foremost, Carolyn, your strength and courage during adversity are absolutely amazing. Thank you for inviting me to be a part of this adventure with you. Your confidence in me has inspired me to accomplish a task I never thought possible. It certainly has been a growing and learning experience. The completion of this text would not have been possible without the direction and assistance of Tony Winkel, Maureen Slaten, Penny Rudolph, and John Casey of Elsevier. Thank you for your professionalism, patience, and perseverance and for helping us to make this book a reality. To all of the authors, your contributions make this text an outstanding resource for practitioners. I feel extremely fortunate to be a colleague of such intelligent and cooperative individuals. Dudley McCaw, your wisdom, continual pursuit of knowledge, and sense of humor are an example to all. Thank you for your support during this entire process. Thank you to my colleagues at Kansas State University for seeing me through the completion of this text. To my colleagues at Auburn University, your involvement in this project has made it all the more sentimental. I thank you all for your friendship; it means the world to me. Mom and Dad, thank you for always encouraging me to pursue my dreams; your unwavering support has helped to make me the individual I am today. Maggie and Jake, you make me smile every day and have taught me the true meaning of unconditional love. And finally, to my husband, Jonathan, words cannot express how fortunate I feel to have you in my life. I look forward to what our life post-editing has to offer.

Mary Lynn Higginbotham

Contents

1 Pathophysiology and Tumor Cell Growth

Barbara E. Kitchell and Nikolaos G. Dervisis

KEY POINTS

- Cancers are complex systems that result from many abnormalities within the cell.
- Cancers involve both genetic predisposition and environmental factors.
- Because of defects in cell physiology, cancers progress from "bad to worse" biologic behavior over time.
- Understanding the basic molecular biology of cancer will facilitate molecularly targeted therapy in the future.

Intricate and complex pathways are involved in the development of a multicellular eukaryotic organism. Each organism originates as a single cell and progresses through rapid proliferation and differentiation, followed by steady state repair and repletion, and ultimately senescence. The genetic information for every part of the mature organism exists in the genome of each cell, yet the individual differentiated cell never expresses the majority of this genetic information. By studying aberrancies in the system, such as the development of neoplasia, mechanisms that control the process of gene activation and repression in health and disease are being elucidated. Consequently, our understanding of what constitutes a "cancer" is becoming increasingly refined.[1-3]

WHAT IS CANCER?

In the normal eukaryotic organism, tissues achieve growth equilibrium, defined as the point at which production of new cells equals the death rate of cells, so that there is no net gain of tissue. In the case of tumors, cell replication exceeds physiologic need. Hyperplasia is the normal tissue's response to certain noxious stimuli, but in contrast to neoplasia, hyperplasia is reversible upon return to the non-stimulated state. When expansion of cell numbers occurs in a locally confined form, the neoplasia is benign. Malignant neoplasia, or cancer, is unambiguously defined as the condition in which abnormal cells invade adjacent normal tissue or successfully colonize distant locations in the body through metastasis.[2]

CANCER AS A GENETIC DISEASE

Cancer is considered a genetic disease because specific changes in the genome are necessary for expression of the malignant phenotype. Initiating changes that lead to malignant transformation typically involves regulation of the G1/S phase transition of the cell cycle.[4] When cell cycle regulation breaks down, increasing genetic errors and progression of the malignant phenotype is evident. The traditional understanding of carcinogenic genetic changes has focused on mutational events, such as point mutations and large rearrangements of chromosome material (translocation, gene amplification, and deletion). These alterations in the coding sequence may occur spontaneously, as seen in somatic gene recombination errors in lymphoma, or through errors in DNA polymerase nucleotide incorporation during DNA replication. In addition to these inherent stochastic risks for genetic alteration, cancer is also caused by the action of external carcinogenic agents such as chemical, physical or viral carcinogens, as will be discussed elsewhere in this book.[1-5] While changes in the coding sequences of DNA are essential to carcinogenesis, cancer also encompasses epigenetic alterations that do not involve mutating the DNA coding sequences. These epigenetic changes include gene silencing through DNA promoter methylation and histone acetylation, as well as through

TABLE 1-1   EPIGENETIC INFLUENCE IN CANCER DEVELOPMENT

Epigenetic Alterations	Cellular Response
DNA promoter methylation	Gene silencing[25]
Histone modification (methylation, acetylation)	Methylation → gene silencing[26] Acetylation → gene expression[27]
MicroRNAs	RNA expression modulation (oncogenic or tumor suppressor function)[28]

regulation of post-transcriptional and post-translational events[6] such as production of small interfering RNA molecules (Table 1-1).

Cancer cells and tissues are generally undifferentiated as compared with normal tissues of the same cellular origin, and the aggressiveness of biologic behavior correlates with the degree of anaplasia. In some senses, the study of cancer is very similar to developmental biology in reverse. In embryogenesis, cells are anaplastic or undifferentiated in the beginning, and subsequently differentiate as they move to the appropriate organ location or site of maturation. In cancer, a primordial stem cell, or a committed or partially committed cell with replicating potential, replicates inappropriately such that the fully mature cellular phenotype is not achieved.[7]

WHICH CELLS ARE SUSCEPTIBLE TO MALIGNANT TRANSFORMATION?

Most researchers believe that cancers result from genetic derangement in a cell that retains replicative potential. The stem cell theory states that pluripotent stem cells, rather than terminally differentiated cells, are the most likely originators of cancer. In this schema, malignant cells generally arise from faulty differentiation of pluripotent or semi-committed cells that retain replicative potential, rather than from de-differentiation of a mature, terminally differentiated cell. However, de-differentiation of mature cells has also been documented to occur in certain malignancies. Cells that replicate more often during the lifetime of the individual are more prone to manifesting aberrant cell replication. Thus, cancers arise most commonly in cells that divide throughout the lifetime of the individual, and carcinomas (cancers arising from cells of ectodermal or endodermal origin) are numerically much more frequent than sarcomas (cancers arising from cells of mesodermal origin).

Some of the events leading to malignant transformation may be related to the environment in which a cell develops. For example, implantation of neural-crest cells from a developing mouse embryo into the testes of a normal mouse results in the development of teratocarcinomas. Conversely, incorporation of malignant teratocarcinoma cells into a developing mouse blastocyst results in the formation of a normal, healthy mouse that contains a mixture of genotypes derived from both the normal cells of the blastocyst and the teratocarcinoma.[8] These experiments demonstrate that epigenetic influences supplied by the tumor cell's microenvironment are involved in cancer development, just as they are in normal cell differentiation in embryogenesis.

CLONALITY, HETEROGENEITY, AND CELL CYCLE REGULATION

Most tumors are clonal in origin; that is, tumors are derived from a single cell that has undergone malignant transformation. However, cells within the cancerous mass are also heterogeneous. Although they originate clonally, by the time a large tumor burden has developed, cancer cells have undergone further mutation and changes in karyotype. Also, cancers that arise from stem cells may have populations of cells representing various stages of differentiation as they attempt to follow more normal maturation pathways. Tumor cell heterogeneity renders treatment of tumors more difficult, since different cells have different growth rates and different sensitivities to chemotherapy and radiation therapy.

Cancers are progressive in nature and undergo what has been called a "bad to worse" phenomenon. This may be because one of the earliest genetic derangements to occur in cancer is the loss of cell cycle regulatory control. In the normal cell cycle, intracellular conditions must be optimum for replication to proceed. Cells that have DNA damage or lack of appropriate precursor nucleotides and proteins for cell replication will halt in progression through the cell cycle, typically at the G1/S phase transition checkpoint. Once DNA has been repaired and protein and nucleotide levels are determined to be sufficient, the cell resumes passage through the cell cycle. Progression through the cell cycle is determined by checkpoint regulators such as cyclins and cyclin-dependent kinases (CDKs), tumor suppressors such as the Rb gene, progression factors, DNA repair enzyme activity, cytoplasmic factors such as mitotic spindle assembly, and regulators of apoptosis (programmed cell death) (Figure 1-1).[9] Defects in any of these systems can result in aberrant cell replication. One of the most common genetic defects detected in human cancers thus far

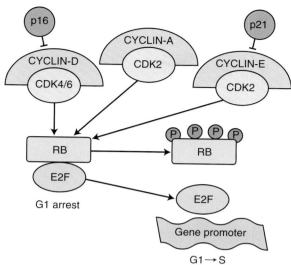

FIGURE 1-1 The RB function in G1 to S phase during cell-cycle progression. Eukaryotic cells have evolved signaling pathways to coordinate cell-cycle transitions and ensure accurate replication of DNA before cell division. Cell-cycle progression is stimulated by protein kinase complexes, which consist of a cyclin and a CDK. The CDKs are expressed constitutively throughout the cell cycle, whereas cyclin levels are restricted by transcriptional regulation and by ubiquitin-mediated degradation. The activation of CDK requires the binding of a cyclin partner and a site-specific phosphorylation. The complexes cyclin-D/CDK4, cyclin-D/CDK6, cyclin-E/CDK2, and cyclin-A/CDK2 all contribute to the regulation of G1 to S phase progression. Unphosphorylated pRb is believed to bind to the transcription factor E2F and prevents E2F-mediated transcription of genes that are responsible for transition from the G1 to the S phase of the cell cycle. Phosphorylation of RB by cyclin-D/CDK4/6 and cyclin-A/-E/CDK2 complexes causes the release of RB from E2F, with subsequent G1 to S progression. Loss of pRb, synthesis of truncated pRb, or mutations that alter the ability of unphosphorylated pRb to bind to E2F, all allow unrestricted progression from G1 to S phase.

is found in the p53 gene pathway. The p53 gene, along with its upstream and downstream signaling partners, is responsible for halting a deranged cell in the G1 phase of the cell cycle. If a normal cell is unable to complete repairs and prepare for replication within a short time, the cell will "commit suicide" (undergo apoptosis) for the benefit of the organism. Because defects occur so commonly in p53 and similar pathway regulation, cancer cells accrue many more mutations over time because they are unable to stop replicating to allow repairs to proceed (Figure 1-2).[10] This phenomenon of early loss of the ability to correct for damaged DNA is referred to as the "mutator phenotype" of cancer cells.

CANCERS GO FROM BAD TO WORSE: THE MULTISTEP NATURE OF CARCINOGENESIS

Over time, cancer cells become more anaplastic, resistant to apoptosis, and more rapidly cycling. An example of this phenomenon is the genetic progression of colon cancer in humans. People who carry the genotype of familial colonic polyposis have a very high predisposition to develop colonic carcinoma. In an important study by Fearon and Vogelstein, [11] progressive genetic changes were mapped in the colon cells of individuals with a familial syndrome referred to as APC (adenomatous polyposis coli). Over time, colon cells of these individuals develop benign adenomatous polyps, premalignant carcinomas *in situ*, locally invasive but non-metastatic colon cancer, and finally aggressive metastatic disease. Sequential and predictable additive mutations are seen in these family members throughout the course of disease progression.

The progression of cancer in an individual may also be viewed as an exercise in Darwinian evolution, in that cells with a selective advantage for survival and replication take precedence in a competitive manner. The addition of sublethal therapy, such as fractionated radiation therapy or chemotherapy, may also increase the selective pressure, so the fittest cancer cell can take over the host organism. Those cells that survive the therapeutic insults we apply are indeed given a selective advantage through the eradication of cells less fit for survival. In this case, the genomic plasticity and adaptability critical to speciation on the planet is clearly detrimental to survival of the individual afflicted with cancer.[12]

CANCER AND AGING

Cancer is a disease of senescence. As an organism ages, the odds of developing an aberrantly dividing cell increase, and the normal immune pathways that detect and eradicate such aberrant cells become less effective. This increased risk of cancer development with age is well documented in human and veterinary medicine. Injury to the genes through exposure to carcinogens, viruses, and physical factors such as UV irradiation can be cumulative. A lifetime of injury may be required for the right combination of events to occur to result in cancer. Thus, malignant transformation occurs late in life. It has also been postulated to take up to two thirds of an individual's lifetime for a single malignant cell to become clinically apparent as a tumor, based on the replication rate of most somatic cells in solid tumors. Aged cells are more susceptible to genetic injury because they are less able to scavenge free radicals and complete

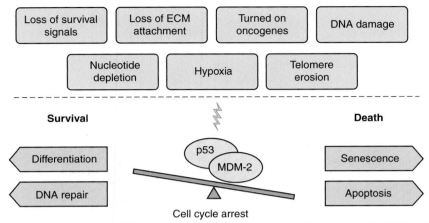

FIGURE 1-2 The p53/MDM-2 balance. The p53 gene, along with its negative regulator MDM-2, mediate the cellular response to various stress signals. Whether the balance leans towards life (differentiation, DNA repair, cell cycle arrest) or death (senescence, apoptosis, cell cycle arrest) depends on several factors, including cell type, extracellular microenvironment, and other damages sustained in the cellular molecular machinery. The point of p53/MDM-2 balance is to favor the preservation of DNA integrity.

DNA repair.[13] For example, aged skin transplanted onto genetically identical young mice developed cancer at the rate of the aged mice, despite the robust metabolism and immune function of the younger graft recipient.

HYPOXIA AND CANCER

Recent interest has focused on hypoxia as a driver of many of the genotypic and phenotypic changes seen in malignant transformation. When tissue oxygen tension (pO_2) drops below the normal tissue level of 10–80 mm Hg, critical signaling pathways are triggered. The most significant of these pathways is mediated by hypoxia inducible factor (HIF-1), which is a heterodimeric basic helix-loop-helix transcription factor that modulates the expression of 130 downstream genes. The HIF-1β subunit of this heterodimer is constitutively expressed in constant levels, while the HIF-1α subunit is expressed but rapidly degraded by hydroxylation of specific proline residues that lead to ubiquitination in the presence of the von Hippel-Lindau (VHL) protein. This event targets HIF-1α for rapid proteosomal degradation. In hypoxic conditions, HIF-1α is not hydroxylated, thus increasing its half-life in the cytoplasm and allowing HIF-1α to dimerize with HIF-1 β. When HIF-1α binds the HIF-1β subunit of HIF-1, HIF-1 translocates to the nucleus and acts as a transcription factor for many essential survival, angiogenesis, and metastasis genes.[14] In addition, the HIF-1 complex mediates expression of genes that allow for survival under acidic and anaerobic

conditions in the unfavorable hypoxic environment. Many of the factors involved in aggressive biologic tumor behavior can be attributed to early onset of tissue hypoxia after uncontrolled cell replication pushes the initiated cell's progeny away from the capillary blood supply. Thus, switch to survival phenotype, anaerobic glycolysis, angiogenesis, epithelial to mesenchymal transition in cell adhesion molecules, increased cell motility to allow migration to more favorably perfused locations, and increased genomic instability are all factors, among many others, that can be attributed to the hypoxic tumor environment. Hypoxic conditions occur as soon as a mass exceeds the 2-mm capillary perfusion radius; hence the angiogenic switch and other factors critical to the malignant phenotype are relatively early events in tumorigenesis (Figure 1-3).[15]

A UNIFIED THEORY: THE HANAHAN-WEINBERG MODEL

In a seminal article entitled "The Hallmarks of Cancer," Hanahan and Weinberg[5] summarized a conceptual overview of cancer biology that has been widely embraced by the cancer research community. Based on the past 25 years of intensive research, six common themes in cancer have emerged. These six factors are detailed in Table 1-2 and will be subsequently discussed below. The acquisition of each of these physical characteristics by the cancer cell represents the successful breaching of an evolutionarily anti-cancer strategy developed to maintain physiologic

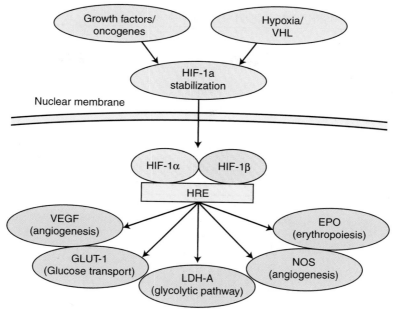

FIGURE 1-3 Regulation of the HIF-1α pathway. Under hypoxic conditions or through oncogene activation, the hypoxia inducible factor 1α (*HIF-1α*) is phosphorylated and stabilized. HIF-1α then enters the nucleus and dimerizes with the hypoxia inducible factor 1β(*HIF-1β*) to induce transcription of genes that favor neo-angiogenesis and glycolysis. *VEGF*, Vascular endothelial growth factor; *GLUT-1*, glucose transporter 1; *LDH-A*, lactic dehydrogenase A; *NOS*, nitric oxide synthase; *EPO*, erythropoietin; *HRE*, hypoxia response element.

homeostasis by the organism. Thus, although each cancer is unique, with a myriad of individual mutations and epigenetic changes manifest, it may be possible in the future to target specific anti-cancer strategies to these common cancer traits. Research in cancer therapy is already honing in on these factors, with dramatic advances being seen in the development of drugs and targeted strategies such as receptor tyrosine kinase inhibitors to block growth signaling, anti-angiogenic drugs, promoters of apoptosis such as antisense therapy for bcl-2 gene over-expression, enzyme inhibitors to block invasion and metastasis, and telomerase inhibition strategies. The future of cancer research will be markedly hastened by the application of important technological breakthroughs, such as genomic, proteomic, and pharmacogenomic screens that will facilitate the practical application of individualized cancer medicine.

SELF-SUFFICIENCY IN GROWTH FACTOR STIMULATION

Aberrancy in growth factor signaling is analogous to a switch that is left in the constant "on" position. Growth factor signaling was implicated in the 1970s by the discovery of viral oncogenes that caused continuous cell cycling. The oncogene theory of cancer was further defined by the 1989 Nobel Prize winners in Medicine, Bishop and Varmus, to state that there exists within all cells normal genes that code for certain products essential to the division and differentiation of cells. These genetic elements are called *proto-oncogenes* in the normal state and *oncogenes* when abnormal. Oncogenes can produce cancer when they are mutated to produce abnormal protein products, or expressed in excess or in a continuous manner. There are hundreds of genes that, when deranged, are capable of functioning as oncogenes.

Oncogenes have also been characterized by their function in the cell replication pathway. A family of oncogenes codes for cell growth factor–related substances. Growth factor genes may code for an extracellular peptide such as platelet-derived growth factor (the *sis* oncogene) or fibroblast growth factor–related protein (*int-2*). These substances signal cell division by making the cell "think" it has received a legitimate command to divide. Cells become autonomously replicating when a cell expressing the receptor for a growth factor

TABLE 1-2   THE HANAHAN-WEINBERG MODEL

Acquired Cancer Traits	Molecular Example	Disease Example
Self-sufficiency in growth signals	Activated *sis* oncogene, IGF-I, GH, SC/HGF	Osteosarcoma[29-32]
Insensitivity to growth-inhibitory (antigrowth) signals	Loss of retinoblastoma tumor suppressor, RAR, RXR, COX-2	Osteosarcoma[33-35]
Evasion of programmed cell death (apoptosis)	Loss of p53 or PTEN tumor suppressor, MDM-2 amplification	Melanoma[36] Osteosarcoma[37] Hemangiosarcoma[38]
Limitless replicative potential	Active telomerase	Carcinomas[39]
Sustained angiogenesis	Induction of VEGF production	Meningioma[40] Carcinomas[41]
Tissue invasion and metastasis	MMPs production	Carcinomas[42] Osteosarcoma[43]

Data from Hanahan D, Weinberg RA: The hallmarks of cancer, *Cell* 100:57, 2000.

IGF-I, Insulin-like growth factor-I; *GH,* growth hormone; *SC/HGF,* scatter factor/hepatocyte growth factor; *RAR,* retinoic acid receptor; *RXR,* retinoid X receptor; *COX-2,* cyclooxygenase-2; *PTEN,* phosphatase and tensin homolog; *MDM-2,* murine double minute oncogene; *VEGF,* vascular endothelial growth factor; *MMPs,* matrix metalloproteinase.

begins producing the growth factor as well (autocrine regulatory signaling). Some oncogenes code for aberrant growth factor receptor molecules that trigger cell division by mimicking normal cell signals. Growth factor receptor type oncogenes are generally kinases that phosphorylate tyrosine, serine, or threonine. Some oncogenes mediate signaling functions from cell surface receptors to intracellular effector molecules. Many oncogenes are intermediate messengers acting by means other than protein kinase function. These signal transduction genes are unable to respond to normal stimuli and are maintained in the constant "on" position. Finally, some oncogenes code for nuclear reactive substances, such as transcription regulators, that bind to DNA and allow gene products to be produced in the cell. In this case, these nuclear binding proteins make it easier for other genes to be turned on. This frequently results in the triggering of cell replication. Oncogenes often complement each other to allow malignant transformation. Some oncogenes (such as *myc, myb,* and p53) may prevent apoptosis so that cells are immortalized. Activation of a second oncogene (such as *ras* or *src*) then induces morphologic transformation of cells by accelerating replication.[16,17] A schematic of such a growth factor pathway is shown in Figure 1-4.

Regardless of the type of oncogene, four mechanisms of activation have been postulated: (1) point mutation, as by chemicals or radiation; (2) chromosomal rearrangements; (3) gene amplification; and (4) retroviral insertion. During the lifetime of an organism, many such "hits" to the genomic DNA of cells occur.

When cells can no longer repair this damage, cancer can occur.

TUMOR SUPPRESSOR GENE DEFECTS

On the other side of gene regulation is the discovery of genes associated with stopping the replication of cells. These tumor suppressor genes or anti-oncogenes include genes that are seen as inherited familial predisposition to specific malignancies, such as mutations in the Rb gene in retinoblastoma and osteosarcoma in people. In this case, a defect in the RB protein causes uncontrolled cell proliferation when both copies of the gene are defective. Thus, Rb genetic defects are considered recessive cancer traits. However, it is now known that other tumor suppressor genes may be haplo-insufficient, in which case loss of only one gene copy results in malignant transformation.[18]

The most commonly defective gene associated with lack of repression of cell growth is the p53 gene. The protein product of p53 plays a complex and pivotal role in oncogenesis. This gene has been found to induce apoptosis. When the p53 gene is non-functional, cells become genetically unstable. With normal cytokine or hormonal stimulation of cell replication in a p53 mutant cell, cell production is not balanced by cell death and tumor formation results. Additional genetic defects then accrue that result in excessive or aberrant replication. Defects of tumor suppressor genes permit replication to move past normal cell cycle check points inappropriately, allowing mutations to accrue in DNA through successive cycles of replication.[19]

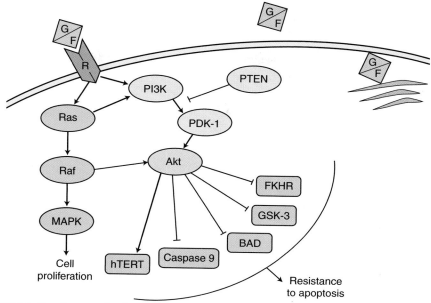

FIGURE 1-4 Signaling cascade of growth factor stimulation. Growth factor receptor stimulation may induce intracellular signaling promoting cellular proliferation and/or resistance to apoptosis. GA, Golgi apparatus; GF, growth factors; R, growth factor receptors; Ras, small GTP-binding protein that acts as binary switch, relaying signals from receptors to cytoplasm signaling molecules; PI3K, phosphoinositide-3-OH kinase; PDK-1, PI3K dependent kinase 1; PTEN, phosphatase and tensin homolog deleted on chromosome 10; hTERT, human telomerase reverse transcriptase; GSK-3β, glycogen synthase kinase 3β; FKHR, forkhead transcription factor; BAD, pro-apoptotic protein.

CANCER CELL IMMORTALIZATION

Normal cells are only capable of a finite number of replications during the lifetime of the individual. A requisite change that permits tumor development is the acquisition of the capacity to continue cell division without limit. This "cancer cell immortalization" is most often accomplished by upregulation of the enzyme telomerase. Telomerase is a specialized ribonucleoprotein reverse transcriptase that functions to extend the telomeres at the end of the chromosomes. Telomerase is developmentally regulated and is normally silent in most adult somatic cells after transition from embryonal development. In normal circumstances, telomerase is constitutively active only in stem cells that retain replicative potential throughout the life of the individual, although conditional upregulation coordinate with cell cycling has been observed in some tissues. The telomeres of the chromosomes act as a "mitotic clock" that determines the number of cell replications a given cell will be able to accomplish during the life span of the individual.

Telomere depletion happens with each round of cell replication, eventually resulting in near total degradation of the telomere. Telomere depletion results in "replicative senescence," permanent exit from the cell cycle, and cell death. Up to 90% of cancers have detectable telomerase enzyme activity. This implies that the critical shortening of the length of the telomere in normal cells acts as a potent tumor suppressor mechanism. Upregulation of telomerase enzyme activity (or alternate mechanisms of telomere length maintenance, which are as yet ill defined) is thus requisite for cancer cells to be able to acquire sufficient mass to result in death of the patient through organ system dysfunction or metabolic derangement.[20]

APOPTOSIS DEFECTS: TOO MUCH CELL REPLICATION OR NOT ENOUGH CELL DEATH?

All cancer cells have a relative survival advantage when compared with homologous normal cells. It is speculated that this relative apoptosis resistance occurs early in the course of tumorigenesis for most solid tumors. Cells are in a constant state of decision between life and death, and the decision for survival is surprisingly tempered in multicellular organisms. Loss of continuous survival signals from neighboring cells results in apoptosis. Cells that are able to survive in transit during metastasis and during tissue invasion evade a form of programmed cell death called *anoikis*, which is triggered by alterations in cell-to-cell contact in normal tissues.

Certain low-grade, well-differentiated cancers have been determined to be largely the result of apoptosis defects. Apoptosis occurs to maintain tissue size equilibrium, control replication of aberrant cells, and allow for normal physiologic activities such as tissue remodeling in embryogenesis. Many non-replicating cells of the body have a predictable life span and die at a physiologically appropriate time. Lymphocytes, particularly antibody-producing B cells and circulating T cells, provide examples of this phenomenon. Lymphocytes circulate or exist in lymphoid tissues for a period of time and then die, to be replaced from stem cell pools. In certain diseases such as chronic lymphocytic leukemia or low-grade lymphoma, the reason for accumulation of lymphocytes to a clinical tumor burden is not excessive cell replication, but, rather, lack of appropriate cell death. Defects in apoptosis regulatory pathways such as alterations in bcl-2 family genes can result in the survival of excessive numbers of cells, with clinical repercussions for the patient. Also, therapeutic interventions for cancer, such as radiation therapy and genotoxic chemotherapy, cause cell death by damaging DNA and triggering apoptotic pathways. Cancer cells that arise because of defects in cell death pathways tend to be resistant to traditional anti-cancer strategies.[21] Worse, these cells can then undergo further malignant transformation and can develop unregulated, rapid cell replication. This results in a rapidly lethal, unstoppable cancer, which is called "blast crisis" in low-grade leukemias.

INVASION, ANGIOGENESIS, AND METASTASIS

The process of metastasis involves a complex biology. Millions of cells are constantly being shed from tumors, yet certainly not all cancers have the capacity to become metastatic. In order for a tumor to metastasize, several sequential steps must occur (Table 1-3). First, cells must be able to survive lack of cell-to-cell or cell-to-extracellular matrix (ECM) signals for survival. These cells acquire motility through a process of gene upregulation and transit toward the adjacent blood supply. Cancer cells respond to trophic signals for cell motility such as lack of cell-to-cell contact, contact with degraded interstitial matrix components, cytokines, and autocrine or paracrine motility

TABLE 1-3 METASTATIC CASCADE

Metastatic Cascade Steps	Physiologic Events
Detachment from the primary tumor	Anoikis/amorphosis resistance
Intravasation	EMT, ECM remodeling
Circulation	Evade immune surveillance, survive mechanical stress
Extravasation	Mechanical restriction in small sinusoids, binding to endothelial cell surface receptors
Angiogenesis	Vascular endothelial growth factor secretion, requirement of vasculature
Survival at metastatic site	Resistance to apoptosis

factors. Cells then intravasate, or enter, into the blood or lymphatic circulation. These cells must be able to survive immune surveillance and the "rough-and-tumble" microenvironment of the circulatory system. Cells are arrested at a new location by aggregation with platelets and fibrin in small blood or lymphatic vessels. Most often, the site of metastasis is the organ containing the first capillary bed that the cells must traverse (e.g., lungs, liver). However, specific cancers have a predilection to spread to selected sites, suggesting a role for recognition and adherence to surface or extracellular molecules in specific organs.[22] Cancer cells must traverse the difficult physical barrier of the basement membrane to leave the primary site and to migrate into the new metastatic site. Many cancers with metastatic potential can be differentiated from non-metastatic tumors of identical cellular origin by their ability to produce proteases capable of digesting basement membrane and other ECM molecules.[23]

Finally, the cancer cell must recruit a blood supply if a new tumor is to be produced. This process must occur at the primary site as well as at the site of distant metastasis. The process of growing a new blood supply is called *angiogenesis*. Cell replication is limited by the distance from the nearest feeding capillary. Normal cells must be within 2 to 5 mm of a feeding vessel in order to have access to sufficient nutrients and environmental conditions to be able to replicate. Cancer cells that are successful in inducing new tumors at distant locations produce angiogenic factors that allow for continued cell replication in the new site. These angiogenic factors include basic fibroblast growth factor and vascular endothelial growth factor among others. The process of angiogenesis is also dependent upon degradation of the extracellular matrix, and the normal signals associated with tissue injury, wound healing, and coagulation. There is mounting evidence that suppressors of angiogenesis exist naturally in the body. Anti-angiogenic factors may, in fact, be elaborated by the primary tumor. When the primary tumor is resected, this angiogenesis inhibiting effect is lost, allowing rapid cell replication in distant metastases.[24]

CONCLUSION

Clearly, the induction of malignant transformation is a highly complex process. The discovery of the specific genetic triggers of malignant transformation and metastasis has made possible the potential for therapy directed at specific molecular intervention appropriate to the individual patient's tumor. Cancer medicine of the future is predicted to be radically different because of these advances in our understanding of basic cancer biology.

Selected References[*]

Balmain A, Gray J, Ponder B: The genetics and genomics of cancer, *Nature Genetics* 33:238, 2003.
An overview of current understanding of molecular genetic events in human cancer.
DeVita VT, Hellman S, Rosenberg SA: *Cancer: principles and practice of oncology*, ed 7, Philadelphia, 2005, Lippincott Williams & Wilkins.
The introductory chapters to this classic oncology textbook cover many fundamental areas of cancer biology in depth, and the remainder discusses individual cancers as seen in human oncology practice with regard to diagnosis, prognosis, and therapy.
Hanahan D, Weinberg RA: The hallmarks of cancer, *Cell* 100:57, 2000.
This is the classic review paper that details the presiding paradigm in cancer research at the present time.
Pelangaris S, Khan M: *The molecular biology of cancer*, Malden, 2006, Blackwell Publishing.
This textbook provides a comprehensive vision of cancer biology and is very comprehensive and easy to read.
Tannock IF, Hill RP, Bristow RG, Harrington L: *The basic science of oncology*, ed 4, New York, 2005, McGraw-Hill.
This book serves as a widely referenced guide to the biology of cancer that is applicable to human and veterinary medicine.

[*]For a complete list of the references cited in this chapter, please go to www.smallanimaloncology.com.

2 Genetic Basis of Cancer

Jaime F. Modiano and Matthew Breen

KEY POINTS

- Cancer is a genetic disease, but it is not always heritable.
- Cancer is a clonal disease (i.e., arises from a single cell) that develops upon the accumulation of somatic mutations that overcome normal mechanisms of growth regulation.
- Tumor-initiating cells or cancer stem cells are responsible for the peculiar features of some or all cancers. It is unclear if these cells arise from transformed multipotent or pluripotent stem cells, or from somatic cells that acquire mutations that endow the capacity for self-renewal.
- Tumor progression follows a Darwinian model of natural selection. This process is intimately tied not only to the tumor's capability to evolve and adapt within its microenvironment, but also to the manner in which the tumor itself can mold the microenvironment to improve its survival.

It is now clear that cancer is a genetic disease.[1,2] Since the discovery and characterization of the Philadelphia chromosome as the first non-random translocation in cancer in the 1960s and 1970s, several hundred genetic abnormalities that are peculiarly associated with specific cancers have been identified. Rather than provide an exhaustive list of genes, here we will focus on contemporary issues that highlight the significance of cancer genetics in diagnosis and treatment, and how interactions between genes and environment impact the origin, progression, and response to therapy of most tumors.

GENES AND CANCER RISK

To understand the implications of cancer, one must first realize that cancer is not a simple disease. Rather, the term *cancer* describes a large number of diseases whose only common feature is uncontrolled cell growth and proliferation. An important concept that is universally accepted is that cancer is a genetic disease, although it is not always heritable. Tumors arise from the accumulation of mutations that eliminate normal constraints of proliferation and genetic integrity in a somatic cell. Among other causes, mutations can arise because of the inherent error rate of enzymes that control DNA replication during each division, which introduces about 1 in 1,000,000 to 1 in 10,000,000 mutations for each base that is replicated during each round of cell division. The genome consists of many millions of base pairs, so each daughter cell is likely to carry at least a few mutations in its DNA. Most of these mutations are silent; that is, they do not present any problems to the cell's ability to function. However, others can disable tumor suppressor genes or activate proto-oncogenes that respectively inhibit or promote cell division and survival. Hence, it can be said that "being alive" is the single largest risk factor for cancer.

However, there is evidence to suggest that in some cases mutations are "directed" because of the presence of a "mutator phenotype," where the factors that control DNA replication and repair are prone to more errors than would be expected by simple random events. This leads to different rates of cancer predisposition, which would be higher than the mean in individuals bearing this "mutator phenotype," and might explain why not all people or animals exposed to similar environmental carcinogens develop the same forms of cancer at the same rate.

This genetic predisposition to cancer is illustrated by the existence of well-defined heritable cancer syndromes.[3] Even though they account for fewer than 5% of all human cancers, studies of families with these syndromes provided many of the initial clues to understand

10

the genetic basis of sporadic (non-heritable) cancers. In most cases, these familial cancer syndromes show dominant patterns of inheritance and have high penetrance, although the mechanism of disease is not due to inheritance of a dominant allele, but rather is generally due to inheritance of a mutant (inactive) allele followed by inactivation of the second allele through a process called *loss of heterozygosity*. A curious observation is worth noting: different mutations in a single gene predispose individuals to distinct cancer syndromes, whereas independent, single mutations of different genes can result in virtually the same disease, or at least diseases with indistinguishable phenotypes.[3] This is less surprising when we consider the fact that commonly affected genes are multifunctional and are parts of complex interactive networks or circuits,[4] so a mutation may only alter gene function along one biochemical pathway, leaving its interactions with other pathways intact. Another intriguing observation is that mutations that contribute to most sporadic cancers are restricted to a small subset of genes,[5,6] many of which are also associated with heritable cancer syndromes. These observations have given rise to competing contemporary theories on the origins of cancer, which are addressed in Table 2-1.

At least one heritable cancer syndrome (renal carcinoma and nodular dermatofibrosis [RCND] of German Shepherd dogs) has been described in dogs.[7] The heritable factor (or *RCND* gene) for this syndrome maps to dog chromosome 5 (CFA 5), and specifically to the folliculin gene, which was recently described as the heritable factor for the corresponding human disease (Birt-Hogg-Dube syndrome). It is probable that other syndromes comparable to those described in humans eventually will be identified in companion and laboratory animals, but it is unlikely these will account for more than 5% to 10% of all cancer cases. Yet, even with the estimated lifetime cancer risk (for humans and for dogs) of approximately 1 in 3, it is incorrect to surmise that most cancers (>90%) are due solely to environmental causes. Heritable influences affect susceptibility, but they are difficult to identify in heterogeneous outbred backgrounds such as those that occur in most human families or mixed breed dogs. On the other hand, highly inbred human populations and families, specific ethnic groups, or purebred dogs may allow for identification of factors that influence both cancer risk and phenotype.[8-10] Outside of these populations, the existence of heritable factors that are modulated by environmental influence will be labor intensive to define. For example, more than 3000 matched cases and controls would be needed to unequivocally identify the multiplicative interaction among two or more genes that increase cancer risk by two-fold when the allele frequency is 5%, and more than 1500 would still be required when the allele frequency is as high as 25%.[11]

Changes in cancer incidence over the course of the 20th century, many reflecting behavior patterns (e.g., lung cancer in smokers), infectious diseases (e.g., stomach cancer in people infected with *Helicobacter pylori*), or exposure to special cultural factors such as urbanization or diet (e.g., increasing breast cancer rates in the second and subsequent generations of Asian-American women),

---

TABLE 2-1   COMPETING HYPOTHESIS FOR GENETIC ORIGIN OF CANCER

Property	Somatic Cell Theory	Stem Cell Theory
Origin	Any somatic cell that acquires the right complement of mutations	Stem cell with a critical transforming mutation or de-differentiated somatic cell with stem cell properties
Self-renewal	Acquired through mutation	Inherent property of stem cells
Genes involved	Does not predict recurrent gene involvement for different cancers—any gene that controls growth, survival, or immortalization of the affected cell can contribute	Predicts that a small number of genes that specifically regulate stem cell self-renewal will disproportionately contribute to all types of cancer
Differentiation	Cells arrest development at a particular stage or undergo limited de-differentiation caused by mutation	Inherent property of stem cell progeny
Metastatic potential	Acquired through mutation	Inherent property of stem cells, but also can be acquired through mutation
Resistance to cytotoxic therapy	Acquired through mutation or selection	Inherent property of stem cells

underscore the significant influence that the environment exerts on the genetic make-up of any individual. We anticipate that the combination of novel molecular and epidemiologic approaches, combined with the judicious use of laboratory animal models and naturally occurring cancers of humans and companion animals, will allow us to tease apart the relative contributions of genes and environment to the process of carcinogenesis in the near future.

IS CANCER A DISEASE OF STEM CELLS?

Unlike diseases that arise from single gene defects, cancer is a complex, multigenic disease. In fact, a sequential progression of mutations is required to produce a *bona fide* tumor cell. In the classical model of initiation, promotion, and progression, a genetic mutation first endows a somatic cell with limitless replicative potential or another growth or survival advantage from other cells in its environment. Alone, this mutation is not sufficient to give rise to a tumor, as the cell remains constrained by environmental factors. A second mutation (or series of mutations) further adds to the cell's ability to outcompete its neighbors in this environment, leading to its potential expansion into a recognizable tumor mass. Finally, a third series of mutations reinforces the cell's malignant potential (invasion, tissue destruction, and metastasis) that leads to clinical disease (see Table 2-1).

This model is useful to illustrate the point that no single gene is universally responsible for transformation, but rather, we can think of many genes contributing to (rather than "causing") the origin and progression cancer.[1] It also provides a basis to set a minimum estimate of five or six mutations that are required before cancer becomes clinically evident, although empirical evidence suggests the actual number required is higher.[6] These mutations provide a cell and its progeny with each of the six hallmarks of cancer,[12] namely (1) self-sufficiency of growth signals, (2) insensitivity to anti-growth signals, (3) the ability to evade apoptosis, (4) limitless replicative potential, (5) sustained angiogenesis, and (6) the capacity to invade tissues and metastasize (Table 2-2). In some instances, mutation of a single gene may provide more than one such property, but more often, mutations of multiple genes are necessary to achieve each of these "milestones." Moreover, since interactive biochemical cascades regulate each of these six steps, mutations of different genes along shared pathways can result in equivalent phenotypes (see http://www.nature.com/nrc/journal/v2/n5/weinberg_poster/). Conceptually, this helps us understand how mutations of different genes can lead to similar cancer phenotypes and outcome, and conversely why mutations of the same gene can result in different cancers with distinct biological behaviors.

This model is consistent with many aspects of the natural behavior of tumors, and to some extent, it can predict risk and outcome. However, if we assume that all cells possess an equal capacity for self-renewal, and that proliferation is a stochastic ("random") process driven entirely by environmental selection of favorable mutations, this model would necessarily predict that cancer is an inevitable outcome for multicellular organisms, and few—if any—long-lived animals would reach reproductive age. Thus, this model by necessity must invoke the existence of protective mechanisms that are independent of cancer risk (e.g., efficient DNA repair mechanisms and immune surveillance).

A competing theory now exists whose main tenet is that self-renewal is limited to a small population of "cancer stem cells," similar in many ways to normal multipotent stem cells that give rise to a population of lineage-committed cells that form organs and tissues,

TABLE 2-2   HALLMARKS OF CANCER

Acquired Property	Examples
Self-sufficiency of growth signals	Activation of oncogenic genes and proteins such as Ras, Kit, EGFR
Insensitivity to anti-growth signals	Loss of tumor suppressors such as Rb, p16, PTEN
Evasion of apoptosis	Production of survival factors such as IGF-1
	Gain of function of survival genes such as Bcl-2
	Loss of function of pro-apoptotic genes such as p53, PTEN
Limitless replicative potential	Induction of telomerase
Sustained angiogenesis	Production of vascular endothelial growth factor
Tissue invasion and metastasis	Inactivation of adhesion molecules such as E-cadherin, upregulation of proteases like MMPs
	Acquisition of survival factors (see evasion of apoptosis)

and cancer is a consequence of malignant transformation of such cells.[13,14] In other words, a small number of self-renewing cells in a tumor generate progeny that comprise the bulk of cells that produce the disease phenotype (see Table 2-1). The origin of these cells is still a matter of debate. Although they might represent transformed stem cells, the preponderance of data now suggest they arise from de-differentiated somatic cells that acquire peculiar stem cell properties of self-renewal and multipotency through mutation. The existence of cancer stem cells is now documented; they are characterized both by peculiar phenotypes and by defined sets of mutations of a small number of genes.[15,16] Other mutations then endow their progeny with limited or extensive capacity to undergo programmed differentiation, hence resulting in distinct clinical phenotypes such as acute and chronic leukemias or high- and low-grade solid tumors. The strongest evidence for cancer stem cells indeed comes from hematopoietic tumors, but cancer stem cells also have been identified in various solid tumors.[17,18]

The cancer stem cell theory is intellectually satisfying in many ways, since it can explain various paradoxical findings.[14] First, this theory accounts for the relatively small number of oncogenes and tumor suppressor genes whose respective activation and inactivation are found in a disproportionate number of different cancers. Second, the cancer stem cell theory accounts for the ability of multicellular organisms to reach reproductive age and attain long lives without cancer. It was recently proposed that stem cells evolved partly as a cancer protective mechanism because even the requirement for a single cell to accumulate several mutations before it becomes cancerous would not be sufficient to prevent long-lived organisms from dying of cancer at a relatively young (pre-reproductive) age. That is, if each of the trillions of cells formed in a complex mammal (such as a dog or a cat) over its lifetime retained the capacity to divide, the probability of a single cell acquiring a complement of mutations leading to cancer would be overwhelming. Thus, an adaptation to limit the number of long-lived cells with self-renewal capacity (and therefore the number of cells that can form tumors) would offer a selective advantage to attain reproductive age. The relatively high incidence of cancer in aged populations reinforces the notion that even with a limited number of susceptible stem cells, the probability to develop cancer over a long life is exceedingly high. Third, the cancer stem cell theory can also explain the observed nature of tumor relapse and metastasis, since cancer stem cells may express drug transporters as a component of their normal phenotype or they might acquire drug resistance over the course of treatment. Because the cells retain high proliferative potential (compared with that of lineage-committed progeny, which is limited), failure to eliminate cancer stem cells after cessation of chemotherapy sets the stage for tumor regrowth and relapse, which would not occur if the remaining cells lacked the capacity for self-renewal. The acquisition of additional mutations (possibly due to the chemotherapy itself) allows cells to generate progeny with enhanced survivability in novel environments, favoring more aggressive, metastatic phenotypes. Our data suggesting that hemangiosarcoma is a disease of stem cells were the first to provide supporting evidence for this theory in a naturally occurring canine tumor.[19]

ADAPTIVE EVOLUTION IN THE TUMOR ENVIRONMENT

Our previous reference to a "selective growth advantage" that is reminiscent of Darwinian selection is not accidental. The clonal evolution theory[20,21] addresses the significance of sequential genetic changes providing growth and survival advantages, but to this we must add the fact that, in addition to these self-sufficient events that influence growth and survival, tumor cells must also evade "predators" (e.g., inflammation and the immune system[22,23]). In essence, the interaction of the tumor with its microenvironment, and ultimately with the host, is in fact subject to Darwinian laws of evolution, albeit in an accelerated time scale.[24] This is evident in the ability of tumors to modulate stromal cells to support their own growth by providing a suitable matrix and an abundance of nutrients, while maintaining antitumor responses at bay.

As is true for other selective environments, tumors that outgrow the capability of their immediate surroundings to support their growth will seek to become established in other favorable locations. The process of metastasis is also strongly influenced by mutations that allow cells to thrive in new environments. Again, the classical model of metastasis proposed by Fidler[25] suggests a step-wise acquisition of assets that enables cells to leave the primary tumor site, travel through blood or lymph, invade stroma in favorable locations, and thus become reestablished at distant sites, but more recent work suggests that most tumors possess the ability to dislodge cells that travel to distant sites, so the ability of such cells to survive in capillary beds may be the most important step in the metastatic process.[26-28]

FROM CONCEPTS TO CLINICS: MOLECULAR GENETICS USHER IN AN ERA OF OPPORTUNITY

Improvements in our fundamental understanding of cancer biology present opportunities to lower the morbidity and mortality associated with this disease. For half a century, conventional cytogenetic approaches provided clues to the genetic basis of cancer. More recently, the introduction of molecular cytogenetics and other molecular genetic tools has revolutionized the way we are able to interrogate changes in chromosome and gene structure or function associated with cancer. Numerical chromosome changes (e.g., whole chromosome aneuploidy, insertions, deletions) represent a deviation from the normal gene copy number, potentially leading to increased or decreased expression of genes associated with regulation of growth or survival. Structural changes (e.g., inversions, translocations) result in genome reorganization, which may cause genes that are separated in the *normal* genome to be brought into close proximity in the *tumor* genome with consequent effects on gene dysregulation. Abnormal patterns of gene expression can also result from mutations that affect single genes. In fact, every tumor will have a multiplicity of mutant genes that will create unique patterns of gene expression and contribute to its pathogenesis.

Clonal chromosome aberrations have been identified in more than 50,000 human neoplasms representing 75 different types of cancer (see http://cgap.nci.nih.gov/Chromosomes/Mitelman). Many of these recurrent chromosome aberrations are associated with histopathological or immunological subgroups and with response to therapy. In addition to directing basic research and the discovery of underlying gene involvement, these associations are now widely used as important diagnostic and prognostic aids during the evaluation of human cancers, with consequent improvements in the clinical management of patients. Patients with good prognosis can be spared unnecessary treatment, and, conversely, those patients whose cytogenetic abnormalities indicate poor prognosis can receive more aggressive treatments to improve the probability of positive outcomes. The World Health Organization recognizes that genetic abnormalities are one of the most reliable criteria for the classification of tumors and has stressed the importance of further research into this area.

Recent progress in molecular cytogenetics of domestic animals, and especially the dog, has allowed us to develop a "toolbox" that will accelerate progress in our understanding of cancer genetics. Specifically, we can now use chromosome-specific fluorescence *in situ* hybridization (FISH) to directly interrogate altered genome organization within individual cells comprising the malignant mass,[29-31] as well as canine comparative genomic hybridization analysis to determine chromosome copy number status across the entire genome.[29,30,32,33] FISH analysis has also enabled the precise definition of structural chromosome aberrations that show a convincing

evolutionary history between homologous cancers of dogs and people.[34] These analyses can be used to predict both tumor origin and response to therapy. For instance, gain of dog chromosome 13 (CFA 13), particularly in a region syntenic to human chromosome 4q (HSA 4q), occurs in ~70% of canine diffuse B-cell lymphoma.[30] This suggests that this region of the genome contains heretofore-unidentified genes that are etiologically and prognostically significant for this disease. There are also indications that gain of CFA 13 is also predictive for chemotherapy response,[30,35] perhaps because amplification of the c-*Myc* and c-*Kit* oncogenes, both of which are encoded in this region of CFA 13, increases the proliferative rate of the malignant cells and consequently their susceptibility to anti-mitotic compounds. These approaches can also be used to define specific chromosomal regions that are associated with heritable risk by identifying unique tumor genomes that segregate with selected breeds or groups, and that can pinpoint new regions for gene discovery.[9]

Although they are at earlier stages of development, tools such as arrays that can be used to analyze global gene expression are making rapid progress toward clinical application. The ability to analyze thousands of genes at once (~36,000 in the case of humans and ~22,000 in the case of dogs) maximizes the efficiency with which we can identify genetic alterations associated with tumor pathogenesis, as well as prognostic "gene signatures."[36-41] In animals, the potential utility of expression arrays has been documented for canine osteosarcoma and canine non-Hodgkin's lymphoma.[42,43] Furthermore, even though ~90% of the genome does not encode proteins, it nevertheless has important functions to maintain homeostasis. As recently as 10 years ago, non-coding DNA was brazenly called "junk DNA" and was thought to be an anachronism inherited from our evolutionary forebears. We now know that this DNA in fact encodes molecules such as micro-RNAs that have important functions in gene regulation.[44] Moreover, gain or loss of function of micro-RNAs may turn out to be no less important in cancer causation than gain or loss of function of traditional protein-coding genes.[45-48] Despite the rudimentary stage of clinical development, we anticipate that the current pace of technological advancement should place these and other technologies at the forefront of cancer management during the next decade.

SUMMARY

We can state with confidence that the genetic basis of cancer is beyond question. It is estimated that five or more mutations are required for overt transformation, and genomic instability seems to be necessary to establish a self-renewing population of cells whose progeny expand to cause clinical disease. In the end, a subpopulation that acquires metastatic properties and is drug resistant will be the cause of death for the cancer patient. A contemporary area of emphasis is to define whether these properties are inherent to cancer stem cells or whether they arise by natural selection and clonal evolution. We can use molecular tools to predict risk, prognosis, and response to therapy in some cancers of companion animals, and we believe the availability and usefulness of such tools in clinical practice will expand rapidly. Therefore, as we improve our understanding of basic mechanisms that account for malignant transformation and tumor progression, we will be able to design better strategies for cancer prevention and therapy.

Selected References*

The following reviews and original manuscript are considered to suitably illustrate our current understanding of cancer genetics.

Nowell PC: The clonal evolution of tumor cell populations, *Science* 194:23-28, 1976.

This paper describes the original hypothesis of clonal evolution in cancer based on the author's experience studying cytogenetics of solid and hematopoietic human tumors.

Hanahan D, Weinberg RA: The hallmarks of cancer, *Cell* 100:57-70, 2000.

This is the quintessential review of the molecular basis of cancer. In it, Hanahan and Weinberg describe the six essential features that define cancer and how these allow cells to thrive as they interact with the microenvironment.

Golub TR, Slonim DK, Tamayo P, et al: Molecular classification of cancer: class discovery and class prediction by gene expression monitoring, *Science* 286:531-37, 1999.

This is one of the first papers showing gene expression profiling can be used to subdivide tumors according to ontogeny and to prognosticate biological behavior in an unbiased fashion.

Sjöblom T, Jones S, Wood LD, et al: The consensus coding sequences of human breast and colorectal cancer, *Science* 314:268-74, 2006.

This is the first paper that completes full transcriptome sequencing of solid human tumors, documenting recurrent mutations that are potentially causal and passenger mutations that might be inconsequential or possibly associated with progression. The data allow the authors to estimate that ~14 to 20 cancer-associated genes must undergo functional mutation in order for a cell to acquire the properties associated with a malignant solid tumor.

Lapidot T, Sirard C, Vormoor J, et al: A cell initiating human acute myeloid leukaemia after transplantation into SCID mice, *Nature* 367:645-48, 1994.

This is the manuscript that revived the interest in a stem cell or stem cell–like progenitor as the single cell that gives rise to cancer.

Johnson CD, Esquela-Kerscher A, Stefani G, et al: The let-7 microRNA represses cell proliferation pathways in human cells, *Cancer Res* 67:7713-22, 2007.

In this paper, Johnson et al describe a role of let-7 miRNA as a master cell cycle regulator that controls stability of anti-proliferative genes and promotes decay of genes that are required for cell cycle progression. The data validate the role of miRNAs as bona fide "tumor suppressor genes."

Breen M, Modiano JF: Evolutionarily conserved cytogenetic changes in hematologic malignancies of dogs and humans—man and his best friend share more than companionship, *Chromosome Res* 16:145-54, 2008.

This manuscript describes the evolutionary relationship between chromosomal abnormalities in naturally occurring tumors of humans and dogs, as well as a potential mechanism to explain the high frequency of rearrangements involving relatively small numbers of genes.

*For a complete list of the references cited in this chapter, please go to www.smallanimaloncology.com.

3 Veterinary Cancer Etiology

In 1978, the U.S. Congress ordered the development of the first Report on Carcinogens (RoC). The report, designed to educate the public and health professionals about potential cancer hazards, is now required by law to be released every 2 years by the Secretary of the Department of Health and Human Services. The most recent RoC, the Eleventh Edition, lists 246 potential carcinogens, of which 58 are categorized as *known to be human carcinogens* and 188 are categorized as *reasonably anticipated to be human carcinogens*.[1] Although no similar report has been developed relative to companion animals, it is reasonable to assume that considerable overlap would exist between such a list and the RoC. The latest RoC is the first to include neutrons, x- and gamma-radiation and viruses (Hepatitis B virus, Hepatitis C virus, and human papillomavirus) as carcinogens. Although the list of carcinogens known to be associated with cancer development in companion animals is somewhat shorter, this chapter will address environmental (chemical and physical), viral, and hormonal factors thought to be associated with carcinogenesis in pet animals.

SECTION A: Environmental, Chemical, and Physical Carcinogens

Carolyn J. Henry

KEY POINTS

- Although causal associations are difficult to prove, there is mounting evidence that environmental factors contribute to development of certain cancers in companion animals.
- Cumulative long-term exposure to ultraviolet-B (UV-B) light can induce skin tumors directly by causing genetic mutations or indirectly by impairing the immune response to tumor antigens.
- While a definitive link between phenoxy herbicides and development of lymphoma or transitional cell carcinoma (TCC) of the bladder in companion animals has not been proven, attempts to minimize the access of pets to these products is warranted based on the data published to date.

PESTICIDES, HERBICIDES, AND INSECTICIDES

In 1991, investigators at the National Cancer Institute (NCI) completed a case-control study to examine the relationship between exposure of dogs to the herbicide 2,4,dichlorophenoxyacetic acid (2,4-D) and development of lymphoma.[2] Dogs diagnosed with lymphoma during a 4-year period were identified through computerized medical records from three veterinary medical teaching hospitals. Each case animal was age-matched with two control animals. The first control group was comprised of dogs diagnosed during the same time period with neoplastic disease other than lymphoma, and the second control group was a non-tumor control group, selected from all other dogs presented to the hospital for conditions deemed unrelated to chemical exposure. Data regarding household use and potential exposure to chemicals including commercial lawn care and owner-applied herbicides were collected and analyzed. The investigators reported a positive association between the use of commercial lawn care services or exposure to owner-applied 2,4-D and the development of canine lymphoma. The risk doubled when owners applied 2,4-D liquid or granules to the lawn four or more times a year. The release of these findings prompted an independent review by an expert panel convened to assess the validity of the study.[3]

The panel raised concerns about the study design, data analysis, and interpretation and concluded that a relationship between 2,4-D exposure and the development of canine lymphoma could not be established based on the data presented by Hayes et al.[2] The original investigators subsequently reanalyzed their data, and addressed many of the concerns raised by the scientific review panel.[4] In their second study, Hayes et al.[4] used a more stringent definition of 2,4-D exposure, including only cases in which the owner applied 2,4-D as the sole herbicide and did not use any other lawn chemicals or lawn care services. Their second report did not show a statistically significant association between exposure to 2,4-D and development of lymphoma. They did, however, conclude that their results indicated a dose-response relationship between disease incidence and the number of yearly 2,4-D applications by dog owners. A fourth report was published in 1999 by researchers from Michigan State University who obtained the original data and reanalyzed it once again.[5] In this last study, a more stringent definition of exposure was applied and a dose-response analysis was completed. The study, which was funded by a grant from a chemical industry task force, showed no dose-response relationship between number of 2,4-D applications and the occurrence of canine lymphoma.[5] Increased urinary excretion of 2,4-D has been demonstrated for dogs exposed to herbicide-treated lawns. However, a direct link between such exposure and development of lymphoma has not been shown.[6] A more recent case-control study conducted in Italy assessed the effect of residential exposure to environmental pollutants on the risk of developing lymphoma.[7] An association between exposure to pesticides (including herbicides) and development of lymphoma was not shown. However, dogs living in industrial areas or with owners who used chemicals such as paints and solvents were shown to be at significantly increased risk of developing lymphoma.

Transitional cell carcinoma (TCC) of the bladder has been linked to insecticide and herbicide exposure beginning with a 1989 case-control study by Glickman et al.[8] In the study, 59 dogs with TCC and 71 age and breed size–matched control dogs with other neoplastic or chronic disease were compared in an effort to assess the effect of obesity, exposure to sidestream cigarette smoke and chemicals, and use of topical insecticides on risk of developing TCC. Dogs treated with topical insecticides were at increased risk of developing TCC, and the risk was enhanced in overweight or obese dogs.

In a study of risk factors for oral SCC in cats, Bertone et al.[9] reported a significantly increased risk of oral SCC in cats that wore flea collars. However, newer topical spot-on flea and tick products have been evaluated in populations of Scottish Terriers, a breed known to be at risk for development of TCC of the urinary bladder, and have not been shown to increase the risk of TCC.[10] Similar studies in Scottish Terriers have suggested that exposure to lawn and garden care products containing phenoxy herbicides, including 2,4-D, 4-chloro-2-methylphenoxy acetic acid (MCPA) and 2-(4-chloro-2-methyl) phenoxy propionic acid (MCPP), is associated with an increased risk of TCC.[11] Although it is difficult to prove a link between phenoxy herbicides and development of lymphoma or TCC, attempts to minimize the access of pets to these products would seem warranted based on the data published to date.

ENVIRONMENTAL TOBACCO SMOKE

Despite ample evidence that secondhand smoke increases the risk of lung cancer in people, there is less compelling evidence for this effect in companion animals.[12,13] A case-control study evaluating canine lung cancer cases from two veterinary hospitals showed only a weak relationship between living with a smoker and the risk of developing lung cancer, and the risk did not increase with an increased level of smoke exposure.[14] However, evidence for a relationship between exposure to environmental tobacco smoke (ETS) and development of other malignancies in companion animals is mounting. Based on evidence that smoking increases the risk of non-Hodgkin's lymphoma development in people,[15,16] Bertone et al.[17] examined the relationship between ETS exposure and development of feline lymphoma. Their case-control study included 80 cats with malignant lymphoma and 114 control cats with renal disease presenting to Tufts University School of Veterinary Medicine (TUSVM) between 1993 and 2000. They reported that the relative risk of lymphoma for cats with any household ETS exposure was 2.4. As is reported for male smokers,[18] the risk of lymphoma increased with both increased duration and quantity of exposure.

Hypothesizing that inhalation and ingestion of carcinogenic compounds in ETS during grooming might also predispose cats in smoking households to develop oral squamous cell carcinoma (SCC), the same group examined ETS, along with other environmental and lifestyle risk factors, in cats with SCC.[9] The study population consisted of 36 cats with oral SCC, and the control population consisted of 112 cats with renal disease, all presenting to TUSVM between 1994 and 2000. Exposure to ETS was associated with a two-fold increased risk of oral SCC, but this was not statistically significant.[9] Interestingly, in a separate report, the investigators showed that SCC tissue from cats exposed to any ETS was 4.5 times more likely to overexpress p53 and cats with 5 years or more of ETS exposure had tumors that were 7 times more likely to overexpress p53.[19] Although the findings did not reach statistical significance, the collective work of this group provides an intriguing suggestion that both ETS and mutations in the p53 gene may play a role in the etiology of feline oral SCC.

CYCLOPHOSPHAMIDE

The chemotherapy drug, cyclophosphamide, has been implicated as an etiologic factor in the development of urinary bladder cancer in people and in dogs.[20-22] Because the drug's metabolite, acrolein, is irritating to the bladder mucosa, sterile hemorrhagic cystitis is a potential side effect of cyclophosphamide therapy. It is thought that chronic inflammation resulting from acrolein exposure is a predisposing event for the development of bladder cancer in patients that have undergone cyclophosphamide therapy. The author has treated a dog for lymphoma that was discovered to have concurrent but clinically occult TCC of the bladder before the initiation of cyclophosphamide chemotherapy. Had an abdominal ultrasound not been performed as part of the initial staging procedures for this dog prior to chemotherapy, the bladder TCC may have been diagnosed at a later date and incorrectly attributed to administration of cyclophosphamide. This exemplifies the fact that one cannot necessarily assume a cause-and-effect relationship for potential carcinogens, especially in animals that have already been diagnosed with another malignancy.

RURAL VERSUS URBAN ENVIRONMENT

Although several reports have noted differences in companion animal cancer incidence between urban and rural settings, the underlying cause for these differences is unclear. An increased incidence of some canine cancers such as nasal carcinoma, lymphoma, and tonsillar SCC[7,23,24] has been reported in urban and industrial settings compared with rural settings. However, because multiple environmental carcinogens may coexist within the same setting, it is often difficult to discern the "smoking gun." Nonetheless, the study of animals as sentinels of environmental health hazards has been recommended and includes the assessment of carcinogenic risk across species.[25-27]

SUNLIGHT

The relationship between sunlight or ultraviolet irradiation and subsequent development of skin cancer is well known in both human and veterinary medicine.

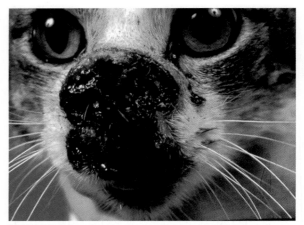

FIGURE 3-1 Invasive squamous cell carcinoma of the nasal planum is an example of a solar-induced malignancy that occurs in lightly pigmented or white areas of the face and ears in cats.

As with the etiology of human SCC, sunlight has been implicated as a cause of SCC in domestic animals and livestock. This implication is strengthened by the clear dose response relationship that has been shown in both epidemiological and experimental studies.[28-31] Specifically, light skin pigmentation and chronic sun exposure are associated with development of facial, aural, and nasal planum SCC in white or partially white cats (Figure 3-1) and may play a similar role in some cutaneous SCC lesions in dogs. Ultraviolet-B (UV-B) light, which is in the range of 280 to 320 nm, is the part of the ultraviolet spectrum that is most likely to be responsible for nonmelanotic skin lesions in people and animals.[28] Cumulative long-term exposure to UV-B may induce skin tumors directly by causing genetic mutations (such as p53) or indirectly by impairing the immune response to tumor antigens.[28,32,33] Companion animals are at greatest risk of UV exposure during the midday hours. Protection from this exposure is warranted, especially in lightly pigmented breeds.

TRAUMA/CHRONIC INFLAMMATION

Chronic inflammation can lead to genetic mutations that ultimately result in neoplastic transformation. In four dogs with chronic pigmentary keratitis, neoplastic lesions of the cornea (three SCC and one squamous papilloma) were reported.[34] Although the underlying etiology of the keratitis could not be confirmed, the neoplastic transformation was thought to be related to chronic inflammation. Earlier reports have linked feline intraocular sarcomas to prior ocular trauma and secondary uveitis and lens rupture.[35] Despite the varied histologies, in both examples the underlying etiology was thought to be related to inflammatory changes (see Chapter 20, Section C, for more detail). Another small animal malignancy thought to be associated with inflammation is vaccine-associated feline sarcoma (VAFS).[36] This tumor type is discussed in Chapter 23, Section E, Vaccine site fibrosarcomas have also been reported in dogs and ferrets.[37,38]

MAGNETIC FIELDS

A potential link between childhood cancer and chronic low-dose exposure to magnetic fields was first proposed more than 25 years ago.[39] Since that time, multiple studies have attempted to identify links between magnetic fields and a variety of human cancers ranging from hematopoietic malignancies to breast cancer. The extremely low–frequency (<60 Hz) magnetic fields in question are ubiquitous in today's society and are generated by household appliances, industrial machinery, and electrical power lines. Because pets share our environment and thus have a similar amount of exposure to magnetic fields, it has been suggested that companion animals are at similar risk of cancer development because of this etiology. A 1995 study found the risk for canine lymphoma was highest in dogs from households with the highest measured exposure to magnetic fields.[40] This risk was related to both the duration and the intensity of exposure. Dogs that spent more than 25% of the day outdoors were found to be at highest risk. A year later, a report was published by the National Research Council (NRC) at the request of Congress and reviewed over 500 studies on the subject of cancer risk and exposure to electromagnetic fields.[41] The report concluded that, although a weak association has been shown between development of childhood leukemia and exposure to electromagnetic fields, no clear evidence exists to suggest that exposure to electromagnetic fields is a true threat to human health. To the author's knowledge, there have been no further reports on the possible link between magnetic fields and cancer in companion animals published since the 1995 report. Still, the magnetic field debate continues in the human oncology literature. The NRC report suggested that other factors including air quality and proximity to high-traffic density are more likely environmental causes of cancer than low-frequency magnetic fields.

RADIATION

The first report of canine cancer developing after therapeutic irradiation dates back almost a quarter century, when orthovoltage radiation was considered state of the art.[42] At the time, the term *malignant transformation* was used to describe the development of epithelial malignancies at the site of prior irradiation for acanthomatous epulides in four dogs. With both the benefit of hindsight and a review of more recent cases, the author of the original report has since suggested that the term *malignant transformation* is misleading, in that the occurrence of second tumors was unlikely due to a true transformation of epulides into carcinomas.[43] Rather, radiation carcinogenesis is the likely cause of second tumors in radiation fields. In human oncology, most tumors that occur in heavily irradiated treatment fields are of mesenchymal, rather than epithelial, origin.[44,45] Several reports of sarcomas occurring at sites of prior radiation may be found in the veterinary literature.[42,46-48] One example is a retrospective review of 57 dogs undergoing definitive megavoltage radiation therapy with ^{60}cobalt photons for acanthomatous epulis.[43] In the report, McEntee et al.[43] described the development of a second tumor (one sarcoma and one osteosarcoma) in two of the 57 irradiated dogs, occurring 5.2 and 8.7 years after the initial treatment, respectively. The overall incidence of second tumors was only 3.5% in the manuscript by McEntee et al.[43] compared with figures of up to 18% in previous reports.[42,49] The fact that no epithelial tumors were reported in this latest paper may indicate that megavoltage radiation therapy used today more efficiently targets an existing subpopulation of malignant epithelial cells than did orthovoltage. The risk of second tumors at sites of radiation therapy is primarily of clinical concern when treating young dogs that are expected to enjoy long-term survival. Second tumors have also been reported in at least six people who have undergone stereotactic radiosurgery.[50] As this radiation technique becomes more commonplace in veterinary medicine, the possibility of second tumors may need to be considered in companion animals as well.

SURGERY AND IMPLANTED DEVICES

Sarcoma development at the site of metallic implants has been reported in people, dogs, and laboratory animal models.[51,52] However, it is often difficult to know if sarcoma development is related to fracture fixation devices or to other factors, including wound-healing complications and osteomyelitis. The largest veterinary study to examine the relationship between metallic implants and tumor development in dogs was published in 1993 by Li et al.[52] The authors reported on 222 dogs that developed tumors of any kind after fracture fixation, compared with 1635 dogs that underwent fracture fixation but did not subsequently develop tumors. The investigators concluded that use of metallic implants was not a risk factor for bone tumor development. Other types of implants and foreign materials related to surgery are sporadically implicated in carcinogenesis in human and veterinary case reports. Published examples include a dog that developed a myxoma at the site of a subcutaneous pacemaker implantation and another that developed a jejunal osteosarcoma associated with a surgical sponge presumably not retrieved during an abdominal surgery 6 years prior.[53,54] More recently, it has been suggested that microchips implanted subcutaneously in companion animals for identification purposes may lead to tumor development at the microchip site.[55,56] This link is yet to be proven but is currently under investigation.

ASBESTOS

Asbestos exposure is an established risk factor for development of human mesothelioma.[57] In fact, between 60% and 88% of all human cases of mesothelioma are estimated to be attributable to asbestos exposure.[57] A similar association has been found for dogs whose owners have an asbestos-related occupation or hobby.[58] Further evidence was provided by a study in which significantly more asbestos bodies were found in dogs with mesothelioma than in control dogs.[59] Pericardial mesothelioma was reported in five golden retrievers with long-term histories of idiopathic hemorrhagic pericardial effusion, suggesting that other factors, including breed predispositions and non-asbestos related causes of chronic inflammation may play a role in the etiology of pericardial mesothelioma.[60]

Selected References*

Bertone ER, Snyder LA, Moore AS: Environmental tobacco smoke and risk of malignant lymphoma in pet cats, *Am J Epidemiol* 156:268, 2002.
This manuscript reports the findings of a case control study demonstrating an increased risk of lymphoma in cats living in households with smokers.
Glickman LT, Raghavan M, Knapp DW, et al: Herbicide exposure and the risk of transitional cell carcinoma of the urinary bladder in Scottish Terriers, *J Am Vet Med Assoc* 224:1290, 2004.
This epidemiological study examining a breed at high risk for transitional cell carcinoma shows a potential link between exposure to herbicides and an increased risk of developing bladder cancer.
Hayes HM, Tarone RE, Cantor KP, et al: Case-control study of canine malignant lymphoma: positive association with dog owner's use of 2,4-dichlorophenoxyacetic acid herbicides, *J Natl Cancer Inst* 83:1226, 1991.
This initial report of a possible link between 2,4-D exposure and risk of canine lymphoma spawned an intense debate and years of investigation into the role of pesticides and herbicides in cancer development in companion animals.
McEntee MC, Page RL, Theon A, et al: Malignant tumor formation in dogs previously irradiated for acanthomatous epulis, *Vet Radiol Ultrasound* 45:357, 2004.
This manuscript discusses the risk of malignant tumor formation within the previous site of therapeutic irradiation for epulides.

*For a complete list of the references cited in this chapter, please go to www.smallanimaloncology.com.

SECTION B: Viral Carcinogenesis

Dennis W. Macy and Kimberly B. Reeds

KEY POINTS

- Canine viral papillomas most frequently occur in the oral or ocular mucous membranes of young dogs, and most will undergo spontaneous regression.
- Feline viral papillomas most frequently occur in older cats and are often located in regions of haired skin, are less likely to spontaneously regress than in dogs, and may transform into carcinoma *in situ* if not removed.
- Transmission of the feline leukemia virus occurs through bite wounds and repeated and prolonged contact by sharing water and food bowls as well as litter pans.

- Tumors that develop in cats infected with feline immunodeficiency virus are thought to be due to immunosuppression.

Cancer may be caused by both DNA and RNA viruses. Malignant transformation of a host cell begins with incorporation of viral DNA or DNA copy of the retroviral RNA into the host genome. Viral oncogenes that lead to malignant transformation of normal host cells have been identified. Overexpression or inactivation of normal host genes can also be initiated by viral integration into the host genome, causing unlimited replication or transformation to a malignant phenotype.[1,2]

PAPILLOMAVIRUSES

Papillomaviruses are DNA viruses that can integrate into cells, activate the expression of normal cellular genes, and ultimately cause overexpression or inactivation of genes that can lead to cellular transformation or uncontrolled growth.[1]

Papillomaviruses are oncogenic, contagious, and infectious and have been described in a number of species.[3] Papillomaviruses are considered species specific, and human, bovine, canine, and feline isolates lack serologic cross-reactivity.[3] However, similar species such as the coyote may be infected with dog isolates.[4] Papillomaviruses of the family Papovaviridae are responsible for producing benign, mucocutaneous, canine papillomas and benign, often multicentric, lesions in cats, some of which may progress to carcinoma *in situ* (Bowen's disease).

The canine and feline papillomaviruses are larger than the parvoviruses of dogs and cats but are similar in structure. Electron microscopy has been used to identify the presence of the virus in infected tissues. Like other papillomaviruses, the canine and feline papillomavirus is resistant, acid stable, and relatively thermostable. Although there is only limited sequence homology between the DNA sequences of papillomaviruses of different species, substantial sequence homology exists between isolates derived from any given species.[3]

Pathogenesis

Papillomas develop after introduction of papillomavirus through breaks in the epithelium. Different virus isolates derived from the same species are believed to correlate with the type of clinical disease produced (i.e., oral isolates vs. cutaneous isolates), although this feature of papillomaviruses is yet to be proven for the dog or the cat. Experimentally, ocular isolates have produced oral papillomas in the dog.[5-9] The presence and location of mature, complete virus on the surface of papillomas are believed to aid in its transmission to adjacent epithelial tissues.[3] In contrast to oncogenic or transforming DNA viruses, papillomaviruses rarely integrate into the cellular genome, but rather remain episomal.[3]

Infections of epithelial cells result in a marked increase in cellular mitosis and hyperplasia of cells with a strand of spongiosum, with subsequent degeneration and hyperkeratinization.[10] Clinical evidence of hyperplasia and hyperkeratinization usually begins 4 to 6 weeks after infection.[10] Canine papillomas generally persist for 4 to 6 months in the mouth and 6 to 12 months on the skin before undergoing spontaneous regression, and multiple warts generally regress simultaneously.[10] Although antibodies are produced against the papillomavirus, antibody levels do not appear to correlate with either growth or regression of the papilloma, and the mechanism of induction or regression remains unknown.[11]

Clinical Features

Papillomas caused by the papillomavirus are usually multiple and frequently infect young dogs. Multiple papillomatosis is most often seen in the oral cavity of the dog, involving the labial margins, tongue, pharyngeal mucosa, hard palate, and epiglottis[11] (Figure 3-2, *A*). Between 4 and 8 weeks after infection, small, pale, smooth, elevated lesions appear and quickly become cauliflower-like in appearance with fine white fronds coming off their surface (Figure 3-2, *B*). Multiple sites of susceptible tissue in the oral cavity appear to be affected early in the course of the disease, with as many as 50 to 100 tumors being present at the time of diagnosis.[11] In most cases, the primary complaints reported by owners of infected dogs are halitosis, ptyalism, hemorrhage, and difficulty eating. Most oral cavity papillomas start regressing after tumors have been present for 4 to 8 weeks. However, some oral lesions may show incomplete regression and some have been known to persist up to 24 months.[11] Ocular papillomas occur less frequently than oral lesions.[11] They are less numerous than oral papillomas and appear on the conjunctiva, cornea, and eyelid margins. Experimentally, the viruses isolated from the ocular lesions may produce oral papillomatosis, although it is unknown if this occurs in nature.[5] Ocular papillomatosis most frequently occurs in dogs 6 months to 4 years of age but is occasionally reported in older dogs. Multiple cutaneous papillomatosis is also thought to be of viral origin. However, experimental evidence suggests that it is not the same strain of papillomavirus that produces oral papillomatosis in the dog.[5]

Multiple skin papillomatosis affects a much broader age range of dogs, and regression of the lesion is prolonged, sometimes taking years.[11] A rare form of cutaneous papillomatosis has been described in greyhounds, with lesions appearing in the interdigital areas of the pad. This form has been described in young greyhounds, 12 to 18 months of age.[9] Although papillomatosis should be considered a benign disease, on rare occasions oral and corneal papillomas have transformed into SCCs.[12,13]

Like canine papillomas, lesions in cats are believed to develop after introduction of the virus through abrasions in the skin. Lesions in cats are often observed at sites of frequent grooming (head and neck and front feet), which may play a role in the clinical distribution of the

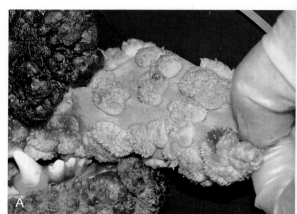
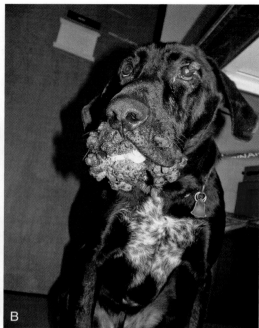

FIGURE 3-2 Note oral papillomas on tongue (**A**) and face (**B**) of this dog.

lesion. Unlike the dog, in which the majority of the cases are seen in animals less than 4 years of age, all feline case reports have been in older cats (6-13 years of age). Table 3-1 provides a species comparison of clinical distribution of papillomas. As in other species, impaired T-cell function likely plays a significant role in lesion formation. Reported feline cases have occurred in cats that are either on immunosuppressive therapy or infected with the feline immunodeficiency virus. The lesions seen in the cat differ from those of the dog by being more plaque-like than wart-like in character. The plaques are several millimeters in diameter and may be white or pigmented, and scaly or greasy (Figures 3-3 and 3-4). An additional difference in the cat is the haired skin location, as opposed to the usual mucous membrane location of oral and ocular papillomas of the dog.

Diagnosis

Definitive diagnosis in both the dog and cat is dependent upon histopathologic, immunohistochemical, or electron microscopic (EM) examination of excised lesions. Intranuclear particles in keratinized cells in the superficial epithelial strata of the plaques are characteristic. Virus-laden keratinocytes, called *koilocytes*, may be

TABLE 3-1 CLINICAL DISTRIBUTION OF PAPILLOMAVIRUS LESIONS

Species	Site	Number	Age
Dog	Oral	Multiple	Young
	Skin	Multiple	Any age
	Ocular	Single	Older
Cat	Oral	Multiple	
	Skin	Multiple	

observed in cytologic samples. Immunohistology can be performed on sections using a band-reactive, genus-specific antiserum.

Treatment

Most clinicians elect not to treat papillomatosis in dogs because of the lack of treatment options with proven efficacy and the expected spontaneous regression of these tumors. However, in canine cases where the number of papillomas increases, or there is significant difficulty in eating, treatment is often requested by the owners. Surgical excision, cryosurgery, laser surgery, and electrosurgery of just a few lesions have resulted

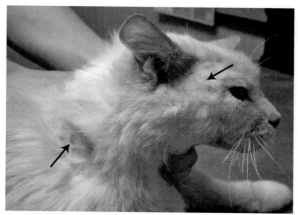

FIGURE 3-3 Multiple skin lesions on both haired and non-haired sites.

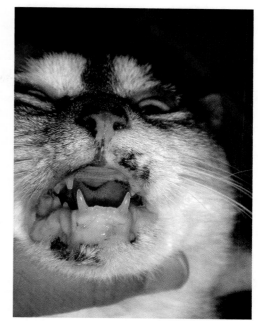

FIGURE 3-5 Pretreatment of lesions carcinoma *in situ*.

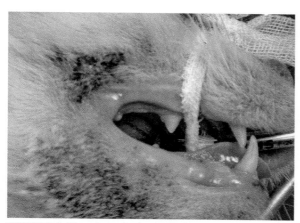

FIGURE 3-4 Note the multiple greasy plaque-like lesions around the mouth.

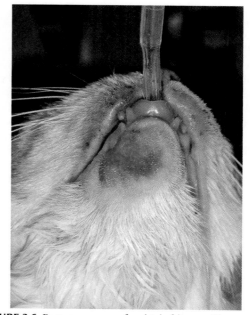

FIGURE 3-6 Post-cryosurgery of multiple feline papillomas.

in regression of the remaining papillomas, presumably through immunologic mechanisms.[11,14] In cats, the lesions are less likely to regress and may transform to carcinoma *in situ* and should be removed. Laser surgery or cryosurgery is often an effective means of management (Figures 3-5 and 3-6). The exact mechanism of regression of papillomas is unknown. Serum from dogs whose papillomas have undergone spontaneous regression not only fails to produce tumor regression when administered to infected animals, but actually enhances existing tumor growth. However, the administration of immune lymphocytes from dogs in which tumors have regressed has been shown to enhance regression in other dogs. Interferon has been used to treat human papillomatosis and, at a dosage of 1 to 3 million IU/m^2 subcutaneously three times a week, has met with some success in dogs.[15] Chemotherapy of resistant lesions has given variable results. 5-Flourouracil has been used in people and dogs but should not be used in cats because of potentially fatal neurotoxicity in this species. Corticosteroids should be avoided, since they have been implicated in the dissemination of papillomas in at least one canine case.[16] In the past, canine autogenous wart vaccines have been tried for the treatment of papillomatosis but have proved of little value in the treatment of resistant papillomatosis.[11] In at least one report, cutaneous neoplasms have been attributed to canine papillomavirus vaccine administration.[8]

RETROVIRUSES

Retroviral infections are responsible for the majority of infectious-related morbidity and mortality in the cat. Both endogenous and exogenous retroviruses exist in the cat. Endogenous retroviruses are non-pathogenic and are genetically passed from parent to offspring. Exogenous retroviruses may be pathogenic or non-pathogenic and include feline leukemia virus (FeLV) and feline immunodeficiency virus (FIV).[17] Feline sarcoma virus (FeSV) is also a pathogenic retrovirus and arises when the exogenous FeLV RNA integrates with the host cat's genome.[18]

Feline Leukemia Virus

FeLV is an RNA virus in the subfamily Oncornavirinae. Important FeLV proteins include the envelope and core proteins. The envelope proteins, P15E and GP70, are involved in the pathogenesis and transmission of FeLV and are important components of FeLV vaccines.[19-21] The core protein, P27, is the antigen detected in the ELISA and IFA tests routinely used to diagnose FeLV.[22] Feline oncornavirus-associated cell membrane antigen (FOCMA) is a protein that may be found on the FeLV virus and in FeLV-induced neoplasms. Antibodies may be produced against FOCMA, and therefore this antigen may protect against the development of lymphoma in some FeLV-positive cats.[23]

The FeLV virus is unstable and is inactivated within 1 to 2 hours in the environment. Heat and disinfectants rapidly inactivate FeLV. Because of its instability, it is unlikely that environmental contamination through cages and examination tables are a source for FeLV infection. Transmission of FeLV occurs through prolonged contact with bodily fluids, especially saliva. Factors associated with the transmission of FeLV are licking,

biting, grooming, and shared water dishes, food bowls, and litter pans.

Virtually every hematopoietic neoplasm in the cat can be caused by FeLV or one of its recombinants. The only hematopoietic neoplasms that have not been associated with FeLV infection are mast cell leukemia, plasma cell tumors, and polycythemia vera.[24] Recently, one case of chronic eosinophilic leukemia in a FeLV-positive cat was reported.[25] This is believed to be the first case of FeLV-associated eosinophilic leukemia. FeLV is diagnosed in 70% to 90% of cats with myeloproliferative disease.[24] Spinal, mediastinal, ocular, renal, and T-cell lymphoma often occur in cats that test positive for FeLV,[26,27] whereas nasal, alimentary, and B-cell lymphoma are often observed in cats that test negative.[24]

Treatment to clear FeLV infection is most often unsuccessful. Although therapies such as interferon, acemannan, and reverse transcriptase inhibitors (suramin, dextran sulfate, phosphonate, etc.) have provided clinical improvement or *in vitro* efficacy, none have been shown to clear viremia. Supportive care is the treatment most often instituted in FeLV-positive cats.[28-32]

The best way to prevent FeLV infection is to eliminate contact with FeLV-positive cats. The test and removal program, described elsewhere, is the most effective means of controlling FeLV in multi-cat households.[33,34] The FeLV vaccine, available since 1985, is not on the American Association of Feline Practitioners (AAFP) list of core vaccinations.[35] The reasons for this include lack of efficacy in adult cats reported in some studies and the risk of injection-associated sarcoma development with adjuvanted vaccines. However, cats at significant risk should be vaccinated for FeLV. Because cats may acquire immunity to FeLV with age and because there is risk of sarcoma development at vaccination sites, the propriety of annual re-vaccination of adult cats has been questioned.

Feline Sarcoma Virus

The FeSV virus is a true hybrid virus, resulting from the combination of FeLV pro-viral particles with parts of the infected cat genome, specifically proto-oncogenes. As such, cats that have FeSV are always positive for FeLV. To date, natural transmission of FeSV between cats has not been observed. FeSV oncogenes cause cancer by transforming fibroblasts and producing fibrosarcomas. Because some cats infected with FeLV can produce FOCMA antibodies, they are capable of rejecting the transformed cells; therefore, FOCMA has been shown to play a role in tumor regression and the prevention of tumor development.[32,36,37] Only 2% of feline fibrosarcomas are virally induced.[18] The tumors that are induced by FeSV are multicentric and occur in young cats.[24,38] They exhibit rapid growth with short doubling times, are often ulcerated, and appear at the sites of previous bite wounds.[24] Metastasis may occur in up to 30% of cases, and spread is usually to the lungs or other organs. As previously mentioned, cats with virally induced fibrosarcomas are always FeLV positive, differentiating them from injection-associated sarcomas. The prognosis for cats with FeSV-associated fibrosarcomas is extremely poor.

Feline Immunodeficiency Virus

FIV is an RNA virus in the subfamily Lentivirinae. High concentrations of viral particles are found in the saliva of infected cats, and transmission occurs through biting during cat fights.[39] The virus itself is not thought to be oncogenic; rather, cancer develops as a result of host immunosuppression and impaired tumor suppression. Lymphoma, myeloproliferative disease, carcinomas, and sarcomas have been associated with FIV infection in cats. Specifically, oral SCC, mammary carcinoma, fibrosarcoma, myeloproliferative disease, and histiocytic mast cell disease[40-43] have been reported in FIV-infected cats. FIV-associated lymphoma usually arises in extranodal sites in older cats (mean age, 8.7 years).[40] Cats co-infected with FIV and FeLV appear to be at a significantly increased risk of developing lymphoid neoplasia compared with non-infected cats.[40]

As with FeLV, treatment consists of supportive care. With any therapy that is attempted, the cat will remain FIV positive because of the inability to clear the viremia. To date, FIV status has not been shown to affect prognosis in cats with lymphoma.

Selected References*

August JR: Husbandry practices for cats infected with feline leukemia virus or feline immunodeficiency virus, *J Am Vet Med Assoc*, 199(10):1474, 1991.
Discussion of the care of FeLV or FIV-infected cats.
Cotter SM: Feline leukemia virus: pathophysiology, prevention and treatment, *Cancer Invest*, 10(2):173, 1992.
Overview of FeLV.
Macy DW: Cancer-causing viruses. In Withrow SJ, Vail DM (eds): *Small animal clinical oncology*, ed 4, St Louis, 2007, Saunders/Elsevier, p 19.
Thorough overview of viral-associated neoplasia in dogs and cats.
Richards J: 2001 Report of the American Association of Feline Practitioners and the Academy of Feline Medicine Advisory Panel on feline retrovirus testing and management, *J Feline Med Surg*. 5(1):3, 2003.
This report cites the most current recommendations on feline vaccinations from the AAFP.

■ *For a complete list of the references cited in this chapter, please go to www.smallanimaloncology.com.

SECTION C: Hormonal Impact on Carcinogenesis

Carolyn J. Henry

KEY POINTS

- Endogenous ovarian hormones and products containing medroxyprogesterone acetate have been linked to an increased incidence of canine mammary tumor development.
- As with dogs, spaying cats at a young age appears to reduce the likelihood of mammary cancer development.
- Perianal adenomas are considered to be androgen dependent, as opposed to perianal adenocarcinomas, which occur in male and female dogs.
- Although neutering is protective against benign prostatic hyperplasia (BPH), evidence suggests that it does not reduce the likelihood of developing prostate carcinoma.

ESTROGEN AND PROGESTERONE

Canine Mammary Cancer

One of the best known examples of hormonally related cancer development in domestic animals is canine mammary cancer. Mammary tumors are the most common neoplasms of female intact dogs, affecting approximately 260 in 100,000 dogs annually in the United States.[1,2] It is well established that spaying dogs before their first estrous cycle greatly reduces their risk of developing breast cancer.[3] The risk of mammary tumor development rises to 26% for dogs spayed after their second estrus.[3,4] Mammary tumors primarily affect middle-aged to older female intact dogs, with an increased incidence beginning at approximately 6 years of age.[5] Steroid sex hormones are thought to have their primary effect on target cells during the early stages of canine mammary carcinogenesis. This idea is supported by the fact that spaying dogs after their second estrous cycle does not confer protection against mammary tumor development as well as by the fact that estrogen and progesterone receptors (PRs) are present in higher proportions in normal breast tissue and benign lesions, compared with breast cancer tissue or metastatic lesions.[5-12] In addition to the influence of ovarian hormones on breast carcinogenesis, the use of products containing medroxyprogesterone acetate (an estrogen and progestin combination) to prevent estrus or to treat pseudopregnancy has been linked to an increased incidence of canine mammary tumor development.[13-15]

It has been shown that progestin-induced growth hormone (GH) excess in dogs originates in the mammary gland. Thus, it is believed that the gene encoding GH may act in an autocrine/paracrine fashion within the mammary gland to cause cyclic epithelial changes and, perhaps, carcinogenesis. Efforts to uncover the mechanism of progestin-induced mammary GH expression in dogs have led to the cloning and cellular localization of the canine PR.[16] It is now believed that within the same mammary gland cell, the activated PR may transactivate GH expression, thus functioning as a prerequisite transcription factor. However, this regulation may be lost during malignant transformation. Because mammary GH expression in women has also been reported, there is reason to believe that understanding the links between GH and mammary carcinogenesis may have implications for both species.[17,18]

Feline Mammary Cancer

Both estrogen and progesterone are thought to play important roles in feline mammary carcinogenesis, although the underlying mechanisms are less clear than in dogs. Intact female cats and cats exposed regularly to progestin are at an increased risk for developing mammary cancer. The literature also suggests that, as is the case for dogs, ovariectomy may protect against feline mammary carcinogenesis.[1,19,20] In one study, cats ovariectomized at 6 months of age had an approximate seven-fold reduction in risk of mammary tumor development compared with intact cats.[1] In a retrospective study comparing a population of 308 cats with biopsy-proven mammary carcinoma to a control population of 400 female cats not diagnosed with mammary tumors, Overly et al.[21] reported a statistically significant reduction in mammary cancer risk for cats spayed prior to 1 year of age. Cats from the two study groups were frequency-matched by age and year of diagnosis. There was

a 91% reduction in risk of mammary tumor development for cats spayed prior to 6 months of age and an 86% reduction in risk for those spayed before 1 year of age, compared with intact cats. Limitations of the study include its retrospective design and the reliance on questionnaire data from a survey with only a 58% response rate. Nonetheless, the manuscript is the first of its kind to age-match controls and evaluate age at the time of spay as a risk factor for feline mammary tumor development. Further epidemiological evaluation and prospective assessment are needed to confirm the findings, but the report provides some justification for recommending ovariohysterectomy prior to 1 year of age in cats.

Lymphoma

According to Surveillance, Epidemiology & End Results (SEER) data, non-Hodgkin's lymphoma (NHL) is approximately 50% more common among men than women.[22] Although a similar male gender predisposition is reported for canine lymphoma, the underlying role of gender in lymphoma etiology remains uncertain. The author and others conducted a population-based study using the Veterinary Medical Database (VMDB) and the Veterinary Cancer Registry (VCR) (www.vetcancerregistry.com) in an effort to determine the relationship between gender and the development of canine lymphoma.[23] Data from a 20-year span (1980–2000) were retrieved from the VMDB and sorted by gender and reproductive status. Spayed or castrated dogs diagnosed with lymphoma were compared to intact dogs seen each year in each gender category. The VCR was also searched for all canine lymphoma cases, and the number of cases in each gender group were compared to the total number of cancer diagnoses per group. The VMDB contained nearly 15,000 lymphoma cases in a population of over 1.2 million dogs. The VCR database included 394 lymphoma cases among 6070 canine cancer diagnoses. In both analyses, intact females were significantly less likely to develop lymphoma than were other gender groups. Based on this initial data, further examination of the role of estrogen in the development or prevention of canine lymphoma appears to be warranted.

ANDROGENS/TESTOSTERONE
Perianal Adenoma

Perianal adenomas are considered to be androgen dependent, occurring primarily in intact male dogs. This is in contrast to perianal adenocarcinomas, which occur in both intact and castrated males. Perianal adenomas may occur in female dogs as a result of secretion of testosterone from the adrenal gland.[24] The majority of perianal adenomas in male dogs resolve following castration, further supporting the assertion that androgens are involved in the etiology of this tumor.[25]

Prostate Cancer

In contrast to the well-established link between testosterone and development of BPH in dogs and humans, prostatic carcinoma occurs in both intact and castrated male dogs.[26] In fact, some studies have demonstrated an increased risk of prostate cancer development in castrated dogs, although castration is not believed to be an initiating event.[26-30] A clear relationship between age at castration and risk of prostate cancer development has not yet been determined.

Selected References*

Bryan JN, Henry CJ, Hahn AW, Caldwell CW: A population study of neutering status as a risk factor for canine prostate cancer, *Prostate* 67:1174, 2007.
This manuscript provides epidemiological evidence that castration is not protective against the development of canine prostate cancer.
Overley B, Shofer FS, Goldschmidt MH, et al: Association between ovariohysterectomy and feline mammary carcinoma, *J Vet Intern Med* 19:560, 2005.
This is the first study to include age-match controls in the evaluation of age at the time of spay as a risk factor for feline mammary tumor development.
Schneider R, Dorn CR, Taylor DON: Factors influencing canine mammary tumor development and postsurgical survival, *J Nat Cancer Inst* 43:1249, 1969.
This was the seminal manuscript demonstrating the relationship between ovariohysterectomy and the risk of canine mammary tumor development.

*For a complete list of the references cited in this chapter, please go to www.smallanimaloncology.com.

4 Cancer Epidemiology and Statistics

Jeff W. Tyler and Jose Armando Villamil

KEY POINTS

- The highest level of evidence is provided by appropriately designed prospective, randomized, blind, clinical trials.
- The larger the sample size, the more likely one is to demonstrate significant differences. Many clinical trials are plagued by inadequate sample size.
- Parametric analyses (t-test, ANOVA, and standard regression models) are inappropriate to analyze the results of most oncologic studies.
- Multiple comparisons increase the likelihood of Type I error.

This chapter reviews some of the epidemiological and statistical concepts related to clinical oncology. Because veterinarians should base their clinical decisions upon advances presented as published, peer-reviewed evidence, an understanding of basic concepts of experimental design and data analysis is essential. For those unfamiliar with statistical terminology, a glossary of terms is provided in Box 4-1.

AVAILABLE STUDY DESIGNS AND QUALITY OF EVIDENCE

Two broad classifications of study design exist: descriptive and analytical. Descriptive studies typically report disease manifestations in a defined group, without comparisons of disease incidence or outcome based on exposure to risk factors. The classic example of a descriptive report is a case series. Descriptive reports provide weaker evidence than analytical studies because no attempt is made to link exposure to a risk factor with causality.

Analytical studies attempt to draw associations between exposure to risk factors and either the incidence of disease or a disease outcome. Among analytical studies, randomized, controlled clinical trials provide the strongest evidence, followed by cohort studies and case-control studies.

Analytical studies may be either experimental or observational. The optimal evidence is provided by experimental studies that are randomized, blind, controlled, clinical trials (see Chapter 5 for more detail). Although this approach provides the strongest evidence, this design is problematic if exposure to a risk factor has either a small or delayed effect on disease outcome. For example, if exposure to a pesticide is postulated to cause an increased incidence of bladder cancer 5 to 10 years after exposure, an experimental study exploring this relationship would entail years of study and effort to answer a single clinical question.

Less rigorous analytical studies include cohort studies and case-control studies. In cohort studies, subjects are placed in groups on the basis of the presence or absence of postulated risk factors or treatments, and disease outcomes are followed over time. This design, like the classic experimental study, is prospective in nature; however, the group assignment and standardization of outcome monitoring is less rigorous. Studies of this type typically assess the impact of a limited number of risk factors, usually treated vs. control, on disease outcome.

In contrast, case-control studies are retrospective. Patients with a specific diagnosis are defined as cases. Controls are drawn from a similar population during the same time interval, but do not have the specific diagnosis. Exposure to risk factors is determined

BOX 4-1 GLOSSARY OF TERMS[1-4]

Bias—A systematic deviation of measured endpoints from true or representative values.

Case-control study—Exposure to risk factors is determined by history or survey data, and differences in exposure to hypothesized risk factors are assessed between cases and controls.

Cohort study—Subjects are placed in groups on the basis of the presence or absence of postulated risk factors or treatments, and disease outcomes are followed over time.

Confounding—An association between a postulated risk factor and a measured outcome, which is the result of some other variable that has not been considered.

Normal—Symmetrically dispersed around a measure of central tendency following a specific pattern of distribution whereby approximately two thirds of observations are located with a single standard deviation of the mean and approximately 95% of observations are within 2 standard deviations of the same mean.

P-value—The likelihood that a difference of the observed magnitude could occur because of chance.

Power—The likelihood of detecting a significant difference among groups or exposures at a given *P*-value, sample size, group means, and standard deviation.

Sensitivity—The likelihood of a positive test result given that a patient has the disease in question.

Specificity—The likelihood of a negative test result given that a patient does not have the disease in question.

Type I error—see *P*-value

by history or survey data, and differences in exposure are assessed between case and control groups. Case-control studies have a number of characteristics which make them attractive. First, because these studies are retrospective, they are relatively inexpensive and can be performed quickly. Secondly, exposure to multiple risk factors can be compared among cases and controls in a single study. These studies provide weaker evidence because owners may have imperfect memory and the owners of case animals may have recollections of risk factor exposures because they have either consciously or unconsciously attempted to determine the cause of their pets' disease.

CONTROLS AND RANDOMIZATION

Clinical observations without controlled comparison groups may be interesting and thought provoking; unfortunately, observations of this type that are erroneous often become accepted, but unproven, dogmas. Examples of publications that lack controls include individual case reports and case series. The limitations of case reports are obvious. Case reports present novel diagnoses, diagnostic approaches and treatments. However, these reports are singular observations, and consequently, lack a control or reference group and fail to provide direct evidence. In some ways, case series are even more problematic. The number of observations in a case series is substantially greater than in a case report, and these manuscripts often include statistics. Thus, they may outwardly appear to carry greater scientific weight, and conclusions may be accepted by the casual reader without appropriate skepticism. Although clinical outcomes are often compared among subjects with differing historical risk factors within a case series, these comparisons are often invalid because historical controls have different parameters and their own set limitations. Consequently, these studies, although more rigorous than case reports, have limited value as direct evidence of diagnostic or therapeutic efficacy. The factor missing from both case reports and case series is the identification of a valid and appropriate comparison or control group. *Controls are the single most important factor determining the validity of a study.*

For studies undertaken to determine the efficacy of a new treatment or intervention, the control group should be comprised of animals that were either left untreated or, preferably, received the current standard therapy.[1] The control group should be as identical to the exposure group or treatment group as possible, except for the particular factor or variable being investigated.[2] Ideally, assignment to either the treatment or control group should be random. Methods of random assignment include coin toss, drawing of a card, or use of a random number table. Regardless of the method used, each subject should have an equal likelihood of being placed in the treatment or control groups, ensuring that treatment and control groups have a similar composition. Examples of non-random and unacceptable group assignment strategies include clinician preference, evolutionary changes in treatment protocols, financial constraints, and owners' preferences. Consequently, owner and clinician willingness to participate in a clinical trial should be determined prior to group assignment. Willingness to participate in a trial that hinges upon group assignment outcome cannot be viewed as a random event. Owners may choose to participate in a trial if given subsidized access to novel treatment that may have the potential to improve clinical outcomes. Likewise, clinicians are likely motivated in a similar manner. These potential biases in group assignment may be accentuated in unsubsidized trials because clients with fewer financial resources may be shuttled into the less-expensive treatment arms of a clinical trial. Another common mistake is the use of a historical population or a population from a previous published study as a control group. The problem with this control group is that diagnostic procedures, standard of care, client expectations, clinician expertise, available drugs, and the definition of the disease in question may have changed over time. Differences over time between groups create the potential for temporal effects in all the identified variables to be misidentified as differences in response to treatment.

Random group assignment will also minimize the impact of extraneous factors associated with the variable in question. *Confounding* has been described as the mixing together of the effect of two or more factors. Thus, when confounding is present, practitioners might think they are measuring the association of an exposure factor with an outcome, but the association measure also includes the effect of one or more extraneous factors.[3] For example, suppose a new chemotherapy agent has become available for treatment of osteosarcoma in dogs but is very expensive. In an effort to maximize the number of patients enrolled, small dogs are given the new, expensive agent and larger dogs receive an older, less-expensive treatment. A significant between-group difference is observed. Unbeknownst to the researcher, the course of disease differs between large and small dogs. The investigator erroneously attributes improved survival in the smaller dogs to improved treatment efficacy when, in fact, the difference is related to patient size.

SAMPLE SIZE

Factors that impact sample size requirements include designated significance threshold *P*-value, power, the rate of the observed event in the control population, and the anticipated reduction in mortality associated with treatment. In general, common events and dramatic treatment effects result in smaller sample size requirements for a study.

Power—the likelihood of recognizing a significant difference between groups—is enhanced by larger sample size. The larger the sample sizes, the more likely significant differences will be demonstrated. Many biological effects are relatively small. Under these circumstances,

only very large sample sizes will be adequate to detect differences. For example, for a procedure or treatment to have demonstrable, statistical significance in reducing a 10% mortality rate by 50%, a study would need to include approximately 500 subjects per group. Proper experimental design and critical examination of research require us to define the minimal relevant difference and then calculate power based on anticipated outcome and sample size. Sample size and power should be calculated before the experiment is started so that the investigator knows how many experimental units are required to find a significant difference between groups. For those studies that fail to demonstrate a significant difference between groups, power should calculated. Large power (>0.80) should suggest the absence of group effects. Very small power suggests an inadequate sample size to demonstrate the significance of the observed between-group difference.

TYPES OF DATA AND CHOICE OF STATISTICAL ANALYSES

In general, there are two broad families of statistical analyses. The first and most familiar are *parametric analyses*. Included are t-tests, Z-tests, analysis of variance, and regression. These parametric techniques are only applicable and appropriate under a series of fairly rigorous conditions. These conditions are referred to as assumptions, because we assume these criteria are satisfied before a statistical analysis is performed. The assumptions include continuous, interval-based data, normal distribution, equal variance across groups, and independence. Interval data imply that a one-unit change in measurement is of equivalent magnitude across the range of measurements. For example, the increase in blood glucose from 40 to 41 is equal to a change from 80 to 81. Continuous data imply that measured endpoints and risk factors span the range from negative to positive infinity. In contrast, discrete data can only take certain values (gender, which is either male or female). Within the discrete data, there are different categories: nominal, binomial, and ordinal. The preceding example of gender is nominal. Binomial data are limited to a "0,1" or "yes, no" scale. Ordinal data demonstrate an order of magnitude but lack a linear, interval scale (small, medium, large). The assumption of an interval-based, continuous scale is rarely met in biological systems. Using our preceding example, one quickly recognizes that blood glucose only spans a limited range of possible values. Both very low and very high measurements are incompatible with life. Normally distributed data are symmetrically distributed around a central value or mean. In addition,

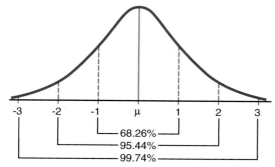

FIGURE 4-1 An example of normally distributed data. The Y-axis represents relative frequency, and the X-axis represents the magnitude of measured outcomes reported as mean, plus or minus various fractions of the standard deviation. Note the central location of the mean.

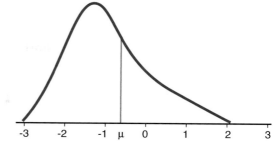

FIGURE 4-2 An example of a skewed or non-normal data distribution.

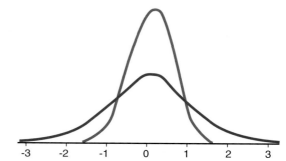

FIGURE 4-3 Examples of data distributions drawn from two populations with identical means, but different standard deviations.

the dispersion of data relative to the mean follows a defined pattern with approximately two thirds of data points within 1 standard deviation (SD) of the mean and 95% of observed data points within 2 SDs of the mean (Figure 4-1). Data that fail to follow this pattern of symmetrical distribution are referred to as skewed (Figure 4-2). The assumption of equal variance across groups implies that data drawn from each group follow a similar pattern of dispersion around a central mean. Figure 4-3 illustrates measured outcomes in two groups with similar means, but unequal variance. The final assumption of independence requires that each and all observations not be related to another observation. Multiple observations derived from one individual cannot be viewed as independent events.

Data derived from clinical oncology studies are particularly problematic. The most common endpoints are disease-free interval, metastasis-free interval and survival times. These endpoints notoriously lack normality. It should be apparent from the preceding discussion that the requirements, or assumptions, for use of parametric statistics are rarely met. Consequently, *any manuscript that uses a t-test, Z-test, analysis of variance, or standard regression analysis without specifically stipulating that the aforementioned requirements have been met should be viewed as suspect.*

Analytical methods appropriate for most oncology studies include *nonparametric methods.* The chi-squared test is typically used to assess the significance of associations between a risk factor exposure and an outcome. Cohort studies assess the strength of association by examination of the relative risk (RR). RR is calculated by dividing disease incidence in the population exposed to a risk factor by disease incidence in a non-exposed population. Case control studies assess the strength of association by use of odds ratios (OR). ORs are calculated by dividing the odds of exposure to a risk factor in cases by the odds of exposure in controls. In either case, RR or OR > 1 indicate increased risk, and RR and OR < 1 indicate decreased risk.

SURVIVAL ANALYSIS METHODS

Survival analysis is the statistical method most commonly used in clinical oncology. Common measured endpoints include survival time, time to disease recurrence, and the time it takes for an examined parameter to exceed a defined threshold value. Survival is binomially distributed (dead vs. living). Survival times are characteristically non-normal in veterinary oncology studies. Even in a referral setting with an affluent clientele and supportive veterinary staff, the diagnosis of cancer is often followed in short order by euthanasia. Many clients perceive quality of life issues and cost as compelling incentives for withholding treatment. In addition, the induction phase of cancer treatment is generally associated with a higher risk of morbidity and mortality than is maintenance chemotherapy. Consequently, large proportions of cancer patients either die or are lost to follow-up in the early time intervals after diagnosis. Thus, survival time of cancer patients typically has either a skewed or bimodal distribution.

Another common characteristic of survival data from veterinary oncology studies is that many data points are censored. Censoring describes the situation where subjects are lost to follow-up in a manner unrelated to the disease of interest. Censored observations may occur because of a variety of reasons; the most obvious one is that the event did not occur before the end of the study period.[1] Other reasons for incomplete data include loss to follow-up (e.g., owner withdraws from the study, treatment was stopped because of side effects, owner moves out of town) and death for other causes (e.g., traumatic accident, any other cause that is unrelated to the disease or treatment being studied). It should be noted, however, that these censoring effects may not be entirely random or equally distributed among experimental groups. For example, suppose a novel chemotherapy agent has unknown negative side effects. This agent causes a delayed-onset, fatal hepatic or cardiac failure in a large number of patients. These deaths are erroneously classified as censored observations, rather than deaths caused by disease. As a direct consequence, the apparent survival times for dogs receiving the new agent appear much better than they in fact are. *When reading and reviewing reports of oncology clinical trials, dramatic differences in either the proportion or pattern of censored observations between groups should raise concerns regarding the propriety of censoring criteria and the validity of study results.*

Some of the commonly used survival analysis methods are Kaplan-Meier, Cox's proportional hazards models, and Weibel models. Kaplan-Meier is by far the most commonly used in veterinary oncology literature; the other two methods are more complicated and have assumptions (i.e., large sample sizes) that are rarely met in veterinary oncology (Figure 4-4). Kaplan-Meier takes censored data into account and does not depend on discrete time intervals constructed by the investigator. The Kaplan-Meier method has the advantage that it avoids the assumption that withdrawals occurred uniformly throughout the interval and that the risk of withdrawal is constant. The only remaining assumption about withdrawals is that they have the same future experiences as those remaining under observation.[4]

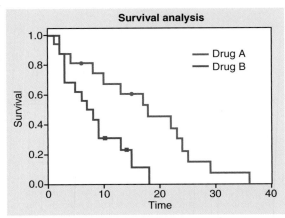

FIGURE 4-4 Hypothetical graph illustrating Kaplan-Meier survival methods. The Y axis represents the proportion of subjects that are still alive and the X axis represents time. The ● and ■ represent censored data. Censored observations are those individuals who were lost to follow-up or died because of an unrelated cause.

One very real disadvantage of the Kaplan-Meier method is that it is only appropriate for univariate analyses in which the effect of a single risk factor on survival time is assessed. Consequently, many veterinary oncology studies will include multiple statistical analyses in which the effects of treatment group, age, weight, breed, and a variety of potential risk factors on survival time are assessed. The first problem raised by this approach is that multiple comparisons, each with the potential for a *type I error* have been performed. The second issue raised by this approach is its inability to identify confounding relationships. For example, in a hypothetical study examining survival time in dogs with mammary tumors, both weight and breed are significantly associated with survival time. These two risk factors are probably closely associated. Multivariate approaches will permit the investigator to differentiate between breed and weight effects. Unfortunately, multivariate approaches generally require larger sample sizes, since each additional risk factor considered increases the size of the sample that must be studied. Most veterinary clinical oncology studies lack sufficient numbers to permit application of these techniques. As we move toward multi-center, cooperative clinical trials, we will likely begin to see multivariate survival techniques more often in the veterinary literature. However, a cautionary note that is appropriate at this juncture is that the study site or practice should probably be considered a risk factor for survival in these studies because the standard of care may vary practice to practice and the behavior or disease itself may vary locally.

MULTIPLE ANALYSES

Each individual statistical test that is performed carries an inherent risk of an erroneously significant result. This risk is referred to as either the type I error or *P*-value. In general, we interpret small *P*-values as indicators of real or significant differences between groups. Perhaps a better way to understand *P*-values is to describe them as the likelihood of observing a difference as large as that observed due solely to chance. Thus, a significance threshold or *P*-value of .05 implies that each statistical analysis carries a 5% probability of an erroneously significant result. If we run a single analysis, there is a 5% risk of a type I error. The second test carries an additional risk of type I error—in this case, 5% + 5% of 0.95. The general formula to determine the likelihood of at least one erroneously significant result is as follows:[4]

$$\text{Cumulative type I error} = 1 - (1-P)^n$$

where P = significance threshold or *P*-value of an individual test and n = the number of statistical tests performed.

To better understand this issue, consider a clinical trial in which the effects of chemotherapy group, completeness of surgical excision, radiation therapy, tumor stage, primary tumor size, patient age, patient weight, and gender are used to predict survival time, disease-free interval, and metastasis-free interval. This proposed analysis has 8 independent variables (risk factors) and 3 dependent variables (outcomes). Most studies would perform 24 separate Kaplan-Meier survival analyses. The cumulative type I error is approximately 70%. Even if there is no significant difference among treatment groups or risk factors, there is a 70% probability of at least one significant result.

The previous example demonstrates why studies with large numbers of endpoints and risk factors should be viewed with skepticism and the results of such studies interpreted with caution. The most common compromise under these circumstances is a more conservative *P*-value. When applying a Bonferroni adjustment, the nominal *P*-value (.05) is divided by the number of multiple comparisons (in this case, 24), yielding a working *P*-value of approximately .002. Only analyses yielding *P*-values less than .002 would then be considered significant. The issue of multiple comparisons is of particular importance in case control studies because a multitude of potential risk factors may be considered.

SYSTEMATIC SOURCES OF ERROR

The two most common sources of error or misleading results are bias and confounding. Bias is a systematic deviation of measured endpoints from true or representative values.[1] Examples of bias include selection bias, detection bias, recall bias, and attrition of susceptible subjects. *Selection bias* occurs when patients are preferentially assigned to a specific treatment arm. In veterinary oncology, a prime example of this bias is when subjects are assigned to specific treatments or admitted to a clinical trial on the basis of clinician preference and perception. Another example is client preference for one treatment over another. This bias is particularly problematic in retrospective studies. *Detection bias* occurs when subjects exposed to a specific risk factor are screened more rigorously than non-exposed subjects and, therefore, disease is detected more frequently and accurately. Consider the following example: An investigator believes that military guard dogs that have been stationed overseas are at greater risk for developing bladder cancer. A screening protocol that includes urinalysis and abdominal ultrasound is instituted. The incidence of neoplasia in this group is compared with a control population that was not exposed to the risk factor; however, this second group only receives routine check-ups. This hypothetical example illustrates how perceptions can create uncontrolled bias in study results. *Recall bias* is of particular importance in case-control studies. Owners of pets with cancer are prone to ask why this happened to their pet. In their personal search for answers, they may unconsciously bias their recollection of exposures in an effort to assign casualty or blame.

The term *confounding* refers to when an association between a postulated risk factor and a measured outcome is actually the result of some other variable that has not been considered.[1] For example, an investigator observes an association between gender and the incidence of a specific tumor. Unbeknownst to the investigator, the actual effect is related to body size, with larger dogs being at greater risk. Because male dogs are consistently larger than female dogs, body size is a confounding influence when evaluating gender as a risk factor. Confounding influences are best detected and accounted for by multivariate analyses. In our hypothetical example when either gender or body weight is considered individually, both are significantly associated with disease incidence. When multivariate analyses are performed, the proportion of risk associated with each variable is defined and apportioned, and the inclusion of body weight in a model eliminates any effect associated with gender. It should be noted that multivariate approaches such as the Weibel or Cox models are infrequently used in veterinary oncology studies because these approaches require much larger sample sizes. As the number of risk factors considered increases, the sample size required to detect significant differences also increases. Unfortunately, a more common approach in veterinary oncology studies is the use of multiple univariate Kaplan-Meier survival analyses. This approach will neither detect nor account for confounding effects. Consequently, *associations between risk factors and outcomes in univariate analyses should be considered suspect, particularly if multiple associations are detected.*

STANDARDIZATION AND DEFINITIONS

Definitions of case inclusion criteria and case outcomes are a critical component of any well-designed study, and these definitions are obligatory components of trustworthy research. Materials and methods sections of manuscripts should specifically define diagnostic criteria, clinical diagnosis, or histology, and the results section should clearly describe cases. These descriptions provide critical assurance to the practitioner that the studied cases are, in fact, representative of patients observed in their practice. Factors such as age, breed, and clinical staging should be reported.

Properly conducted clinical trials require patients to be reassessed at defined intervals. This scheduled follow-up may be at defined and consistent intervals, or it may be based on the investigators' perceptions regarding behavior of the disease. Regardless, the follow-up intervals must be standardized for all enrolled subjects. To illustrate the importance of this concept, consider the following example: Dogs with tumor A either receive surgery only or receive surgery and monthly adjunctive chemotherapy. Dogs with surgery only require no additional treatment, so these dogs are re-evaluated at 6-month intervals. Dogs receiving chemotherapy are re-evaluated in conjunction with scheduled treatment visits. In this example, all enrolled dogs in both groups experience profound (100%) mortality between 4 and 5 months after enrollment. No dogs receiving only surgery survive to their 6-month recheck. Dogs receiving chemotherapy all survive through their 3- or 4-month follow-up examination and then succumb before 6 months after enrollment. Analysis of these data would suggest a longer survival time in dogs that received chemotherapy. *Practitioners should view with inherent skepticism studies in which (1) defined follow-up schedules are not presented, and (2) the follow-up schedule is not identical in all patients and all treatment groups.* This standardization of follow-up is difficult if not impossible in retrospective studies. Consequently, *results of retrospective studies should be considered less trustworthy than those from well-designed prospective studies.*

Selected References[*]

Reeves MJ, Reeves NP: Epidemiology and the veterinary oncologist—evaluation and critical appraisal of the scientific oncology literature, *Vet Clin North Am Sm Anim Pract* 25(1):1, 1995.
This article describes the process of critical evaluation of the scientific literature with an emphasis on the experimental design and data analysis.
Smith RD: *Veterinary clinical epidemiology: a problem-oriented approach,* ed 2, Boca Raton, 1995, CRC Press LLC; www.crcpress.com.
This book describes the standard statistical and epidemiological methods and illustrates basic calculations.

[*]For a complete list of the references cited in this chapter, please go to www.smallanimaloncology.com.

5 Clinical Trial Design and Access to Clinical Research Studies

Melissa C. Paoloni and Chand Khanna

KEY POINTS

- Clinical trials are becoming a more readily available option for the treatment of pets with cancer.
- Clinical trials are prospectively designed by stringent ethical guidelines and aim to answer specific scientific objectives.
- Comparative oncology clinical trials will shape the future of cancer care for companion animals and people by providing data about both the efficacy and mechanisms of novel therapies.
- The role of primary care veterinarians is crucial in providing clients with information and access to clinical trials and facilitating patient follow-up.

Clinical trials in veterinary oncology are growing in scope and importance. Trials that evaluate novel therapies for pet animals with cancer have the opportunity to improve the outcome and quality of life for veterinary patients, as well as human patients with cancer. The demand for clinical trials has been fueled by a sustained increase in the number of pet animals diagnosed with cancer and the pet-owning public's interest in finding effective and well-tolerated treatments for their pets. Interest from the human cancer drug development industry is based on a need for more reliable ways to evaluate new cancer drugs and the strong similarities between veterinary and human cancers.[1-5] Accordingly, well-designed clinical trials in veterinary oncology offer the opportunity to develop new drugs for use in both companion animals and people, a field known as comparative oncology.

Interestingly, the outcome for patients who are managed within a clinical trial has been consistently shown to be superior to that of patients who receive the same agents outside the setting of a clinical study. This suggests that clinical trials are of value not only for improving care of future patients, but also for those patients enrolled in a study. Through the conduct of clinical trials, our opportunities to prevent, diagnose, and treat cancer will continue to improve. It is likely that the availability of clinical trials in veterinary oncology will continue to expand. This expansion will require and will welcome greater direct and indirect participation from both primary care veterinarians and veterinary specialists. The goals of this chapter are to introduce concepts of clinical trial design and conduct and to focus on the types of questions that these trials have the capability to address.

TRIAL DESIGNS

The first step in clinical trial design is to articulate the questions that the trial should address. This is generally done by asking: what are the study objectives? Based on a combination of primary and secondary objectives, investigators will define the optimal trial design for a specific study. There are three general types of clinical trials:

Therapeutic trials test new therapies, including new drugs, radiation protocols, combination therapies, or novel technologies such as gene therapy or cancer vaccines.

Prevention trials assess new approaches to reduce the risk of developing certain types of cancer. These are less common in veterinary medicine but can be thought of as those that involve lifestyle changes for pets, such as diet changes or supplement administration. In the future, these trials may assess the ability of an intervention to reduce the risk of cancer development in high-risk animals (i.e., breeds at high risk for specific cancers).

Screening trials evaluate novel tests that diagnose or define the stage of a cancer. These tests may involve new imaging techniques, such as positron emission tomography (PET) scans, magnetic resonance imaging (MRI), or new molecular tests like polymerase chain reaction (PCR) to confirm a diagnosis of leukemia in a patient with lymphocytosis.

Irrespective of the intent of the trial, clinical trials are conducted in a prospective fashion and are distinctly different from retrospective studies that are commonly reported in the veterinary literature. *Retrospective* studies are those in which patients have already received a specified treatment or undergone a specific test, and then data are collected from their medical records for analysis. *Prospective* trials involve the deliberate design of a clinical trial intended to answer a specific objective or question. Patients entered into a prospective trial are managed within the constraints of a carefully designed study protocol.[6,7] This protocol design ensures accuracy and consistency of results and provides an opportunity to verify and validate results. A clinical trial protocol provides the background, specifies the objectives and describes the design and organization of the trial. All participants in a study follow the same protocol in the conduct of the clinical trial. In general, the results from prospective clinical trials are considered to be more valuable and reproducible than results from retrospective studies. Prospective trials are those most likely to make inferences about effectiveness of a new treatment. These trials are the basis of subsequent discussion.

The simplest prospective trial design in oncology is a *case-series* that assesses the ability of a drug to reduce the size of a measurable tumor (objective response) as the primary study endpoint. *Objective response* refers to an unequivocal reduction in tumor burden and is usually defined by > 50% reduction in tumor volume via World Health Organization (WHO) criteria or >30% reduction in tumor longest diameter via Response Evaluation Criteria in Solid Tumors (RECIST). Such trials allow each patient to be assessed before treatment, usually through measurement of tumor burden and then after treatment in an open-label setting, where all patients receive the active treatment or intervention. Patients are then re-evaluated at subsequent time points to determine if there has been a response (reduction in size) in the measurable tumor. Prospective clinical trials are usually included early in the development of a clinical intervention (see the next section for phases of study). Examples of such trials include the evaluation of the activity of a xenogeneic DNA vaccine for treatment of canine melanoma and of SU11654, a tyrosine kinase inhibitor in tumor-bearing dogs.[1,3,8]

PHASES OF CLINICAL TRIALS

Most clinical research in human oncology is very well defined, and the testing of new therapies proceeds in a step-wise process. Clinical trials are broken up into three phases so that the questions they answer are distinct. Table 5-1 outlines the most traditional phases.[9] Phase IV trials, not included in this table, are those that evaluate a drug for possible new uses or assess its market impact after it is already approved by the Food and Drug Administration (FDA). The FDA generally assesses new indications, dosages, or delivery methods of a drug. Although the named phases of clinical trials are not always used in veterinary oncology trials, many of our studies aim to answer the same questions of safety, efficacy, and comparison to conventional therapy.

RANDOMIZATION AND STRATIFICATION

Randomization is the process of assigning patients to a treatment group within a clinical trial by chance, rather than by choice. Treatment groups may include the standard of care, the standard of care plus a new therapy, a new

TABLE 5-1   CONVENTIONAL PHASES FOR PROSPECTIVE CLINICAL TRIALS

	Phase I	Phase II	Phase III
Aim	Toxicity Dose finding	Efficacy Responding histologies	Comparison to standard of care
Patient number	Small	Large	Large
Dose	Escalating in cohorts	Fixed	Fixed
Single therapy	Yes	No	Yes or No—can be combination therapy
Randomization	No	Yes or No	Yes

Phase I trials define a maximally tolerated dose (MTD) of a new drug/regimen through dose escalation. In these trials, toxicities associated with a new therapy can be defined. If a phase I trial is successful, its discovered dose moves into a phase II trial to assess efficacy and identify responding histologies. Phase III trials enroll a larger number of patients to compare the dose of the new therapy to standard of care treatment. Phase III trials can also assess if a new treatment is less toxic or less expensive with equal/improved efficacy to current standards.

therapy alone, or, in some cases, a placebo. The goal of randomization is to reduce bias (i.e., influence) for known and unknown characteristics (e.g., age, stage of disease, previous treatments) that may influence a response to the study therapy. Random allocation can be achieved by various methods described in Chapter 4. It is important that the sequence for randomization is concealed from clinical investigators *(allocation concealment)* in order to not bias the review of patient data as the study is ongoing. Therefore, during group assignment, treatment, assessment, and follow-up, it is common for the randomization of patients to be "blinded" or left unknown to participants, investigators, and statisticians. Randomization tends to produce comparable treatment groups in terms of those factors (i.e., confounders) that are not necessarily part of a study, but that may affect a treatment outcome.[9-11]

Depending on the study, treatment group randomization may be balanced 1:1, where a patient has an equal chance of being assigned to one study group over another, or skewed. Skewed or weighted randomization strategies allow more patients to enter one group versus another. This strategy is most often used in placebo-controlled studies where a 3:1 randomization structure would result in 3 patients being randomized to receive the active treatment for every 1 patient that receives placebo. Randomization allows treatment and control arms to be compared as equally as possible. However, historical controls are sometimes used as a "control" arm instead of a new patient group. Historical controls are confounded by many variables that cannot be balanced between groups, as described in Chapter 4.

In some cases, a patient characteristic (age, breed, past treatment, stage, etc.) is known or suspected to have an effect on the outcome of patients included in a clinical trial. For example, dogs with T-cell lymphoma are known to have a poorer outcome compared with dogs with B-cell lymphoma. To ensure that this variable is equally distributed across treatment groups, the strategy of patient *stratification* for these known prognostic variables occurs before randomization (Figure 5-1),[12-15] thus allowing patients with a known confounding variable (i.e., T-cell lymphoma) to be randomized to the two study treatment groups separately from patients without the confounding variable.

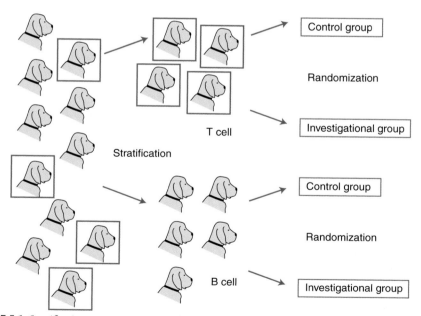

FIGURE 5-1 Stratification can prevent potential bias from known prognostic factors, such as immunophenotype in canine lymphoma. For example, it may appear that a treatment arm is doing poorly, hence concluding that the treatment is ineffective. But this cohort had a majority of dogs with T-cell lymphoma. Therefore, the immunophenotypic effect could mask the would-be positive benefits of the new therapy. Stratifying dogs by immunophenotype prior to randomization would allow researchers to look at separate subgroups and see if differences exist between "equal" treatment and control arms.

POWER

Power is a measure of the ability of a study to identify statistically significant differences between treatment groups.[16,17] This and other statistical parameters are explained in more detail in Chapter 4. The size of the patient population is a primary determinant of its power. By increasing the statistical power in a study, the chance of demonstrating statistically significant differences among treatment groups is increased. Thus, it is important to define the size of a study (e.g., number of participants) before a clinical trial is initiated.

ENDPOINTS

Endpoints are selected to answer the primary and secondary objectives of a trial and reflect the specific measures that will be followed in a study. Common endpoints in clinical trials include defining a *maximally tolerated dose (MTD)* to assess safety and evaluating *tumor response* to measure activity.[18,19] Criteria for *safety* and *toxicity* have been established recently for veterinary patients through the Veterinary Cooperative Oncology Group (VCOG) and are described in Chapter 13.[20] These criteria provide a means by which safety and toxicity endpoints may be consistently reported.[21,22] The effectiveness of a new cancer agent can be measured in several ways. These include *response rates* in measurable/macroscopic disease, *disease free interval* (DFI), overall *survival time* (ST), and *quality of life* (QOL) assessments.[16,23] Endpoints differ depending on the type and objectives of a study and are defined prospectively in the study protocol.

Biological endpoints, such as pharmacokinetic and pharmacodynamic assessments, are becoming increasingly important in veterinary oncology clinical trials. These biologic endpoints have been incorporated into study designs to better understand the mechanisms and biological effects of novel therapies and interventions.[24-27] *Pharmacodynamic (PD)* effects describe changes that occur in target tissue (such as the tumor), or within other tissues or fluids from the patient (surrogate tissues) after the patient receives a drug. An example of a pharmacodynamic endpoint is the measurement of a specific protein in a tumor following treatment with an agent that blocks the expression of that protein. *Pharmacokinetic (PK)* measurements define what the body does to a drug, such as absorption, metabolism, and excretion. It is most useful to concurrently assess PK and PD endpoints. Biological endpoints such as PK/PD analysis allow for a much broader understanding of how new drugs work and whether they should proceed to future clinical trials. This is especially important for new cancer agents that may not cause an early and immediate response to therapy (such as is conventionally seen with cytotoxic chemotherapy). Measurement of PD changes occurring in a tumor as a result of therapy may be readily measured in veterinary oncology trials, thus affording the opportunity to answer biological questions about a new drug that are otherwise difficult to answer.

FLEXIBILITY OF VETERINARY CLINICAL TRIALS

Clinical trials in companion animals with cancer allow for a level of flexibility that may not exist in human clinical trials. This is due to the lack of true *"gold-standard"* medical treatments in veterinary medicine. Although there are treatment protocols considered to be optimal or "best offerings," a requirement for a particular cancer to be treated with a standard of care therapy does not exist. Thus, in veterinary clinical trials there is the opportunity to treat animals with cancer earlier in the course of their disease, including at initial diagnosis. The ability to treat naïvely diagnosed patients, as well as those with recurrent disease, can be more informative than treating patients with advanced disease, as is most commonly the case in human trials. In veterinary oncology clinical trials there is a greater opportunity for serial sampling of tumors and/or blood than in human clinical trials, again adding to the cache of information about a new drug (especially important is PK/PD and biomarker data collection).[14] Samples collected in such studies may be preserved in a variety of different media conditions, including formalin, frozen in liquid nitrogen, RNA-preserving liquids (e.g., RNAlater), or they may be held in tissue culture media. For most studies, DNA, RNA, and proteins will be purified from these samples for biological analysis.

ETHICAL CONSIDERATIONS

There are key ethical standards used in clinical trial design, and it should be the goal of all clinicians to ensure these standards are met when presenting the option of a trial to a client or enrolling a patient in a clinical trial. The motivation for clients to consider clinical trials includes the lack of other effective treatments for their pet's cancer, side effects that may limit their interest in pursuing conventional treatments, or cost of conventional therapy. For the most part, clinical trials are provided at no cost or at limited cost to clients. In almost all trials, the cost of the study drug is not the responsibility of the client. It is increasingly important to include the option of clinical trials when presenting the medical options available for a specific patient. In many instances, owners are motivated to choose a clinical trial influenced by their desire to help their pet and to improve outcomes for future pets or people with cancer.

Informed consent is required for all patients to enroll in a clinical trial.[9,28-30] This is a written acknowledgement created by a trial's principal investigators and signed by a client, indicating that both the potential benefits and the *adverse effects* associated with clinical trial participation have been discussed. This informed consent defines a trial's purpose and the requirements of the client to return with their pet for future follow-up procedures/appointments. It ensures that the relationship and responsibilities of all parties involved in the trial are clear. Although adverse events outside of those described are always possible, informed consent ensures that clients understand that in many trials the outcome/side effects are yet unknown.

It is important to protect from harm all patients who enter clinical trials. *Stopping rules* within a trial protocol are used to remove participants in a trial if severe side effects are seen or if there is evidence that the patient's cancer is progressing in the face of treatment.[31,32] Stopping rules are particularly important in clinical trials that include placebo treatment arms and that allow patients whose cancer is progressing to move on to alternative treatments if they exist. Also, if a patient fails to respond or progresses while in one treatment arm, it can be possible for them to *cross over* into another treatment arm. In addition to stopping rules for patients in a trial, the entire trial might be stopped prematurely if there is strong evidence that the new intervention/agent is very effective or if the overall incidence of side effects is higher than expected. More recent innovative trial designs, referred to as Bayesian or outcome adaptive randomization trials, assign more patients to the treatment arm that appears to be most effective.[33,34] The increased use of such adaptive trials will increase the benefit and reduce the likelihood of side effects for study participants. *Compassionate use* of an investigational agent is a mechanism for patients to continue on a therapy or have access to a therapy outside of the original clinical trial objectives or design. An example of this would be to allow a dog who has experienced a treatment response or significant disease stabilization to continue to receive a study treatment beyond the defined study duration. Collectively, these measures ensure that patients' best interests are maintained during their participation in a trial.

PRACTITIONER INVOLVEMENT IN CLINICAL TRIALS

The active engagement of veterinary general practitioners in conducting oncology clinical trials is vitally important. These clinicians are the ones who first diagnose a pet with cancer and can act as the front line to educate clients about the availability of clinical trials. Reassuring clients about the myriad of treatment options available today to pets with cancer and removing the mystery surrounding clinical trials is one of the most important steps in developing new techniques to fight cancer in companion animals. It is also proven that

TABLE 5-2 **ELECTRONIC RESOURCES PROVIDING INFORMATION REGARDING ONGOING VETERINARY CLINICAL TRIALS**

Institution/Organization	Website Address
American College of Veterinary Internal Medicine	http://www.acvim.org
Animal Clinical Investigation (multi-institutional)	http://www.animalci.com/index.php
Animal Medical Center	http://www.amcny.org/technology/clinicaltrials.aspx
Colorado State University	http://www.csuanimalcancercenter.org/wbswebpage.cfm?pagetextid=Trials
Comparative Oncology Program, National Cancer Institute (multi-institutional)	http://ccr.cancer.gov/resources/cop/
North Carolina State University	http://www.cvm.ncsu.edu/vth/clinical_services/onco/studies.html
Purdue University	http://www.vet.purdue.edu/pcop/what.html
University of California-Davis	http://www.vetmed.ucdavis.edu/
University of Minnesota	http://www.cvm.umn.edu/accr/clinicalstudies/home.html
University of Missouri-Columbia	http://www.cvm.missouri.edu/oncology/current.htm
University of Pennsylvania	http://www.vet.upenn.edu/departments/csp/oncology/trials/
University of Tennessee	http://www.vet.utk.edu/studies/oncology.shtml
University of Wisconsin-Madison	http://www.vetmed.wisc.edu/data/news/trials.html
Veterinary Cancer Society	http://www.vetcancersociety.org/index.php?c=1

involving patients in clinical trials provides the best care to patients in both the short and long term.

Clinical trials are often conducted through academic veterinary teaching hospitals or referral centers, and they increasingly include direct involvement from private practitioners. It may not be feasible for patients to return to tertiary care centers for recheck examinations; hence, these are often handled locally by their referring veterinarians. The timely reporting of these rechecks to the study center site and detailed record-keeping are essential for accurate assessment of clinical trial results. This includes all possible long-term adverse events (side effects) from a new therapy, as well as outcome data.

There are a number of resources available to practitioners to find information regarding oncology clinical trials (Table 5-2). As suggested previously, it is certain that the availability of clinical trial options for pet owners will expand in the coming years. These options will in many cases be the "desired" option for a client/family to pursue for their pet. As a trusted source of information, the primary care veterinarian plays an important role in describing the advantages and disadvantages of all treatment options available for a pet with cancer. In many cases these options will include clinical trial participation.

Selected References*

Brown DC: Control of selection bias in parallel-group controlled clinical trials in dogs and cats: 97 trials (2000-2005), *J Am Vet Med Assoc* 229(6):990-993, 2006.

This manuscript aims to determine how selection bias was controlled in a number of published veterinary clinical trials.

Giacinti L, Lopez M, Giordano A: Clinical trials, *Front Biosci* 11:2918-2923, 2006.

This paper reviews the principal phases of clinical trials and discusses the basic requirements needed to ensure a well-conducted experimental study.

Green SJ, Pauler DK: Statistics in clinical trials, *Curr Oncol Rep* 6:36-41, 2004.

Statistical developments in clinical trial analysis over the past several years are described in this review. These include the incorporation of multiple endpoints, randomization, methods to use the sample size more efficiently, and associated biological endpoint evaluation.

Paoloni M, Khanna C: Translation of new cancer treatments from pet dogs to humans. *Nat Rev Cancer* 8:147-156, 2008.

This review discusses the use and integration of spontaneous cancer models into a comprehensive and comparative approach to preclinical drug development. Examples of their successful use and an outline of their relative strengths and weaknesses is provided.

Vail DM: Veterinary co-operative oncology group, *Vet Compar Oncol* 2:194-213, 2004.

Description of the grade and scale of a myriad of toxicities in the dog is provided in this manuscript. The text provides a uniform standard to adverse event reporting in veterinary clinical trials.

■ *For a complete list of the references cited in this chapter, please go to www.smallanimaloncology.com.

6 Methods of Tumor Diagnosis: Fine-Needle Aspiration and Biopsy Techniques

Carolyn J. Henry and Eric R. Pope

KEY POINTS

- Fine-needle aspirates can be diagnostic for tumors that exfoliate well. Using larger-gauge needles on solid masses facilitates retrieval of larger numbers of cells.
- Needle-core biopsies are very accurate and can often be obtained without general anesthesia.
- Harvesting multiple biopsy samples increases the likelihood of obtaining a definitive diagnosis.

Accurate determination of tumor type and, in many cases, tumor grade is important for determining the most appropriate treatment regimen for companion animal cancer patients.[1] Fine-needle aspiration (FNA), needle core biopsy (NCB), punch biopsy, and open (surgical) biopsy can provide that information for soft tissue tumors. Open biopsy is considered the gold standard for most solid tumors but is invasive and in most instances requires either heavy sedation and local anesthesia or general anesthesia. FNA can usually be performed without any anesthesia in cooperative patients. NCB may require local anesthesia, with or without sedation.

FNA and NCB of easily palpable tumors can usually be accomplished by immobilizing the mass with the nondominant hand and directly guiding the biopsy instrument into the mass. The ability to obtain representative samples with FNA or NCB of deeper masses or those located within body cavities is increased when imaging guidance techniques such as ultrasonography or computed tomography are used.[2,3]

Bone biopsy samples are usually collected using a Jamshidi needle or Michelle trephine instrument, although FNA may be possible with lytic lesions. This section outlines the techniques commonly used to obtain diagnostic samples from tumor tissue.

FINE-NEEDLE ASPIRATION (FNA)

FNA is an excellent technique for collecting samples for cytologic evaluation of cytoplasmic and nuclear detail.[4] Since only single cells or small sheets of cells are obtained, details concerning tumor architecture cannot usually be assessed. Examination of FNA samples is useful for differentiating neoplastic from inflammatory lesions. A tumor diagnosis can be made if the cells exfoliate well and have characteristic morphology. Cellular morphology may also allow neoplastic lesions to be classified as benign or malignant.

Materials

- 22- to 25-gauge hypodermic needles (25-gauge needles are used with vascular appearing lesions, whereas 22-gauge needles facilitate collection of more cellular samples in solid tumors)
- 5- or 10-ml syringe
- Microscope slides

Technique

- Scrub the skin over the lesion with antiseptic solution or alcohol.
- Immobilize mass between fingers with nondominant hand.
- Zajdela technique (without aspiration)[5]
  - Pass the needle percutaneously into the mass.
  - Move the needle back and forth rapidly within the mass multiple (5–20) times and redirect the needle into different areas of the mass every few strokes. Sampling should be halted if blood appears in the needle hub, since further sampling will only result in blood contamination that may dilute the sample and obscure the cytologic diagnosis.

- Withdraw the needle from the mass.
- Attach the needle to an air-filled syringe and expel the specimen onto a microscope slide, ensuring that the beveled edge is oriented toward the slide.
- The procedure can be repeated multiple times until an adequate specimen is obtained.
- Aspiration technique
  - Attach the needle to a 5- to 10-ml syringe.
  - Pass the needle percutaneously into the mass.
  - Apply suction by pulling back on the plunger multiple times in rapid succession.
  - The needle may be redirected within the mass and the above procedure repeated before withdrawing the needle from the mass.
  - Release the plunger before withdrawing the needle from the mass.
  - Remove the syringe from the needle and fill it with air.
  - Expel the sample onto a microscope slide.
- Slide preparation
  - Expel the sample onto the microscope slide near the frosted end.
  - Use a second slide to spread the sample into a monolayer before staining. Simply allowing the weight of the second slide to spread the sample is generally sufficient. Applying additional pressure when dispersing the sample on the slide will only result in disruption of the cell membranes and make interpretation of the cells difficult.

Interpretation

- Should be interpreted by a trained cytopathologist (Chapter 7)
- Sensitivity, specificity, and accuracy of cytology are similar to histology when performed by a trained cytopathologist.
- The diagnostic accuracy of FNA of deep thoracic and abdominal masses in dogs and cats is reported to be between 70% and 90%.[3]
- In a study of FNA samples from malignant tumors, the cellular line of origin was correctly determined in 72% and 87% of dog and cat tumors, respectively.[6]
- The sampling and processing technique can have a significant effect on diagnostic accuracy.[7]

NEEDLE CORE BIOPSY (NCB)

NCB instruments can be used to collect intact tissue samples from soft tissue tumors. The accuracy of diagnosis is enhanced when larger-gauge biopsy needles are used and when multiple samples are collected from different areas of the mass.[1,8]

Materials

- NCB needles
  - 14- to 16-gauge recommended
  - Manual, spring-loaded, automated models
- Hypodermic needles to facilitate removal of specimen from biopsy needle
- Microscope slides for touch preps (impression smears)
- Specimen cassettes
- Fixative solution(s)
- Suture material, skin staples, or tissue adhesive

Technique (Figure 6-1)

- Sedation and local anesthesia (general anesthesia may be necessary for deep lesions or uncooperative patients)
- Clip hair and routinely prep skin.
- Superficial lesions can be sampled by direct insertion of the biopsy needle.

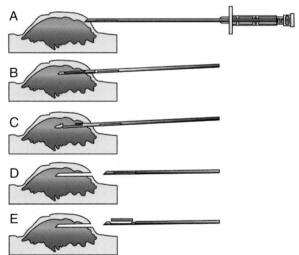

FIGURE 6-1 Needle core biopsy technique. **A,** A small skin incision is made with a No. 11 blade to allow insertion of the instrument. With the instrument closed, the outer capsule is penetrated. **B,** The outer cannula is fixed in place and the inner cannula with the specimen notch is thrust into the tumor. The tissue then protrudes into the notch. **C,** The inner cannula is held steady while the outer cannula is moved forward to cut off the biopsy specimen. **D,** The entire instrument is removed closed with the tissue contained within it. **E,** The inner cannula is advanced to expose the tissue in the specimen notch. (From Withrow SJ, Vail DM: *Withrow & MacEwen's small animal clinical oncology,* ed 4. St Louis, 2007, Saunders/Elsevier, p 148.)

- A small skin incision can be made when deeper lesions are present.
- Read and carefully follow manufacturer's directions for use of the biopsy needle.
- Collecting multiple samples with the needle directed in different planes is recommended with larger masses.
- Retract the outer cannula to expose the specimen.
- Tease the specimen from the biopsy needle onto a slide for cytopathology or place directly into fixative.
- If a skin incision was made, close it with a simple interrupted suture, skin staple, or tissue glue.

Interpretation

- Impression smears can be made for immediate evaluation. This is especially useful when the results are used to guide intraoperative decision-making.
- The remaining tissue should be fixed for histopathologic examination.
- The diagnostic accuracy of NCB is excellent with high sensitivity, specificity, and positive predictive value.[9]
- In one study, correlation with surgical biopsy was 100% for epithelial tumors and 94% for mesenchymal tumors.[9]

PUNCH BIOPSY

Dermal biopsy punches can be used to collect larger biopsy samples than can be obtained with the NCB instruments yet can still be performed through a minimal incision. Surface lesions can be biopsied without making an incision. This technique is also useful for obtaining biopsy samples from internal organs such as the liver during exploratory celiotomy.

Materials

- Punch biopsy—available in 1- to 8-mm diameter sizes
- Thumb forceps
- Scissors or scalpel with no. 11 blade
- Microscope slides for touch preps
- Specimen cassettes
- Fixative solution(s)
- Suture material or skin staples

Technique (Figure 6-2)

- Sedation and/or local anesthesia (may not be necessary for ulcerated surface lesions)
- Dermal lesions can be sampled directly through the intact skin.
- Biopsy of deeper lesions should be planned in order to not alter definitive surgery (i.e., any biopsy tract will need to be excised at the time of the definitive surgery).

- Incise skin over mass with scalpel blade.
- Immobilize mass between fingers.
- Insert punch biopsy instrument into lesion.
- Rocking the tip of the biopsy instrument back and forth may avulse the sample from friable masses.
- Withdraw the biopsy punch.
- If specimen is still attached, grasp it with thumb forceps and retract.
- Cut off specimen at base with scissors or scalpel.
- Multiple specimens can be collected by inserting the biopsy punch instrument from different directions.
- Digital pressure is generally sufficient to control bleeding.
- Close the skin incision with suture or skin staple.

Interpretation

- Touch preps can be made for immediate evaluation.
- The remaining tissue should be fixed for histopathologic examination.

OPEN BIOPSY

Open biopsy samples may be collected by an incisional or excisional technique.[1] Excisional biopsies are generally performed on small accessible lesions when a sufficient margin of normal tissue can be removed with the mass and when the excision will not likely result in increased morbidity if further surgery is necessary. Excisional biopsy is usually diagnostic and therapeutic. Incisional biopsies are indicated when knowing the type of tumor is important in planning the definitive resection or when knowing the tumor type might influence the treatment protocol. The following description is for incisional biopsy; excisional biopsy is covered in Chapter 14.

Materials

- Surgical pack appropriate for the procedure
- Specimen cassettes and containers
- Fixative solution(s)
- Suture material or skin staples

Technique

- Sedation and local anesthetic or general anesthesia
- Routine clipping, skin preparation, and draping
- Surface and ulcerated lesions can be directly biopsied. Be sure to get a deep enough biopsy of ulcerated lesions to sample beyond the inflamed tissue.
- Incise the skin over the mass when deeper lesions are present. Avoid opening new tissue planes that might alter the definitive surgery.
- Harvest a deep narrow wedge of tissue from the mass. This type of biopsy facilitates wound closure, especially with surface lesions.

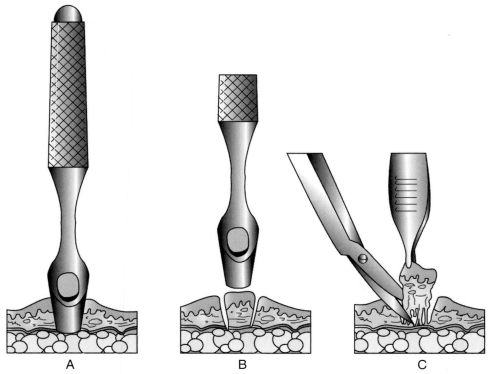

A   B   C

FIGURE 6-2 Punch biopsy technique. **A,** Punch biopsy instrument is rotated clockwise and counterclockwise into the lesion until sufficient depth has been penetrated. **B,** Punch is removed or angled across base to sever deep attachments. **C,** Specimen may be gently grasped with thumb forceps (do not use rat tooth forceps) and cut off deeply. (From Withrow SJ, Vail DM: *Withrow & MacEwen's small animal clinical oncology*, ed 4. St Louis, 2007, Saunders/Elsevier, p 149.)

- Close the biopsy site with sutures. Cruciate sutures work well for this.
- Routinely close tissue layers.
- Place the specimen in the appropriate fixative solution.

BONE BIOPSY

Bone biopsy samples are typically collected using a coring instrument such as the Jamshidi needle or Michelle trephine.[1] Pre-biopsy radiographs are useful for identifying the most appropriate biopsy site. Intraoperative fluoroscopic (C-Arm) or CT guidance may be helpful, particularly for lesions surrounded by muscle. In general, *the periphery of a bone lesion should be avoided* since the biopsy specimens from this area are frequently read out as reactive bone on histopathological examination. Collecting multiple biopsy specimens increases the likelihood

of getting an accurate diagnosis but may predispose the bone to pathologic fracture.

Materials

- Jamshidi needle or Michelle trephine (3/16 or ¼ inch) with stylet
- Scalpel handle and no. 11 blade
- Thumb forceps, hemostats, needle holder
- Specimen container and fixative
- Suture material or skin staples

Technique (Figure 6-3)

- General anesthesia is preferable, but heavy sedation and local anesthetic block could be considered in cooperative patients.
- Routine clipping, skin preparation, and draping
- Incise the skin over the lesion.

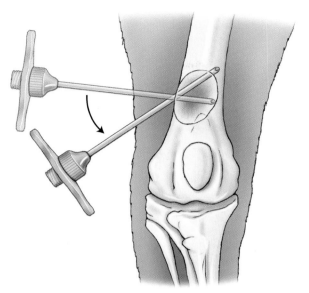

FIGURE 6-3 Bone biopsy technique. Note that the biopsy instrument enters the center of the lesion, not the periphery. Additional samples may be collected using the same entry site, but with the instrument redirected to sample from other areas within the lesion.

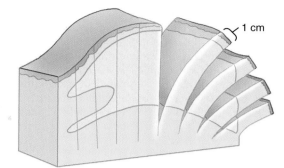

FIGURE 6-4 Excised mass prepared for processing. The surgical margins have been marked with dye. The mass has been "bread-loafed" to ensure adequate tissue preservation, but the mass remains intact to facilitate examination by the pathologist.

- Insert the Jamshidi needle through the soft tissues down to the bone surface; a hemostat can be used to bluntly separate soft tissues to facilitate introduction of the Michelle trephine instrument.
- Remove the stylet and advance the needle or trephine into the bone, using a twisting motion.
- The biopsy should include the near cortex and medullary cavity but should not exit the far cortex.
- Withdraw the biopsy needle and use the stylet to expel the biopsy into the fixative.
- Repeat the process, entering through the same entrance into the near cortex but angling the instrument in different directions. Three biopsies—one central, one directed proximal, and one directed distal—increase the likelihood of obtaining a diagnosis.
- Multiple holes in the cortex increase the likelihood of iatrogenically induced pathologic fracture.
- Control bleeding with digital pressure.
- Close the skin with suture material or skin staple.

SAMPLE HANDLING AND PROCESSING

The samples should be placed in fixative as soon as possible. Consultation with a pathologist concerning the most appropriate fixative to use is highly recommended, especially if special stains or other diagnostic techniques may be needed. For formalin fixation, the ratio of formalin solution to sample volume should be at least 10:1. Samples greater than 1 cm thick should be "bread-loafed" to ensure adequate penetration of the fixative (Figure 6-4). Once the specimen has been fixed, it can be placed in a smaller volume of fixative to reduce shipping weight.

The ability to evaluate surgical margins is as important as proper fixation when processing excisional biopsies. Since it is likely that most samples will be too large to fit on a single slide, the specimen will be divided during preparation for evaluation by the pathologist. Differentiating sectioning margins and the actual surgical margins is of utmost importance in assessing completeness of excision. Identifying surgical margins and areas of interest can be accomplished in several ways.[10] If there are areas where the completeness of excision is of particular concern, those areas can be identified with suture material or metallic clips. Another option is to harvest additional tissue from the adjacent wound bed to determine whether neoplastic tissue was left in the wound.

Various dyes may be used to mark the surgical margins prior to fixation of the tissue.[10-12] Commercial dye kits providing several colors are available, but India ink can also be used for most tissues. After the mass is removed, swab off excess fluids with a sponge. Apply the dye to all of the cut surfaces or to any surface of particular interest. Allow the dye to dry thoroughly before "bread-loafing" it or placing it in the fixative. The dye will remain on the tissue after processing, making it easy to differentiate a surgical margin from a sectioning margin. If tumor is visible at the dyed edge or very close to it, the excision should be considered incomplete. How close is too close has not been clearly determined and probably varies with the tumor type and grade. Interpretation of a report indicating "close, but clean" surgical margins must be made in light of the fact that tissue shrinkage during fixation decreases some of the margins compared with the fresh tissue.[13] Ideally, the surgeon should account for the shrinkage in planning the surgery, but the amount of shrinkage that will occur has not been determined for most tissues in animals.

Selected References[*]

Aitken ML, Patnaik AK: Comparison of needle-core (Trucut) biopsy and surgical biopsy for the diagnosis of cutaneous and subcutaneous masses: a prospective study of 51 cases, *J Am Anim Hosp Assoc* 36:153-157, 2000.
This manuscript demonstrates that needle-core biopsies correlate well with surgical biopsies. Using larger-gauge needles and taking multiple samples increases the accuracy of needle-core biopsies.

Ehrhart N: Principles of tumor biopsy, *Clin Tech Small Anim Pract* 13:10-16, 1998.
A good review of biopsy techniques and sample handling procedures.

Reimer BS, Séguin B, DeCock HE, et al: Evaluation of the effect of routine histologic processing on the size of skin samples obtained from dogs, *Am J Vet Res* 66:500-505, 2005.
This study shows that the tissue shrinkage that occurs as a result of preserving tissues can significantly affect the apparent width of histologic margins. Pinning the samples to reduce the amount of shrinkage during fixation minimizes this potential artifact.

Seitz SE, Foley GL, Marretta SM: Evaluation of marking materials for cutaneous surgical margins, *Am J Vet Res* 56:826-833, 1995.
This manuscript describes how various dyes can be used to mark surgical margins of excised masses. Multiple color systems aid the identification of specific areas of concern about completeness of excision.

[*]For a complete list of the references cited in this chapter, please go to www.smallanimaloncology.com.

7

The Cytology of Neoplasia

Marlyn S. Whitney and Linda M. Berent

KEY POINTS

- Cytology is a rapid and inexpensive procedure, but some experience is required if one is to obtain diagnostic samples and properly evaluate them.
- Cytology is often sufficient for diagnosis of the round cell tumors.
- Cytology is often equivocal in lesions complicated by inflammation or necrosis.
- Although it is a useful tool in veterinary oncology, cytology cannot completely replace the histopathologic examination of tumors.

Cytologic examination of masses, effusions, and lymph nodes can aid in the diagnosis and staging of neoplastic processes. It is a rapid and relatively inexpensive procedure. However, it does have its limitations. Although cytology has excellent sensitivity and specificity for the round cell tumors, it is often equivocal in lesions complicated by inflammation or necrosis. Even when cytologic evaluation indicates that malignancy is present, it is often not possible to determine the specific type of carcinoma or sarcoma that is present.[1,2] Immunocytochemistry is not widely available and tumor grading cannot be accomplished using cytology alone. For these reasons, cytology is a useful tool in veterinary oncology but cannot completely replace histopathology. This chapter is intended to serve as an overview of common cytologic findings in neoplastic lesions and is not intended to be a stand-alone resource. A practitioner must be versed in the normal cytology for each tissue before he or she can competently diagnose neoplastic lesions. The reader is directed to any one of the excellent atlases available for a complete review of normal, inflammatory, and neoplastic cytology.[3-5]

GENERAL APPROACH TO THE INTERPRETATION OF CYTOLOGIC SPECIMENS

Adequate samples are essential for optimal cytologic evaluation (see Chapter 6). The first step in slide evaluation is to locate an area with adequate cellularity and good quality of cells. The next step is to determine if the specimen is comprised primarily of inflammatory cells, non-inflammatory cells, or a mixture of both. Inflammatory cell populations are further classified according to the types of cells present, since this helps to narrow the list of etiologic possibilities. Non-inflammatory cell populations are categorized as one of the following: (1) normal cells for the given anatomic site, (2) hyperplasia or benign neoplasia (these often cannot be cytologically differentiated from one another), or (3) malignant neoplasia. Mixed cell responses are quite common and present as inflammatory cells mixed with normal, hyperplastic, or neoplastic cells. When cells are suspected of being neoplastic, the next step is to determine the general cellular category: epithelial cells, mesenchymal cells, or one of the discrete round cell neoplasms. Epithelial cells are round to polygonal and have a tendency to arrange in cohesive clusters. Mesenchymal cells often have one or more cytoplasmic tails. Those with one cytoplasmic tail may be described as flame shaped, those with two as spindle shaped, and those with more than two as stellate shaped. In some mesenchymal neoplasms, such as the lipoma, the cells may be round to oval. Mesenchymal cells tend to appear as single forms, but aggregates of cells may be present. The discrete round cell neoplasms, which are technically of mesenchymal origin, are usually placed into a separate category because they are made up of round cells that do not form cohesive clusters. Melanomas are of neuroectodermal origin and do not fit well into the above morphologic classification system, since their cells may exhibit round, epithelial and mesenchymal characteristics. The key to diagnosing a melanoma is to find melanin granules in the cytoplasm of the tumor cells.

CYTOLOGIC CRITERIA OF MALIGNANCY

Cytologic criteria of malignancy are primarily used to determine if an epithelial or mesenchymal population is abnormal enough to be considered malignant (Box 7-1). These criteria often relate to the variability in the cell population and are less useful for monomorphic round cell neoplasms. General criteria of malignancy include anisocytosis (variable cell size in a population that would normally consist of cells of similar size), higher cellularity than expected, and presence of cells in an abnormal location. Nuclear criteria of malignancy include variable nuclear size (anisokaryosis), increased nuclear to cytoplasmic volume ratios (N:C ratios), variable N:C ratios in a cell population not normally expected to exhibit this feature, multiple nucleoli, variable size of nucleoli, presence of abnormally shaped nucleoli, coarse and irregular chromatin clumping, thickening of the nuclear margin, large numbers of mitotic figures, mitotic figures of abnormal configuration, presence of multiple nuclei, and nuclear molding. Nuclear molding is characterized by the wrapping of a nucleus from one cell around an adjacent cell, or the wrapping of one nucleus around another in a multinucleated cell. Cytoplasmic criteria of malignancy are the least useful and include increased cytoplasmic

basophilia and vacuolation. As a rule, at least four general or nuclear criteria of malignancy should be observed before assigning the term *malignant*, although there are exceptions to this rule. One can be most confident in assessing malignancy when many criteria are present, or when one or more very strong criteria are present. The presence of cells in an abnormal location, such as sheets of epithelial cells within a lymph node aspirate, is such a strong criterion of malignancy that it can be used to make the assessment of malignancy even when few or no other criteria are present.

Some of the criteria of malignancy just mentioned can also be found in hyperplastic cell populations. These include high cellularity, anisocytosis, anisokaryosis, increased N:C ratios, presence of multiple nuclei and/or nucleoli, increased mitotic figures, and increased cytoplasmic basophilia. Some types of epithelial cells, including squamous and transitional epithelial cells, normally exhibit variability in N:C ratios, because nuclei become smaller as the cells mature. When multiple nuclei are present in hyperplastic cells, they should be present in even numbers and should all be of equal size. While multiple nucleoli are often present in hyperplastic cells, they should remain small and round.

CYTOLOGIC APPEARANCE OF MESENCHYMAL TUMORS (FIGURE 7-1)

As a rule, mesenchymal neoplasms do not exfoliate well, often resulting in suboptimal cytology preparations.[6,7] Lipomas are the most common mesenchymal tumor in older dogs and often yield poorly cellular, oily material that will not dry when placed on slides. Rarely, mature adipocytes can be found and are characterized by large round cells with a large amount of clear cytoplasm and a small condensed oval nucleus at one pole. This cytologic appearance is identical to that of subcutaneous fat and should, therefore, always be correlated with the clinical presentation of the lesion. Liposarcomas are rare and have small clear cytoplasmic vacuoles in cells with features similar to the soft tissue sarcomas described in subsequent sections.

Soft Tissue Sarcomas

Soft tissue sarcomas are characterized by flame- to spindle- or stellate-shaped cells with a tendency to appear as individualized cells, rather than in cohesive groups. Multiple criteria for malignancy are usually present in sarcomas, differentiating them from the benign connective tissue tumors such as a fibroma. Cytologic examination may narrow the diagnosis to sarcoma, but it is often insufficient to further classify these lesions into subtypes of tumor (e.g., fibrosarcoma vs. hemangiopericytoma).

BOX 7-1 CYTOLOGIC CRITERIA FOR MALIGNANCY

Strong Criteria for Malignancy
- Cells in an abnormal location
- Nuclear molding
- Abnormal mitotic figures
- Odd numbers of nuclei
- Anisokaryosis within a multinucleate cell
- Variability in nucleolar size
- Abnormally large and/or irregularly shaped nucleoli

Weak Criteria for Malignancy (Often Also Seen in Hyperplastic Populations)
- Anisocytosis
- Anisokaryosis
- Cytoplasmic basophilia
- Normal mitotic figures
- Binucleation

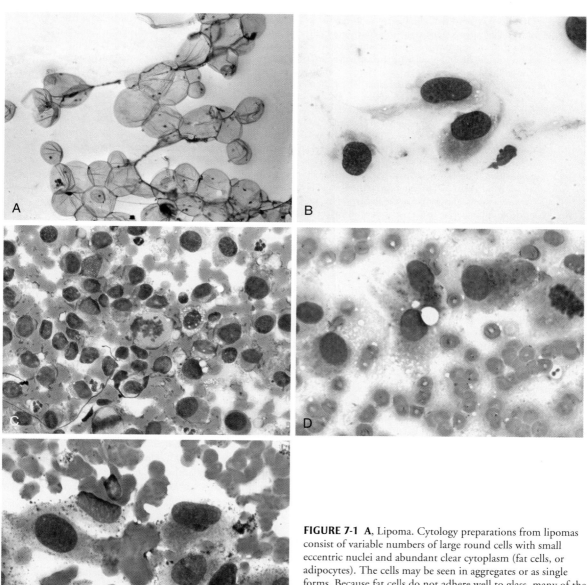

FIGURE 7-1 A, Lipoma. Cytology preparations from lipomas consist of variable numbers of large round cells with small eccentric nuclei and abundant clear cytoplasm (fat cells, or adipocytes). The cells may be seen in aggregates or as single forms. Because fat cells do not adhere well to glass, many of the cells may be lost from the slide during the staining process and stained preparations thus may be quite hypocellular (Wright-Giemsa stain, 100×). **B,** Sarcoma. Sarcomas tend to be made up of cells with cytoplasmic tails that appear as individual forms rather than in cohesive sheets (Wright-Giemsa stain, 1000×).

Continued

FIGURE 7-1, cont'd C, Malignant histiocytosis, splenic aspirate, dog. Malignant histiocytic neoplasms may have highly variable appearance. Discrete round cells that exhibit morphologic criteria of malignancy and that lack cytoplasmic granules often predominate, and such cells may exhibit phagocytosis of erythrocytes or other cells (not seen here). Spindle-shaped cells may also be present in some forms of malignant histocytic tumors. The lymphocytes seen here are most likely a component of the normal splenic tissue that remains (Wright-Giemsa stain, 600×). **D,** Osteosarcoma. The cells in osteosarcoma may vary from round to flame, spindle, or stellate shaped. Nuclei are round to oval, and the variably abundant basophilic cytoplasm may contain fine pink to red granular material, as seen here. The cells usually exhibit cytologic criteria of malignancy. Here, note anisocytosis, anisokaryosis, variability in N:C ratios, and multiple nucleoli (Wright-Giemsa stain, 1000×). **E,** Malignant melanoma. The cells in a melanoma may be epithelioid, spindle-shaped, appear as discrete round cells, or there may be a mixture of cell types, as seen here. The key to diagnosis is the presence of intracytoplasmic melanin granules. In benign melanomas and well-differentiated malignant ones, heavy granulation may obscure cellular detail. In malignant melanomas, granulation may range from heavy to scant to nearly non-existent (amelanotic melanoma). This melanoma has scant to moderate granulation. Note the anisocytosis, anisokaryosis, variability in N:C ratios, coarsely stippled chromatin patterns, and multiple nucleoli. A binucleate cell is present near the right margin of the field (Wright-Giemsa stain, 1000×).

Thus, a biopsy is necessary for definitive diagnosis. Care must be taken when assessing mesenchymal cells via cytology because reactive connective tissue cells may be misinterpreted as neoplastic.[8]

Histiocytic Neoplasia

The nomenclature for histiocytic neoplasms is evolving based on new information generated almost daily. As of this writing, the most current information can be found at http://www.histiocytosis.ucdavis.edu. In addition to benign histiocytomas of young dogs, there are several highly aggressive malignancies of histiocytic origin. Cytologic features include bizarre spindle or polygonal cells with marked criteria of malignancy. Erythrophagocytosis is a unique feature of these malignant cells but is not consistently found in all cases.

Osteosarcoma

The cells of osteosarcoma (OSA) may vary from round to flame to spindle shaped. Nuclei are generally round to oval, and the cells usually exhibit numerous cytologic criteria of malignancy. The cytoplasm is usually moderately abundant and basophilic and may contain variable numbers of small pink to red granules. The cells sometimes appear to be embedded in a bright pink-staining matrix material, which may represent osteoid. Tumor cells may contain two or more nuclei, and nuclei of disparate size may be present in a single cell. Low numbers of multinucleate cells in which all nuclei are of equal size may be present, typical of normal osteoclasts that are admixed with the tumor cells. OSAs

may be differentiated from other mesenchymal tumors by staining the air-dried slide for alkaline phosphatase activity.[9] This stain will react with the cytoplasm of the osteoblast, producing a dark brown to black reaction. The stain must be applied to unstained air-dried preparations of sufficient cellularity. Reactive bone formation, which might occur, for example, following a fracture or other damage to the bone or periosteum, can falsely mimic OSA in cytology preparations and will also stain positively for alkaline phosphatase activity. As such, it is critical that the cells are scrutinized for criteria of malignancy prior to the decision to use this stain. Radiographic findings and clinical history will often help prevent mistaking reactive bone for OSA.

Melanomas

Melanomas are difficult to classify based on cell shape, since they may appear round, spindle, polygonal, or in epithelial-like sheets on the same slide. When the cellular classification for a cytologic preparation is difficult to discern, melanoma should top the differential diagnosis list. The key to diagnosing a melanoma is to find melanin granules within the cytoplasm. Even tumors classified as "amelanotic" on histopathology will often exhibit rare fine granulation on cytology. Malignant melanoma cells have a round to oval or irregularly shaped nucleus with fine light chromatin and classically contain a single large nucleolus. They exhibit many criteria for malignancy. Benign melanomas (sometimes called melanocytomas) generally contain more abundant pigment granules and have a more uniform appearance than their malignant counterpart.

CYTOLOGIC APPEARANCE OF EPITHELIAL NEOPLASMS (FIGURES 7-2 AND 7-3)

Epithelial cells most often appear as round to oval or polygonal cells in cohesive sheets, clusters, or acinar patterns. Although some individualized forms may be present, the overall tendency is usually toward cohesive groups of cells. Some common benign epithelial neoplasms such as sebaceous adenomas may not exfoliate well and are difficult to distinguish from normal skin structures. Cytology preparations made from the various benign cystic follicular tumors (pilomatrixoma, trichoepithelioma, etc.) contain various proportions of normal mature keratinized squamous epithelial cells and keratin flakes, sometimes with cholesterol crystals and/or inflammatory cells admixed.

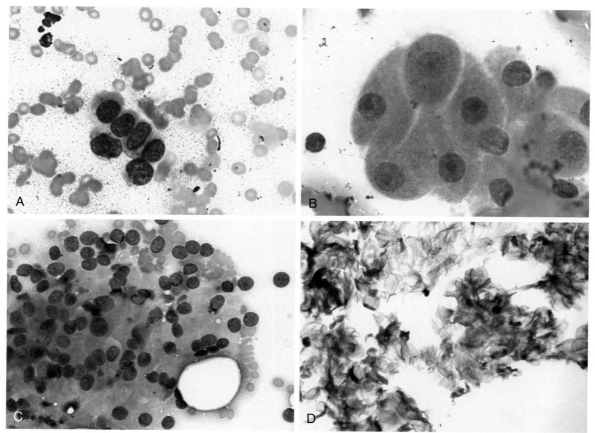

FIGURE 7-2 A, Basal cell tumor. Basal cells appear as small epithelial cells with oval nuclei and high N:C ratios. They are often arranged in rows in cytology preparations, as seen here. The cells are uniform in size and appearance (Wright-Giemsa stain, 1000×.) **B**, Perianal gland tumor. The cells are polygonal and tend to appear in cohesive sheets. Nuclei are small and round, often with a single prominent central nucleolus, and the abundant pinkish-blue cytoplasm has a somewhat granular appearance (Wright-Giemsa stain, 1000×.) **C**, Anal sac carcinoma. The cells have round to slightly oval nuclei and moderately abundant pale basophilic cytoplasm with indistinct borders. The cells are fragile, so many free nuclei are present in cytology preparations. Other nuclei appear embedded in a "sea of cytoplasm" as a result of the indistinct borders of the intact cells. Note the presence of anisokaryosis (Wright-Giemsa stain, 600×.) **D**, Epidermal inclusion cyst. Epidermal cysts are not neoplasms, but may resemble neoplasms grossly. They are made up of varying proportions of mature keratinized squamous epithelial cells and keratinaceous debris. Some such cysts contain sebaceous epithelial cells (Wright-Giemsa stain, 200×).

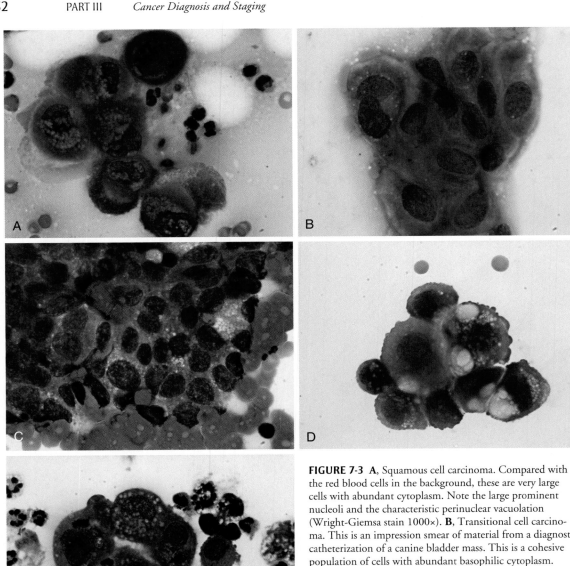

FIGURE 7-3 A, Squamous cell carcinoma. Compared with the red blood cells in the background, these are very large cells with abundant cytoplasm. Note the large prominent nucleoli and the characteristic perinuclear vacuolation (Wright-Giemsa stain 1000×). **B,** Transitional cell carcinoma. This is an impression smear of material from a diagnostic catheterization of a canine bladder mass. This is a cohesive population of cells with abundant basophilic cytoplasm. Note the large nucleoli and binucleate cells (Wright-Giemsa stain 1000×). **C,** Anaplastic carcinoma. Fine-needle aspirate of a canine liver mass. This cohesive population of cells is not consistent with either a biliary or hepatocellular population and is likely a metastatic lesion. Note the anisokaryosis and binucleate cells. The lack of normal hepatocytes makes tissue identification difficult (Wright-Giemsa stain 1000×).

FIGURE 7-3, cont'd **D**, Metastatic mammary carcinoma. In this direct smear of canine thoracic fluid, the neoplastic cells can appear rounded and may mimic a reactive mesothelial population (Wright-Giemsa stain 1000×). **E**, Reactive mesothelial cells and neutrophils from a dog with bile peritonitis. Note the similarity to the cells in **D**. The bile pigment and the inflammation should make a reactive population your first thought.

Basal Cell Tumors

Basal cell tumors (also called *basal cell carcinomas*) are common low-grade epithelial malignancies of the dog and cat. Small basophilic cuboidal cells may exfoliate as single cells (mimicking a round cell tumor), but there are usually some cells that line up in rows, forming small sheets with ribbon-like arrangements of uniform hyperchromatic nuclei. The cytoplasm is generally scant and deeply basophilic, and strong criteria of malignancy are usually lacking. Basal cells may contain cytoplasmic melanin pigment, but this is generally coarser than that seen in melanocytes. Some basal cell tumors display sebaceous or squamous differentiation and, thus, may share some cytologic characteristics with the follicular tumors.

Perianal Gland Tumors

Perianal gland tumors are common in the dog and may be present anywhere in the perineal region, prepuce, thigh, or tail head. These cells are characterized by abundant eosinophilic granular cytoplasm and a round, centrally located nucleus containing a single prominent nucleolus, giving them a "hepatoid" appearance. Occasional small, darker cuboidal cells with scant basophilic cytoplasm may be present and represent the "reserve cell" portion of the tumor. The majority of these neoplasms are benign in cytologic appearance and behavior. Malignant forms are uncommon and usually exhibit typical criteria for malignancy. Rarely, perianal gland tumors appear cytologically benign despite exhibiting invasive or other malignant behavior.

Adenocarcinoma of the Anal Sac Gland

Adenocarcinoma of the anal sac gland is distinct from perianal gland tumors, both cytologically and behaviorally. Anal sac adenocarcinomas have round to oval nuclei with coarse chromatin and a small amount of basophilic cytoplasm. Acinar structures may be seen, but cell margins are often indistinct, giving the impression of many nuclei in a sea of cytoplasm.

Squamous Cell Carcinoma

Squamous cell carcinoma is unique among the carcinomas in that it is characterized by individualized angular cells that only infrequently form small sheets. The cells are typically large but exhibit marked anisocytosis. The nuclei are round with prominent nucleoli. The abundant cytoplasm is the distinguishing feature, since it is often angular and deeply basophilic, with abundant perinuclear vacuoles that sometimes obscure the nuclear detail. These tumor cells are often mixed with inflammatory cells, and skill is needed to differentiate reactive from malignant squamous cells. Correlation with the clinical presentation is essential, and biopsy may be necessary for definitive diagnosis.

Mammary Tumors

Mammary tumor cytology is often unrewarding because of concurrent inflammation and the propensity for mammary tumors to be cytologically bland, yet behaviorally invasive. The main incentive for performing cytology on a tumor in the mammary region is to rule out a different disease such as a mast cell tumor (MCT) or other nonmammary lesion.[10]

Transitional Cell Carcinoma

The transitional cell epithelium of the urinary bladder exhibits marked dysplasia in response to prolonged inflammation or irritation (i.e., urinary tract infections or urolithiasis), and a clinical correlation is essential for proper interpretation of bladder cytology. Malignant transitional cells are often arranged in small sheets and exhibit marked variation in N:C ratio and overall cell size. Some cells may contain a prominent pink-staining cytoplasmic secretory vacuole. Although transitional cell carcinomas may exfoliate into the urine, a urine sediment examination may be unrewarding because of rapid degeneration of the cells in the urine, which makes evaluation for criteria of malignancy difficult.

CYTOLOGY OF EFFUSIONS

Although effusions are often associated with neoplastic disease in the abdominal and thoracic cavities, the presence of the neoplastic cells in the effusion is uncommon. Lymphoma and carcinomas are seen most frequently. Identification of neoplastic cells may be obscured by the presence of concurrent inflammation, or they may be misinterpreted as reactive mesothelial cells. Likewise, reactive mesothelial cells can appear markedly dysplastic and are often misinterpreted as neoplastic cells by inexperienced cytologists.[11]

CYTOLOGIC IDENTIFICATION OF DISCRETE ROUND CELL NEOPLASMS (FIGURE 7-4)

There are five discrete round cell tumors: lymphoma, histiocytoma, MCT, plasmacytoma, and transmissible venereal tumor (TVT). These mesenchymal neoplasms are made up of cells that appear as individualized round forms. Although the cells are not cohesive, they may be pushed together on the slide, making it possible to mistake them for epithelial cells. Given some experience, the discrete round cell neoplasms are distinctive enough in appearance that they can be correctly identified regardless of their arrangement on the slide.

Lymphoma

Lymphoma (also called *malignant lymphoma* or *lymphosarcoma*) commonly affects lymph nodes or other lymphoid tissue but can be found in virtually any tissue. Primary lymphoid neoplasia is generally a monotonous population of lymphoid cells, all at a similar stage of

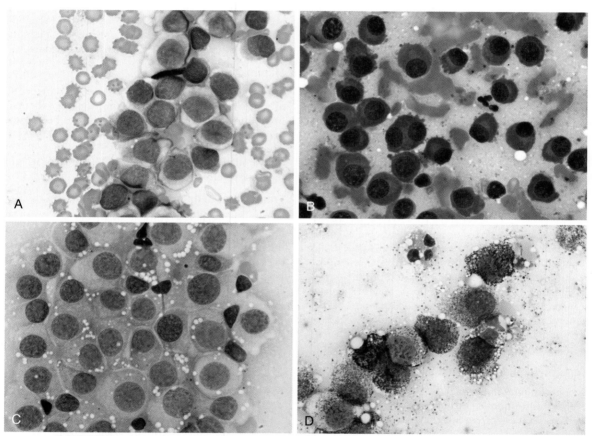

FIGURE 7-4 A, Canine histiocytoma. These round cells have a centrally located nucleus and indistinct nucleoli. There is a moderate amount of pale blue cytoplasm (Wright-Giemsa stain 1000×). **B,** Cutaneous plasmacytoma. These round cells have an eccentrically placed dark condensed nucleus with a moderate amount of deep blue cytoplasm. Some cells exhibit the characteristic perinuclear clear zone, and one binucleate form is seen (Wright-Giemsa stain 1000×). **C,** Transmissible venereal tumor. These cells are in a thick preparation, making the round cell nature a challenge to detect. The nuclei are centrally located with a single prominent nucleoli. The pale pink cytoplasm contains many clear distinct small vacuoles which help to identify this tumor type (Wright-Giemsa stain 1000×). **D,** Mast cell tumor. These cells have a moderate amount of cytoplasm filled with varying numbers of dark purple granules. The nuclear characteristics are often obscured if the tumor is highly granulated. Note the eosinophils in the background (Wright-Giemsa stain 1000×).

development. Disrupted cells are common, and variably sized cytoplasmic fragments known as "lymphoglandular bodies" may be present. Neoplastic lymphoid cells are usually two to three times larger than normal mature small lymphocytes. The cytoplasmic volume varies, but N:C ratios are high. Cytoplasm color ranges from pale to very deep blue, sometimes with a faint Golgi zone and/or mild cytoplasmic vacuolation. Chromatin patterns are often more finely stippled than in normal, mature lymphocytes. One or more nucleoli may be present. The neoplastic cells may vary in size. Macrophages containing engulfed debris are often present. Rarely, lymphomas consist of small well-differentiated lymphocytes and are difficult to differentiate from normal lymphoid tissue in cytology preparations.

Histiocytoma

The cells that make up the common benign solitary canine cutaneous histiocytoma have round to oval to slightly indented nuclei and scant to moderately abundant pale blue cytoplasm, which may have indistinct margins. They have finely stippled chromatin patterns. One or more rather indistinct nucleoli may be visible. Mitotic figures are rare. Variable numbers of small lymphocytes may be admixed with the tumor cells, particularly in lesions undergoing regression.

Mast Cell Tumor

MCTs (or mastocytomas) consist predominantly of mast cells, but variable numbers of eosinophils and mesenchymal cells are often admixed. The mesenchymal cells are most likely of fibrocyte origin, representing cells that have become hyperplastic in response to irritating chemical substances released by the mast cells. They may appear so dysplastic as to falsely mimic malignant mesenchymal cells. Heparin release from mast cells may cause the tumor to bleed readily, so that aspirates of MCT often contain large numbers of red blood cells. Mast cells have round eccentric nuclei and abundant pale blue or bluish-pink cytoplasm that contains variable numbers of reddish-purple granules when stained with the common Wright-Giemsa-type stains. Granulation can range from scant to heavy, and cells with variable degrees of granulation may be present within the same MCT. In occasional poorly differentiated MCT, granules may be difficult to find, but a few cells with scant granulation can usually be found. It has been reported that mast cell granules sometimes fail to stain with the rapid dip stains commonly used in veterinary medicine. Heavy granulation can obscure nuclear detail and make assessment of nuclear criteria of malignancy difficult. Because mast cell granules

are better evaluated via cytology than histopathology, cytology may be superior to routine histopathology for diagnosing poorly granulated MCT. However, biopsy is needed to determine tumor grade for canine cutaneous MCT. The common stains for histopathology may not stain mast cell granules well, but provide superior nuclear detail. Histopathologic grading of MCT relies heavily on nuclear detail, mitotic index, and tissue invasion.

Plasmacytoma

Plasmacytomas can occur as extramedullary solitary masses in the skin or oral cavity. Most solitary cutaneous or oral plasmacytomas behave benignly even if they exhibit cytologic criteria of malignancy. These lesions are not associated with hyperglobulinemia. Occasional extramedullary plasmacytomas are found in other sites including the rectum, gastric mucosa, esophagus, spleen, and kidney. These lesions often metastasize to local lymph nodes and sometimes to more distant locations, and they may be associated with hyperglobulinemia.[12] Extramedullary plasma cell tumors may also be a component of multiple myeloma, in which the bone marrow is affected by neoplastic plasma cells. Multiple myeloma is associated with hyperglobulinemia and is a systemic malignancy. Plasmacytoma cells exhibit varying degrees of differentiation, and binucleate or multinucleate cells are a common feature. Most of these tumors contain at least some cells that strongly resemble normal plasma cells. Poorly differentiated plasmacytomas consist largely of discrete round cells that exhibit criteria of malignancy and may be difficult to identify as plasma cells. In this case, histopathologic evaluation with immunohistochemical staining for immunoglobulin light chains may facilitate diagnosis.

Transmissible Venereal Tumor

The cell of origin of TVTs (sometimes called *transmissible venereal sarcoma*) is uncertain. TVTs contain discrete round cells with round nuclei and moderately abundant basophilic cytoplasm with distinct borders. Chromatin patterns are moderately coarse to coarsely stippled. The cytoplasm often contains low numbers of small discrete round clear vacuoles, and, in some cells, these have a tendency to line up along the cytoplasmic margin. Small lymphocytes, plasma cells, and other inflammatory cells may be admixed with tumor cells, since TVTs are often ulcerated and have secondary bacterial infections.

CYTOLOGY OF LYMPH NODES (FIGURE 7-5)

Familiarity with normal lymph node cytology is essential in order to recognize abnormal features. Lymph nodes may become hyperplastic and reactive in response

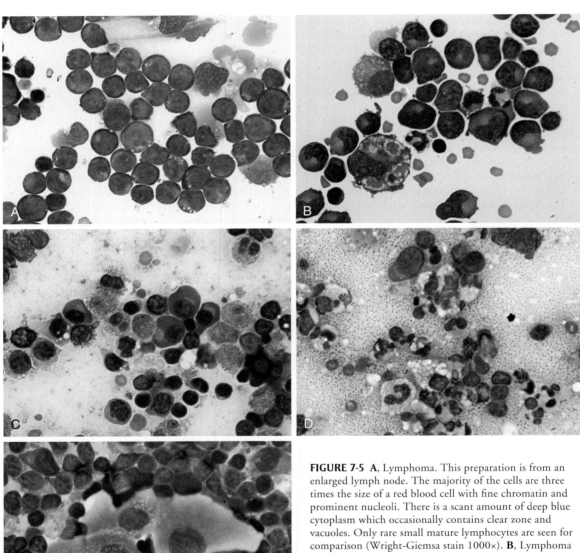

FIGURE 7-5 A, Lymphoma. This preparation is from an enlarged lymph node. The majority of the cells are three times the size of a red blood cell with fine chromatin and prominent nucleoli. There is a scant amount of deep blue cytoplasm which occasionally contains clear zone and vacuoles. Only rare small mature lymphocytes are seen for comparison (Wright-Giemsa stain 1000×). **B**, Lymphoma present in thoracic fluid from a dog. When tumor cells are present in fluid, the nuclei are sometimes distorted. Also, note the macrophage containing phagocytized red blood cells, indicating true hemorrhage into the thoracic cavity (Wright-Giemsa stain 1000×). **C**, Eosinophilic lymphadenitis with plasma cell hyperplasia. This aspirate from a feline lymph node contains many eosinophils and plasma cells mixed with normal small lymphocytes (Wright-Giemsa stain 1000×).

FIGURE 7-5, cont'd D, Pyogranulomatous lymphadenitis. This canine lymph node contains many degenerate neutrophils and macrophages. Blastomyces yeast was present in other areas of the slide (Wright-Giemsa stain 1000×). **E,** Metastatic squamous cell carcinoma in a reactive lymph node. Three large neoplastic squamous cells are surrounded by normal and reactive lymphocytes (Wright-Giemsa stain 1000×).

to inflammation or neoplasia within the area they drain. Lymph nodes may themselves become inflamed (lymphadenitis), they may develop primary neoplasia (lymphoma), or they may contain metastatic foci of non-lymphoid neoplastic cells. Cytology specimens from normal lymph nodes consist predominantly of small lymphocytes (75%-95%), but some lymphoblasts, prolymphocytes, and plasma cells are usually present. Small mature lymphocytes should be about the size of a canine RBC or just a bit larger. Reactive lymph node hyperplasia is a response to antigenic stimulation. The proportion of immature lymphoid cells (prolymphocytes) and plasma cells is increased, but small mature lymphocytes still predominate. The line of demarcation between normal and slightly reactive lymph nodes is not strong. Lymphadenitis is characterized by excessive numbers of inflammatory cells. Lymph nodes are subject to the same types of inflammation as most other tissue, and the makeup of the inflammatory cell population will vary according to the type of inflammation present. Infectious organisms may be present. If inflammation is severe, the inflammatory infiltrate may obliterate the lymphoid population. Otherwise, evidence of reactive lymphoid hyperplasia is also often present. Metastatic neoplasia is characterized by the presence of cells not normally found in lymph nodes, or excessive numbers of cells, such as mast cells, which are usually only present in low numbers. The neoplastic cells may resemble their counterparts in the primary site of the neoplasm, or they may be less well-differentiated. Metastatic lesions may be focal and, thus, missed by lymph node aspiration. The lymphoid population is often reactive and hyperplastic; in some instances, metastatic neoplastic cells completely efface the normal lymphoid populations.

The general description of lymphoma was provided in the section on round cell tumors. When lymphoma is well advanced within a lymph node, most of the normal lymphoid cells will have been effaced, and the sample will consist predominantly of a monotonous population of lymphoid cells all at a similar stage of maturation. In early cases of lymphoma within lymph nodes,

considerable numbers of normal lymphoid cells may be admixed with the neoplastic lymphocytes, making cytologic diagnosis difficult. The knowledge that multiple lymph nodes are enlarged should increase suspicion of lymphoma. Aspiration of additional nodes may allow diagnosis (other nodes may contain fewer normal lymphoid cells).

LIMITS OF CYTOLOGY IN THE ASSESSMENT OF NEOPLASMS

Mixed cell responses can be very difficult to evaluate definitively via cytology alone. Neoplasms can become inflamed, and when this happens the presence of the inflammatory cells may dilute the number of neoplastic cells that are present in the specimen, making them more difficult to identify and evaluate for criteria of malignancy. In lesions that are inflammatory in nature, the inflammation may cause the affected tissue cells to become hyperplastic or even dysplastic in response, and reactive hyperplasia can falsely mimic malignant neoplasia in cytology specimens. The assessment for criteria of malignancy in a tissue cell population must be especially stringent when inflammation is present. The animal's clinical history, a description of the lesion, supporting information such as radiographic findings, etc. can all be very helpful for deciding which of the possibilities is most likely, but sometimes it is simply not possible to make a definitive decision regarding the presence of neoplasia or its malignant potential when inflammation is present.

WHEN TO SUPPLEMENT THE CYTOLOGIC ASSESSMENT WITH HISTOPATHOLOGIC EVALUATION

Cytology is a very useful procedure, but there are times when neoplasms should be evaluated via histopathology. Sometimes cytologic collection procedures do not result in recovery of sufficient numbers of cells to allow an adequate assessment. This is especially likely to happen when tumors of connective tissue (mesenchymal) origin are aspirated, since the cells often will not readily exfoliate. Oftentimes it is not possible to differentiate the various types of sarcomas via cytologic evaluation alone. If treatment is anticipated, the cytologic assessment of sarcoma should be supplemented with histopathologic evaluation of the lesion to better determine the specific type of sarcoma. As has been discussed previously, when inflammation is present, reactive tissue hyperplasia can falsely mimic neoplasia. Histopathologic evaluation provides an evaluation of overall tissue architecture and, thus, may be very helpful for determining if one is dealing with an inflamed neoplasm, or a primary inflammatory lesion that has incited secondary reactive hyperplasia and/or dysplasia. For some neoplasms, degree of invasiveness and tumor grade are important prognostic indicators, and this cannot be adequately assessed via cytologic assessment. Perianal gland tumors and mammary tumors are examples of neoplasms for which invasiveness is an important indicator of malignant behavior, even when cytologic criteria of malignancy are not present.

Selected References*

Cowell RL, Tyler RD, Meinkoth JH, DeNicola DB: *Diagnostic cytology and hematology of the dog and cat,* ed 3, 2008, St. Louis, Mosby/Elsevier.

This comprehensive hardcover atlas provides a thorough review of cytology from the basics of specimen acquisition to the interpretation of samples by organ system. It covers both inflammatory and neoplastic cytology of fluids and solid tissues with an additional section on blood and bone marrow findings. There are color photomicrographs in each chapter.

Raskin RE, Meyer DJ: *Canine and feline cytology: a color atlas and interpretation guide,* ed 2, 2009, Philadelphia, Saunders.

This comprehensive hardcover atlas also provides a thorough review of cytology from the basics of specimen acquisition to the interpretation of cytology samples by organ system. Extensive color photomicrographs illustrate the cytologic appearance of normal and abnormal tissue. Each organ system chapter contains histologic and histopathologic correlates. Histochemical and immunohistochemical stains are discussed, as well as diagnostic techniques such as electron microscopy, flow cytometry, and PCR for antigen receptor rearrangements (PARR).

*For a complete list of the references cited in this chapter, please go to www.smallanimaloncology.com.

8

Histopathology, Immunohistochemistry, and Tumor Grading

Elizabeth M. Whitley

KEY POINTS

- Handle tissue samples gently during surgery to help prevent crushing, stretching, and electrocautery artifacts.
- Mark sites of concern with suture material or marking inks; mark surgical margins with India or other tissue marking ink.
- Incise the resected tissues to approximately {3/8}-inch thick. Perform a partial-thickness incision of a dermal mass beginning at the epidermal surface.
- Immerse tissues in 10× volume of 10% neutral buffered formalin in a wide-mouthed container immediately after excision.
- Immediately after surgery, complete the histopathology submission form, including signalment, history, previous treatments and responses, previous biopsy case numbers, and a description of the lesions found in the submitted tissues. If the form is prepared by an assistant, it should be reviewed by the surgeon.
- Develop a collaborative relationship with your pathologist and include them as part of the oncology care team.

PRACTICAL ASPECTS OF BIOPSY SUBMISSION

History

The signalment and historical narrative given at the time of sample submission provide the framework in which the pathologist views a case. A complete, concise history is a tremendous aid to the pathologist and, in some cases, is critical for arriving at an accurate diagnosis. A gross description and diagram of the anatomic location and shape of the mass help provide a mental image of the lesion. A short description of any previous treatments and the response to treatment should also be included.

A comment regarding the etiologic agent or pathologic process suspected is a valuable addition to the history, since it summarizes the clinical impression of the practitioner. Comments regarding any additional tests being performed, such as bacterial or fungal culture, or adjunctive therapies, such as post-surgical cryotherapy, are also useful to the pathologist. Providing case numbers or a copy of the report of previous submissions helps the pathologist follow the disease progression. Finally, if any legal actions are being considered related to the case, it is helpful to alert the pathologist to this fact.

Sample Collection

From the pathologist's perspective, the larger the sample size, the better the chance of examining an area that will yield an accurate diagnosis. Submission of the entire lesion is preferable. Surgical excisions with wide normal tissue margins will provide more tissue for histologic examination, will allow margins to be examined for presence of tumor cells, and may be curative. If an incisional or core biopsy is to be performed, selection of the biopsy site is crucial. It is critical to avoid areas of necrosis, often found within the center of the mass and characterized by soft, friable, or ulcerated tissue. Instead, multiple samples from the edges of the lesion are preferred and will provide tissue that is more likely to contain viable, proliferating cells with diagnostic architectural features. An exception is when a mass within bone is to be sampled. In these cases, the tissue most useful for biopsy is usually situated near the center of the mass.

Decision-Making for "Difficult" Tumor Types

Splenic Hemangioma and Hemangiosarcoma

Accurate sample site selection for the diagnosis of splenic hemangiosarcoma is notoriously difficult because the major portion of most splenic masses consists of hematoma or necrotic tissue. When sectioning a spleen that contains a hemorrhagic mass, tissue samples from multiple sites should be submitted. The most useful samples typically come from areas that are moderately firm, white to gray-tan (indicating high cellularity), and often at the margins between grossly normal or moderately congested splenic parenchyma and more bloody tissue. Metastatic nodules of hemangiosarcoma are also very useful to the pathologist.

Bony Neoplasms

Failure of core or needle biopsies from suspected bony neoplasms to provide diagnostic quality specimens is usually due to not coring deeply enough into the hard mass to reach the tumor, and instead collecting reactive fibrous or bony tissue. Including a description of the radiographic findings is particularly helpful to the pathologist.

Very Small Sample Size

Samples collected via endoscopy or needle biopsy are very susceptible to crushing artifact and, in some cases, may not be representative of the disease process. Therefore, collection of multiple samples enhances the probability of obtaining useful information by these techniques and will increase diagnostic accuracy. Because of their small size, pieces of mucosal tissues collected by endoscopy are difficult to orient during embedding, sometimes requiring that the paraffin block be melted and the tissues rolled and sectioned again. To facilitate orientation of small samples, they may be placed on a solid support, such as a tongue depressor or thin piece of cardboard, before fixation.

Biopsy Tissue Handling

Handling biopsy samples gently helps to preserve normal tissue architecture. Samples that have had excessive pulling or crushing forces applied will have distorted tissue architecture that may prevent accurate diagnosis or margin evaluation. The use of electrocautery or laser energy causes coagulation of tissues, which results in loss of the fine features of cells.

Identification of Tissues and Margins

Ideally, when multiple samples are submitted, individual specimens should be placed in separate, labeled containers of formalin. Containers should be labeled on the side, instead of the lid, to help avoid mix-up of specimens.

Surgical margins are examined by the pathologist to determine the degree of invasiveness of neoplastic cells and to determine if complete excision was accomplished.

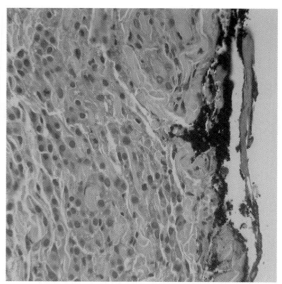

FIGURE 8-1 India ink may be used to delineate surgical margins as shown here. The black border of India ink on the right margin differentiates surgical borders from artifactual borders created by tissue sectioning when slides are prepared.

To aid in this examination, surgical margins of resected tissue may be marked using a tissue dye, such as waterproof India ink (available at art and office supply stores) or colored inks (Davidson's Marking System, Bradley Products, Inc., Bloomington, MN). Different-colored inks may be used to mark individual regions of a biopsy sample or to aid in orientation. Surgical margins are easily differentiated from cuts made at the time of sectioning by the thin black line of carbon particles of India ink that line a true surgical margin (Figure 8-1). Suture material may be used to mark areas of interest, but the ends of the sutures sometimes are difficult for the pathologist to find. Leaving long ends of suture material and using colored suture material make these markers easier to locate.

Sample Fixation and Shipping

If portions of the tissue are to be submitted for testing by other modalities (i.e., bacterial or fungal culture), those tissues must not be fixed and should be reserved before the sample is placed in formalin. Otherwise, any infectious agents in the sample may be fixed and will not grow in culture.

For optimal penetration of fixative, the maximal thickness of tissue should be {3/8} inch (about 1 cm).

Once a biopsy sample is obtained, incisions into the neoplasm at intervals of approximately 1 cm ("bread loafing") will allow the fixative to permeate the tissues, resulting in better tissue preservation. For cutaneous neoplasms, it is preferable to keep the deep margins intact, so that the margins are easily identifiable at the time of tissue sectioning and the architecture of the deep margin is undisturbed.

The goal of fixation for routine histopathology is to preserve tissues so that they retain normal cellular and tissue architecture. Immediately after excision, the surgeon should hand off the excised tissues to an assistant for marking of surgical margins, followed quickly by immersion in the fixative. For routine histologic examination, tissues should be fixed in 10% neutral buffered formalin, using a volume of formalin that is at least 10 times the volume of the tissue being fixed. For ophthalmic specimens, globes are optimally fixed by slow injection of 0.1 ml of Davidson's fixative into the vitreous chamber of the resected globe, using a small-gauge needle and syringe, followed by immersion in a 10× volume of Davidson's fixative. Fixation in Davidson's solution, which contains formalin plus acetic acid and alcohol, has the advantage of optimal preservation of morphologic detail.[1] If Davidson's solution is not available, globes should be fixed in formalin.

The selection of a proper container for transport is important. Unless the tissue is completely fixed before transport, the container must provide sufficient volume to hold the formalin. When the tissue is completely fixed, it may be transported in a smaller volume of fixative. For ease of removal of the tissues from the container once at the histopathology laboratory, avoid using a container with a narrow opening. If the fresh tissue is just able to slide into the container, then, when the tissues are fixed, they will become more rigid and will not be able to be removed from the container without aggressive manipulations that may tear tissues or break the container.

Unstained cytology samples on glass slides should be mailed to the clinical pathology laboratory in a separate container that does not also contain formalin-fixed tissues. Cytologists report altered staining of cells that have been exposed to formalin fumes during transport, which limits the accuracy of cytologic diagnoses.

Freezing of tissues is not a good way to preserve samples intended for histopathologic examination. During freezing, ice crystals form within cells, disrupting the cellular and tissue architecture and resulting in artifacts. If a necropsy is anticipated but not imminent, refrigerate, but do not freeze, the body. Sometimes biopsy collection from tissues that have been frozen is unavoidable, and a

message to that fact accompanying the tissues will alert the pathologist. To avoid artifacts caused by freezing during transportation of tissues during the winter, the fixative may be diluted by the addition of isopropanol or ethanol in a ratio of 1 part alcohol and 9 parts neutral buffered formalin.

Selection of a Pathology Laboratory

The selection of a pathologist and histopathology laboratory is sometimes based on convenience and cost. However, consideration of several other factors will aid the practitioner in developing a collaborative relationship with a veterinary pathologist that will maximize the quality of medical care for the veterinary oncology patient.[2,3] Reliably correct results reported quickly are essential for proper decision-making for oncology patients. Since effective information transfer is paramount to high-quality medical care, the ability and willingness to communicate easily and to seek second opinions should be valued. Board certification by the American College of Veterinary Pathologists ensures that the veterinary pathologist has a well-rounded and complete pathology education.

Overview of Tissue Processing

When a tissue arrives at the histopathology laboratory, the history is read and the tissue is examined, making sure that the submitted tissues correlate with that described in the history. Small sections of tissue are cut and placed in a plastic cassette. The tissues are then dehydrated and infiltrated by paraffin in a process that takes several hours, and this is accomplished overnight in many histology laboratories. After that, the tissues are embedded in paraffin blocks and very thin sections are cut using a microtome, adhered to a glass slide, and stained, usually with hematoxylin and eosin. Subsequently, the glass slides are examined by the pathologist using light microscopy. The tissue changes are interpreted, and a report is written and submitted. Calcified tissues must be demineralized before they can be sectioned. Demineralization is accomplished by immersion of the tissues in solutions composed of acids for several hours to days, depending on the density of the tissues and amount of mineral to be removed.

The time from tissue submission to the laboratory until the report is generated may be from one to several days, depending upon many factors, including invariable times for fixation (24 hours), tissue processing and staining (18–24 hours), and a more variable amount of time for the analysis of slides and generation of the report. The time that it takes for the pathologist to produce the report includes reviewing the history, examining the tissues microscopically, and composing the histologic description, morphologic diagnosis, and comments. On more difficult or unusual cases, the pathologist will also spend time reading the literature, sharing the slides with colleagues, requesting and reviewing specially stained tissue sections, and contemplation of differential diagnoses before rendering an opinion. Diagnoses can be provided for fresh frozen samples much more rapidly because of the reduced processing time. However, very few veterinary diagnostic laboratories routinely provide this service.

INTERPRETATION OF HISTOPATHOLOGY RESULTS

Reading and Interpreting the Histopathologic Description

For many non-pathologists, the paragraphs from a biopsy report describing the histopathologic findings seem to be filled with confusing terms and boring details. However, the information in this description forms the basis for the morphologic diagnosis and contains useful information for the practitioner. The description will usually begin with a statement of the tissues examined, which should match the tissue submitted by the practitioner. The description also communicates the features of anaplasia, invasiveness, and numbers of mitotic figures, all information that can be used to help predict the clinical aggressiveness of a neoplasm. With experience in reading these descriptions, and perhaps the use of a medical dictionary or consultation with the pathologist or oncologist, the description will provide added value to the care of the oncology patient.

Limitations of Histopathology

Biopsy findings should be interpreted in the context of the entire body of information collected from the case. When a biopsy report does not correlate well with the rest of the clinical picture, the practitioner and pathologist should work together to reevaluate the case information and histopathology results, sometimes using additional procedures. A limitation of histopathology is that it is an inexact science, reflecting a combination of technology and the art of interpretation.[2,4-8] Pathologists render opinions based on observing cellular and tissue architecture and deducing the pathologic processes that are occurring in the tissues. Unfortunately, all tumors do not demonstrate all of the features classically associated with their tumor type, and, thus, the pathologist may not be able to interpret the changes and make a morphologic diagnosis with complete confidence.

An important limitation of histopathology is in discriminating between a purely inflammatory process and an inflammatory or immune response within a neoplasm. Some types of neoplasia are known to arise from inflammatory foci. In particular, because feline vaccine-associated fibrosarcomas originate in foci of chronic inflammation, it can be very difficult to discriminate between intense, chronic inflammation with fibroplasia and the early stages of fibrosarcoma. Likewise, differentiating hyperplastic fibroblastic responses in wound healing from neoplastic proliferation of fibroblasts can be problematic.

Diagnostically useful tissue changes are not always uniformly distributed within a resected piece of tissue. Although it may be tempting to divide a tissue sample and submit it to two laboratories to obtain two opinions, this practice may lead to confusion when different diagnoses are rendered. In many cases, both diagnoses may be accurate, but the discordant results may simply be a reflection of the different sections of tissue examined by each pathologist. A better approach is to submit all tissue to one laboratory and to request a second opinion as needed. Multiple pathologists may interpret the same lesion differently or may use different nomenclature to describe the same change.[7] In this case, communication with the pathologists or the performance of additional studies such as immunohistochemistry (IHC) may be required to achieve a definitive diagnosis.

Interpreting the Morphologic Diagnosis—Histologic Grading

Besides assessing if a lesion is neoplastic and determining the cell type of origin, the pathologist may be able to assign a histologic grade to a tumor as a measure of the predicted clinical outcome. Research that correlates histologic features with clinical aggressiveness has been used to develop clinically useful histopathologic grading systems.

Cutaneous mast cell tumors in dogs are usually graded according to a system developed by Patnaik et al.[9] that is based on features of tissue architecture, cellular differentiation, and numbers of mitotic figures. Tumors that contain well-differentiated mast cells are assigned a grade of I, whereas poorly differentiated, clinically aggressive tumors are assigned a grade of III. In the system by Bostock et al.,[10] canine soft tissue sarcomas (STSs) are graded according to the number of mitotic figures per ten 400× microscope fields, with the designation of high grade given to a mitotic index of greater than 9 and correlating with a reduced lifespan. More information on grading of STS is provided in Chapter 23, Section E. Grading systems based on histologic criteria are available for several other tumor types and, with continued research, more systems will be validated.[11-13]

TABLE 8-1   COMMON VETERINARY IMMUNOHISTOCHEMICAL MARKERS

Immunohistochemical Marker	Cell Type	Tumor Type
Cytokeratin	Epithelial cells	Adenoma, carcinoma
Vimentin	Mesenchymal cells	Benign mesenchymal tumors, sarcoma
Desmin	Muscle	Rhabdomyoma, rhabdomyosarcoma, leiomyoma, leiomyosarcoma
Smooth muscle actin	Smooth muscle	Leiomyoma, leiomyosarcoma
Glial fibrillary acid protein	Glial cells of the central and peripheral nervous systems	Astrocytomas, ependymomas, some peripheral nerve sheath tumors
S-100	Cells of neuroectodermal origin, such as melanocytes, and cells of the nerve sheath	Melanoma, peripheral nerve sheath tumor
Melan A	Melanocytes	Melanoma
Factor VIII or Factor VIII–related protein	Vascular endothelial cells	Hemangioma, hemangiosarcoma
CD31	Vascular endothelial cells	Hemangioma, hemangiosarcoma
CD3	T lymphocytes	T-cell lymphoma
CD79a, CD20	B lymphocytes	B-cell lymphoma
Lysozyme, Alpha-1–anti-trypsin, MAC387, CD68	Macrophages, histiocytes	Benign cutaneous histiocytomas, malignant histiocytic neoplasms
Thyroglobulin	Thyroid follicular epithelium	Thyroid follicular adenomas and adenocarcinomas
Synaptophysin	Neuroendocrine cells	Neuroendocrine and neuroectodermal tumors
Chromogranin A	Neuroendocrine cells	Neuroendocrine and neuroectodermal tumors

Immunohistochemical Staining

Immunohistochemical (IHC) staining allows the identification of antigens that are relatively specific for one cell type.[14] Many of the antigens are intermediate filaments, which are structural proteins within the cytoplasm, and are specific to different cell lineages. Other markers, such as the cluster of differentiation (CD) antigens, are cell surface proteins that are also lineage specific. The identification of intracytoplasmic or secretory products is useful for identifying cell populations that synthesize those products. IHC staining is especially useful for the diagnosis of poorly differentiated neoplasms. For example, a panel of antibodies and other special stains directed against populations of lymphocytes, plasma cells, histiocytes, melanocytes, and mast cells is used to discriminate between the various round cell tumors of the skin.[15] Other stains commonly used in the diagnosis of neoplasia include toluidine blue to identify mast cell granules, periodic acid-Schiff to stain mucin and mast cell granules, Alcian blue to stain cartilaginous extracellular matrix, and Masson trichrome to identify collagen and muscle. Common IHC markers are listed in Table 8-1.

Like all diagnostic techniques, there are limitations to the use of IHC. Some tumor types are so poorly differentiated that they fail to express the appropriate marker. If tissues remain in formalin for more than a few days, the success of IHC staining is reduced because of extensive cross-linking of proteins. Autolysis may result in the degradation of antigens, rendering their identification by immunostaining impossible. Histopathology laboratories vary widely in the use of special stains, including IHC staining.

Selected References*

Meuten DJ: *Tumors in domestic animals*, ed 4, 2002, Ames, Iowa State University Press.
This is a comprehensive, well-written textbook covering the pathology and clinical pathology of neoplasms of domestic animal species.
Ramos-Vara JA: Technical aspects of immunohistochemistry, *Vet Pathol* 42:405, 2005.
This article describes in depth the strategies and techniques used in IHC staining.

▌ *For a complete list of the references cited in this chapter, please go to www.smallanimaloncology.com.

9 Imaging Methods in Cancer Diagnosis

SECTION A: Radiography

Jimmy C. Lattimer

KEY POINTS

- Three radiographic views (right and left lateral recumbent and ventrodorsal) of the thorax are essential to assess for pulmonary metastasis.
- Calcified nodules in the lung field are typically granulomas or benign osteomas and should not be misinterpreted as metastatic lesions.
- Radiographic interpretation of bone changes may be more accurate than histopathological evaluation of bone biopsy specimens for diagnosing skeletal neoplasia.

Over the years, the discipline of radiology has expanded in scope to include images generated by ultrasound, computed tomography (CT), magnetic resonance imaging (MRI), gamma cameras, and lasers. Thus, the field is perhaps more appropriately termed *imaging* and is often referred to in this way. The use of x-rays to project shadows onto film is no longer the predominant method for generating medical images in many radiology departments. Radiographic film is now being replaced by electronic detectors that produce digital images stored in a file on a computer. Nonetheless, radiography is still the quickest and easiest way to evaluate for the presence of a neoplastic process in veterinary patients. It is not the most sensitive or accurate method, but it does provide a large amount of data at a reasonable cost. Frequently, the importance of the radiographic examination is not so much in what is detected, but in what is not detected. For instance, in the evaluation of the thorax in a cancer patient, it is important to *not* find evidence of pulmonary metastasis. It is also important to *not* find intercurrent disease such as pneumonia or heart disease.[1]

Screening radiographs can and should also guide the use of more sophisticated imaging studies such as CT. For instance, the presence of a nodule in the lung of a cancer patient is frequently viewed as a metastasis—and it may well be. However, a CT scan should be performed to determine the true nature of the nodule and in an attempt to find other smaller nodules not seen on the radiographs. Radiographs of the abdomen provide a more global view of the abdomen than does ultrasound. Diseases of the GI tract in particular are often more easily detected on radiographs, and the presence of GI tract disease on the radiographs can direct attention of the ultrasonographer to a specific portion of the bowel. Mass lesions in the abdomen may be difficult to characterize with respect to organ of origin on ultrasound, but the relative position of other organs to the mass on the radiographs provides guidance in making this determination. Radiographic detection of vertebral lysis in a patient with paresis could indicate that the patient would be more appropriately imaged using CT rather than MRI. These are but a few examples of how radiography can be used to guide the choice of more advanced imaging techniques.

THORACIC RADIOGRAPHS

Three radiographic views of the thorax should be made in all cancer patients.[2,3] The reason for this is twofold. The primary objective of this examination is detection of pulmonary metastasis, disease extension into the mediastinal or hilar lymph nodes, or some other extension of the neoplastic process into the thorax. The secondary objective is to detect any concurrent disease process that would have a negative impact on treatment of the cancer. Examples of the types of diseases that might be detected are heart disease, pulmonary diseases, mediastinal and pleural disease, or diseases of the skeleton. Advanced disease of any of these types could either alter or delay treatment or could obviate it altogether. For example, treatment of a patient with an enlarged heart using doxorubicin may be ill advised or a protracted course of radiation therapy would have little therapeutic value in a patient with advanced pulmonary metastatic disease.

It is essential that the radiographic examination of the thorax consist of both the right and left lateral recumbent views as well as a ventrodorsal (VD) view.[2,3] Because of the recumbent nature of the radiographs generally taken in dogs and cats, there is rapid migration of fluid within the lung to the down side, as well as compression of the down lung lobes by the overlying heart and upper lung. There is also reduced motion of the chest wall and diaphragm on the dependent side, owing to the compressive effects of the animal's weight. The down side of the diaphragm is also displaced forward by the weight of the abdominal viscera. All of this results in a marked increase in the density of the dependent lung, which can hide not only metastatic lesions but also other lung pathology (Figure 9-1). These effects take place rather quickly and are increased as the animal spends more time on its side before the radiograph is made. Sedation or anesthesia advances the rate and severity of these changes. Radiographs of the thorax taken with an animal under anesthesia should be made with the thorax in a state of forced inhalation by inflating the lungs with a ventilation device. Radiographing the lung field from both sides with a short period of accommodation between allows examination of both sides of the lung field in a relatively aerated state. This facilitates detection of pulmonary lesions, particularly those in the periphery.

The orthogonal view should generally be a VD view rather than a dorsoventral view, in order to allow more of the lung field to be seen. The same type of density changes that occur for the lateral positions also occur for the VD view but are generally minimized by the fact that animals are not usually held on their backs for extended periods. Again, anesthesia or sedation will exacerbate the effects. Dorsoventral views are acceptable as orthogonal views and may be preferable if the lateral views detect suspect lesions in the dorsal part of the lung field.

Typical metastatic lesions and other small opacities within the lung are frequently more difficult to detect on the VD view than on the lateral views. This is due to the larger amount of tissue through which the x-ray beam must pass on its way to the film or detector. The heart occupies a relatively larger proportion of the lung field in the VD view, and mediastinal structures obscure the portions of the lung field that cross it. However, the VD view is important for demonstrating that a lesion seen on the lateral view is not located on or in the chest wall (see Figure 9-1). A lesion seen over the lung field on orthogonal views is quite likely to actually be within the lung field.

Radiographic detection of metastatic lesions on chest radiographs has a substantial negative impact on the prognosis of a cancer patient. Owners may opt not to proceed with treatment if pulmonary nodules are identified. For this reason it is very important that suspected metastatic nodules be confirmed. Metastatic lesions in the lung field share the general characteristics of any soft tissue nodular lesion in the lung field. Namely, they are single or multiple, round to ovoid, poorly to moderately circumscribed, and of a wide range of sizes and soft tissue in opacity. These characteristics are also those of cysts, abscesses, granulomas and primary neoplasms, and there is essentially no way to specifically differentiate one from the other on the basis of plain radiographs (see Figure 9-1). A diagnosis of metastasis should be confirmed by aspiration or at least by demonstrating growth on sequential films. However, the presence of large numbers of nodules of uneven size coupled with the known metastatic potential of the primary neoplasm allows a tentative diagnosis of metastatic disease with a high level of confidence. Likewise, development of new lung nodules in a cancer patient is highly suggestive of neoplasia. However, a diagnosis of metastasis should not be made when the nodules are calcified.[4] Pulmonary metastatic disease, even that arising from bone tumors, essentially never calcifies in dogs and cats, to the extent that it appears calcified on radiographs. On occasion, primary lung tumors may faintly calcify, but even this is rare. Calcified nodules in the lung field are typically calcified granulomas or benign osteomas (see Figure 9-1). Thus, any calcified lung lesion must be biopsied to confirm a tentative diagnosis.

SKELETAL RADIOGRAPHS

Radiographs are extremely useful in the diagnosis of osseous neoplasia. It would seem that every oncologist has obtained biopsies of osseous lesions thought to be neoplasia, only to receive a biopsy diagnosis of reactive or inflammatory bone despite a typical clinical presentation. Biopsy only yields a small part of the lesion for histological examination, and bone tumors vary widely in the phenotype of the neoplastic cells from one side of the lesion to the other. There is also usually an inflammatory component in advanced tumors that may obscure the underlying disease. Radiographs depict the entire lesion, and some radiographic lesions very reliably indicate the lesion in question is a neoplasm (Figure 9-2). It has been shown in human oncology that radiographic diagnosis of bone

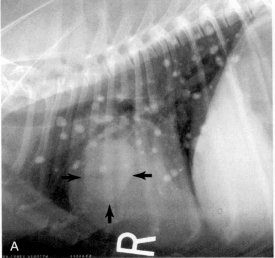

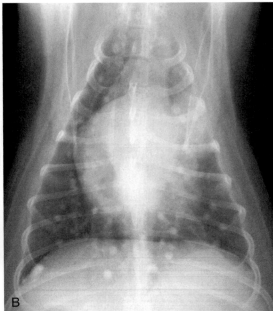

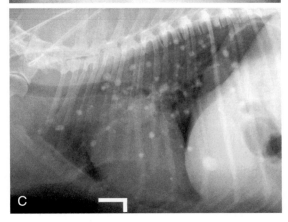

FIGURE 9-1 Right lateral (**A**), ventrodorsal (**B**), and left lateral (**C**) radiographs of the thorax. Multiple, well-defined 3- to 12-mm, smoothly marginated, calcified nodules are seen in all lung lobes. These represent calcified granulomas and are a benign change. The right lateral view also reveals the presence of a 3- × 4-cm moderately circumscribed, soft-tissue opaque mass lesion superimposed over the cranial part of the heart shadow *(arrows).* The ventrodorsal view indicates the presence of a poorly defined opacity in the left cranial lung lobe corresponding to the mass lesion seen on the right lateral. The left lateral radiograph (**C**) does not indicate the presence of the mass lesion due to increased opacity of the left side of the lung field by positional atelectasis and fluid shifting. Bronchogenic carcinoma was confirmed after surgical removal of the left cranial lung lobe.

tumors is up to 20% more specific than biopsy.[5] Although improvement in biopsy techniques has closed this gap somewhat, the reliability of a radiographic diagnosis of bone neoplasia by a radiologist in the face of a negative biopsy indicates that the biopsy should be repeated.

SPECIAL PROCEDURES

Radiographic special procedures involving contrast media are still appropriate for diagnosis and characterization of some neoplastic diseases. This is especially true when assessing involvement of the gastrointestinal (GI) and genitourinary (GU) tracts. Small lesions in the GI or GU tracts may be missed by imaging systems with less intrinsic resolution than radiographs, and it may be easier to evaluate extent of involvement on contrast radiographs than on other imaging systems.[6] The functional impact of the disease in these tubular organ systems is easier to assess on radiographs when the variable of anesthesia can be avoided.

LIMITATIONS

Radiographs have historically been used to assess response to therapy or progression of neoplastic diseases. Although this is still appropriate and useful in some

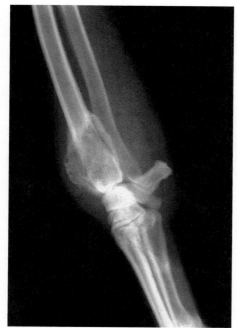

FIGURE 9-2 Dorsal palmar view of the carpus in a dog with a chronic lameness and a lump on the leg. The presence of a large zone of lysis that is indistinctly marginated accompanied by a fragmentation and displacement of the medial radial cortex allows a tentative diagnosis of medullary osteosarcoma with a high degree of confidence.

cases such as with thoracic or bony lesions, follow-up of other lesions may be more appropriately performed with another imaging modality. Radiography lacks the specificity to evaluate tumor viability and may be quite insensitive to the presence or absence of tumors such as in nasal and brain tumors. Newer nuclear medicine procedures can image tumor metabolism and viability on a time schedule far ahead of that which radiographs indicate simply by reduction or increase in size. Radiography is perhaps the last imaging modality to indicate a response to treatment. This is not to say that radiographic imaging does not have a place in the management of the oncologic patient. However, its role has changed substantially in recent years. This change has occurred dramatically in human medicine but is just as applicable in veterinary medicine.

INTERVENTIONAL RADIOGRAPHY

Interventional radiography is one of the fastest growing fields in imaging. This method uses radiographic imaging, usually fluoroscopy, to guide local non-sur-

gical therapy of neoplastic diseases.[7] Fluoroscopy, in combination with contrast media, can allow the radiologist to guide a vascular catheter into a tumor for local therapy of that lesion. Several such local therapies may be used.

A catheter may be directed into the arterial supply of many tumors. Chemotherapy agents may then be infused directly into the tumor bed, increasing the exposure of the tumor to the agent relative to that of the rest of the body.[8] Tumors with isolated arterial blood supplies such as those of the liver, kidney, thyroid, and spleen are especially suited to this treatment. For example, the arterial blood supply to the liver accounts for only about 10% of the blood supply to the normal liver parenchyma but for greater than 90% of the blood supply of the typical liver tumor. Administration of chemotherapy into the hepatic artery, therefore, should result in a ten-fold increase in drug exposure to the tumor over that seen by the normal liver tissue.

Transvascular embolization of tumors can also be used to control tumor hemorrhage in patients that are poor surgical candidates. A catheter is guided into the vessel feeding the bleeding lesion, and some form of embolus is induced directly into the vessel feeding the tumor. The procedure also defines the blood supply to the tumor by default, which may be of some benefit in planning a subsequent surgical procedure.

One additional method of transvascular therapy of tumors is the introduction of radioactive microspheres into the vasculature of a tumor or organ bearing a tumor. Microspheres made of glass and containing ^{90}yttrium have been in use for treatment of liver tumors in humans for a number of years.[9] Microsphere therapy may be used for treating any tumor where an isolated vascular supply can be identified. The treatment supplied by this method is twofold: (1) the microspheres deliver radiation directly to the tumor, and (2) they occlude the capillaries of the tumor, thus robbing it of its blood supply. Because the radioactive agent is limited to the tumor, the radiation dose to the lesion can be astronomical relative to the rest of the body or the organ in which the tumor is located. A similar approach to local administration of chemotherapy has also been described.

Fluoroscopy can also be used to guide biopsy procedures to ensure that the sample is obtained from the appropriate part of the lesion (as with bone tumors) or to avoid sensitive surrounding structures (as with lung nodules). Other imaging modalities can be used to do this as well, but in some cases using fluoroscopy is far easier and quicker.

CONCLUSIONS

Although the role of radiography in the diagnosis and management of neoplastic diseases has undergone a dramatic change in the last couple of decades, it remains a mainstay of cancer management. Its repeatability and the quickness with which it can be performed make it the most suitable way to screen for the presence of pulmonary metastasis or suspected skeletal lesions. New and emerging uses of fluoroscopy have added to the scope of radiographic imaging, which holds promise for improved delivery of therapy that increases the impact of therapy while decreasing its side effects. Radiographic imaging will play an important role in the diagnosis and management of cancer for the foreseeable future.

Selected References*

Biller DS, Myer CW: Case examples demonstrating the clinical utility of obtaining both right and left lateral thoracic radiographs in small animals, *J Am Anim Hosp Assoc* 23:381-386, 1987.
This paper gives good examples of why three views of the thorax should be considered the standard of care when evaluating a cancer patient for disease of the lungs.
Moser RP Jr, Madewell JE: An approach to primary bone tumors, *Radiol Clin North Am* 25(6):1049-1093, 1987.
An excellent article describing the approach to evaluating lesions of bone for malignancies. Dr. Madewell is a recognized authority on this subject in human radiology and has written many articles on this subject.
Singh H: Interventional radiology in the gynaecological oncology patient, *Best Pract Res Clin Obstet Gynaecol* 15(2):279-290, 2001.
Good article on basic principles and techniques used in interventional radiographic procedures for treatment of cancer.

▌ *For a complete list of the references cited in this chapter, please go to www.smallanimaloncology.com.

SECTION B: Ultrasound

Stephanie C. Essman

KEY POINTS

- Sonographic changes are non-specific—*biopsy and aspirate*!
- Lack of sonographic changes does not rule out neoplasia!
- Target lesions have a high incidence of being neoplasia.
- GI tumors usually result in wall thickening and loss of layering.

Ultrasound is commonly used in veterinary medicine as a complimentary modality to radiographs, especially when evaluating abdominal masses. Advantages of ultrasound include that it is noninvasive, is well-tolerated by the patient, and allows examination of organ parenchyma. The site of origin of a mass can often be determined by ultrasound, and other organs may be evaluated for concurrent abnormalities or metastases. Sometimes, changes noted on ultrasound are non-specific such that neoplastic lesions cannot be distinguished from non-neoplastic diseases without the aid of aspirates or biopsies. In these cases, ultrasound-guided aspirates and biopsies can generally be obtained rapidly and by minimally invasive techniques.

Several patient-related factors can affect the usefulness of ultrasound examinations. Lack of patient compliance, excessive bowel gas, and obesity can all result in a suboptimal examination. Ultrasound is also a highly operator-dependent technique. A thorough examination of the abdomen as well as a basic understanding of ultrasound physics and artifacts is required to perform a high-quality examination.

CHARACTERIZATION OF PARENCHYMAL LESIONS

Echogenicity refers to the relative brightness of a structure.[1] Anechoic structures lack the presence of internal echoes and appear black. When comparing the echogenicity of two organs, the brighter organ is hyperechoic and the darker organ is hypoechoic.[1] Organs that are similar to each other in echogenicity are referred to as isoechoic. Because neoplasia and other types of diseases can result in a change in tissue brightness, knowledge of the relative echogenicity in commonly imaged organs is imperative (Box 9-1).[1]

Parenchymal lesions of abdominal organs can be characterized as either focal or diffuse.[2] Diffuse disease is characterized by changes in echogenicity. Focal or multifocal abnormalities are characterized by lesions with well-defined margins compared with the surrounding parenchyma.[2] The architecture of these lesions may be cystic, solid, or complex. It is important to remember that sonographic appearance is usually not pathognomic and overlap is seen between benign and neoplastic diseases.

LIVER

Diffuse Disease

The normal hepatic parenchyma has a uniform, slightly coarse echogenicity that is interrupted by visualization of hepatic and portal veins.[3] The normal liver is more coarse and slightly less echogenic than the spleen. A number of diseases can result in non-specific changes in the echogenicity of the liver. Malignant diseases that commonly cause the liver to be *decreased* in echogenicity include lymphoma and leukemia.[3,4] Non-neoplastic diseases that result in decreased liver echogenicity include chronic passive congestion resulting from right heart failure and acute hepatitis.[3] Malignant diseases that may cause the liver to be *increased* in echogenicity include lymphoma and mast cell tumor.[3,5] Non-malignant diseases that result in an increased echogenicity include fatty infiltration, steroid hepatopathy, and cirrhosis.[3] It is important to remember that a normal sonographic appearance to the liver does not rule out neoplastic disease. In one study, sensitivity of ultrasound in detection of hepatic lymphoma was only 21%.[6] An aspirate and/or biopsy is usually required to reach a diagnosis in cases of diffuse hepatic disease. A list of differentials for diffuse liver disease is summarized in Box 9-2.

Focal/Multifocal Disease

Metastatic or primary neoplasia should be considered in the differential diagnosis list for animals with focal or multifocal parenchymal changes. Primary liver tumors commonly seen with ultrasound include hepatocellular carcinoma, hemangiosarcoma, malignant histiocytosis, and mast cell tumor. The most common appearance of hepatocellular carcinoma is a solitary hyperechoic mass; however, multifocal hyperechoic masses or masses of mixed echogenicity or "target" lesions have also been reported.[7,8] Target lesions have hypoechoic rims with hyperechoic or isoechoic centers. The finding of one or more target lesions in the liver or spleen has a positive predictive value for malignancy of 74%.[9] Mast cell tumor has been reported to be diffuse or multifocal with one or more hypoechoic nodules. Malignant histiocytosis may be characterized by multiple hypoechoic nodules with well-defined borders.[10] In the dog and cat, hepatic metastases are more common than primary liver tumors and should always be considered as a differential for focal/multifocal disease.[8] Benign diseases that can cause a similar appearance include nodular regeneration, abscess, steroid/drug-induced hepatopathy and hepatic necrosis.[3] A list of differentials for focal/multifocal hepatic disease is provided in Box 9-3.

SPLEEN

Diffuse

The normal splenic parenchyma is homogenous and hyperechoic relative to the liver and kidney.[11] Diffuse, focal, and multifocal lesions originating from the spleen are not pathognomonic for benign or neoplastic disease.

BOX 9-1	COMMONLY IMAGED TISSUE IN ORDER OF INCREASING ECHOGENICITY

- Bile, urine
- Renal medulla
- Renal cortex
- Liver
- Spleen
- Prostate
- Structural fat and vessel walls
- Bone, gas, organ boundaries

BOX 9-2	DIFFERENTIALS FOR DIFFUSE LIVER DISEASE

Differentials for a Hypoechoic Liver
- Lymphoma
- Leukemia
- Chronic passive congestion
- Acute hepatitis

Differentials for a Hyperechoic Liver
- Lymphoma
- Mast cell tumor
- Fatty infiltration
- Steroid hepatopathy
- Chronic hepatitis

Diffuse neoplastic disease may be a result of lymphoma, mast cell tumor, malignant histiocytosis, or leukemia and can result in a decreased echogenicity.[10-12] Lymphoma of the spleen may have a variety of appearances but is often described as having a "honeycomb" pattern as a result of multiple, small (1-2 cm) hypoechoic nodules (Figure 9-3).[11,12] Benign diseases that can result in a change in splenic echogenicity include lymphoid hyperplasia, extramedullary hematopoiesis, and inflammation.[11] As with other organs, normal splenic echogenicity does not rule out the possibility of neoplasia.

BOX 9-3   DIFFERENTIALS FOR FOCAL/MULTI-FOCAL HEPATIC DISEASE

Primary Neoplasia
• Hepatocellular carcinoma
• Hepatocellular adenoma
• Mast cell tumor
• Hemangiosarcoma
• Malignant histiocytosis

Non-neoplastic Disease
• Hepatic cysts
• Hematoma
• Nodular regeneration
• Hepatic abscess
• Steroid hepatopathy
• Hepatic necrosis

Focal/Multifocal

Focal and multifocal diseases of the spleen may be easy to detect, but a definitive diagnosis is usually not possible without the aid of biopsies and aspirates. Hemangiosarcoma and lymphoma are the most common primary splenic tumors; however, other types of tumors have been reported. Hemangiosarcomas usually are mixed in echogenicity with a variable amount of anechoic to hyperechoic material throughout the mass.[13] Benign lesions such as a hematoma may have a similar appearance. A list of differentials for diffuse and focal diseases of the spleen is given in Table 9-1.

KIDNEY

It is important to compare the normal relationship of the echogenicity between the kidney, spleen, and liver in order to recognize parenchymal abnormalities. Diffuse abnormalities can be caused by numerous diseases such as neoplasia, inflammatory diseases (glomerulonephritis), and infectious diseases (feline infectious peritonitis).[14] Biopsies are usually required for definitive diagnosis. Focal mass lesions that cause distortion of the renal parenchyma are easily recognized, but the only lesion that can be definitively diagnosed from an ultrasound examination is a renal cyst. Focal lesions with complex echogenicity and concurrent disruption of the renal parenchyma are a common finding with neoplasia.[14] Primary renal tumors include renal adenocarcinoma and lymphoma.

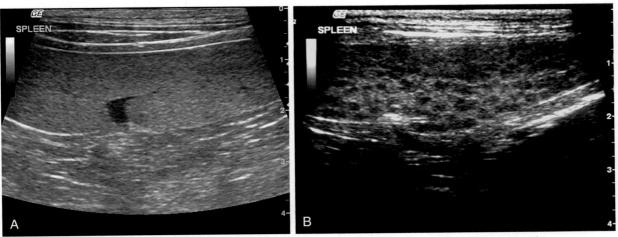

FIGURE 9-3 A, Normal spleen. **B,** Spleen with multiple hypoechoic nodules characteristic of lymphoma. This is often called a "honeycomb" appearance.

GASTROINTESTINAL TRACT

Using ultrasound to evaluate the GI tract is advantageous because it allows evaluation of intestinal wall thickness and layering, both of which may be altered with neoplasia.[15] Usually the layers of the gastric and intestinal wall can be seen as alternating hypoechoic and hyperechoic layers corresponding to the mucosa, submucosa, muscularis propria, and serosa.[16] Intestinal tumors are characterized by moderate to severe thickening of the wall with concurrent loss of layering (Figure 9-4).[15-17] Lymphoma tends to involve multiple bowel segments and regional lymph nodes. Adenocarcinomas usually affect a short or single bowel segment and appear as transmural thickening with loss of layering.[15,17] In a recent study of 150 dogs with intestinal disease, 99% of the patients with intestinal neoplasia had loss of wall layering.[15] In GI tumors, the ultrasonographic characteristics of loss of layering and wall thickening can result in a presumptive diagnosis and encourage further investigation.

PROSTATE

The prostate gland is usually evaluated in both neutered and intact male dogs as part of a complete ultrasound examination. The prostate is similar in echogenicity to the spleen.[18] Although numerous disease conditions affect the prostate, focal or multi-focal areas of increased echogenicity, or a heterogenous complex appearance to the parenchyma is generally seen only with bacterial prostatitis and neoplasia.[19] Concurrent mineralization can also be seen with these two conditions. Biopsies and aspirates are the procedure of choice for further differentiation.

BLADDER

Female dogs and male cats have a higher incidence of bladder neoplasia, with the dog affected more commonly than the cat.[14] The most common tumor is transitional cell carcinoma, which typically appears as an irregular sessile mass arising from the bladder wall and extending into the bladder lumen.[14] These masses often occur in the trigone area and can extend into the urethra and

TABLE 9-1   DIFFERENTIALS FOR DIFFUSE AND FOCAL/MULTIFOCAL DISEASES OF THE SPLEEN

Diffuse/ Multifocal	Neoplastic	Benign
Diffuse	Lymphoma	Lymphoid hyperplasia
	Mast cell tumor	Extra-medullary hematopoiesis
	Malignant histiocytosis	Inflammation
	Leukemia	
Focal/ Multifocal	Hemangiosarcoma	Hematoma
	Lymphoma	Myelolipomas Hyperplastic nodules

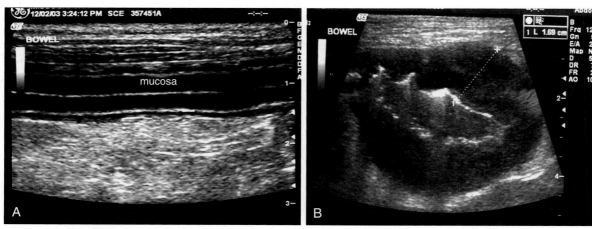

FIGURE 9-4 A, Normal small bowel showing layering corresponding to alternating hypoechoic/hyperechoic layers. **B,** Intestinal lymphoma with thickening of the bowel wall and complete loss of layering.

prostate. Bladder neoplasia can also result in a mechanical ureteral obstruction with secondary hydronephrosis. An aspirate or biopsy is not recommended because of the possibility of seeding the abdomen with tumor cells, but ultrasound-guided traumatic catheterization can aid in diagnosis.

In conclusion, ultrasound is valuable in helping to identify and characterize abdominal masses. Certain ultrasonographic characteristics can help lead to a tentative diagnosis of neoplasia. However, biopsies and aspirates are usually required for definitive diagnosis, since numerous benign conditions can have similar appearances. Because of an increase in the use of ultrasound in veterinary medicine and the improved availability of this modality, becoming familiar with the wide variety of sonographic appearances of neoplastic and benign diseases is important for practitioners. Ultrasound is a valuable tool in veterinary oncology to guide aspirate and biopsy procedures, assist in tumor staging, and provide important prognostic information about the patient.

Selected References*

Drost WT: Basic ultrasound physics, In Thrall DE (ed): *Textbook of veterinary diagnostic radiology*, ed 5, St Louis, 2007, Saunders/Elsevier, pp 38-49.
This is a good basic review of the principles of ultrasound including artifacts. This outlines the minimal knowledge base that is needed prior to beginning an ultrasound examination.
Lamb CR, Hartzband LZ, Tidwell AS, et al: Ultrasonographic findings in hepatic and splenic lymphosarcoma in dogs and cats, *Vet Radiol Ultrasound* 32:117, 1991.
This is an excellent review paper on the types of sonographic patterns that may commonly be seen in hepatic and splenic lymphoma in small animals.
Nyland TG, Mattoon JS, Herrgesell EJ, et al: Liver. In Nyland TG, Mattoon JS (eds): *Small animal diagnostic ultrasound*, ed 2, Philadelphia, 2002, WB Saunders.
This is a good book chapter on the appearance of both the normal and diseased liver in small animals. Both diffuse and focal liver abnormalities are described.
Nyland TG, Mattoon JS, Herrgesell EJ, et al: Urinary tract. In Nyland TG, Mattoon JS (eds): *Small animal diagnostic ultrasound*, ed 2, Philadelphia, 2002, WB Saunders.
This is a well-written book chapter describing a variety of disease conditions that can be diagnosed with ultrasound. Ultrasound of the normal urinary tract is also described.
Paoloni MC, Penninck DG, Moore AS: Ultrasonographic and clinicopathologic findings in 21 dogs with intestinal adenocarcinoma, *Vet Radiol Ultrasound* 43:562, 2002.
This review details the common sonographic changes seen in intestinal adenocarcinoma in small animals and is a good review of the types of appearances that should alert the sonographer to the high probability of intestinal neoplasia.

■ *For a complete list of the references cited in this chapter, please go to www.smallanimaloncology.com.

SECTION C: Endoscopy

William G. Brewer, Jr.

KEY POINTS

- Endoscopy is a minimally invasive technique that can play an important role in diagnosis and treatment of disease.
- Endoscopy instruments are fixed focus and require a distended hollow organ for proper visualization.
- When used appropriately, endoscopy is complementary to other diagnostic and therapeutic modalities.

The word *endoscopy* means to look inside a hollow organ.[1] This diagnostic modality offers what is frequently a less-invasive means of evaluating hollow organs than possible with surgery. For most endoscopic procedures, however, general anesthesia is necessary. This chapter will discuss GI endoscopy, rhinoscopy, bronchoscopy, and cystoscopy. Obviously, none of these are stand-alone procedures but may complement other diagnostic and therapeutic modalities.

GASTROINTESTINAL ENDOSCOPY

Upper Gastrointestinal Endoscopy

Upper GI endoscopy (Box 9-4) facilitates visual assessment of the oropharynx, esophagus, stomach, and proximal duodenum. The technique for upper GI endoscopy

BOX 9-4   PRACTICE TIPS: UPPER GI ENDOSCOPY

- Although the gastroesophageal sphincter may appear slightly reddened compared with the rest of the esophageal mucosa, this is a normal feature where the transition from esophageal to gastric mucosa occurs.
- Repeated stimulation of the pyloric sphincter (either with the endoscope or during biopsy acquisition) causes it to tighten, making entrance more difficult.
- Passing the endoscope into the duodenum before complete evaluation and sampling of the gastric mucosa may eliminate the artifacts created by biopsy-induced hemorrhage and scope redirection with the stomach.
- By sampling perpendicular to the edge of a rugal fold, one is more likely to get a deeper biopsy sample of greater diagnostic quality.
- Prior administration of barium may cause the gastric mucosa to appear edematous.

is outlined in Box 9-5. As the endoscope (Figure 9-5) is passed aborally, all structures are observed for abnormalities and to ensure correct placement of the endoscope. Other than finding an inflamed distal esophagus resulting from repeated vomiting or reflux, it is uncommon to see esophageal lesions. As shown in Figure 9-6, the gastroesophageal sphincter may appear slightly reddened compared with the rest of the esophageal mucosa, but this is a normal feature where the transition from esophageal to gastric mucosa occurs. The stomach may be evaluated immediately as the endoscope is passed through the gastroesophageal sphincter or, as is the author's preference, may be bypassed initially and evaluated after the duodenum is explored. The latter approach allows for visualization of the pyloric sphincter and proximal duodenum before any mucosal damage or bleeding that may occur as a result of redirection of the endoscope or biopsy of the gastric mucosa. The normal duodenal mucosa is smooth and a light moist pink. Frequently, the mucosa is grossly normal, but it is important to obtain multiple biopsies. A study by Willard et al.[2] demonstrated a minimum of eight biopsies are required for a reasonable chance of obtaining a

BOX 9-5   UPPER GASTROINTESTINAL ENDOSCOPY TECHNIQUE

1. The patient should have fasted for 8-12 hours prior to the procedure and should be anesthetized and placed in left lateral recumbency. A flexible 8- to 12-mm diameter endoscope of 100- to 150-cm length is appropriate for most small animal patients.
2. With a mouth gag in place to protect the endoscope, the endoscope is advanced through the mouth, pharynx, and esophagus. While advancing through the esophagus, continuous insufflation is applied for visualization of esophageal size, color, and texture. The normal wall is a dull pink (see Figure 9-6).
3. The endoscope is next passed through the lower esophageal sphincter into the stomach. The author prefers to first pass the endoscope through the pyloric sphincter into the proximal duodenum before viewing the stomach. Repeated stimulation of the pyloric sphincter (either with the endoscope or during biopsy acquisition) causes it to tighten, making entrance more difficult.
4. To enter the duodenum, the stomach is partially insufflated for visualization of the pyloric region, being sure not to flatten the incisura. The endoscope is guided to the pyloric sphincter and then is quickly moved up and to the right to enter the duodenum. This is confirmed as insufflation demonstrates the parallel walls of a continuous tube. The area is observed and evaluated for masses or foreign bodies. Even if the mucosa is normal in appearance, multiple biopsies should be obtained.
5. Once evaluation of the duodenum is complete, the endoscope is pulled back into the stomach and the pyloric sphincter is visually assessed.
6. To fully evaluate the stomach, the endoscope is completely retroflexed and advanced. This allows visualization of the body of the stomach, which is confirmed by visualization of the portion of the scope that is entering through the lower esophageal sphincter into the cardia. These areas are evaluated for the presence of foreign bodies, masses, ulceration or mucosal thickening. Multiple samples should be collected, with deeper tissue facilitated by directing the biopsy cups perpendicular to the edge of the rugal folds.
7. Biopsy samples should be placed in cassettes according to sampling site within the upper GI tract and labeled accordingly.

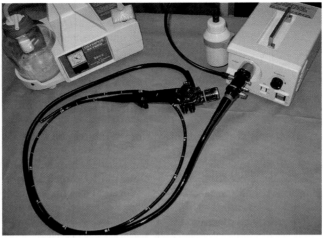

FIGURE 9-5 Olympus 140 cm pediatric gastroscope and light source (Olympus America, Center Valley, PA).

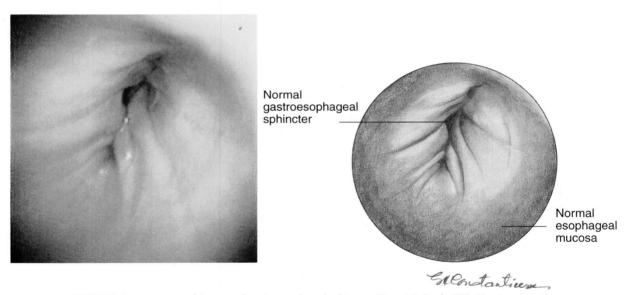

Normal
gastroesophageal
sphincter

Normal
esophageal
mucosa

FIGURE 9-6 Appearance of the normal canine esophageal sphincter. (From McCarthy TC: *Veterinary endoscopy for the small animal practitioner*, St Louis, 2005, Saunders/Elsevier.)

diagnostic sample. After evaluation of the duodenum, the endoscope is pulled back into the stomach. Normal gastric mucosa is a glistening light pink, and the rugal folds can be visualized depending on the degree of insufflation (Figure 9-7). Because the biopsy cups are small and tend to obtain only mucosal samples, diseases that are deeper in the GI wall, such as a gastric adenocarcinoma, may be missed. The diagnostic quality of gastric

biopsy samples can be enhanced by sampling perpendicular to the edge of a rugal fold.

Lower Gastrointestinal Endoscopy

Lower GI endoscopy (Box 9-6) permits visual evaluation and biopsy of the rectum, colon, cecum, and, in some cases, the ileum. The technique for lower GI endoscopy is outlined in Box 9-7. The cecum is a blind pouch off

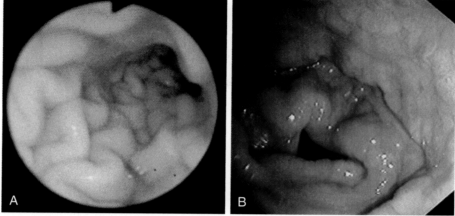

FIGURE 9-7 **A**, Normal stomach with whitish-pink glistening mucosa and rugal folds. **B**, Gastric antrum and pylorus of a dog with gastrointestinal lymphoma. Note the granularity of the mucosa as compared to normal gastric mucosa *(A)*. (From Tams TR: *Small animal endoscopy*, ed 2, St Louis, 1999, Mosby/Elsevier.)

BOX 9-6   PRACTICE TIPS: LOWER GASTROINTESTINAL ENDOSCOPY

- Spurious hemorrhagic mucosal lesions can be created by insertion of an enema tube during patient preparation.
- Because it is difficult to distend the rectum for optimal lesion evaluation, some lesions are best evaluated by palpation.

BOX 9-7   LOWER GASTROINTESTINAL ENDOSCOPY TECHNIQUE

1. Prepare the patient with an 18- to 24-hour fast.
2. Administer an oral osmotic cathartic, 20 mg/kg twice, 1 to 2 hours apart on the evening before endoscopy. Administer metoclopramide, 0.2 mg/kg IV 30 minutes after the first dose of oral cathartic.
3. A warm-water enema may be administered on the morning of the procedure.
4. Place the patient in left lateral recumbency. While insufflating, insert the endoscope into the rectum and advance it up the descending colon to the transverse colon. If masses are identified within the rectum, the entire lower GI tract that is accessible via endoscope should still be evaluated to rule out the possibility of multifocal or diffuse disease.
5. Once at the level of the transverse colon, flex the endoscope up at 90 degrees and advance into the transverse colon.
6. Flex the endoscope caudally to advance it into the ascending colon to the level of the cecum and ileum. Frequently, the endoscope can be advanced into the cecum and sometimes the ileum. The normal colonic mucosa is a glistening pale pink and somewhat rough in texture (see Figure 9-8). Multiple biopsies should be obtained from each section of the colon, even if the mucosa is grossly normal.

---

the end of the ascending colon, and the terminal portion of the ileum protrudes into the cavity of the colon. This is normal and serves as a functional sphincter for the terminal ileum when the colon contracts. Frequently, the endoscope can be advanced into the cecum and sometimes the ileum. Normal colonic mucosa is a glistening pale pink with a somewhat rough texture (Figure 9-8). Multiple biopsies should be obtained from each section of the colon, even if the mucosa is grossly normal.

RHINOSCOPY

With a rigid 2- to 4-mm diameter rhinoscope (Figure 9-9) or a flexible 2- to 3-mm fiberoptic scope, rhinoscopy can be performed in order to evaluate patients with chronic sneezing, congestion, epistaxis, nasal discharge, or nasal swelling (Box 9-8). In addition to a transnasal approach, a flexible scope can also be introduced through the oral cavity and retroflexed to visualize the

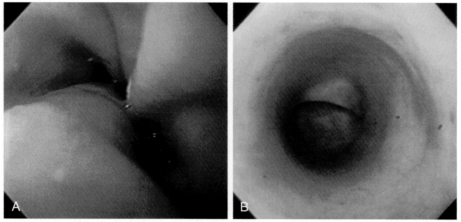

FIGURE 9-8 Normal appearance of the canine colon before (**A**) and after (**B**) insufflation. Without adequate insufflation, it is not possible to assess the entire mucosal surface. (From Tams TR: *Small animal endoscopy*, ed 2, St Louis, 1999, Mosby/Elsevier.)

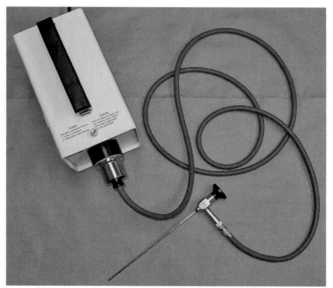

FIGURE 9-9 Rigid arthroscope and light source suitable for rhinoscopy (Endoscopic Support Services, Brewster, NY).

caudal nasopharyngeal region. If a flexible scope is not available, a spay hook may be used to retract the soft palate, allowing visualization of a portion of the nasopharynx. As described in Box 9-9, the rhinoscope is passed all the way through the nasal cavity and then withdrawn, while observing for abnormal tissue. In particular, the nasal cavity is observed for white fluffy plaques that may indicate fungal infection (Figure 9-10, *A-D*), smooth clear glistening nodular areas that may represent cryptococcosis, masses suggesting neoplasia (Figure 9-10, *E-F*) or foreign bodies. Biopsy samples are collected, regardless of the gross appearance of the nasal tissue.

BOX 9-8 PRACTICE TIPS: RHINOSCOPY

- CT or MRI should be performed prior to rhinoscopy. Otherwise hemorrhage resulting from rhinoscopy will distort the appearance of the nasal cavity.
- The entire nasal cavity should be visualized prior to biopsy, such that biopsy-induced hemorrhage does not obscure the visualization of important lesions.
- Any gauze used to pack the oropharynx during nasal flushing should be examined for foreign body material or tissue that would be useful to submit for histopathology.
- Culture of nasal exudate is generally of little value, since it often results in growth of contaminants, rather than revealing the etiology of underlying clinical signs.
- Hemorrhage frequently accompanies nasal biopsy. Phenylephrine hydrochloride (Neo-Synephrine®, Bayer Health Care, Tarrytown, NY) nose drops may be instilled directly into the nasal cavity or placed onto a long cotton-tipped swab that is then directed into the nasal cavity.

BOX 9-9 RHINOSCOPY TECHNIQUE

1. Place the patient in ventral recumbency with its head elevated on a rolled towel or other support.
2. Direct the scope into the nasal passage medially and ventrally, carefully advancing through the nasal cavity.
3. Guide the scope to the caudal portion of the nasal cavity and then view the entire nasal cavity as the scope is withdrawn. This technique decreases the chance of inadvertently striking the mucosa with the scope and inducing hemorrhage.
4. The normal nasal mucosa is a glistening bright pink. If visualization is obscured by discharge, flush with copious volumes of normal saline via a syringe and soft rubber catheter of appropriate diameter. The cuff of the endotracheal tube should be tightly inflated, and the nose should be pointed downward during flushing. Gauze may also be used to pack the oropharyngeal area during flushing.
5. If no abnormalities are noted, representative biopsies should still be obtained. Biopsy samples should be placed in appropriately labeled formalin jars. Cultures of the nasal cavity, regardless of how obtained, frequently result in the growth of contaminants and, therefore, are not reliable.

BRONCHOSCOPY

Using a 3.7- to 5-mm diameter endoscope of 100- to 150-cm length, the practitioner can gain visualization of the upper respiratory tract through bronchoscopy (Box 9-10). This method is indicated to assess patients presenting with cough, laryngeal, tracheal, and pulmonary diseases, including but not limited to changes in airway diameter, inflammatory, infectious, or neoplastic disease. This method also facilitates brush cytology, culture, direct bronchoalveolar lavage, biopsy, and foreign body removal. Bronchoscopy must be well planned in advance such that the procedure can be completed rapidly and without unnecessary respiratory compromise caused by prolonged placement of the endoscope into the airway. The technique for bronchoscopy is outlined in Box 9-11. Radiographs, ultrasound, CT, and MRI images may help guide the procedure, identifying areas of interest in advance of bronchoscopy.

CYSTOSCOPY

Cystoscopy allows visualization of the urethral mucosa, ectopic ureters, the prostatic urethra, the area of the trigone where urine can be seen entering through the ureters, and the bladder mucosa (Box 9-12). It can be performed either transurethrally or by a prepubic percutaneous approach. See Box 9-13 for details regarding cystoscopy technique. If intraluminal masses are visualized, tissue should be obtained for both histopathological examination and bacterial culture and sensitivity testing. For patients thought to have renal infections, the ureters can be catheterized via cystoscopy to obtain urine samples from each kidney individually. With the prepubic percutaneous approach, tumor seeding within the abdomen or cutaneous tissues is a risk. Owners should be advised of this risk in advance of the procedure, and every attempt should be made to minimize the risk of tumor seeding. After cystoscopy procedures, antibiotics should be administered only when a urinary tract infection is present, and they should be chosen based on results of bacterial culture and sensitivity testing whenever possible.

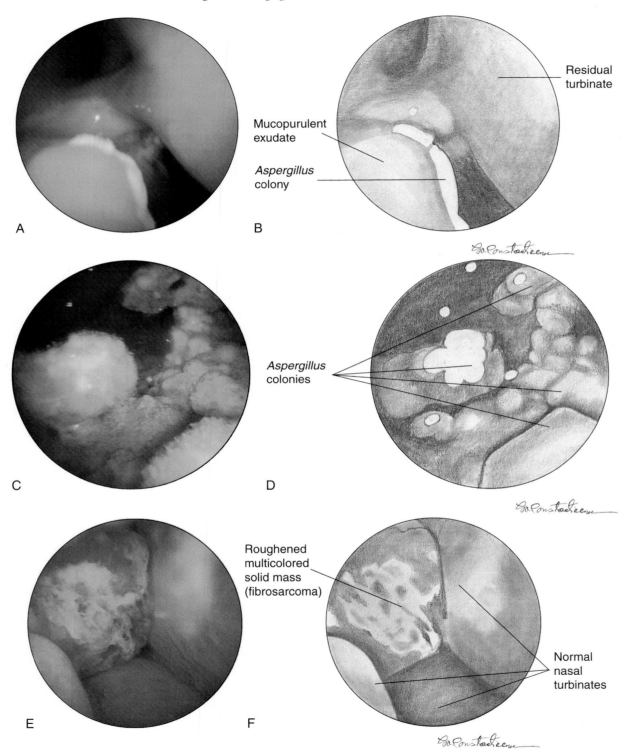

FIGURE 9-10, cont'd **A-D**, Nasal aspergillosis plaques can vary from flat white, non-glistening forms (**A**, **B**) to larger, firm structures seen in more advanced disease (**C**, **D**) and must be differentiated from neoplastic disease, such as the nasal fibrosarcoma shown in **E** and **F**. (From McCarthy TC: *Veterinary endoscopy for the small animal practitioner*, St Louis, 2005, Saunders/Elsevier.)

BOX 9-10   PRACTICE TIPS: BRONCHOSCOPY

- Because of the multiple branches of the airways and the need to quickly perform the procedure in order to maintain appropriate oxygenation and anesthesia, it is recommended that training in bronchoscopy be pursued before performing the procedure.
- Before inducing anesthesia, it is important to have all equipment and supplies ready. This includes sampling tubes and syringes preloaded with saline for bronchoalveolar lavage.
- The use of Dopram at 2.2 mg/kg IV has been recommended to increase laryngeal motion and thus aid in demonstrating laryngeal dysfunction.[3]
- Samples obtained from the airways should be labeled appropriately as to location in the tracheobronchial tree to help guide further procedures such as surgical excision of tissue involved with a neoplastic process. Maps of the tracheobronchial tree to assist in this are available.[4]

BOX 9-11   BRONCHOSCOPY TECHNIQUE

1. Anesthetize the patient with IV anesthesia such as Propofol and place in left ventral recumbency.
2. Attach pulse oximetry and ECG monitoring equipment for continuous monitoring during the procedure.
3. Pre-oxygenate the patient via face mask before beginning bronchoscopy. During the procedure, O_2 is delivered via the biopsy port or through a separate catheter placed into the trachea.
4. With a mouth gag in place to protect the bronchoscope, the bronchoscope is advanced to visualize the oropharynx and larynx.
5. The scope is advanced down the trachea to evaluate for size, shape, and mucosal appearance (which should be a smooth light pink with an underlying bed of capillaries). The C-shaped rings should be visible under the tracheal capillary bed. Lack of visualization of the capillary beds supports the presence of a mucosal infiltrative process. The dorsal membrane should be relatively tight and not veil down into the tracheal lumen. Any suspect lesions should be biopsied.
6. Once the distal end of the trachea is reached, the V-shaped bifurcation of the carina is noted. Distal airway bifurcations are also V-shaped. If the carinal bifurcation is U-shaped, this suggests encroachment by enlarged perihilar lymph nodes. U-shaped bifurcations of the more distal airways can be seen with chronic bronchitis. As the airways are entered, abnormal appearing mucosa or nodules can be biopsied, secretions can be sampled for analysis and culture, foreign bodies can be removed, and directed bronchoalveolar lavage can be performed through the biopsy port for fluid analysis and culture.

BOX 9-12   PRACTICE TIPS: CYSTOSCOPY

- Tumor seeding into the abdominal cavity is a potential risk of prepubic cutaneous cystoscopy; thus, transurethral approaches are preferable when feasible (small female dogs).
- It is important to remember that urine is an excellent culture media for bacteria, especially in the presence of urinary tract abnormalities, and the utmost sterility must be maintained during cystoscopy. Infection of the bladder can lead to seeding of the kidneys and other organs.

BOX 9-13   CYSTOSCOPY TECHNIQUE

Transurethral approach (using rigid cystoscope in females and flexible bronchoscope in males)
1. Place female dogs in dorsal or ventral recumbency. Medium and large male dogs are placed in lateral recumbency.
2. Sterile prep the urethral opening and empty the bladder via urethral catheter.
3. Advance the cystoscope through the urethral opening while saline is infused via the side port. The normal bladder mucosa is pale pink.
4. Biopsy intraluminal masses (see Chapter 22, Section I) and mucosa for both histopathology and culture.
5. If indicated, catheterize the ureters to obtain urine samples from each kidney individually.

Prepubic percutaneous approach (using rigid arthroscope)
1. Place patient in dorsal recumbency.
2. Clip and sterile prep the abdomen.
3. Catheterize and empty the bladder; then, distend the bladder with sterile saline.
4. Make a small incision through the skin overlying the distended bladder and insert the arthroscope cannula containing a trochar through the ventral bladder wall via the skin incision.
5. Remove the trochar and pass the scope through the cannula.
6. Infuse saline through the cannula side port. The saline is allowed to drain via the urethral catheter.
7. Evaluate the bladder in a manner similar to the transurethral method.
8. Take biopsies through a second puncture site.
9. Once the procedure is completed, drain the bladder via the urethral catheter and remove all instrumentation.
10. Close the skin incision and leave the urethral catheter in place for 2-3 days to allow the bladder to remain decompressed and allow the bladder wounds to heal.
11. Administer antibiotics only if a urinary tract infection is present.

Selected References*

For a thorough discussion of veterinary endoscopy, the reader should see one of the following texts:

McCarthy TC: *Veterinary endoscopy for the small animal practitioner*, St Louis, 2005, Saunders/Elsevier.
This reference offers a comprehensive, up-to-date discussion of small animal endoscopy including equipment selection, equipment handling, and endoscopic procedures. The discussions are enhanced by numerous quality photographs taken at various stages of endoscopic procedures.

Tams TR: *Small animal endoscopy*, ed 2, St Louis, 1999, Mosby/Elsevier.
This reference is a second edition of the original complete volume on small animal endoscopy, which offers a comprehensive, up-to-date discussion of small animal endoscopy, including equipment selection, equipment handling, and endoscopic procedures. The discussions are enhanced by numerous quality photographs taken at various stages of endoscopic procedures.

■ *For a complete list of the references cited in this chapter, please go to www.smallanimaloncology.com.

10 Advanced Imaging Modalities

SECTION A: Positron Emission Tomography (PET)

Amy K. LeBlanc

KEY POINTS

- Positron emission tomography (PET) and fused PET/computed tomography (CT) are widely used as non-invasive imaging techniques for staging and management of human cancer.
- [18]FDG is the most common PET tracer used in clinical practice, which can readily identify areas of increased glucose utilization within the body, such as malignancy and inflammation.
- PET will be used for staging and management of veterinary patients with cancer as access to necessary equipment and radiopharmaceuticals improves, representing an important step forward in the practice of veterinary oncology.

POSITRON EMISSION TOMOGRAPHY

Positron emission tomography (PET) is a nuclear medicine technique that uses a radiopharmaceutical tagged with a positron-emitting isotope to map distribution of radioactivity throughout the body.[1] Distribution of the radiopharmaceutical is dependent on specific cellular function(s), providing an assessment of physiologic and/or metabolic processes in the body. Recent advances in scanner design and performance, in addition to PET/CT fusion, have moved PET to the forefront of oncologic imaging. PET technology was first used in the 1980s for study of neurologic and cardiac diseases through mapping of glucose metabolism with a commonly used positron-emitting tracer, 2-[^{18}F]-fluoro-2-deoxyglucose ([18]FDG).[2] PET is now widely used for the staging and management of human cancer patients, based on the increased glucose transport and metabolism in tumors compared with surrounding normal tissues.[3,4]

Physics of Positron Emission and Detection

The images produced with PET use unique physical properties of positron-emitting radionuclides, which are "neutron-deficient" unstable isotopes that decay by emission of positrons (e+), or positively charged electrons with mass equivalent to an electron.[5] The positron emitted from the nucleus loses energy through collision with electrons in the surrounding tissue until it annihilates with an electron from an adjacent atom. The energy produced by the annihilation reaction is in the form of two 511 keV photons that are emitted about 180 degrees apart.[5,6] Detection of these two photons, and not the positron itself, is the foundation of PET imaging.

PET Scanners

The PET camera is designed to detect the pair of annihilation photons from the decay of the positron-emitting isotope and is comprised of a ring of block detectors that encircles the patient. The two annihilation photons produced by positron emission are captured in coincidence by opposing detectors around the patient, meaning that detectors record "true" coincidence events.[6] A true coincidence is defined by a pair of unscattered photons arising from a single annihilation that arrive within the coincidence time window.[5] Detection of the photons by opposing detectors means that the annihilation reaction, and thus the location of the radiopharmaceutical, occurred somewhere along a line between the detectors, which is referred to as the line of response (LOR). These paired events are stored in matrices or sinograms where each row in the matrix represents a projection of the activity distribution in the patient at a specific angle and axial position.[6] An image reconstruction algorithm is applied to recover the radioactivity distribution, thus using LORs to indirectly map

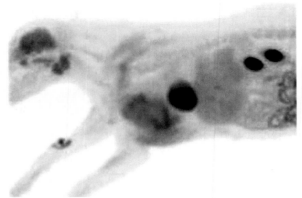

FIGURE 10-1 This image depicts a dog in right lateral recumbency with a large tumor involving the left axilla within which significant uptake of radionuclide is visible. The site of FDG injection is visible on the right antebrachium. Note normal uptake of radionuclide within the brain, salivary glands, myocardium, and kidneys.

the functional process that created the distribution of positron emitter. The resulting images represent radiopharmaceutical accumulation in specific areas of the body, representative of the underlying biologic process of interest (Figure 10-1).

The recent fusion of PET with computed tomography (CT) has been an important step in maximizing the attributes of both modalities.[6-8] The fused scanner design allows anatomy and function to be assessed in a one-scan session with single positioning of the patient. This minimizes organ movement with no requirement for labor-intensive image registration algorithms as when the scans are obtained separately.[7,8] Accurately aligned fused images of anatomy and function obtained with PET/CT offer advantages to the study interpreter through accurate localization of tracer accumulation, the distinction of normal uptake of tracer within certain organs/tissues from pathologic uptake, and the verification that a suspicious finding on one modality can be confirmed by the other.[7,8]

POSITRON EMITTERS AND PRACTICAL ASPECTS OF PET IMAGING

FDG and the Glycolytic Pathway

The most common radiopharmaceutical used in modern PET imaging is FDG. Developed in 1976 for the purpose of mapping regional cerebral glucose metabolism, this molecule is an analogue of glucose that is used to quantify

the rate at which the hexokinase reaction of glycolysis is occurring in a tissue or an organ.[9] The development of FDG is based on the intracellular fate of 2-deoxyglucose (2-DG), an analogue of glucose that is phosphorylated in a similar manner by the hexokinase enzyme, the first step of glycolysis. However, once phosphorylated, 2-DG-6-P is trapped within the cell, unable to undergo the ensuing steps of glycolysis or the pentose phosphate shunt. Phosphorylated FDG, as with 2-DG-6-P, cannot be further metabolized, so all accumulated radioactivity over time is proportional to the rate of the hexokinase reaction in the observed tissue. At steady state conditions, this represents the rate of glycolysis in the tissue.[9]

Scanning Technique

Patient Preparation

In human oncology, routine patient preparation involves fasting for approximately 6 hours before FDG injection to maximize uptake of the tracer by the tumor. After injection, it is important that the patient remain still and quiet for 90 minutes while FDG uptake occurs to avoid active skeletal muscle uptake of FDG as an interpretive pitfall.[10] For veterinary patients, fasting and use of a sedative premedicant with cage confinement is recommended after FDG injection to minimize aberrant uptake of FDG in skeletal muscle. Generally PET scans, similar to CT or MRI, are performed under general anesthesia in veterinary patients.

Image Interpretation and Standardized Uptake Value

When evaluating a static PET image, the most common way to assess tracer uptake is with the standardized uptake value (SUV).[5] With the use of computer software, a region of interest (ROI) is drawn around a lesion or an organ of interest and the activity of the tracer in this area is measured. The SUV is calculated to determine the relative tracer uptake within the ROI. As with other nuclear medicine techniques, visual inspection of the images is also used to characterize suspect areas of increased tracer uptake.

Uptake of FDG is not specific to malignancy. Organs such as brain, liver, spleen, tonsils, thymus, salivary glands, urinary system, and bone marrow are known to have varying degrees of normal FDG uptake.[10] Inflammatory processes are known to exhibit increased glucose metabolism through chemotaxis and phagocytic activity of inflammatory cells. Most malignant diseases produce lesions with higher SUVs than inflammatory conditions, but a few exceptions, specifically diseases causing granulomatous inflammation, do exist.[11]

FDG-PET IN ONCOLOGY

Human Applications

Applications of PET and PET/CT are numerous and widely visible in human oncologic practice.[1,3] The unique ability of PET to non-invasively assess the likelihood of malignancy based on the SUV value has resulted in improved detection and management of, for example, solitary pulmonary nodules that may represent adenoma, granulomas, or neoplasia.[12] However, PET is more often applied in the staging of malignancy and assessment of response to therapy than in the initial diagnosis of human cancers. FDG-PET has been applied to the staging and follow-up of cancer of the breast, lung, colon, brain, and Hodgkin's disease (HD) and non-Hodgkin's lymphoma (NHL), becoming the test of choice in the staging, assessment of response to therapy, and detection of recurrence in both human HD and NHL.[12-18]

Veterinary Applications

Lack of available equipment and high cost of PET radiopharmaceuticals have limited the use of PET as a diagnostic tool in veterinary oncology. Reports of PET in animals are sparse in the veterinary literature.[11,19,20] PET was used to characterize experimentally induced and naturally occurring blastomycosis and was compared with cases of canine lymphoma.[11,20] A recent study of whole-body PET in normal dogs demonstrates patterns of [18]FDG distribution and SUVs for parenchymal organs to assist in lesion interpretation in disease states.[21] Currently, the availability of PET for staging and evaluation of response to therapy in clinical patients is limited to a few locations in the United States. Applications in veterinary oncology will increase as this technology becomes more widely available, aided by regional cyclotron distribution networks for radiopharmaceuticals. As studies are published that validate its use as a non-invasive whole-body staging method, PET will become a useful and innovative tool in the management of veterinary oncology patients.

Selected References*

Cook GJR, Wegner EA, Fogelman I: Pitfalls and artifacts in [18]FDG PET and PET/CT oncologic imaging, *Semin Nucl Med* 34:122, 2004.
In response to increasing use of PET in human oncologic imaging, this paper does a very good job of detailing the potential artifacts and pitfalls in image interpretation for optimization of PET interpretation.
Friedberg JW, Chengazi V: PET scans in the staging of lymphoma: current status, *Oncologist* 8:438, 2003.
A clinician-friendly review of the current accepted usage of PET in the diagnosis and management of human lymphomas.
Juweid ME, Cheson BD: Positron-emission tomography and assessment of cancer therapy, *N Engl J Med* 354:496, 2006.
This is a recent review of the common applications of PET and PET/CT in human oncology.
LeBlanc AK, Jakoby B, Townsend DW, et al: Thoracic and abdominal organ uptake of 2-deoxy-2-[18F]fluoro-D-glucose (18FDG) with positron emission tomography in the normal dog, *Vet Radiol Ultrasound* 49(2):182, 2008.
The first report of dynamic organ [18]FDG uptake in normal dogs to aid in lesion interpretation in future studies of canine diseases imaged with PET.
Townsend DW: Physical principles and technology of clinical PET imaging, *Annals Acad Med Singapore* 33:133, 2004.
This comprehensive review of PET covers both basic physics and technical factors influencing image quality. It contains an in-depth discussion of scanner design and technical aspects of PET/CT fusion.

*For a complete list of the references cited in this chapter, please go to www.smallanimaloncology.com.

SECTION B: Computed Tomography (CT) and Magnetic Resonance Imaging (MRI)

Craig A. Clifford, Anthony J. Fischetti, Justin M. Goggin, and E. Scott Pretorius

KEY POINTS

- CT and MR images are two-dimensional tomographic slices, which allow the observer to evaluate an area of interest without interference from overlying structures that would be summed in planar radiographs.
- CT imaging is usually performed in the transverse (axial) plane, whereas MR images are routinely made in multiple planes.
- MR provides superior anatomic detail of the nervous system and is considered the modality of choice for neuroimaging.
- For thoracic imaging, CT is superior to MRI because of an overall lower cost, more widespread availability, faster imaging with fewer artifacts associated with cardiac and respiratory motion, and generally shorter anesthesia time.

- Both CT and MRI are considered the standard of care in human oncology for diagnosis, staging, and assessment of response to therapy for many malignancies, including those of the liver, as well as of the spleen, adrenal gland, kidney, and pancreas.
- High accuracy of CT for diagnosis of dogs with different sources of chronic nasal disease (neoplasia, non-specific rhinitis, fungal rhinitis) has been reported.

The use of CT and MR imaging in veterinary practice has grown rapidly over the past few years. Although standard radiography and ultrasound remain important in diagnostic evaluation, CT and MR have emerged as important tools for evaluation of patients in whom diagnosis, disease stage, or tumor response to therapy are not well-evaluated by other means.

CT and MR images are two-dimensional tomographic slices that allow the observer to evaluate an area of interest without interference from overlying structures that would be summed in planar radiographs.[1-3] CT images are generally made in the transverse plane, whereas MR images are made in any plane. CT's spatial resolution is greater than that of MRI, although MRI has the highest intrinsic contrast resolution of the three cross-sectional imaging modalities (ultrasound, CT, and MRI).[3] CT attenuation values are reported on the Hounsfield scale, which ranges from −1000 to +1000, with water assigned the value of 0.[3-5] There is no similar absolute scale for MR, since MR signal intensity values depend upon a large number of scanner and pulse sequence parameters. Valid comparisons between signal intensity measurements can therefore only be made within a given pulse sequence acquisition, or between two data acquisitions (such as pre- and post-contrast datasets) obtained with exactly the same scan parameters as one another.

The basic physical principles of radiography apply to CT image acquisition, although a volume of tissue receives a larger radiation dose in CT than with radiography.[5] Differential X-ray absorption by tissues is used to generate an image on a radiograph or, in CT, these absorption/transmission data can be mathematically interpolated by a computer, which then assigns a value in Hounsfield Units (HU) to each voxel within a CT slice. Since the human eye cannot distinguish 2000 shades of grey, CT data may be viewed in different "windows," allowing the observer to assign visible shades of grey to a clinically useful range of HU. A window width is assigned to encompass all clinically relevant HU values, and a window "level" is the central HU value within the window. Window-level combinations in common clinical use include those for evaluation of the abdomen, brain, bones, and lungs.

MR imaging takes advantage of the magnetic properties of certain atomic nuclei, primarily protons (hydrogen ions), that are abundant within the body. At rest, the body's protons are aligned randomly in space. Within the strong magnetic field of the MR scanner, protons line up either parallel or anti-parallel to the main magnetic field. A series of radio-frequency pulses—a "pulse sequence"—perturbs the protons from their equilibrium. When the radio waves are removed, the body's protons tend to relax back to their alignment with the scanner's magnetic field. They do so, however, at different rates within different chemical environments. These differential proton relaxation rates are monitored by detectors and are used to form the MR image.[3]

NEUROIMAGING

Loss of symmetry, changes in tissue density (CT) or signal intensity (MR), displacement of normal structures, and changes in contrast enhancement are evaluated in the diagnostic evaluation of the brain or vertebral column.[5-7]

MRI vs. CT

Both CT and MRI can assess loss of symmetry and displacement of normal tissues (a mass effect, termed like a "falx cerebri shift" in the brain).[5,6] However, MRI provides superior anatomic detail of the nervous system and is considered the modality of choice for neuroimaging.[5,8] Small lesions and lesions lacking contrast enhancement are less likely to be identified on CT.[9,10] Resolution is especially compromised when CT is used to assess the caudal fossa because of the dense surrounding petrous temporal bone, causing unwanted black streaking artifacts, called *beam hardening*.[11] CT-guided brain and retrobulbar biopsies have high diagnostic accuracy and low complication rates in dogs.[12-14]

Brain and Spinal Tumors

Correlations between imaging characteristics and tumor types have been reviewed extensively.[6,7,15,16] Some claim excellent agreement between histologic diagnosis and imaging diagnosis.[16] Others express caution in defining tumor type based on imaging characteristics alone (Table 10-1).[17,18] This hesitation is primarily due to the overlap of imaging signs for different tumor types and between neoplastic versus non-neoplastic diseases.[18,19] Disease prevalence, clinical presentation, and CSF analysis are often used in conjunction with imaging signs to support an imaging diagnosis.[20]

TABLE 10-1   MAGNETIC RESONANCE IMAGING SIGNS THAT CORRELATE MOST WITH A SPECIFIC TUMOR TYPE

	Meningioma	Choroid Plexus Tumor*	Pituitary Neoplasia	Gliomas	Metastases
Location	• Broadly based along calvarium, falx, or tentorium ossium • In cats, most common in the tela choroidea of the third ventricle • C2 and C3 more common than lower cervical • "Golf tee" sign in vertebral column • Retrobulbar	• Intraventricular • Most common at fourth ventricle (lateral aperture) • Interventricular septum	• Pituitary fossa • Macroadenomas tend to grow dorsally to displace thalamus	• Anywhere within the brain or spinal cord (intra-medullary)	• Often at gray-white matter junction • Meningeal metastasis is also reported
Number	• Single, although multiple can be seen, especially cats	• Single, although carcinomas may seed to multiple locations in the CSF, including the meninges	• Single	• Single	• Single or multiple
Enhancement	• Often highly contrast enhancing. • "Dural tail" sign	• Highly contrast enhancing	• Contrast en-hancing	• Variable	• Variable
Peri-tumoral changes	• Adjacent hyperostosis • Edema • Hemorrhage • Possibly cystic	• Obstructive hydrocephalus • Edema	• Possible edema	• Edema, more so than other tumors	• Edema

Note: "Dural tail"[22] sign; most specific for meningioma on contrast-enhanced T1-weighted MR images.[18] The dural tail is strong linear contrast-enhancement at the border of the tumor with the adjacent meninges because of vascular congestion in the dura mater, and not necessarily because of tumor invasion[23] (see Figure 10-2, *A*).

The "Golf tee" sign is characteristic of intradural-extramedullary lesions of the vertebral column. The differential diagnosis for this sign includes but is not limited to meningiomas, nerve sheath tumors, and, depending on location/signalment, nephroblastoma.[23]

Edema is non-specific and often peritumoral. Seizure-related edema can be seen with brain neoplasia. The edema is not restricted to the peritumoral region, can be symmetric, tends to affect the piriform/temporal lobe region, has variable contrast enhancement, and most importantly, will resolve once the seizure activity is resolved. Do not misinterpret seizure-related edema in a patient with a brain tumor as a multi-focal inflammatory or neoplastic disease process.[24]

The intensity or density of the lesions has been purposefully omitted since this generally does not define a tumor type. Most lesions are isodense to hypodense on CT prior to contrast administration. Most lesions are hyperintense on T2-weighted MR with isointense to hypointense on T1-weighted MR. Variations in these generalities depend on the amount of edema, hemorrhage, mineralization, and cellular content.[6,7,9,10,18,25]

*Choroid plexus tumors include papillomas and carcinomas. Ependymoma should also be in the differential diagnosis for these imaging characteristics.[7,21]

THORACIC IMAGING

CT is the imaging method of choice for thoracic cancer detection and staging. The anatomy of the normal canine and feline thorax on CT images has been described.[26,27] The greater sensitivity of CT over radiographs in detection of pulmonary nodules and mass lesions is well established in human medicine and more recently in veterinary medicine.[28-34] Advantages of CT over conventional radiography for thoracic oncologic imaging include its superior contrast resolution and the ability to create multiplanar and 3D reconstructions of complex anatomy.[28]

Studies in humans and animals have shown that helical CT can detect smaller and more numerous pulmonary nodules than radiographs or conventional CT.[31,32] With radiographs, soft-tissue nodules less than 5 mm are typically not visible in dogs and cats, whereas micrometastatic lesions between 1 and 5 mm are detectable with helical CT (Figure 10-2, B).[33-38] Intravenous contrast augments thoracic CT imaging by increasing soft-tissue contrast and is especially useful in differentiating mediastinal lymph nodes and mass lesions from adjacent vascular structures.

CT is much more widely used than MRI in the chest, since it has several important advantages. In addition to overall lower cost and more widespread availability,

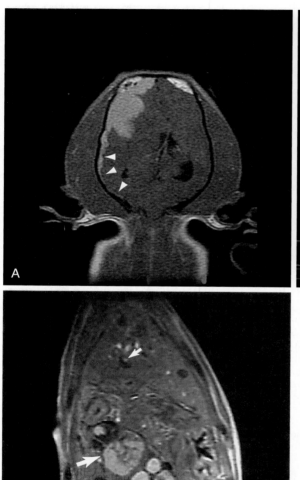

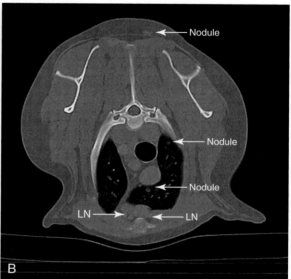

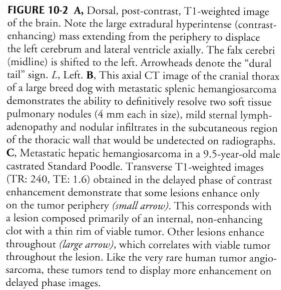

FIGURE 10-2 A, Dorsal, post-contrast, T1-weighted image of the brain. Note the large extradural hyperintense (contrast-enhancing) mass extending from the periphery to displace the left cerebrum and lateral ventricle axially. The falx cerebri (midline) is shifted to the left. Arrowheads denote the "dural tail" sign. *L*, Left. **B,** This axial CT image of the cranial thorax of a large breed dog with metastatic splenic hemangiosarcoma demonstrates the ability to definitively resolve two soft tissue pulmonary nodules (4 mm each in size), mild sternal lymphadenopathy and nodular infiltrates in the subcutaneous region of the thoracic wall that would be undetected on radiographs. **C,** Metastatic hepatic hemangiosarcoma in a 9.5-year-old male castrated Standard Poodle. Transverse T1-weighted images (TR: 240, TE: 1.6) obtained in the delayed phase of contrast enhancement demonstrate that some lesions enhance only on the tumor periphery *(small arrow)*. This corresponds with a lesion composed primarily of an internal, non-enhancing clot with a thin rim of viable tumor. Other lesions enhance throughout *(large arrow)*, which correlates with viable tumor throughout the lesion. Like the very rare human tumor angiosarcoma, these tumors tend to display more enhancement on delayed phase images.

CT imaging is faster than MR imaging. Because of its shorter imaging times, CT generates fewer artifacts associated with cardiac and respiratory motion than does MRI, and anesthesia time is generally shorter.[31,39]

Further, although some fast MR pulse sequences have been used in the chest, this modality is of limited utility in evaluating pulmonary parenchyma in that, by volume, the lung is mostly composed of airspaces and therefore has relatively fewer protons to create MR signal than do other soft tissues.[31,39]

Use of CT and MRI for non-pulmonary thoracic imaging is evolving. MRI has been used for evaluation of the heart in dogs and cats and appears to have use in evaluating heart base mass lesions.[40] For either thoracic CT or MRI, respiratory gating and/or ECG gating can be used to minimize imaging artifacts associated with cardiac and respiratory motion.[31,40,41] However, use of ultrasound generally overshadows CT and MRI in evaluation of the canine/feline heart, because of lower cost, lack of need for anesthesia, wide availability of equipment and experienced sonographers, well-established standard cardiac chamber size measurements, the ability to characterize blood flow with Doppler ultrasound, and display cardiac anatomy in real-time through repeated cycles of contraction.

ABDOMINAL IMAGING

CT and MRI of canine/feline abdomen are not yet widely clinically used. They are firmly established, however, as the standard of care in human oncology for diagnosis, staging, and assessment of response to therapy for many malignancies, including those of the liver,[42] as well as of the spleen, adrenal gland, kidney, and pancreas.

MRI vs. CT

As imaging modalities, MRI and CT have different strengths. CT is capable of greater spatial resolution than MRI. MRI generates greater contrast between soft tissues than does CT or ultrasound, and, in characterization of focal lesions of abdominal organs, this often proves to be an important factor.

MRI's lack of ionizing radiation, the overall safety of gadolinium agents as contrast agents, and the inherently greater soft-tissue contrast associated with MRI represent three important considerations for preferential use of MRI over CT. Factors favoring the use of CT for abdominal oncologic cross-sectional imaging include its relatively wider availability, shorter examination times, greater spatial resolution, and the overall greater familiarity among the veterinary radiology community with this modality. The greater availability and familiarity of CT over MRI are longer true for some institutions and specialists.

In general, abdominal or pelvic MRI studies in the cat and dog are best performed on high-magnetic-field strength scanners (1.0 Tesla and 1.5 Tesla), using respiratory-triggered techniques when possible. Field-of-view choices are highly dependent upon the size of the animal and upon whether or not a surface coil is available. High-resolution MR images can be acquired using respiratory trigger, if available, allowing the patient to breathe on the ventilator while imaging is performed only during relatively motion-free portions of the respiratory cycle.

Pre- and post-contrast imaging may be acquired as either 2D or 3D T1-weighted gradient echo images. The use of gadolinium provides further information regarding a lesion's vascularity, the presence of internal necrosis, resectability, and the presence of non-necrotic tumor. Three-dimensional imaging is increasingly used in the human population and is therefore presented here. Delayed post-contrast images can be acquired in any plane, and coronal post-contrast images are often useful, especially in renal or adrenal imaging. For direct comparison, pre- and post-contrast images must be performed with identical imaging parameters or else valid comparison of pre- and post-contrast signal intensities cannot be made.

CT scanning of the abdomen is best performed on a multidetector-row scanner, but it can be done on any scanner. Pre-contrast images are generally helpful, especially if the issue is focal mass characterization. Multiphasic imaging in the arterial and portal venous phases allows improved lesion detection and characterization, and it is the standard of care in human abdominal oncologic imaging. In general, pre-contrast imaging can be performed in 5-mm sections, whereas arterial and portal venous phase imaging is performed at 3 mm. The dose of iodine-based contrast is 2 ml/kg, up to 100 ml, with injection rates of 2-3 ml/sec. Selected kV is generally 120, whereas mAs of 80 is generally sufficient for a patient of 30 kg; mAs can be lowered for smaller animals, or raised for larger patients, whereas kV is generally kept at 120.

Veterinary Experience

MRI

An early study using a low-field MR characterized several abdominal tumors in eight dogs.[43] Overall MR was in agreement with ultrasound findings; however, in two patients MR enabled further identification of lesions and better depiction of tumor margins than ultrasound.

In a recent study performed on a high-field scanner, 35 focal lesions of either the spleen (n = 8) or the liver (n = 27) were characterized as malignant or benign in

23 dogs.[3] An accuracy of 94% was noted with an overall sensitivity and specificity of 100% (95% CI, 78%-100%) and 90% (95% CI, 68%-99%) (Figure 10-2, *C*).[44] Pertinent MRI characteristics that were used to differentiate malignant from benign lesions are listed in Tables 10-2 and 10-3.

CT

A recent study documented the use of CT to accurately distinguish benign (n = 14) from malignant (n = 10) splenic masses in 21 dogs.[45] Malignant lesions had significantly lower attenuation than non-malignant lesions. It was suggested that a threshold of 55 HU could be used to determine benign vs. malignant, since values greater than 55 were associated with benign lesions and values less than 55 were associated with malignant lesions. With this threshold, a sensitivity of 100% and specificity of 78.6% were noted.

CT/MRI EVALUATION OF NASAL TUMORS

CT and MRI were compared for assessing nasal tumor invasion into the central nervous system in four dogs.[46] MRI was superior for evaluating peritumoral edema, displacement of normal tissues, and in one dog, extension through the cribriform plate. However, the scanning technique and equipment used may have influenced these differences.[1] The optimal scanning plane for evaluating tumor extension into the cribriform plate is the dorsal imaging plane. In CT, dorsal reformatting of thinly sliced transverse images can also be performed.[47,48]

CT imaging signs that are most helpful in differentiating nasal tumors from rhinitis in dogs and cats are as follows:

- Patchy areas of increased density within a soft tissue dense mass[49]
- Severe destruction of nasal turbinates, ethmoturbinates, maxillae, and/or nasal bones[49-51]
- Hyperostosis of the lateral maxilla[49]
- Lysis of the nasal septum[50,52]
- Extension of soft tissue density to the orbit or facial soft tissues[52]

Note: mild to moderate turbinate destruction with scattered areas of soft-tissue density can be identified with rhinitis. Destruction tends to be more severe with neoplasia.[49,50,52]

TABLE 10-2 HEPATIC LESION CHARACTERIZATION RELATIVE TO NORMAL LIVER

	T1	T2	Post-Gd	Other
Malignant				
HCC	Isointense to liver	Isointense to mildly ↑	↑↑↑	Capsule; abnormal hepatic architecture
Hemangiosarcoma	↓↓	↑↑	↑↑	Multiplicity; continuous rim enhancement, progressive enhancement in delayed phase
Metastatic disease	↓↓	↑	↑	Multiplicity; continuous rim enhancement
Benign				
Regenerative nodules	Isointense	Isointense	Isointense	Nodular contour to liver
Pseudolesion	Isointense	Isointense	Isointense	No lesion present

Up arrows represent lesion hyperintensity relative to normal organ; down arrows represent lesion hypointensity relative to normal organ.
Gd, Gadolinium; HCC, hepatocellular carcinoma.

TABLE 10-3 SPLENIC LESION CHARACTERIZATION RELATIVE TO NORMAL SPLEEN

	T1	T2	Post-Gd	Other
MALIGNANT				
Metastatic disease	↓	↑	↑↑	Heterogeneous enhancement
BENIGN				
Lymphoid hyperplasia	↓	↓↓	↓↓	

Down arrows represent hypointensity; up arrows represent hyperintensity.
Gd, Gadolinium.

High accuracy of CT for diagnosis of dogs with different sources of chronic nasal disease (neoplasia, nonspecific rhinitis, fungal rhinitis) has been reported.[51] The accuracy, sensitivity, specificity, positive predictive value, and negative predictive value of CT in dogs with nasal neoplasia was 96%-98%, 89%, 98%-100%, 94%-100%, and 96%-97%, respectively.[51]

Nasal tumor staging based on CT findings has been described. The World Health Organization (WHO) system for clinical staging of neoplasms of the nasal and paranasal cavities of dogs did not have prognostic relevance for management.[53,54] A modified staging scheme based initially on radiographic evaluation held promise for prognosis.[53] When modified staging schemes were extrapolated to CT as the imaging modality, no difference in survival was found between stages.[54,55] Finally, and most recently, a four-category modification of the WHO system showed a significant difference in relapse-free interval as well as survival based on staging.[56] The categories are as follows:

T1: confined to one nasal passage, paranasal sinus or frontal sinus, with no bone involvement

T2: any bone involvement, but with no evidence of orbit, subcutaneous, or submucosal mass

T3: involvement of orbit, or a subcutaneous or submucosal mass

T4: tumor extension into nasopharynx or cribriform plate

CT/MR images target specific areas of the nose for guiding biopsy tools. This decreases the likelihood of attaining an unrepresentative biopsy sample. CT/MR are superior to rhinoscopy alone in the ability to evaluate the extent of disease.[50] Dynamic CT measurement of contrast medium wash-in kinetics (perfusion) of canine nasal tumors has been used as a way to measure tumor oxygenation for assessing local tumor control following radiation therapy. No identifiable pattern of perfusion alteration was detected.[57]

MUSCULOSKELETAL IMAGING
Osteosarcoma

- T1-weighted imaging is most useful for estimating the intramedullary extent of disease.[58,59]
- MRI may be less accurate at defining true length of disease, but in one report, it never underestimated extent of disease.[58] In another report, MRI underestimated four of eight cases.[59] Both reports recommend MRI in the preoperative assessment of a limb-sparing procedure.[58,59]
- In people, transient MR changes consistent with bone edema can mimic bone marrow–replacing lesions such as neoplasia.[60]

Nerve Sheath Tumors

- CT and MR have been described for nerve sheath tumors in dogs, primarily originating from the brachial plexus. Early detection is critical.[61-64]
- Detectable masses in dogs with clinical signs of nerve root disease are generally larger than 1 cm with contrast-enhanced CT; enhancement is typical (20 of 24 dogs) and often rim enhancing (13 of 24 dogs).[62]
- Few studies describe the MR imaging features of nerve sheath tumors in dogs; T2-weighted images appeared to increase lesion conspicuity relative to T1-weighted images. Contrast-enhanced T1-weighted images and fat saturation techniques are also helpful.[63,64]
- Contrast enhancement of denervated muscle is described; the pattern of enhancement is appropriate for the distribution of the nerves affected and this may help identify small tumors.[65]
- In the cat, lymphoma of the brachial plexus was identified with MR.[66]
- In people, MR evaluation of brachial plexus abnormalities is superior to CT.[67,68]

Selected References*

Cherubini GB, Mantis P, Martinez TA, et al: Utility of magnetic resonance imaging for distinguishing neoplastic from non-neoplastic brain lesions in dogs and cats, *Vet Radiol Ultrasound* 5:384-387, 2005.
This is a pivotal study to evaluate benign and malignant brain lesions with MRI in both dogs and cats.
Clifford CA, Pretorius ES, Weisse C, et al: Magnetic resonance imaging of focal splenic and hepatic lesions in the dog, *J Vet Intern Med* 18:330-338, 2004.
This prospective study determined MRI had a high sensitivity and specificity in determining malignant vs. benign splenic and hepatic lesions.
Nemanic S, London CA, Wisner ER: Comparison of thoracic radiographs and single breath-hold helical CT for detection of pulmonary nodules in dogs with metastatic neoplasia, *J Vet Intern Med* 20:508-515, 2006.
This study confirmed the superiority of CT to evaluate pulmonary nodules vs. radiographs.
Saunders JH, Van Bree H, Gielen I, de Rooster H: Diagnostic value of computed tomography in dogs with chronic nasal disease, *Vet Radiol Ultrasound* 44:409-413, 2003.
An excellent review of CT characteristics associated with a variety of nasal diseases in dogs.
Thomas WB, Wheeler SJ, Kramer R, et al: Magnetic resonance imaging features of primary brain tumors in dogs, *Vet Radiol Ultrasound* 37:20-27, 1996.

This is an excellent review on lesion characterization of brain tumors in dogs.

Troxel MT, Vite CH, Massicotte C, et al: Magnetic resonance imaging features of feline intracranial neoplasia: retrospective analysis of 46 cats, *J Vet Intern Med* 18:176-189, 2004.

A large retrospective study evaluating brain lesions in cats via MRI.

■ *For a complete list of the references cited in this chapter, please go to www.smallanimaloncology.com.

SECTION C: Nuclear Scintigraphy

Cristi R. Cook

KEY POINTS

- Nuclear scintigraphy is an important imaging procedure for the oncologic patient.
- Scintigraphy is useful in determining the functional and physiologic evaluation of a variety of organs.
- Scintigraphy is an important procedure for determining the extent of a disease, including ectopic tissues and areas of metastasis.
- Radiopharmaceuticals are available for both diagnosis and treatment of a variety of neoplastic conditions.
- Technetium-99m is the radioisotope of choice for many diagnostic techniques in scintigraphy, but other commonly used agents in human medicine are becoming more widely used in veterinary medicine in recent years.

Nuclear scintigraphy is an important imaging modality in oncology. Nuclear scintigraphy provides both physiologic and anatomic data. As such, it allows for diagnosis, staging, treatment planning, and prognostication. Nuclear scintigraphy in oncology involves the use of technetium-99m (^{99m}Tc) pertechnetate labeled to various agents to be excreted, secreted, or taken up by the organ of interest.[1,2]

THYROID SCINTIGRAPHY

Thyroid scintigraphy is one of the most commonly performed procedures in veterinary nuclear medicine. Technetium pertechnetate, which concentrates within active thyroid tissue in feline hyperthyroidism and canine thyroid carcinomas, is the isotope of choice. Other agents, such as ^{123}I and ^{131}I, also concentrate in active thyroid tissue, but are less frequently used for diagnostic imaging because of cost, availability, and radiation safety concerns.[3]

Indications for thyroid scintigraphy include the following:

1. Evaluate thyroid function
2. Determine extent of involvement of pathology
3. Determine benign versus malignant disease
4. Determine presence and location of ectopic thyroid tissue
5. Evaluate for functional metastatic lesions
6. Determine efficacy of therapy[1-6]

The recommended dose for ^{99m}Tc is 1 to 4 mCi (37 to 148 MBq) in cats and 2 to 5 mCi (74 to 185 MBq) in dogs. Following injection of ^{99m}Tc, right and left lateral and ventral views of the neck and thorax are obtained using a general purpose (e.g., LEAP) collimator.

The isotope is primarily eliminated in the urine, with a small amount secreted from the salivary glands and gastric mucosa and eliminated in the feces. The secretion of the ^{99m}Tc in the salivary glands is used as a reference to evaluate the thyroid tissue uptake (normal range 0.6:1–1.03:1, thyroid to salivary).[3,6,7]

A normal thyroid scan (Figure 10-3, A) reveals uniform uptake in symmetrical, elliptical, or oval thyroid lobes. The margins of the lobes should be smooth and regular.

Thyroid hyperplasia is the most common cause of hyperthyroidism in cats. When hyperplastic, the thyroid lobes have increased uptake of ^{99m}Tc compared with the salivary glands. They are smooth, with a regular border with homogeneous uptake. One or both lobes may be enlarged. Unilateral disease accounts for approximately 30% of the cases. Adenomas may be single or multiple, resulting in one or both lobes showing a multifocal increase in uptake within the lobe(s) (Figure 10-3, *B*). These are best seen using a pinhole collimator.

Thyroid carcinomas occur in 2% to 5% of the cases of feline hyperthyroidism (Figure 10-3, *C*).[3,8,9] Carcinomas typically have a heterogeneous uptake pattern with irregular margins or a linear or tail-like appearance along the pole. However, this appearance may also be seen with multifocal adenomas. Uptake may also be seen in the cranial mediastinum from ectopic or metastatic disease or within the lung from metastatic disease. If irregular and enlarged lobes are seen on the scan, biopsy should be performed to confirm malignancy.

Canine thyroid tumors account for approximately 1% to 4% of all tumors in dogs and are typically carcinomas

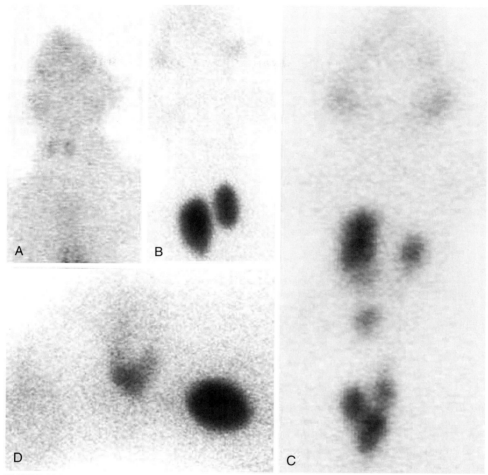

FIGURE 10-3 A, Ventral view of head and neck, normal feline thyroid scintigraphy. **B**, Ventral view of neck, bilateral thyroid enlargement with discrete margins consistent with a thyroid adenoma. **C**, Ventral view of neck, thyroid enlargement with extension of multiple nodes and ectopic tissue into the cranial mediastinum, consistent with a thyroid carcinoma. **D**, Lateral view of head and neck, canine thyroid carcinoma (functional).

(63%–88%).[3,8,10] There are functional (Figure 10-3, *D*) and nonfunctional thyroid carcinomas with heterogeneous, unilateral uptake or no uptake, respectively, within the thyroid parenchyma. The majority of canine thyroid carcinomas are euthyroid with an estimated 10% considered hyperfunctional.[8]

Isotope therapy with ^{131}I can be an effective method of treatment for hyperplasia and for some functional tumors. When ectopic thyroid tissue is present, it is the preferred method of therapy.

Complications with ^{131}I for benign disease are uncommon, with iatrogenic hypothyroidism being the most commonly reported.[8,11] Complications of high-dose ^{131}I for thyroid carcinoma include a transient myelosuppression, radiation pneumonitis, thyroiditis, or sialodenitis.[9,11] Other medical, surgical, or radiation therapy treatments for thyroid adenomas or carcinomas may also be indicated.

BONE SCINTIGRAPHY

Bone scintigraphy is one of the most common nuclear scintigraphy procedures performed in small animals.[12,13] For oncology cases, it is commonly used to determine presence and extent of pathology, detect metastases, and aid in treatment planning.

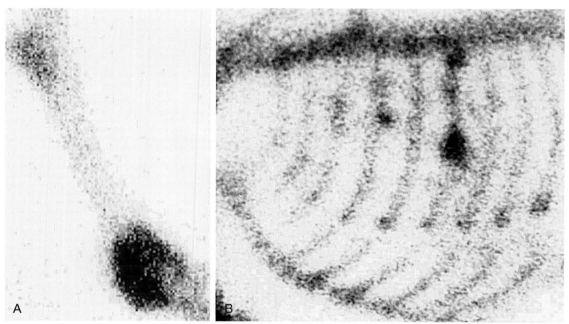

FIGURE 10-4 **A**, Distal radial metaphyseal osteosarcoma. **B**, Pulmonary metastasis with radiopharmaceutical uptake.

The isotope used in bone scintigraphy is ^{99m}Tc labeled to a phosphonate, either methylene diphosphonate (^{99m}Tc-MDP), hydroxyethylene diphosphonate (^{99m}Tc-HEDP), or hydroxymethylene diphosphonate (^{99m}Tc-HMDP). Recommended doses are 3 to 5 mCi for cats and 5 to 20 mCi for dogs. Three imaging phases can be assessed. The vascular phase occurs immediately; the soft tissue phase at 5 to 10 minutes, and the bone phase at 2 hours after injection. For oncologic imaging, the bone phase is the most commonly used, with acquisition starting at 1 hour (HDP) or 2 hours (MDP) after injection. Multiple lateral and dorsal or palmar/plantar views of the whole body are obtained.[2,12]

The major factors that influence uptake of these isotopes are increased osteoblastic activity and, to a lesser degree, increased blood flow.[2,12,13] Normal areas of increase in radiopharmaceutical uptake include the epiphyses, costochondral junctions, temporomandibular joints, ventral skull, and actively growing physes in immature patients.[12] Lesions are identified by finding focal, asymmetrical areas of uptake. Neoplastic bone lesions are primarily metaphyseal and occasionally diaphyseal in origin (Figure 10-4, A). Bone tumors tend to show marked increases in intensity. The entire skeleton should be carefully evaluated for areas of increased uptake. Neoplastic lesions must be differentiated from non-neoplastic lesions. Osteoarthrosis of a joint typically has mild to moderate uptake in the bone on either side of the joint.[13] Rarely, pulmonary metastatic disease will have uptake of the radiopharmaceutical (Figure 10-4, B). To determine if these areas are within the parenchyma and not along the rib or costochondral junctions, lateral, dorsal, and ventral views of the thorax are performed. Comprehensive assessment is important for staging disease, planning treatment, and determining prognosis.

OTHER ONCOLOGIC IMAGING

Renal morphology and function can be determined with ^{99m}Tc-dimercaptosuccinic acid (DMSA). The isotope will accumulate within the normal parenchyma and not within the mass (cyst, tumor, or abscess).[14,15] ^{99m}Tc sulfur colloid (SC) is used to image hepatic and splenic masses. The mass is identified by a photopenic region within the parenchyma and is not specific for an etiology. However, this technique is not commonly used based on the advantages of ultrasound and CT.[16] Similarly, brain scintigraphy is rarely used based on the availability and advantages of MRI and CT. When used, ^{99m}Tc-diethylenetriaminepentaacetic acid (DTPA) or glucoheptonate (^{99m}Tc-GHA) are the preferred agents.[17,18] A normal study would be void of radiopharmaceutical within the calvarium. Increased uptake within the calvarium indicates disruption of the blood brain barrier.[2,17,18] Location, pattern, and intensity of the uptake aid in suggesting the type of lesion (neoplastic, inflammatory, or cerebrovascular). Pheochromocytoma imaging has been accomplished in a dog with the use of ^{123}I-labeled metaiodobenzylguanidine (^{123}I-MIBG). This is used commonly in people to image tumors of neural crest origin. The MIBG structure is similar to norepinephrine. Therefore, it is taken up and stored by the neurosecretory granules in neural crest cells and can be used to image the adrenal medulla. Since pheochromocytomas are rare in dogs, this technique has limited use in veterinary medicine.[19]

Daniel GB, Berry CR, (eds): *Textbook of veterinary nuclear medicine*, Raleigh, 2006, North Carolina State University.
This is a comprehensive textbook of nuclear medicine protocols, normal imaging, as well as findings in various diseases.
Daniel GB, Mitchell SK, Mawby D, et al: Renal nuclear medicine: a review, *Vet Radiol Ultrasound* 40:572, 1999.
This is a comprehensive review of the anatomy and physiology, radiopharmaceuticals, and imaging protocols and interpretations of renal scintigraphy.
Henrikson TD, Armbrust LJ, Hoskinson JJ, et al: Thyroid to salivary ratios determined by technetium-99[m] pertechnetate imaging in thirty-two euthyroid cats, *Vet Radiol Ultrasound* 46:521, 2005.
This is a prospective study on the scintigraphic thyroid appearance in normal, middle-aged to geriatric cats with comparison of thyroid to salivary ratios.

Selected References*

Adams WH, Walker MA, Daniel GB, et al: Treatment of differentiated thyroid carcinoma in 7 dogs utilizing ^{131}I, *Vet Radiol Ultrasound* 36:417, 1995.
This is an article on the treatment and safety of treating canine thyroid carcinomas with high-dose ^{131}I therapy.

*For a complete list of the references cited in this chapter, please go to www.smallanimaloncology.com.

11 Paraneoplastic Syndromes

Ruthanne Chun

KEY POINTS

- Paraneoplastic syndromes (PNS) are caused by tumor-produced substances that have a systemic effect.
- Effective treatment of most PNS requires control of the underlying malignancy.
- The PNS may cause more morbidity and mortality than the tumor itself.
- The PNS may precede clinically detectable tumor, and monitoring for recurrence of the PNS can be a sensitive and specific way to monitor for tumor relapse.
- Hypercalcemia is the most common of the PNS.

Paraneoplastic syndromes (PNS) are systemic disorders resulting from substances produced by a tumor. According to the strictest definition, PNS are caused by the production and release of substances not normally produced by the tumor cell of origin or in amounts not normally produced by those cells. Hypoglycemia resulting from an insulinoma, hyperglobulinemia resulting from multiple myeloma, and hyperestrogenism resulting from testicular tumors are mentioned in this chapter because of their effects on multiple systems in the body. Pathologies caused by PNS, as opposed to the finding of a tumor, may be the factor that prompts the client to pursue veterinary attention. Other etiologies of PNS aside from production of metabolically active substances include autoimmune disease induction, immune complex formation, immunosuppression, and ectopic receptor production/competitive blockade of normal hormones. PNS may also arise because of substances produced by normal cells caused by presence of the tumor (e.g., tumor necrosis factor production contributing to cancer cachexia). Many PNS in veterinary medicine are of unknown etiology.

PNS are common in human cancer patients. The PNS may precede identification of the cancer by weeks to years. Thus, recognition of PNS is important for many reasons. A PNS may be the first sign of disease, facilitating work-up and diagnosis. Monitoring the PNS can be an effective means of evaluating response to anticancer therapy and tumor relapse.

Clinically, PNS can cause greater morbidity and mortality than the primary tumor, thus greatly impacting patient quality and quantity of life. While resolution of the underlying tumor is the best way to eliminate the PNS, symptomatic therapies may control the PNS and improve quality of life. PNS, the tumors that cause them, clinical signs, and frequency are summarized in Table 11-1.

ENDOCRINOLOGIC PARANEOPLASTIC SYNDROMES

Hypercalcemia

Hypercalcemia of malignancy is most commonly caused by production of parathyroid hormone-related peptide (PTH-rp) by tumor cells.[1-3] It is most often associated with lymphoma, anal sac adenocarcinoma, multiple myeloma, thymoma, and, especially in cats, squamous cell carcinoma; however, many other tumors have been linked with hypercalcemia.[4-14] Hypercalcemia may also be caused by primary hyperparathyroidism and excessive production of parathyroid hormone (PTH).[1,2] Although serum 1,25-dihydroxycholecalciferol (calcitriol) plays a role in hypercalcemia of malignancy in people, it does not appear to play a significant role in veterinary patients.[15-18] Other differentials for hypercalcemia are listed in Box 11-1.[19-21]

The most common clinical sign associated with this PNS is polyuria resulting from calcium interfering with

TABLE 11-1   SUMMARY OF PARANEOPLASTIC SYNDROMES, THE TUMORS WITH WHICH THEY ARE ASSOCIATED, THEIR SYSTEMIC EFFECT, AND FREQUENCY

Paraneoplastic Syndrome	Associated Tumor(s)	Systemic Effect	Frequency
Endocrinologic paraneoplastic syndromes			
Hypercalcemia	LSA, MM, thymoma, anal sac adenocarcinoma, parathyroid tumors, miscellaneous other	Polyuria/polydipsia, renal failure, arrhythmias, seizures, coma, death	Common
Hypoglycemia	LSA, intestinal and hepatic tumors, insulinoma	Behavioral changes, seizures, death	Uncommon
Hyperestrogenism	Testicular tumors	Alopecia, gynecomastia, skin changes, pancytopenia	Uncommon
Hematologic paraneoplastic syndromes			
Anemia	LSA, MM, thymoma, HSA	Weakness, inappetence, or anorexia	Common
Polycythemia	Renal and nasal tumors	Polydipsia, dark red mucous membranes, inappetence/anorexia, seizures, death	Rare
Thrombocytopenia and coagulopathies	HSA, LSA, MM, multiple others	Petechiation, bleeding tendencies	Common
Hyperglobulinemia	LSA, MM	Increased susceptibility to infection; hyperviscosity that is associated with heart failure, bleeding tendencies, renal failure, behavioral changes, seizures, polyuria	Uncommon
Neutrophilic leukocytosis	Renal tumors, HSA	None	Rare
Neurologic Paraneoplastic Syndromes			
Myasthenia gravis, peripheral neuropathy	LSA, thymoma, miscellaneous other	Regurgitation, weakness, depends upon affected site	Rare
Cutaneous Paraneoplastic Syndromes			
Alopecia	Pancreatic or biliary CA, thymoma—cats	Easily epilated hair or alopecia	Rare
Superficial necrolytic dermatitis	Glucagonoma or glucagon-secreting tumors, liver CA, pancreatic CA—cats	Alopecia, skin erosions and crusts, pad hyperkeratosis	Rare
Miscellaneous Paraneoplastic Syndromes			
Hypertrophic osteopathy	Intrathoracic and intra-abdominal tumors	Lameness (often shifting leg lameness), limb edema	Uncommon
Fever	Any	Lethargy, anorexia	Rare
Cachexia	Any	Weight loss and anorexia	Rare

CA, Carcinoma; *HSA*, hemangiosarcoma; *LSA*, lymphoma; *MM*, multiple myeloma.

renal tubule cell response to anti-diuretic hormone. Other signs may include polydipsia, inappetence, vomiting, weakness, bradycardia, obtundation, and death.

Because ionized calcium is the biologically active fraction, animals with elevated total calcium should be evaluated with measurement of ionized calcium. If the ionized calcium is high, serum should be submitted for PTH and PTH-rp measurement. It is important to note that not all animals with hypercalcemia of malignancy have persistently elevated serum calcium; values may

---

BOX 11-1   NON-NEOPLASTIC DIFFERENTIAL DIAGNOSES FOR HYPERCALCEMIA[19-21]

Laboratory error
Primary renal disease
Primary hyperparathyroidism
Hypervitaminosis D
    Cholecalciferol rodenticides
    Plant ingestion such as calcitrol glycosides
    Iatrogenic
Hypervitaminosis A
Hemoconcentration
Hyperproteinemia
Skeletal lesions
    Hypertrophic osteodystrophy
    Osteomyelitis
    Disuse osteoporosis
Factitious
    Lipemia
    Post-prandial samples
    Young animal <6–12 mos
Thiazide diuretics
Granulomatous disease
Hypoadrenocorticism
Idiopathic hypercalcemia of cats

---

fluctuate. If the PTH is normal or high in the face of hypercalcemia, primary hyperparathyroidism is likely. If the PTH-rp is normal or high in the face of hypercalcemia, malignancy is likely.

Therapy for hypercalcemia of malignancy is two-fold: treatment of the hypercalcemia if necessary and, more importantly, of the underlying malignancy. Animals with clinical signs of hypercalcemia beyond polyuria (e.g., weak, vomiting, bradycardic), typically those with total calcium ≥18 mg/dL, should be hospitalized and treated with aggressive fluid therapy using a calcium-replete solution (e.g., 0.9% NaCl at >66 ml/kg/day with urine output goal of 2 ml/kg/hr). Furosemide (2–4 mg/kg PO, SC, or IV bid) may be administered to promote calciuresis, provided the patient is well hydrated. Aside from serious clinical signs, other indications for treatment include a calcium phosphorus product (total calcium × phosphorus) ≥60. Other pharmacologic options for decreasing calcium include prednisone (1–2 mg/kg PO, SC, or IV bid), calcitonin (4-6 IU/kg SC bid to tid) or bisphosphonates.[22] The use of prednisone is ill-advised unless the patient has been screened for lymphoma, since steroid use may induce remission of this disease and can make

subsequent diagnosis impossible. Calcitonin use may fall out of favor now that bisphosphonates are available and have been used in veterinary patients. Patients with unresolved hypercalcemia after saline-induced diuresis and furosemide should be treated with pamidronate at 1 mg/kg given over 2 hours in 250 ml 0.9% saline.[22,23] Effective treatment of the underlying malignancy is the approach most likely to resolve the hypercalcemia.

Hypoglycemia

Hypoglycemia is defined as a blood glucose of <60 mg/dL. The most common malignant cause is insulinoma.[24-26] It is also reported as a result of lymphoma, hepatocellular carcinoma and hepatoma, smooth-muscle intestinal tumors, hemangiosarcoma, salivary gland adenocarcinoma, renal adenocarcinoma, and oral melanoma.[27-33] Non-neoplastic differentials include liver dysfunction, hypoadrenocorticism, breed-related causes (e.g., hunting dog hypoglycemia or hypoglycemia of young toy or miniature breeds), or sepsis. Rarely, artifactual hypoglycemia occurs with prolonged storage of blood samples before processing.

Early clinical signs of hypoglycemia are subtle and include behavioral changes, polyphagia, polyuria, and polydipsia. More obvious later signs are muscle fasciculations, lethargy, weakness and collapse, and seizures. Diagnosis of hypoglycemia is straightforward; patients may have profound hypoglycemia (<30 mg/dL) at presentation.

Treatment of hypoglycemia in the severely symptomatic patient is administration of a 1- to 5-ml bolus of 50% dextrose given slowly intravenously. Since this may result in rebound release of insulin and worsening of clinical signs, it is important to treat patients to effect only. Once the animal is sternal, it should be fed a small meal. If the pet is seizing at home, the client can pour a sugar solution (i.e., syrup) over the pet's gums and then attempt to feed the pet once it is sternal. Intractable seizures can be managed preoperatively in hospital with a constant rate infusion of glucagon (starting at 5–10 ng/kg/min), or the animal may be managed with diazepam or other anticonvulsant therapy.[5,34]

Ideally the causative tumor should be surgically debulked.[35] If this is not feasible because of cost or metastatic disease, medical management may reduce the severity of clinical signs for a period of weeks to months (see Chapter 26, Section D, for more information).

Hyperestrogenism

Sertoli cell tumors of the testicle are the most common cause of hyperestrogenism. In particular, tumors in cryptorchid testicles are more likely to be associated with excessive estrogen production.[36]

Clinical signs and physical examination findings associated with hyperestrogenism include non-pruritic symmetric alopecia, hyperpigmentation, gynecomastia, asymmetrically enlarged prostate, and a pendulous prepuce.[37] Clients may report that their dog is attractive to intact male dogs and that the dog squats to urinate.[36] Significantly, hyperestrogenism can cause bone marrow toxicity, which results in pancytopenia and manifests clinically as lethargy, hemorrhage resulting from thrombocytopenia, petechiae, vomiting, anorexia, fever, and pale mucous membranes.[36] A complete blood count (CBC) shows pancytopenia; bone marrow evaluation indicating hypocellularity confirms decreased production. Diagnosis of hyperestrogenism is often presumptive based on typical history, clinical signs, physical examination or ultrasound, and clinicopathologic findings.

Successful treatment of hyperestrogenism resulting from a Sertoli cell tumor relies on tumor removal.[36,37] Animals with marrow suppression may be treated supportively with broad-spectrum antibiotics and red blood cell transfusions; there is no effective way to increase platelet count, and the prognosis for marrow recovery is usually poor. If the marrow does recover, it can take weeks to months before the blood count normalizes.

HEMATOLOGIC PARANEOPLASTIC SYNDROMES

Anemia

Anemia is a commonly recognized PNS in veterinary patients.[38] It can occur because of hemorrhage, destruction (immune mediated or as a result of microangiopathic disease), or decreased production (associated with anemia of chronic disease or myelophthisis). Hemorrhage is commonly associated with hemangiosarcoma, gastric tumors, and mast cell tumors (bleeding from the primary tumor or from gastric ulcers), but any neoplasm can erode through blood vessels and result in bleeding.[39-42] Immune-mediated red blood cell destruction occurs as a PNS with lymphoma and multiple myeloma. Microangiopathic disease is typically linked with hemangiosarcoma, but any metastatic tumor causing disseminated intravascular coagulation (DIC) will have a component of microangiopathic hemolytic anemia.[43,44] Anemia of chronic disease rarely causes significant morbidity in cancer patients. This anemia is due to disordered iron storage and metabolism, shortened red blood cell life span, and, potentially, decreased marrow responsiveness.[38] Likewise, the anemia resulting from chemotherapy rarely causes clinical signs. Myelophthisis, most common with lymphoma and other leukemias, can be a major cause of patient morbidity and mortality. Because red blood cells circulate longer than all other blood cells, animals with myelophthisis-related anemias generally have other life-threatening cytopenias. As noted, hyperestrogenism can also cause anemia.

Clinical signs of anemia include weakness, lethargy, and inappetence or anorexia. Pale mucous membranes and tachycardia are common physical examination findings. Particular attention should be paid to red blood cell morphology to help classify the anemia as regenerative or non-regenerative and to determine if hemolysis is present.

Treatment of anemia depends on the cause. If hemorrhage is the underlying cause, transfusions (see Chapter 13, Section C) and tumor removal are indicated. Bleeding ulcers are treated with oral anti-acids (H2 blockers such as famotidine at 0.5 mg/kg/day or omeprazole at 0.5–1 mg/kg/day, dose should not exceed 20 mg/day) and gastric protectants (sucralfate at 0.5–1 gm orally every 8–12 hours or misoprostol at 2–5 µg/kg every 8–12 hours). Resolution of hemolytic anemia requires control of the primary tumor, but therapy with immunosuppressive doses (2 mg/kg/day) of prednisone is also indicated. Unless it is caused by lymphoma, myelophthisis is difficult to resolve; the long-term prognosis for any animal with myelophthisis is grave. Exogenous administration of erythropoietin is not indicated in the majority of cases, since therapies directed at the primary tumor typically result in resolution of the anemia.

Polycythemia

This uncommon PNS is reported with renal tumors, lymphoma, liver tumors, schwannoma, nasal fibrosarcoma, and transmissible venereal tumors.[45-51] Excessive erythropoietin production by tumor cells, or as a result of renal hypoxia, is the most common cause. Other underlying causes include arteriovenous shunts and polycythemia vera (a myeloproliferative disorder in which there is excessive normal red blood cell production and decreased erythropoietin production).[52,53]

Clinical signs and physical examination findings with polycythemia include erythema of the mucous membranes, polydipsia, and neurologic signs such as disorientation, ataxia, and seizures resulting from hyperviscosity or hypervolemia. Polycythemia is readily apparent on a CBC, but every attempt should be made to elucidate the cause, since therapies differ depending upon etiology. Relative polycythemia is seen with hemoconcentration from dehydration, splenic contraction, or hypovolemia. In this case, the absolute red blood cell mass is not increased. Absolute polycythemia is characterized by an increase in red blood cell mass as a result of tissue hypoxia, increased erythropoietin production, or a myeloproliferative disorder. Diagnostic evaluation should include a CBC, chemistry profile, thoracic radiographs, arterial blood gas, and abdominal ultrasound. Erythropoietin levels can be measured, and a bone marrow aspirate may be necessary.[49]

Relative polycythemia is treated with rehydration. Therapeutic phlebotomy and volume replacement are indicated for absolute polycythemia with a hematocrit >65%. Removal of 20 ml of blood/kg body weight, and replacement of that volume with crystalloid fluids, should bring the hematocrit down by approximately 15%. This procedure may be repeated every 2 to 4 weeks if necessary. Resolution of the underlying tumor is essential for complete resolution of polycythemia. In the case of polycythemia vera, therapy with hydroxyurea (30 mg/kg/day for 10 days followed by 15 mg/kg/day) may maintain the red blood cell mass close to normal.[54]

Thrombocytopenia and Coagulopathies

A wide range of tumors have been associated with thrombocytopenia and other coagulopathies, including lymphoma, melanoma, hemangiosarcoma, osteosarcoma, mast cell tumor, and various carcinomas.[55-57] Like anemia, thrombocytopenia arises with increased utilization, destruction, or decreased production. Increased utilization is associated with hemorrhage (hemangiosarcoma, mast cell tumors) or coagulopathies such as DIC seen with metastatic tumors and hemangiosarcoma.[43,55] Immune-mediated destruction of platelets is seen with lymphoma or multiple myeloma. Decreased platelet production resulting from myelophthisis can occur with hematologic malignancies.

Clinical signs and physical examination findings in thrombocytopenic animals includes petechiation and, potentially, hemorrhage. Signs vary depending upon the body cavity into which the bleeding is occurring.

Treatment of thrombocytopenia varies depending upon the cause. As with all PNS, resolution of the underlying tumor is ideal. Hemorrhage-related thrombocytopenia is best managed by surgical resection of the bleeding tumor. Because these patients are often anemic and thrombocytopenic, administration of fresh whole blood immediately before or during surgery may be indicated. Animals that are not anemic but that are actively bleeding because of thrombocytopenia would benefit from a transfusion of either platelet-rich plasma or platelet concentrate. Patients with paraneoplastic DIC and thrombocytopenia have a poor prognosis. Fresh or fresh-frozen plasma will replace depleted coagulation factors; the only way to supply functional platelets is through a fresh

whole blood transfusion. Unless the cause of DIC can be reversed, the patient is unlikely to survive. Immune-mediated thrombocytopenia is managed with immunosuppressive dosages of corticosteroids and chemotherapy to treat the tumor.

Neutrophilic Leukocytosis

Neutrophilic leukocytosis is a rare PNS associated with renal carcinomas (both transitional cell and tubular), lymphoma, metastatic fibrosarcoma, and rectal adenomatous polyp.[58-62] This PNS is thought to occur because of tumor production of colony-stimulating factors (CSFs) such as granulocyte monocyte (GM)-CSF or granulocyte (G)-CSF.[63] This PNS is an incidental finding and should resolve upon successful treatment of the underlying tumor.

Hyperglobulinemia

Hyperglobulinemia is most commonly associated with multiple myeloma, although it has been reported with lymphoma and may occur with any neoplasm.[7,13,64,65]

Signs of hyperglobulinemia are often very non-specific, but excessive globulin production can cause multiple problems for the patient. Frequent infections can occur because excessive globulin production by the tumor inhibits production of normal immunoglobulin. Hyperviscosity syndrome arises as a result of the massive hyperproteinemia. Increased perfusion pressure and hypervolemia increase the cardiac workload and cause cardiomegaly. Poor perfusion results in cardiac and/or renal failure and retinopathies, as well as neurologic abnormalities including lethargy, ataxia, and seizures. Increased bleeding tendencies are also common. These are caused by (1) decreased adhesion of platelets to damaged surfaces, (2) interference with the normal clotting cascade including fibrin plug formation, (3) consumption of coagulation factors following multiple bleeding episodes, and (4) hypervolemia and vascular over-distention.[7,64]

Treatment of hyperglobulinemia relies heavily upon resolution of the underlying tumor. Plasmapheresis, a process in which the patient's plasma is removed and replaced with donor plasma, colloidal, or crystalloid solution, may provide immediate relief from hyperviscosity if necessary.[66,67]

NEUROLOGIC PARANEOPLASTIC SYNDROMES
Myasthenia Gravis

This rare PNS is most often seen in thymoma patients but has also been reported with cholangiocellular carcinoma, lymphoma, and osteosarcoma.[68-72] It occurs because of production of antibodies to nicotinic acetylcholine receptors by the tumor.

Clinical signs of myasthenia gravis include mild to severe muscle weakness, dysphagia, regurgitation, and aspiration pneumonia as a result of megaesophagus.

Supportive management of patients with myasthenia gravis includes amelioration of muscle weakness with anticholinesterase agents (pyridostigmine bromide at 1–3 mg/kg every 8–12 hours or neostigmine at 0.04 mg/kg every 6 hours IM) that prolong acetylcholine interactions with available receptors. Immunosuppressive therapy with prednisone (2 mg/kg/day) or azathioprine (1–2 mg/kg/day) is controversial, but may control signs.[73] At minimum, providing food and water in an elevated position decreases the risk of aspiration. This PNS may not resolve with primary tumor control.[69,74]

Other Peripheral Neuropathies

Peripheral neuropathies are rare PNS reported as a result of a variety of neoplasms including anaplastic sarcoma, fibrosarcoma, insulinoma, lymphoma, prostatic adenocarcinoma, pancreatic adenocarcinoma, and pulmonary carcinoma.[75-78]

Clinical signs vary depending on the nerves affected. Focal to whole body weakness is most common. Electromyography shows increased insertional activity, fibrillation potentials, and positive sharp waves.[77] Motor nerve conduction velocities tend to be slower than normal.

Aside from removal of the inciting tumor, there is no treatment for PNS peripheral neuropathy. However, prognosis for resolution of the neuropathy is good with primary tumor control.

CUTANEOUS PARANEOPLASTIC SYNDROMES

Alopecia

A striking PNS causing alopecia through an unelucidated mechanism is seen in cats with pancreatic carcinoma (Figure 11-1). The hair is very easily epilated; the skin underneath is glossy and smooth.[79,80] The prognosis for cats with pancreatic carcinoma is poor; if the tumor is unresectable, there is no treatment for the alopecia.

Superficial Necrolytic Dermatitis

This rare PNS is associated with liver and pancreatic tumors in dogs. It may be related to hypoaminoacidemia. Skin lesions have a characteristic appearance of erythema, crusting, exudation, ulceration, and alopecia.[81-83] The distribution is typically along the footpads, periocular and perioral regions, anal and genital regions, as well as pressure points along the trunk and limbs. The

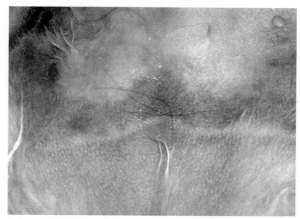

FIGURE 11-1 Close-up image of the ventral abdomen of a cat with a pancreatic adenocarcinoma, showing the characteristic glistening appearance of the epilated skin. (Courtesy of Dr. Laura Garrett.)

prognosis for these patients is poor. If the tumor is unresectable, there is no treatment for the skin lesions.

MISCELLANEOUS PARANEOPLASTIC SYNDROMES

Hypertrophic Osteopathy

This PNS is characterized by periosteal proliferation along the shafts of long bones. It is most often associated with intrathoracic tumors, but occurrence with renal, adrenal, metastatic Sertoli cell tumors and urinary bladder tumors have also been reported.[84-91] The etiology of hypertrophic osteopathy (HO) is unclear, but it is thought to result at least in part from afferent neurologic stimulation. Animals with HO have shifting leg lameness or reluctance to move. Physical examination typically reveals warm, edematous limbs. Irregular periosteum may be palpable along the long bones. Radiographs of the affected limbs show a unique 90-degree periosteal reaction (Figure 11-2).

Resolution of the primary tumor resolves HO.[84,85,91] If the primary tumor is untreatable, reported therapies for HO range from anti-inflammatory doses of steroids and pain management to vagotomy. Although vagotomy did resolve HO in one dog, it is not routinely recommended because of the poor prognosis associated with the primary tumor in many cases.[92]

Fever

Although fever is a common human PNS, it is not a well-documented PNS of dogs and cats. Production of cytokines such as IL-1, IL-6, tumor necrosis factor-alpha

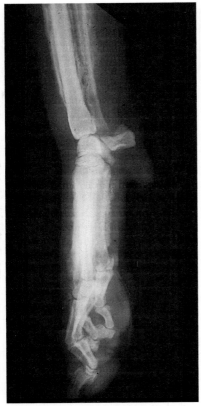

FIGURE 11-2 Radiographic image of hypertrophic osteopathy along the metacarpals, radius, and ulna of a dog with a primary pulmonary carcinoma.

and interferons by the tumor is the cause of paraneoplastic fever in people. Cancer is an important differential for dogs or cats with fever of unknown origin.

Cachexia

Cachexia is a complex PNS of weight loss, with or without anorexia, and loss of lean body mass. This PNS is a common problem in people with cancer and is a major cause of morbidity. A study investigating cachexia in veterinary cancer patients did not identify this as a major issue.[93] However, cachexia can occur with any tumor.

Clinical signs of cachexia are weight loss and anorexia. Aggressive nutritional support is recommended (see Chapter 18, Section B). Resolution of the underlying tumor is the best management, although some treatment options are not well tolerated in these patients because of their debilitated state.

SUMMARY

Paraneoplastic syndromes are a diverse group of systemic effects of cancer. Because they are often associated with dramatic clinical signs, the PNS may be the presenting complaint. Management of the underlying tumor is the best way to resolve PNS, although there may be therapies that help manage some PNS. Some PNS, such as hypercalcemia and hyperglobulinemia, may be monitored and used as indicators for relapse of the cancer.

Selected References*

Fischer JR, Smith SA, Harkin KR: Glucagon constant-rate infusion: a novel strategy for the management of hyperinsulinemic-hypoglycemic crisis in the dog, *J Am Anim Hosp Assoc* 36:27, 2000.
A case-based discussion of the medical management of hypoglycemia.
Giraudel JM, Pages JP, Guelfi JF: Monoclonal gammopathies in the dog: a retrospective study of 18 cases (1986-1999) and literature review, *J Am Anim Hosp Assoc* 38:135, 2002.
A discussion of 18 dogs with monoclonal gammopathy and a review of the literature regarding gammopathies.
Hostutler RA, Chew DJ, Jaeger JQ, et al: Uses and effectiveness of pamidronate disodium for treatment of dogs and cats with hypercalcemia, *J Vet Intern Med* 19:29, 2005.
A review of the clinical signs of hypercalcemia and medical management of this problem with a focus on the use of bisphosphonates.
Madewell BR, Feldman BF: Characterization of anemias associated with neoplasia in small animals, *J Am Vet Med Assoc* 176:419, 1980.
A comprehensive review of anemia resulting from neoplasia in dogs and cats.
Milner RJ, Farese J, Henry CJ, et al: Bisphosphonates and cancer, *J Vet Intern Med* 18:597, 2004.
A thorough review of bisphosphonate mechanism of action and indications.

*For a complete list of the references cited in this chapter, please go to www.smallanimaloncology.com.

12 Chemotherapy

SECTION A: Basic Chemotherapy Principles

Carlos O. Rodriguez, Jr.

KEY POINTS

- Tumor cells are most sensitive to chemotherapy before they are clinically detectable. Cytoreduction is recommended for maximum efficacy, with the exception of lymphoma, in which chemotherapy is the primary treatment.
- By the time tumors are clinically detectable, they contain a significant number of mutations, rendering those cells inherently resistant to many chemotherapeutic agents.
- Cytotoxic drugs should be given at their maximally tolerated dose as often as possible to maximize their efficacy.

The goal of chemotherapy is to reduce the number of malignant cells in a patient to zero. Two theories have been developed predicting cell kill with cytotoxic therapy: the fractional cell kill hypothesis, and the Norton-Simon hypothesis. The Norton-Simon hypothesis relates the effect of cytotoxic therapy to the growth dynamics of the tumor. In other words, the response of a tumor to chemotherapy is proportional to the tumor growth rate.[1] According to the fractional cell kill hypothesis, a given drug will kill a constant fraction of the cell population, regardless of the absolute number of cells in that population.[2-4] Putting this into clinical context, if a patient with an average-sized tumor of 10^{11} cells is treated with a drug that will reduce the number of tumor cells by 99%, 1% or 0.01 of the tumor cells will survive. *Theoretically* after the first dose of chemotherapy, the remaining number of tumor cells will be $10^{11} \times 0.01$, or 10^9 cells. If five more doses of chemotherapy are given ($10^9 \times 0.01 \times 0.01 \times 0.01 \times 0.01 \times 0.01$), the remaining neoplastic population will be 10^7, 10^5, 10^3, 10^1 (one cell), and 10^{-1} (one tenth of one cell, or zero cells), respectively.[2-4] Experience amply demonstrates that this theory rarely translates into clinical reality, but why? There are myriad factors. These can be divided into tumor-related and pharmacological considerations.

TUMOR-RELATED CELL KILL CONSIDERATIONS

The kinetics of the cell cycle plays a role in determining the sensitivity of a population of cells to chemotherapeutic agents. Neoplastic and normal cells that are actively proliferating are considered to be "in the cell cycle." The cell cycle is divided into four phases: G_1, S, G_2, and M phase.[5,6] See Figure 12-1 for an illustration of the cell cycle. Terminally differentiated cells (such as neurons or small lymphocytes) are considered to be in a resting phase outside of the cell cycle termed G_0. Poorly oxygenated tumor cells are often in this phase as well. The growth of tumors has been characterized by Gompertzian growth kinetics[4] (Figure 12-2). According to this model, the fraction of proliferating, and therefore drug-sensitive, cells is not constant. A 1-cm, clinically detectable tumor contains 10^9 tumor cells.[7] At low population numbers, $<10^9$ cells, the cells are most likely to be in the cell cycle and therefore most sensitive to chemotherapy. By the time a tumor is clinically detectable, the tumor cell population is actually entering a phase of decelerating growth. Because chemotherapeutics are most effective against rapidly dividing cells, having cells in the G_0 phase of the cell cycle results in poor cell killing by the administered chemotherapeutics.[2-4]

Cellular biochemistry is another important determinant of cellular sensitivity to chemotherapy. Because

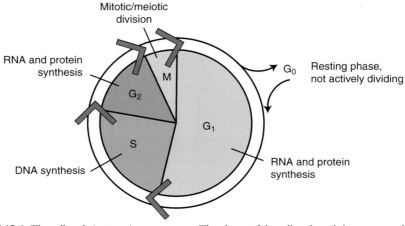

FIGURE 12-1 The cell cycle is a continuous process. The phases of the cell cycle and the corresponding activities of each phase are shown.

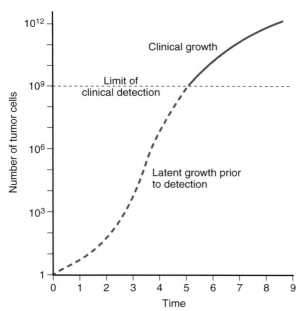

FIGURE 12-2 Gompertzian growth kinetics. According to this model of tumor growth, the fraction of proliferating tumor cells is not constant. A clinically detectable tumor is approximately 1 cm in diameter and contains 10^9 tumor cells. Tumors experience exponential growth prior to this, and once they contain more than 10^9 cells, their growth decelerates as shown by the plateau on the growth curve. Tumor cells are most sensitive to chemotherapy and radiation therapy since they are rapidly dividing prior to becoming clinically detectable. (From Slingerland JM, Tannock IF: Cell proliferation and cell death. In Tannock IF, Hill RP [eds]: *The basic science of oncology*, ed 3, New York, 1998, McGraw-Hill.)

of genetic instability, the mutation rate in a tumor is expected to be high. These mutations lead to a heterogenous population of tumor cells, which likely account for the outgrowth of resistant tumor cells. The clinical reality is described by the Goldie-Coleman hypothesis,[8] which states that at the time of clinical detection (10^9 cells) the tumor contains within it a population of cells (10^3–10^4) that is resistant to chemotherapy. During relapse of tumors, which were initially sensitive to chemotherapy, there is a proliferation of these resistant cells. Additional forms of resistance may also occur once chemotherapy has been started.[2] Examples of these phenomena found in both veterinary and human neoplasms include mutations in the tumor suppressor gene, p53; perturbations of balance between pro- and anti-apoptotic bcl-2 family members; activation of cellular growth factors such as epidermal growth factor or insulin-like growth factor-1; alterations in death receptor pathways, such as Fas/FasL; and resistance to chemotherapeutic molecules by upregulation of the multidrug resistance gene.

PHARMACOLOGICAL CELL KILL CONSIDERATIONS

The response of the tumor to chemotherapy also depends upon pharmacokinetic factors such as drug absorption, metabolism, and elimination. These parameters are extremely important in guiding the dose, schedule, and route of administration of the drugs. Few drugs used in veterinary oncology have undergone rigorous clinical pharmacological investigations. One parameter that has been determined for many of the useful drugs is the maximally tolerated dose (MTD). The MTD is the maximum recommended dose of an agent that can be administered safely based on toxicity. The MTD is then administered as often as allowable, which is determined by the recovery of the normal tissues (e.g., bone marrow and gastrointestinal lining). Maximizing the exposure of the tumor to the MTD is important in achieving desired clinical results.

The expected response of a tumor to chemotherapy also depends on the way in which the agent is used. Chemotherapeutic agents may be used in a neoadjuvant or adjuvant setting and can be divided into induction, consolidation/maintenance, or salvage/rescue protocols. *Neoadjuvant chemotherapy* refers to the use of chemotherapy *before* primary treatment for the disease. An example is the use of chemotherapy in an effort to cytoreduce a bulky tumor in advance of the definitive local treatment with surgery or radiation therapy. Complete resolution of a bulky tumor with chemotherapy is unlikely because a large tumor is likely to contain only a small fraction of cycling cells that are sensitive to chemotherapy and many cells that have acquired chemotherapy resistance through mutation. *Adjuvant chemotherapy* is applied after definitive local therapy (surgery, radiation therapy) but where the risk of local recurrence (incompletely excised malignancies) or the likelihood of metastasis (e.g., apocrine gland adenocarcinoma of the anal sac or osteosarcoma) is high. *Induction therapy* most often applies to the use of chemotherapy to treat lymphoid malignancies. These protocols are intensive because they involve short dosing intervals and aggressive drug combinations. The goal of induction therapy is to achieve a complete remission, or complete resolution of clinically measurable disease. *Consolidation therapy* is less intensive than induction therapy and may or may not use the same drugs as the induction phase. The goal of consolidation therapy is to continue the cytoreduction of the tumor burden when induction resulted in only a partial response. *Maintenance therapy* is a continuation of chemotherapy when a complete remission has been achieved in an effort to maintain remission and, thus, prevent relapse. *Salvage/rescue protocols* are used in patients where standard protocols no longer maintain complete (or partial) remission. In general, the drugs in these protocols are not considered front-line treatments and occasionally have more severe toxicity profiles. Recalling the Goldie-Coleman hypothesis, this population of tumor cells has been subjected to multiple rounds of chemotherapy and, consequently, are likely to have acquired mutations that result in their continued survival.

Most chemotherapy protocols combine multiple drugs at minimal intervals. The Goldie-Coleman hypothesis

TABLE 12-1   CELL CYCLES AND CHEMOTHERAPY DRUGS*

Cell Cycle Phase	Chemotherapy Drug Class
G_1	L-Asparaginase
S	Antimetabolites
G_2	
M	Vinca alkaloids

*Some classes of chemotherapy drugs exert their mechanisms of action during specific phases of the cell cycle. The alkylating agents, anthracyclines, and platinum agents are non-cell cycle phase–specific exerting their effects throughout the cell cycle. Cell cycle phase specificity is considered when developing multi-agent chemotherapy protocols.

again provides the rationale for combination chemotherapy: *at the time of clinical detection,* the presence of drug resistance is almost assuredly guaranteed. When choosing agents for combination chemotherapy protocols, three principles should be applied: (1) each drug should have known cytotoxic activity against the intended tumor, (2) overlapping toxicities should be avoided between drugs, and (3) each drug should be used as near its MTD as possible.[9] In addition, each drug should possess different mechanisms of action from one another. Table 12-1 lists chemotherapy drugs and the phase of the cell cycle within which they function, which is also an important factor when combining chemotherapy drugs. *Dose intensity,* the amount of drug delivered over time (mg/m^2/week), should be maximized by administering the MTD as often as possible for each drug so there is a greater chance of killing both sensitive and moderately resistant cells in the heterogeneous tumor population.

It is the hope of the author that the above concepts, theories, and discussions will translate into an increased appreciation of what is happening (or not happening) when a chemotherapy drug is administered. These concepts are crucial to the understanding of the theory of chemotherapy and its application and are as important as the properties of the individual chemotherapy drugs.

Selected References*

DeVita VT, Schein PS: The use of drugs in combination for the treatment of cancer: rationale and results, *N Engl J Med*, 288:998, 1973.
This publication describes the rationale to choose cytotoxic agents for combination chemotherapy protocols.

Goldie JH, Coldman AJ: A mathematical model for relating the drug sensitivity of tumors to their spontaneous mutation rate, *Cancer Treat Rep* 63:172, 1979.
This publication provides the rationale behind the hypothesis that each tumor contains mutations making them inherently resistant to chemotherapy.
Skipper HE, Schabel FM Jr, Mellet LB, et al: Implications of biochemical, cytokinetic, pharmacologic and toxicologic relationships in the design of optimal therapeutic schedules, *Cancer Chemother Rep* 54:431, 1950.
This publication was the first to describe the fractional cell kill hypothesis of tumors with the application of chemotherapy.

■ *For a complete list of the references cited in this chapter, please go to www.smallanimaloncology.com.

SECTION B: Chemotherapy Drug Interactions

Wendi Velando Rankin and Carolyn J. Henry

KEY POINTS

- Chemotherapy drugs can interact with other drugs *in vitro* (such as during mixture or administration) and *in vivo*.
- Drug interactions can enhance or decrease activity of the chemotherapy drug.
- Drug interactions can result in beneficial effects, severe toxicities, or no detectable clinical change.
- Laboratory tests can be altered with some chemotherapy drugs.

Treatment of a cancer patient with chemotherapy drugs can be complex, since patients may be receiving supportive therapy or other drugs for treatment of concurrent disease conditions, including systemic and topical therapies (ophthalmic and otic preparations). In addition, chemotherapy often requires multiple drug therapy (polypharmacy) for more efficacious treatment of neoplastic diseases; therefore, knowledge of drug interactions is important for safe drug administration.

Chemotherapeutics can interact with other drugs both *in vitro* (outside the body) and *in vivo* (inside the body). The results of these drug interactions may vary from beneficial to severely adverse reactions, or there may be no detectable clinical change. To prevent detrimental effects of drug interactions, it is important to be familiar with potential adverse reactions, since some reactions are unpredictable.

MECHANISMS OF DRUG INTERACTIONS

In vitro interactions may occur when incompatible drugs are mixed together before administration, such as in the same intravenous fluids. This can result in alteration of the chemical nature of one or more of the drugs, leading to decreased activity of the drug. Some of the incompatibilities manifest as visible changes, including a precipitate or haze from the drug reactions, an increase or decrease in the natural turbidity of the drug, gas evolution, or color change of the solution (Figure 12-3). For example, consecutive injections of doxorubicin and heparin into a fluid line without flushes between them results in immediate precipitation.[1-9] In addition, mixtures of paclitaxel and amphotericin B *in vitro* result in a decrease in the natural turbidity of the solution,[8,9] and fluorouracil in a solution with doxorubicin results in an immediate color change from red to purple.[3-5,6,9] A mixture of carmustine and allopurinol in a fluid line results in gas formation.[9] On the other hand, the reactions can be more subtle and result in a change in drug activity without visible signs; some drug interactions will change the spectrophotometry of a drug solution as a result of altered drug activity, and this will not be an overtly visible change. Chemical decomposition of the drug can also occur in a mixture without detectable visible changes, and sometimes can only be detected by purification of the agent. Fluorouracil combined with methotrexate *in vitro* results in a change in the spectrophotometry of both agents,[3-7] and this is not visibly apparent. In addition, cisplatin in solutions with low chloride content (<0.2% sodium chloride) will result in a displacement of the chloride ions by water, resulting in inactivation of the agent[3,5,7-9] as a result of the addition of a positive charge (Figure 12-4). The positive charge prevents the movement of cisplatin into cells. Many drug interactions can go unnoticed if there is no visible color change or precipitate; therefore, avoid mixing drugs for which there are no compatibility data.

In vivo drug interactions may enhance or decrease drug activity and toxicity depending on various factors. These drug interactions depend on factors that affect the administration route, absorption, distribution of the drug, metabolism and activation, or excretion of drugs. For example, intravenous melphalan may reduce the threshold for carmustine-induced pulmonary toxicity[8];

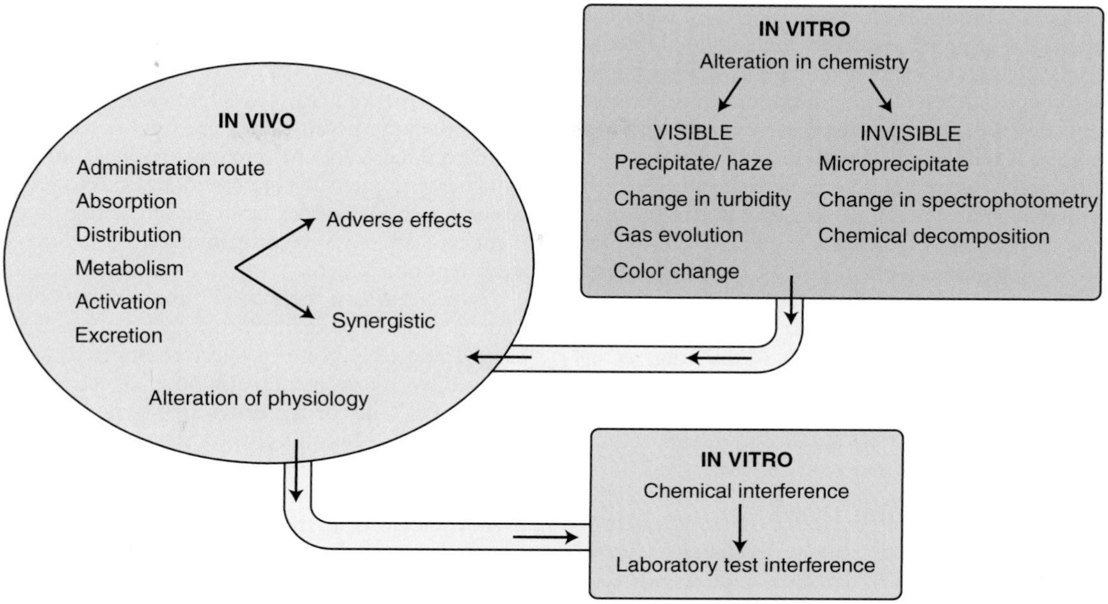

IN VITRO

Alteration in chemistry

VISIBLE	INVISIBLE
Precipitate/ haze	Microprecipitate
Change in turbidity	Change in spectrophotometry
Gas evolution	Chemical decomposition
Color change	

IN VIVO

Administration route
Absorption
Distribution
Metabolism
Activation
Excretion

Adverse effects

Synergistic

Alteration of physiology

IN VITRO

Chemical interference

Laboratory test interference

FIGURE 12-3 Mechanisms of drug interactions.

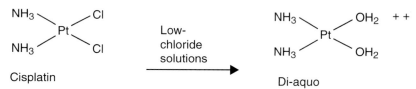

Cisplatin

Low-chloride solutions

Di-aquo

FIGURE 12-4 Cisplatin in low-chloride solutions (e.g., dextrose 5% in water, <0.2% sodium chloride) will allow chloride groups to leave. They are replaced by water, and the resulting compound has a charge and cannot enter cells for its anti-tumor effects. *Pt*, Platinum; *Cl*, chloride; *NH3*, ammonia.

however, this is not reported with oral melphalan and carmustine. In addition, food given with oral methotrexate will result in decreased absorption of methotrexate and therefore decreased bioavailability and efficacy of the chemotherapeutic.[10] Therefore, methotrexate should not be given with food. Cyclosporine decreases doxorubicin clearance and allows better distribution inside cells because of inhibition of the P-glycoprotein drug efflux pump.[5] Although this can allow better anti-tumor effects, it can also potentiate hematologic toxicity and neurotoxicity.[8,11] One drug can affect the metabolism or excretion of another, as with cyclophosphamide and barbiturates. Patients receiving concurrent barbiturates and cyclophosphamide can have increased metabolism of cyclophosphamide to its active metabolites because of barbiturate

induction of hepatic microsomal enzymes[2,4,5,7,8]; this increases cyclophosphamide toxicity. Cimetidine can decrease the hepatic degradation of 1-(2-chloroethyl)-3-cyclohecyl-1-nitrosurea (CCNU) resulting in increased myelosuppression of the chemotherapeutic.[5,11] Cimetidine inhibits hepatic microsomal enzymes, decreases hepatic blood flow, and results in increased bioavailability of drugs (such as CCNU) with high hepatic excretion.[8] Cisplatin given concurrently with methotrexate results in increased nephrotoxicity because of cisplatin decreasing the renal clearance of methotrexate.[5,7] Although many interactions can have adverse effects as described previously, the interactions can also be used to our advantage for anti-tumor effects, including fluorouracil and cisplatin,[7,8] chlorambucil and prednisone for leukemia,[4,7,8] and cisplatin and bleomycin given together.[8] However, note that some drug combinations have both synergistic as well as adverse effects. For example, whereas cisplatin and bleomycin have synergistic anti-tumor effects,[8] cisplatin decreases the renal clearance of bleomycin[5] and can increase bleomycin toxicity.[7,12]

Lastly, some interactions are *in vitro* as well as *in vivo*. Drugs may interact with laboratory tests due to the drug effects on the analysis method *(in vitro)* or altering the body's physiologic response *(in vivo)*, resulting in false results (Table 12-2). For example, patients receiving mercaptopurine can have falsely elevated blood glucose and uric acid measurements because of the drug's interference *in vitro* with the laboratory analyzer.[8] In addition, patients who recently received L-asparaginase may have falsely low-serum thyroxine measurements because of decreased synthesis of thyroxine *in vivo*.[8]

SPECIFIC DRUG INTERACTIONS

Tables included on the website (www. smallanimaloncology.com) list drug interactions with various chemotherapy agents used in veterinary clinical oncology. The information focuses on agents applicable to veterinary medicine but is not an exhaustive list of all possible interactions. Chemotherapy drugs with no known incompatibilities are not discussed. Although herbal medications and nutritional supplements are increasing in popularity as alternatives or adjuncts to cancer therapy, because they are not currently used as standard therapy for our veterinary patients, interactions with these supplements are not included. However, veterinarians should understand that any drug or supplement can have potential drug interactions and may affect treatment of a patient.

Table 12-A1 on the website summarizes interactions with chemotherapy agents; drugs are listed based on drug class. Table 12-A2 on the website summarizes reported physical *in vitro* incompatibilities of chemotherapy agents with other drugs; drugs are listed based on drug class. Table 12-2 in this chapter is a summary of known laboratory test interferences of which clinicians should be aware; drugs are in alphabetical order. Although the interactions listed in these tables summarize the reported interactions, much of the data is obtained from human pharmacology books; therefore, the clinical relevance to veterinary patients is unknown. In addition, the clinical effects of some *in vitro* drug incompatibilities listed have not been evaluated in veterinary patients.

TABLE 12-2   LABORATORY TEST INTERFERENCES

Drug	Laboratory Test Abnormalities	Comments
Actinomycin D	Interference with antibacterial drug levels[8,11]	Actinomycin D may interfere with bioassay
Carboplatin	Abnormal liver function tests[8]	With high doses of carboplatin (>four times dosage)
Hydroxyurea	Increased serum uric acid, blood urea nitrogen, creatinine[8]	
L-Asparaginase	Rapid and marked reduction in serum thyroxin-binding globulin, reduction in total serum thyroxine[8]; leads to increased thyroxine-binding globulin index[11]	Occurs within 2 days after first dose; serum concentrations of thyroxine-binding globulin returned to pre-treatment values within 4 weeks[8]; may result from asparaginase-induced inhibition of serum thyroxine synthesis in liver[11]
Mercaptopurine	Falsely elevated serum glucose and uric acid levels[11]	Mercaptopurine interferes with sequential multiple analyzer 12/60 determinations
Mitotane	Decreased protein-bound iodine[8,11]	Mitotane competitively binds thyroxine-binding globulin and decreases serum protein-bound iodine[11]
	Decreased urinary 17-hydroxycorticosteroids[8,11]	Increased extra-adrenal metabolism of cortisol to 6-β-hydroxycortisol; may not reflect decrease in cortisol secretion rate or plasma cortisol concentration
Phenytoin	Interference with dexamethasone-suppression tests[11]	
Prednisone	Decreased ^{131}I uptake and protein-bound iodine concentrations[11]	

Selected References*

Chabner BA, Longo DL: *Cancer chemotherapy and biotherapy: principles and practice*, ed 3, Philadelphia, 2001, Lippincott, Williams & Wilkins.
A textbook on principles of chemotherapy and chemotherapy drug information.

Dorr RT, Von Hoff DD: *Cancer chemotherapy handbook*, ed 2, Norwalk, 1994, Appleton & Lange.
A textbook on administration of chemotherapy in human patients and individual drug information, including drug interactions for each drug.

Fisher DS, Knobf MT, Durivage HJ: Drug interactions with antineoplastic agents. In Fisher DS, Knobf MT, Durivage HJ (eds): *The cancer chemotherapy handbook*, ed 4, St Louis, 1993, Mosby.
A manual on chemotherapy principles, administration, and drug interactions.

Henry CJ, Brewer WJ: Drug interactions with antineoplastic agents. In Bonagura J: *Kirk's current veterinary therapy XII*, Philadelphia, 1995, WB Saunders.
This chapter lists chemotherapy agents and drugs with which they interact in vivo as well as in vitro incompatibilities focusing on drugs more commonly used in veterinary medicine.

McEvoy GK (ed): *Antineoplastic agents*. In *American Hospital Formulary Services (AHFS) Drug Information*, Bethesda, 2005, American Society of Health-System Pharmacists.
A pharmaceutical manual providing details of individual drug information, including pharmacology, use, toxicities, drug interactions, incompatibilities, stability, and chemistry of agents.

■ *For a complete list of the references cited in this chapter, please go to www.smallanimaloncology.com.

SECTION C: Safe Handling of Chemotherapy Drugs

Natalie S. Royer

KEY POINTS

- Appropriate personal protective equipment should be worn by all persons handling chemotherapy and patients receiving chemotherapy.
- Patient excrement should be handled as contaminated waste for 48 hours after chemotherapy administration.
- Dogs should be walked in low-traffic sunlit areas for 48 hours after chemotherapy.
- Litter box liners should be used and litter changed daily for 48 hours after chemotherapy.

Safety is of utmost importance when handling cytotoxic agents. The cytotoxic agents used in veterinary medicine are primarily human-approved drugs used off label in the veterinary setting. Therefore, toxicity is possible if these drugs are absorbed or ingested by veterinary personnel. Because of this, the clinical use of cytotoxic agents requires an understanding of associated risks by all personnel involved with chemotherapy preparation, administration, and patient handling. The Occupational Safety and Health Administration (OSHA) has developed guidelines for handling of cytotoxic agents, and these guidelines—available at www.osha.gov/dts/osta/otm/otm_vi/otm_vi_2.html—should be available for all personnel to review prior to their involvement in chemotherapy administration.

PERSONAL PROTECTIVE WEAR

All personnel involved with chemotherapy administration should wear protective clothing. Chemotherapy gloves or a double layer of powder-free latex gloves, eye protection, and a closed-front, elastic-cuffed, nonpermeable, lint-free gown are recommendations of OSHA for personal protective equipment for individuals handling hazardous drugs, including cytotoxic agents (Box 12-1). These recommendations should be followed not only by those administering chemotherapy, but also by those restraining animals for treatment. Chemotherapy gloves that are powder free and are thicker than typical examination gloves are commercially available. The thickness of the gloves is most important, and latex has been found to be the least permeable glove material. Powder-free gloves are recommended, since powder may absorb contaminants and thereby potentially

---

BOX 12-1   RECOMMENDED PERSONAL PROTECTIVE EQUIPMENT FOR HAZARDOUS DRUG HANDLING

Powder-free latex gloves
Closed-front disposable gown of lint-free, low-permeability fabric with long sleeves and cuffs
Chemical-barrier face and eye protection

increase exposure to cytotoxic drugs. Double-gloving is recommended if specific chemotherapy gloves are not used. Hands should always be washed before gloves are put on and immediately after they are removed. Gowns should be disposable with a closed front and made from low-permeability fabric. The sleeves should be long with elastic or knit cuffs. Gloves should be placed over the cuff unless double gloves are used; then the inner layer of gloves should be under the cuff and the outer over the cuff. Personal protective equipment should also be worn when cleaning up accidental spills or patient waste during the first 48 hours after administration of chemotherapy medications. If clients are to administer chemotherapy such as oral cyclophosphamide or chlorambucil at home, powder-free latex gloves should be dispensed for the client to wear to administer the tablets.

CHEMOTHERAPY ADMINISTRATION SAFETY

Administration of chemotherapy should always be done in a low-traffic, controlled airflow area such as an examination room or radiology room with a sign on the door warning personnel that chemotherapy is being administered. No food storage, eating, drinking, gum-chewing, smoking, or make-up application should be performed in the area. Heavy make-up wearers and smokers need to be especially cautious, since chemotherapy will adhere to make-up and nicotine on hands and faces.

Equipment necessary for chemotherapy administration is listed in Box 12-2. Before drug infusion, a plastic-backed absorbent pad should be placed under the animal and injection site to absorb any drug that may be lost accidentally during the administration procedure. When IV administration is performed, the use

---

BOX 12-2　CHEMOTHERAPY ADMINISTRATION EQUIPMENT

Personal protective equipment
Alcohol wipes
Disposable, plastic-backed absorbent pad
Clearly labeled chemotherapy drug
Infusion equipment (catheter, tape, T-port adaptor, etc.)
Non-heparinized 0.9% NaCl to flush the catheter before and after chemotherapy infusion
Bandage for venipuncture site after catheter removal
Disposable container for chemotherapy administration waste

---

of an alcohol-soaked gauze around the injection connection will help to trap any chemotherapy that may leak from the connection. Removal of needle caps with your teeth or recapping needles should be avoided at all times. Luer-Lok syringes are recommended for cytotoxic drugs as they help to reduce leakage of drugs and accidental disconnections during drug administration, thus, decreasing the potential for personnel exposure. Using Luer-Lok fittings will decrease the need for needles during chemotherapy administration and significantly decrease the potential for personnel exposure. See Section E for discussion of chemotherapy administration techniques.

DISPOSAL OF CHEMOTHERAPY WASTE

All materials that have been in contact with chemotherapy during administration should be disposed of in a specified chemotherapy waste container. All catheters, infusion ports, tape, plastic-backed absorbent pads, alcohol pads, plastic transportation bags, gloves, and gowns should be placed in a designated chemotherapy waste bag. This bag should then be placed in a clearly labeled leak-proof container. Chemotherapy waste should be handled separately from other hospital trash and disposed of in accordance with Environmental Protection Agency (EPA), state, and local hazardous waste disposal regulations. Each municipality has its own regulations for disposal of hazardous waste; therefore, each clinic should check with its local officials for proper disposal guidelines in the area.

HANDLING OF PATIENT EXCREMENT

Linens contaminated with bodily wastes (e.g., blood, vomitus, urine, or feces) within 48 hours of chemotherapy administration may be contaminated with active drug or metabolites and should be placed in clearly marked laundry bags. Personnel or owners handling this laundry should wear latex gloves and a gown if possible. This laundry should be pre-washed separately from other laundry and then washed again before re-entering general use. The second wash may be with other items. The area where the excrement was found should be thoroughly cleaned once the excrement is removed. The use of a spray nozzle to apply water or cleaning agents is discouraged since this could aerosolize drug in the excrement, thereby exposing any persons in the area. The preferred method of cleaning includes wearing latex gloves and using a paper towel soaked with water or a cleaning agent, such as a dilute bleach solution, to wipe the floor or table that was contaminated. The area should be cleaned two to three times to ensure complete removal of the potential contaminants. Gloves and paper towels used for cleaning should be bagged separately and placed in a hospital chemotherapy waste container or double bagged before being placed in the trash at home.

Regarding patient urination and defecation after chemotherapy, sunlight deactivates chemotherapy agents. Practitioners should encourage clients to walk their pet after chemotherapy in a part of the yard that receives sunlight and not where children play. With regard to cat excrement, daily litter box changing is recommended for the 48 hours immediately after chemotherapy. Using litter box liners helps to significantly decrease the potential of aerosolization of active chemotherapy metabolites in the excrement while changing the litter. It is not necessary to separate cats in multi-cat households after chemotherapy, and using the same litter box poses no known threats to untreated cats in the household.

CHEMOTHERAPY SPILLS

With careful and proper chemotherapy handling, the potential for chemotherapy spills is minimized. However, plans for chemotherapy spills should be devised and posted in all areas where chemotherapy is handled. Chemotherapy spill kits are commercially available and are recommended for clinics routinely using cytotoxic agents. Should contamination to personnel occur, these steps should be followed:

1. Immediately remove the gloves or gown that are contaminated.
2. If the skin is contaminated, the affected skin should immediately be cleansed with soap and water for 15 minutes.
3. If the eye is contaminated, the eye should be rinsed with an eyewash station or designated eyewash for at least 15 minutes.

Small spills should be cleaned immediately by personnel wearing appropriate personal protective equipment. All liquids should be wiped with absorbent pads, and the spill area should be cleaned three times using a soap solution followed by clean water. For large spills, an absorbent pad should be used to soak up the liquid spilled. Any broken glass should be swept up, not picked up by hands, and placed in a sharps container. All material used to clean chemotherapy spills should be bagged and placed in the chemotherapy waste containers for appropriate disposal.

Selected References*

Lucroy MD: Chemotherapy safety in veterinary practice: hazardous drug administration, *Compend Contin Educ Pract Vet* 24:140, 2002.
This article reviews safe chemotherapy administration in the private practice setting.
Henry CJ: Safe handling of chemotherapy drugs. In August JR (ed): *Consultations in feline internal medicine*, ed 3, Orlando, 1996, WB Saunders.
This chapter reviews procedures and tips for safe handling of chemotherapy in a feline practice setting.

*For a complete list of the references cited in this chapter, please go to www.smallanimaloncology.com.

SECTION D: Chemotherapy Preparation

Helen P. Gill

KEY POINTS

- Preparation of chemotherapy doses should be performed in a low traffic area with appropriate equipment and personal protective wear.
- Venting devices, preferably a closed-system device, should be used when preparing chemotherapy to reduce the risk of drug aerosolization and personnel exposure.
- Care should be taken when transporting chemotherapy doses through the hospital by placing the dose within a bag or other leak-proof transporter.

WHERE TO PREPARE CHEMOTHERAPY DOSES

Cost is often the major factor that determines the extent of chemotherapy preparation facilities used in a veterinary practice. Regardless, safety of personnel should be a priority for practices using chemotherapy as treatment for their cancer patients. Standards have been established by the National Institute for Occupational Safety and Health (NIOSH) for chemotherapy preparation in a "Clean Room Setting." Such standards may be unrealistic in veterinary medicine because of space and cost; however, recommendations exist as to how to safely prepare cytotoxic agents in practice situations. The standard is to use a Class II, Type B biological safety cabinet (BSC) contained in a separate room with venting to the outside. Personal protective equipment should be worn by all personnel handling chemotherapy and is discussed in Section C. Box 12-3 presents *minimal* requirements that should be used in a practice setting.[1,2] Box 12-4 lists items that should be within reach of the work area.

PREPARATION TECHNIQUE

Gloves should be donned *before* touching the packages of chemotherapy drugs. Studies have shown that during manufacturing and packaging, drug residue may remain on the outer packaging of vials or bottles.[3] Everything that will be needed should be taken into the preparation

---

BOX 12-3   MINIMAL REQUIREMENTS FOR CHEMOTHERAPY PREPARATION IN A VETERINARY PRACTICE

Room
Enclosed room in a low traffic area
Uncluttered counter to prepare doses
Washable counter and floor that can be disinfected with bleach

Preparation Site
Protective mat on counter (vinyl side down and absorbent side up)
Work with drugs inside a large plastic bag (to reduce contamination to environment)
Ziploc-style bag nearby to quickly dispose of empty vials, contaminated syringes, and outer gloves

Personal Protective Equipment (see Section C)
Mask and protective goggles
Gown
Double gloves
Shoe covers
Hair covering

BOX 12-4   ITEMS NEEDED WITHIN REACH OF THE WORK AREA

Chemotherapy-dedicated sharps container; closed when not in use
Hazardous waste container
All items to prepare dose: needles, Luer-Lok syringes, syringe caps, labels, bags for transport, etc.
Chemotherapy spill kit
Chair or stool, completely washable

---

area at one time to avoid having to leave to get them. This reduces the chance for contaminating the areas outside the Clean Room/prep area or the need to don gown and gloves multiple times.

Drugs that must be reconstituted pose the most risk to the preparer since needle entry into and withdrawal from the vial can allow the release of drug into the environment. Because of this, devices are available that help to prevent drug aerosolization during this process. Chemotherapy dispensing pins are commercially available venting devices that reduce the internal pressure within a bottle during reconstitution and dispensing and therefore decrease the risk of drug exposure (Figure 12-5). Closed-system drug transfer devices (such as the PhaSeal [Carmel PharmaLab, Columbus, Ohio] or ONGUARD [BBraun, Bethlehem, Penn] systems) can also be used to reduce the release of drug during reconstitution and administration. The PhaSeal device has a double membrane that captures powder or spray released from the vial during reconstitution. The PhaSeal device should be used if working outside a BSC. Studies have not shown it to be advantageous if working within a BSC. Another safety measure, if preparing chemotherapy without a hood, is to place an alcohol-soaked gauze pad around connection sites to reduce the risk of aerosolization when disconnecting a syringe from a dispensing pin, for instance. The usual method of displacing a solution with air injected from a syringe is *not* used with chemotherapy drugs because the pressure introduced may cause drug to leak or spray from the vial.

Many drugs must be diluted before administration. Using aseptic technique, prepare the diluent in a syringe or infusion bag and set it aside, then prepare the drug. If a drug will be administered via an infusion, attach the infusion set to the bag of IV fluid with no drug added, prime the line, and clamp it off *before the drug is added to the fluid.* This eliminates the possibility of a chemotherapy spill while priming the line because there is no drug in the fluid. When preparing a drug in a syringe, do not fill the syringe more than three fourths of its total volume. A syringe filled over three-fourths full poses a risk of spilling because the barrel may be pulled inadvertently from the syringe. This may require the total dose to be divided in multiple syringes. Once the dose is prepared in the syringe(s), the volume in the hub should be pulled back into the syringe. The plunger should then be gently pushed up so that the drug reaches the tip of the syringe, and then it should be capped with a Luer-Loking syringe cap to reduce spills in transit. The amount of drug contained in a needle and hub is approximately 0.05 ml, which is usually insignificant but may indeed be significant if the dose of an undiluted drug is very small. If a needle will be left on the syringe,

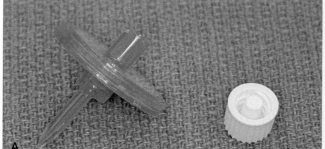
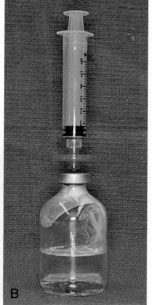

FIGURE 12-5 **A**, Chemotherapy dispensing pin. **B**, Use of chemotherapy dispensing pin.

the hub-filled volume should be drawn into the syringe and the needle replaced. The drug should be pushed back carefully into the hub and needle. Label the dose and place it inside a Ziploc-style bag and seal it. The outer gloves can then be removed and placed in the Ziploc-style "disposal" bag. Place the bag containing the chemotherapy dose inside a second bag for extra safety. This bag should be kept outside the BSC or the immediate work area to reduce any possibility of contamination from the work surfaces.

Orally administered drugs pose the same potential hazards as injections (drug residues on the package, as well as from capsules and tablets) and therefore should be handled in a BSC if possible. Specific trays and spatulas should be set aside for use *only* with those drugs. If a BSC is not available, a specific isolated handling area should be designated. Counting on a tray within a large clear plastic bag will reduce contamination from dust or spillage. Cleaning counting trays and spatulas by briefly soaking in a diluted bleach solution between uses is advised. If an oral drug is to be divided into smaller doses, this should *only* be done within a BSC because of the significant risk of drug aerosolization. In cases where a protocol calculation requires splitting tablets or capsules for exact doses, the regimen should be altered if at all possible. For example, if the calculated dose of cyclophosphamide in a protocol is

12.5 mg daily for 4 days, the regimen could be changed to 25 mg daily for 2 days to deliver the entire dose without having to split tablets. In instances where oral medication schedules cannot be altered, the dose of the drug should be rounded down to the nearest tablet or capsule size to prevent overdosing the patient. Table 12-3 lists frequently used chemotherapy drugs, available formulations, and special instructions for handling or dispensing.

DISPOSAL OF "TRASH" ASSOCIATED WITH CHEMOTHERAPY PREPARATION AND CLEAN-UP

The Chemo Sharps container should be used to contain anything that may have been in contact with chemotherapy drugs. This includes all needles; syringes with drug residue; outer gloves; vials with drug remaining in them; clear plastic bags in which drugs were prepared or drawn up; the disposal bag containing empty vials, syringes, etc.; and gown if it is known to have been contaminated. Inner gloves and non-contaminated gowns can go into a separate hazardous waste container.

CLEANING OF PREPARATION AREAS

Cleaning of surfaces should be carried out wearing a gown, chemotherapy thickness gloves or double gloves (powder-free latex) and eye protection. Cleaning of a BSC should

TABLE 12-3   COMMONLY PREPARED CHEMOTHERAPY DRUGS, DILUTIONS, AND STABILITY

Drug Name(s), Strength(s), and Formulation	Storage Prior to Reconstitution or Use	Usual Preparation of Basic Drug Dose	Stability and Storage[4,5]
L-Asparaginase 10,000 IU vial powder (Elspar)	Refrigerate	5 ml SWFI Do *not* shake vial; if necessary, gently swirl to mix	Use immediately Discard remainder*
Bleomycin 15 and 30 unit vials powder (Blenoxane)	Refrigerate	Dilute with saline or SWFI to 3 U/ml	In saline, 4 wks refrigerated 2 wks at room temperature*
Carboplatin 10 mg/ml solution or powder (Paraplatin)	Room temperature Protect from light	Powder-SWFI to 10 mg/ml. May further dilute with saline before administration Do not use aluminum-containing needles	14 days at room temperature* after reconstitution (10% loss of potency) Protect from light
Chlorambucil 2mg tablet (Leukeran)	Refrigerate		Store refrigerated Package in glass
Cisplatin 1 mg/ml solution (Platinol-AQ)	Room temperature Protect from light	Dilute with saline for infusions Mix with medical grade, sterile sesame oil for intralesional injection Do not use aluminum containing needles	Discard 28 days after vial entry† Protect from light
Cyclophosphamide 500 mg and 1 g powder 25 and 50 mg tablets (Cytoxan)	Room temperature	Dilute to 20 mg/ml with SWFI	Solution: 6 days refrigerated or 24 hr at room temperature
Cytarabine 100 and 500 mg solution or powder (Cytosar-U)	Room temperature	Dilute with BWFI For intrathecal use, use saline and reconstitute to 5 mg/ml	In BWFI, stable 5 days at room temperature In saline for intrathecal use, discard remainder immediately*
Dacarbazine 100and 200 mg powder (DTIC-Dome)	Refrigerate Protect from light	Dilute to 10 mg/ml with SWFI	Refrigerated 72 hr Room temperature 8 hr
Dactinomycin 0.5 mg (500 µg) powder (Actinomycin D, Cosmegen)	Room temperature Protect from light	Dilute with 1.1 ml SWFI to final concentration of 500 µg/ml	24 hr at room temperature*
Doxorubicin 2 mg/ml solution: SDV/MDV powder: SDV/MDV (Adriamycin)	Refrigerate Protect from light	Dilute powder with saline	Reconstituted MDV: 7 days at room temp 15 days refrigerated Reconstituted SDV: 24 hr at room temperature 48 hr refrigerated
Fluorouracil 500 mg/10 ml (5-FU, Adrucil)	Room temperature	No dilution required	
Gemcitabine 200 mg and 1 g vials powder (Gemzar®)	Room temperature	Dilute with saline 5 ml/200 mg or 25 ml/1g 38 mg/ml final concentration	Reconstituted stable for 24 hr at room temperature

(Continued)

TABLE 12-3   COMMONLY PREPARED CHEMOTHERAPY DRUGS, DILUTIONS, AND STABILITY—CONT'D

Drug Name(s), Strength(s), and Formulation	Storage Prior to Reconstitution or Use	Usual Preparation of Basic Drug Dose	Stability and Storage[4,5]
Lomustine 10 mg and 40 mg capsules (CeeNU)	Room temperature		
Mechlorethamine 10 mg powder (Mustargen)	Room temperature Protect from light	Dilute with 10 ml SWFI	Use immediately Remaining drug must be neutralized before disposal—see package insert
Melphalan 2 mg tablet (Alkeran)	Refrigerate Package in glass		
Mitoxantrone 2 mg/ml solution (Novantrone)	Room temperature		Room temperature: Discard vial 7 days after entry Refrigerated: 14 days
Vinblastine 1mg/ml MDV Solution or powder (Velban)	Refrigerate	Powder: dilute with BSFI to 1 mg/ml	Reconstituted: 28 days refrigerated Solution: 2 months refrigerated Stable in syringe for 30 days refrigerated
Vincristine 1 mg/ml solution (Oncovin)	Refrigerate	No dilution needed	Contains no preservative*

BSFI, Bacteriostatic saline for injection; *BWFI*, bacteriostatic water for injection; *MDV*, multi-dose vial; *saline*, non-preserved 0.9% sodium chloride for injection; *SDV*, single-dose vial; *SWFI*, sterile water for injection.

*Most sources do not recommend prolonged storage of products that do not contain preservatives.

†Oxygen introduced into vial eventually reduces strength of drug, so storage beyond recommended time may not provide adequate therapeutic effects.

be done routinely and after any spill. Non-BSC prep areas should be cleaned after every chemotherapy preparation. All work surfaces should be washed with a diluted (40% or higher) bleach solution (equal to a 2% sodium hypochlorite content) and allowed to air dry. This inactivates most chemotherapy drugs and makes the preparation area relatively safe again. If cleaning a BSC, a 1% thiosulfate solution applied to the surface after the bleach has been removed will prevent "pitting" of the BSC's stainless steel surfaces.

Selected References*

Centers for Disease Control and Prevention, National Institute for Occupational Safety and Health, and Department of Health and Human Services: *NIOSH Alert: Preventing occupational exposures to antineoplastic and other hazardous drugs in health care settings,* DHHS (NIOSH) Publication No. 2004-165, 2004.
This alert offers a recent review of recommendations for hazardous drug, including chemotherapy drug, handling in the workplace.
Lucroy MD: Chemotherapy safety in veterinary practice: hazardous drug preparation, *Compend Contin Educ Pract Vet* 23:860, 2001.
This is a good review in the veterinary literature that discusses chemotherapy safety in the practice setting.

▌*For a complete list of the references cited in this chapter, please go to www.smallanimaloncology.com.

SECTION E: Chemotherapy Administration

Jamie D. Steffy-Morgan

KEY POINTS

- Dosages, dose calculations, and drug concentration and volume should always be verified before administration of chemotherapy drugs.
- Route of chemotherapy administration is based on physical properties of the drug being used, as well as patient and tumor characteristics; in some cases intralesional or intracavitary chemotherapy may be appropriate.
- Venous access ports may be implanted in dogs, cats, and exotic animals receiving chemotherapy and can be used for blood collection and fluid administration in addition to chemotherapy administration.

Most chemotherapy agents are administered intravenously. Other routes of administration include intramuscular, subcutaneous, intralesional, intracavitary, and oral. The route of administration is dependent upon the chemotherapeutic agent used, the disease being treated, and the patient receiving the medication. Table 12-4 lists routes of administration for commonly used agents.

It is important to become familiar with the recommended and safe routes of administration for each prescribed agent and to double check dosages and dose calculations before administration. Agents may be prescribed on a mg/kg, mg/m^2, IU/kg, or IU/m^2 basis. The formula for calculating m^2 is shown in Box 12-5. Miscalculation of drug dose can lead to life-threatening over-dosage. Emergency procedures related to chemotherapy drug overdose situations are provided on the website (www.smallanimaloncology.com). Care must be exercised when writing and interpreting prescriptions for chemotherapy drugs, since some agents have similar names. For example, vincristine, which is commonly dosed at 0.5 to 0.7 mg/m^2, has a name very similar to vinblastine, which is dosed at 2 mg/m^2. Obviously, calculating a dose of vinblastine, but accidentally pulling up vincristine could lead to a lethal overdose. It is advisable to record the dose, route of administration, and site of administration whenever chemotherapy is given. This will serve as a reference to which subsequent dose calculations can be compared, and it may help with decisions regarding choice of sites for catheter placement. In addition, guidelines for the safe handling of chemotherapy agents should be reviewed by all personnel involved with administration. See Section C for a review of chemotherapy safety information.

TABLE 12-4   METHODS OF CHEMOTHERAPY ADMINISTRATION

Route of Administration	Chemotherapy Drugs
Intravenous	Actinomycin D
	Carboplatin
	Cisplatin
	Cyclophosphamide
	Doxorubicin
	Gemcitabine
	Mechlorethamine
	Mitoxantrone
	Vinblastine
	Vincristine
	5-Fluorouracil
Intramuscular	L-asparaginase
Subcutaneous	L-asparaginase
	Cytosine arabinoside
	Bleomycin
Intracavitary	Cisplatin
	Carboplatin
	Mitoxantrone
	5-Fluorouracil
Intralesional	Cisplatin
	5-Fluorouracil
	Bleomycin
Oral	Cyclophosphamide
	Chlorambucil
	Lomustine (CCNU)
	Procarbazine

BOX 12-5   FORMULA FOR CALCULATION OF BODY SURFACE AREA (M^2)

$$m^2 = \frac{weight(kg)^{2/3} \times constant*}{100}$$

*Constant = 10.1 for dogs; 10.0 for cats

INTRAVENOUS ADMINISTRATION

Peripheral veins are preferred for intravenous drug administration. These vessels are easily monitored to prevent drug extravasation. The injection site should be clipped and scrubbed using aseptic technique before venipuncture and chemotherapy administration. It is a good rule of thumb to alternate legs on the patient if multiple doses of chemotherapy are given to allow previous injection sites time to recover.

Butterfly Catheter

Certain types of intravenous chemotherapy drugs may be given with a butterfly catheter. Drugs given as a bolus of a small volume may be given through a butterfly catheter; however, appropriate patient selection is vitally important. Calm, non-fractious patients are candidates for the use of butterfly catheters. Animals that are of unknown temperament or that are likely to move during venipuncture should not be considered as candidates for drug administration via a butterfly catheter, since sudden movement may cause the needle end to lacerate the vessel and drug extravasation could also occur. Recommended steps for drug administration through a butterfly catheter are shown in Box 12-6.

Intravenous Catheter

If the chemotherapy drug is a vesicant or is infused over time, an indwelling catheter should be used. It is important that chemotherapy drugs be administered through catheters that are freshly placed with one clean attempt at venipuncture. If catheter placement is unsuccessful, another limb or a location clearly proximal to the site of the failed placement should be used. T-port extensions should be connected to the catheter to allow for the attachment of the Luer-Lok syringe containing the chemotherapy dose. The catheter and T-port should be flushed using heparin-free 0.9% saline to ensure patency. Some chemotherapy agents bind with heparin and therefore heparinized flush should be avoided. The catheter should be secured in place, keeping in mind not to obstruct visualization of the entry of the catheter into the skin, and then administration can begin. The catheter site and leg should be constantly monitored for drug leakage or swelling to avoid extravasation (Figure 12-6).

INTRAMUSCULAR, SUBCUTANEOUS, OR INTRALESIONAL ADMINISTRATION

The caudal thigh region or lumbar regions are popular sites for intramuscular injection and the intrascapular region for subcutaneous injection. Personal protective equipment should be worn as with any chemotherapy administration, as discussed in Section C. One should aspirate and assess the needle hub and syringe for blood to ensure that a vessel has not been accessed before injecting the drug.

Intralesional administration is used occasionally for treatment of cutaneous or soft tissue masses that are not amenable to surgical excision. Cisplatin and 5-fluorouracil are two agents that have been administered in this fashion in companion animal oncology practice. The selected drug should not be a vesicant, nor should it require metabolism to its active form (such as cyclophosphamide, which must be metabolized by the liver). Chemotherapeutic agents to be administered intralesionally can be formulated into sustained-release gel implants for surgical implantation[1-3] or mixed with medical-grade sesame seed oil[4] to be injected into the tumor. It is important to

---

BOX 12-6	PROCEDURE FOR ADMINISTRATION OF CHEMOTHERAPEUTIC AGENTS THROUGH A BUTTERFLY CATHETER

1. Assemble all necessary supplies in a drug administration site that is free of clinic traffic.
2. Clip and aseptically prep the venipuncture site.
3. Place the butterfly catheter and flush thoroughly with non-heparinized 0.9% saline to check for swellings or leakage.
4. Detach the saline syringe and attach the Luer-Lok syringe containing the chemotherapy.
5. Pull back the syringe plunger to ensure blood flow and then depress the plunger to administer the drug.
6. Once the chemotherapy has been given, kink the tubing and reattach the 0.9% saline syringe, then unkink the tubing and flush thoroughly.

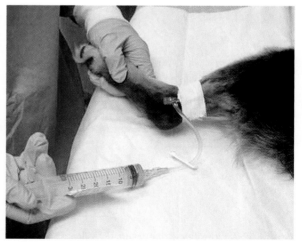

FIGURE 12-6 Example of intravenous chemotherapy administration. This patient is receiving chemotherapy in the left lateral saphenous vein.

distribute the drug as evenly as possible throughout the lesion and to watch for any leakage during administration. If leakage occurs, the area should be washed thoroughly with soap and water and all cleaning materials disposed of in the proper hazardous materials area.

INTRACAVITARY ADMINISTRATION

Intracavitary chemotherapy is indicated for treatment of tumors causing effusion. Certain chemotherapy agents (e.g., cisplatin, 5-fluorouracil, carboplatin, and mitoxantrone) can safely be administered into body cavities.[5-7] If cisplatin is the drug used, saline diuresis protocols are necessary to prevent renal toxicity. The dose of drug recommended is typically that of intravenous administration. The drug should be further diluted with the recommended diluent to 250 ml/m^2 before intracavitary administration (e.g., at a dosage of 300 mg/m^2, a 1-m^2 dog would receive 300 mg or 30 ml of carboplatin, and that volume would be further diluted to a total of volume of 250 ml). The cavity to receive the chemotherapy should be drained of effusion before drug infusion. Personal protective equipment should be worn by all personnel involved with intracavitary administration. Equipment necessary for intracavitary chemotherapy includes a self-sealing thoracocentesis catheter such as an Argyle catheter (Covidien, Mansfield, Mass.) or surgically implanted PleuralPort (Norfolk Vet Products, Skokie, Illinois) as shown in Figure 12-7, an IV extension set, three-way stopcock, sterile 20- to 60-ml syringe

for removal of effusion, and the chemotherapy drug. A thoracocentesis catheter or PleuralPort are recommended over a traditional IV catheter for thoracic administration to prevent induction of a pneumothorax when the stylet is removed from the catheter. There is a significant risk for laceration of the lung, liver, or spleen when using a butterfly catheter, should the patient become agitated during the infusion. Therefore, they are not recommended for intracavitary chemotherapy administration. Steps for administering intrathoracic chemotherapy are outlined in Box 12-7. Half of the volume may be given into each hemi-thorax to help maximize surface exposure if so desired. The same steps are taken for abdominal administration as thoracic administration, except the patient is placed in dorsal recumbency and the injection site is generally a midline site caudal to the umbilicus. The urinary bladder should be emptied before starting

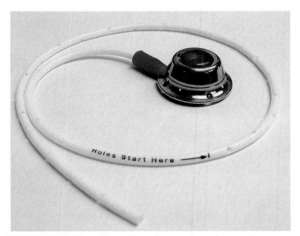

FIGURE 12-7 PleuralPort. Note fenestrations along catheter that allow for removal of fluid from body cavities, as well as instillation of intracavitary chemotherapy. (Courtesy of Norfolk Veterinary Products, Skokie, Illinois.)

BOX 12-7   STEPS FOR INTRATHORACIC CHEMOTHERAPY ADMINISTRATION

1. Place patient in standing or lateral recumbency position.
2. Determine the thoracocentesis site (7th–9th intercostal space).
3. Aseptically prep the region.
4. Infiltrate the skin at the chosen site with lidocaine if necessary.
5. Insert thoracocentesis catheter.
6. Attach IV tubing and three-way stopcock to thoracocentesis catheter.
7. Attach empty, sterile syringe to three-way stopcock and remove effusate from thorax.
8. Flush catheter to ensure patency.
9. Attach chemotherapy to three-way stopcock and infuse over 15 minutes. (Note: Volume may be divided in half to divide dose between thoracic cavities.)
10. When complete, close three-way stopcock to the patient and remove chemotherapy syringe.
11. Attach flush to three-way stopcock and flush IV tubing to insert remainder of drug into the thorax.
12. Remove thoracocentesis catheter from chest and apply gentle pressure to the entry site using a gauze sponge until no fluid is absorbed.
13. Once complete, remove personal protective equipment and dispose of properly.

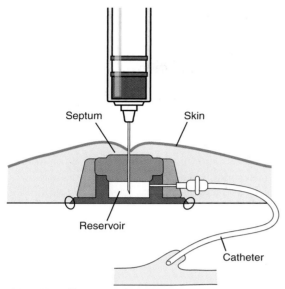

FIGURE 12-8 Illustration of vascular access port. Note proper placement of Huber point needle within the port. (Courtesy of Norfolk Veterinary Products, Skokie, Illinois.)

the procedure to avoid accidental infusion of the drug into the bladder. The chemotherapy is typically infused over 15 minutes per site, and the solution is left in the body cavity. To help ensure adequate contact with all surfaces, some advocate rotating the animal on all sides (dorsal, lateral, sternal, and opposite lateral) for 5 to 15 minutes per side after infusion.

ORAL ADMINISTRATION

Oral chemotherapy administration is done in the same manner as any other pilling procedure. Latex gloves should be worn. Owners giving oral drugs at home should be provided with latex gloves and instructed to wash their hands before and after administration. It is important to place the pill(s) in the back of the mouth to avoid crushing of the pill by the animal. This could result in drug loss or aerosolization of the agent, risking exposure to the person administering. A pill dispenser may be helpful for some animals. Tablets should never purposefully be crushed, and capsules should never be opened as this, too, will result in drug aerosolization and exposure.

VASCULAR ACCESS PORTS

A vascular access port is a subcutaneously implanted device (Figure 12-8) that allows for administration of medications (including chemotherapy), blood donation, and sampling.[8-10] The most common vessel catheterized

BOX 12-8 BASIC VENOUS ACCESS PORT PRINCIPLES

1. Palpate the port's location under the skin and aseptically prep the site.
2. Stabilize the port using your thumb and finger.
3. Insert a Huber needle through the skin and septum at a 90-degree angle to the port.
4. Advance the Huber needle through the septum to the bottom of the port. When you reach the bottom of the port, you will feel the needle abruptly stop on a metal surface (see Figure 12-8).
5. Hold the needle securely against the base of the port while aspirating or flushing.
6. When drawing blood samples from a VAP, remove 1.5 ml (for cats) and 5 ml (for average-sized dogs) of discard blood and then remove the blood needed for sampling.
7. Chemotherapy should be delivered following recommendations for peripheral intravenous administration.
8. The port should be flushed with 0.9% saline and a heparin lock placed as per specific port instructions before removal of the Huber needle.

for the port is the jugular vein, but the femoral vein may also be used. The access port is implanted under the skin of the dorsolateral neck/scapula region for jugular vein access and in the subcutaneous tissue at the caudal aspect of the ribs or the ilial wing for femoral vein access.[8-10] Accessing the port is achieved by penetrating the skin and port septum using a non-coring Huber point needle. It is important to use only Huber needles when accessing venous access ports, since the use of regular needles risks lacerating the port, rendering it non-functional. The port septum can accept at least 1500 punctures without losing its integrity. It is unnecessary to remove the port after completion of a chemotherapy protocol. The port may safely and indefinitely remain implanted. Basic steps involved in the use of venous access ports are outlined in Box 12-8.

Selected References*

Cahalane AK, Flanders JA, Steffey MA, et al: Use of vascular access ports with intrathoracic drains for treatment of pleural effusion in three dogs, *J Am Vet Med Assoc* 230:527, 2007.

This report presents the use of vascular access ports with an associated Jackson-Pratt drain for the infusion of intracavitary chemotherapy in three dogs.

Charney SC, Bergman PJ, McKnight JA, et al: Evaluation of intracavitary mitoxantrone and carboplatin for treatment of carcinomatosis, sarcomatosis and mesothelioma, with or without malignant effusions: a retrospective analysis of 12 cases (1997-2002), *Vet Comp Oncol* 3:171, 2005.

This retrospective study reports on the use of intracavitary mitoxantrone and carboplatin for treatment of various neoplastic effusions in dogs.

Henry CJ, Russell LE, Tyler JW, et al: Comparison of hematologic and biochemical values for blood samples obtained via jugular venipuncture and via vascular access ports in cats, *J Am Vet Med Assoc* 220:482, 2002.

This study reports on the use of vascular access ports in cats and compares results of hematologic and biochemical parameters obtained with that of traditional jugular venipuncture.

Moore AS, Kirk C, Cardona A: Intracavitary cisplatin chemotherapy experience with six dogs, *J Vet Intern Med* 5:227, 1991.

This retrospective study report on the use of intracavitary cisplatin for the treatment of neoplastic thoracic and abdominal effusion. The response to therapy and overall survival of six dogs are reported.

■ *For a complete list of the references cited in this chapter, please go to www.smallanimaloncology.com.

SECTION F: Formulary and Sources of Chemotherapeutic Agents

Carlos O. Rodriguez, Jr., Mary Lynn Higginbotham, and Carolyn J. Henry

See Table 12-5 for a formulary of chemotherapy drugs and Table 12-6 for a list of chemotherapy drugs and safety equipment sources.

TABLE 12-5   FORMULARY OF CHEMOTHERAPY DRUGS

Generic Drug Name	Trade Names or Acronyms	Available Formulations	Reported Dog Dosages	Reported Cat Dosages	Route of Administration	Unique Toxicities or Other Considerations	Relative Cost
Asparaginase	Elspar L-Asparaginase	10,000 or 20,000 IU vials	400 IU/kg; 10,000 to 20,000 IU/m^2	400 IU/kg; 10,000 IU/m^2	SQ, IM, IP	Pancreatitis, hypersensitivity reaction (pretreat with diphenhydramine)	$$$
Carboplatin	Paraplatin	10 mg/ml in 50, 150, and 450 mg solution or powder vials	300 mg/m^2 q21d; Some recommend dose reduction for dogs <15 kg to 250 mg/m^2	240 mg/m^2 or 10 mg/kg q21d	IV, intracavitary	Use D$_5$W for reconstitution, rather than saline	$$
Chlorambucil	Leukeran	2 mg tablets	40 mg/m^2 or 1.4 mg/kg q21d; 2-6 mg/m^2 q24-48hr	2 mg q2–3d	PO		$$

(Continued)

TABLE 12-5   FORMULARY OF CHEMOTHERAPY DRUGS–CONT'D

Generic Drug Name	Trade Names or Acronyms	Available Formulations	Reported Dog Dosages	Reported Cat Dosages	Route of Administration	Unique Toxicities or Other Considerations	Relative Cost
Cisplatin	Platinol-AQ	1 mg/ml in 50, 100, and 200 mg MDV	50–70 mg/m^2	LETHAL	IV, intra-lesional, intracavitary	**Dogs:** acute vomiting*; nephrotoxic (requires saline diuresis†), ototoxic **Cats:** fatal pulmonary edema	$$
Cyclophosphamide	Cytoxan	500 mg and 1 g bottles; 25 and 50 mg tablets	200–250 mg/m^2 per treatment week; (50–62.5 mg/m^2 for 4 days)	50 mg/m^2 × 3 days; 10 mg/kg per treatment week (2.5 mg/kg for 4 days)	IV, PO	Sterile hemorrhagic cystitis (discontinue use if occurs)	$$
Cytarabine	Cytosar-U; ara-C; cytosine arabinoside	100 mg, 500 mg, 1 g, and 2 g vials solution or powder	100 mg/m^2 daily for 4 days; may divide into 2 daily subQ injections due to short t$^{1/2}$; 300–600 mg/m^2 once weekly	100mg/m^2 daily for 2–4 days or 300mg/m^2 once weekly	IV, SQ, intrathecal	Crosses the blood–brain barrier	$$
Dacarbazine	DTIC-Dome	100 and 200 mg bottles	800 mg/m^2 IV as 6- to 8-hour infusion q3wk or 200 mg/m^2 IV for 5 days	Not assessed	IV		$$$
Dactinomycin	Actinomycin-D; Cosmegen	0.5 mg bottle	0.6 to 0.8 mg/m^2 q21d; 0.75 mg/m^2 q21d	Not assessed	IV	Vesicant	$$$$$
Doxorubicin	Adriamycin; Rubex; Doxorubicin HCl	2 mg/ml MDV	30 mg/m^2; 1 mg/kg if ≤10 kg q21d	1 mg/kg q21d	IV	Vesicant **Dogs:** cumulative cardiotoxicity >180–220 mg/m^2 **Cats:** nephrotoxic	$$
Epirubicin	Ellence	50 mg/ 25 ml & 200 mg/ 100 ml SDV	30 mg/m^2 q21d	Not assessed	IV	Vesicant	$$$
Fluorouracil	5-FU; Adrucil Efudex cream	500 mg/ 10 ml bottle	150 mg/m^2; 5-10 mg/kg per treatment week	LETHAL	IV	Fatal neurotoxicity in cats	$$

(Continued)

TABLE 12-5 FORMULARY OF CHEMOTHERAPY DRUGS—CONT'D

Generic Drug Name	Trade Names or Acronyms	Available Formulations	Reported Dog Dosages	Reported Cat Dosages	Route of Administration	Unique Toxicities or Other Considerations	Relative Cost
Gemcitabine	Gemzar	200 mg and 1 g vials (powder)	250–1000 mg/m²	Same as dog	IV, SQ		$$$$
Lomustine	CCNU; CeeNU	10, 40, and 100 mg capsules	60–90 mg/m² q21d	10 mg/cat; 50–60 mg/m² q3-6wk	PO	Hepatotoxic; cumulative thrombocytopenia; delayed myelosuppression	$$
Mechlorethamine	Mustargen	10 mg vial (powder)	3 mg/m²	Same as dog	IV	Vesicant	$$$
Melphalan	Alkeran	2 mg tablets	2 mg/m² q48h; 1.5 mg/m² daily for 10 days on, 10 days off each cycle	0.2 mg/kg or 2 mg/m² q48h	PO		$$
Mitoxantrone	Novantrone	2 mg/ml solution	5 mg/m² q21d	6–6.5 mg/m² q21d	IV over 20 min		$$$$
Piroxicam	Feldene	10 mg capsules	0.3 mg/kg QD	0.3 mg/kg q24–48h	PO	Gastric ulceration; cats: nephrotoxicity	$
Prednisone/ Prednisolone			0.5–2 mg/kg; 20–40 mg/m² daily	5 mg q12–24h	PO, SQ		$
Procarbazine	Matulane	50 mg capsule	50 mg/m²	10 mg/cat	PO		$$$$$
Temozolomide	Temodar	5, 20, 100, 250 mg capsule	125 mg/m² once; 60 mg/m² daily for 5 days	Not assessed	PO		$$$$$
Vinblastine	Velban	1 mg/mL MDV	2 mg/m² q7d or q14d	Same as dog	IV	Vesicant	$
Vincristine	Oncovin	1 mg/mL solution	0.5–0.7 mg/m² per treatment week	Same as dog	IV	Vesicant; peripheral neuropathy	$
Vinorelbine	Navelbine	10 mg/1 ml or 50 mg/5 ml vial	15 mg/m²	Not assessed	IV		$$$

IM, Intramuscular; *IP*, intraperitoneal; *IU*, International Units; *IV*, intravenous; *PO*, by mouth; *MDV*, multi-dose vial; *SDV*, single-dose vial; *SQ*, subcutaneous; $t^{1/2}$, half-life.

*Butorphanol 0.4 mg/kg SQ 20 minutes before cisplatin administration *or* maropitant 1 mg/kg SQ 1 hour before cisplatin administration.

†Diuresis protocol: 4-hour pre-treatment saline diuresis; 20-minute infusion of cisplatin; 2-hour post-treatment saline diuresis.

(1) 0.9% NaCl at 18.3 ml/kg/hr for 4 hr.

(2) cisplatin diluted in 6.1 ml/kg of 0.9% NaCl given over 20 minutes.

(3) 0.9% NaCl at 18.3 ml/kg/hr for 2 hr.

TABLE 12-6   CHEMOTHERAPY DRUGS AND SAFETY EQUIPMENT SOURCES IN THE UNITED STATES[*,†]

Company	Phone Number	Website	Product Notes
Amatheon	1-800-300-8387	www.amatheon.com	Drugs and safety equipment
ClienTails	1-888-546-8245	www.biologicstoday.com	Oral drugs in less than whole bottle quantities; prescribe for patient or office use
Diamondback Drugs	1-866-646-2223	www.diamondbackdrugs.com	Compounding pharmacy
Florida Infusion	1-800-407-9900	www.floridainfusion.com	Drugs and safety equipment
Health Care Logistics	1-800-848-1633	www.healthcarelogistics.com	Safety equipment
Red-X Medical	1-866-406-9385	www.redxmedical.com	Drugs
South Pointe Wholesale	1-866-541-4995	www.southpointe.us	Drugs
TW Medical Veterinary Supply	1-888-787-4483	www.twmedical.com	Commonly used chemotherapy drugs

[*]Other sources may include local hospitals treating cancer patients.

[†]Retail pharmacies may be able to order a specific drug from a wholesaler.

13 Managing Oncologic Emergencies

SECTION A: Tumor- and Treatment-Related Complications

Ravinder S. Dhaliwal

KEY POINTS

- Chemotherapy targets rapidly dividing cells including cells of the bone marrow, mucous membranes (e.g., gastrointestinal lining cells), and hair follicles, as well as malignant cells.
- Chemotherapy toxicities can be acute or delayed and are potentially life threatening if not appropriately treated.
- Chemotherapy-induced neutropenia is a life-threatening condition when a secondary infection develops. Prompt identification and treatment with broad-spectrum antibiotics is crucial for survival of the patient.

TREATMENT-RELATED COMPLICATIONS

Chemotherapy is widely used in the management of veterinary cancer patients. In addition to the cancer cells, virtually all chemotherapeutic drugs also have an effect on normal replicating cell populations. Rapidly dividing normal cells that are vulnerable to damage include cells of the bone marrow, mucous membranes (including the gastrointestinal [GI] tract), and hair follicles. Current veterinary chemotherapy protocols generally produce minimal toxicity, and side effects are medically manageable.[1-5] It is rare that a patient will experience toxicities necessitating protocol alteration or discontinuation.[6-11] This chapter discusses oncologic emergencies and toxicities associated with chemotherapy and the possible pathogenesis of these complications. Because of their importance, in-depth discussion of drug extravasations is covered in Section B, and the management of nausea and vomiting is covered in Chapter 18, Section A. Radiation-related toxicities are addressed in Chapter 15, Section C.

Drug Hypersensitivity and Anaphylaxis

Type I hypersensitivity reactions can occur with any chemotherapeutic agent. Doxorubicin, L-asparaginase, and paclitaxel (Taxol) are among the most commonly used cytotoxic drugs in veterinary medicine that have a potential for hypersensitivity reactions.[12,13] These reactions characteristically occur during or up to 1 hour after injection. Possible clinical manifestations include urticaria or hives and facial pruritus. Respiratory distress, bronchoconstriction (particularly in cats), vomiting, diarrhea, hematochezia, and circulatory collapse could occur with a systemic anaphylactic reaction. Medical management of an acute hypersensitivity drug reaction is illustrated in Box 13-1. Most hypersensitivity reactions associated with doxorubicin infusion will rapidly resolve with appropriate intervention, and doxorubicin treatment may be resumed at a slower rate at that point in time. Because of the antigenic nature of L-asparaginase, which is derived from *Escherichia coli* bacteria, the potential for hypersensitivity reaction increases with each subsequent dose. Premedication with diphenhydramine (2.2 mg/kg SQ) is warranted for animals receiving more than one treatment with this drug. Hypersensitivity reactions are reported to occur in the majority of dogs receiving paclitaxel because of an agent called Cremophor EL, which is present in the drug formulation in order to solubilize the drug. Premedication with prednisone (1 mg/kg PO) 12 to 24 hours before and diphenhydramine (4 mg/kg IM), cimetidine (4 mg/kg IV), and dexamethasone sodium phosphate (2 mg/kg IV) 30 to 60 minutes before paclitaxel administration enabled the use of this agent in dogs[13] with various types of cancer. Regardless of the drug, should an animal exhibit hypersensitivity, they are likely to develop reactions with subsequent doses and pretreatment with diphenhydramine

BOX 13-1   MEDICAL MANAGEMENT OF HYPERSENSITIVITY REACTIONS TO CHEMOTHERAPEUTIC AGENTS

1. Discontinue chemotherapy infusion.
2. Ensure that airway is patent.
3. Administer short-acting steroid such as dexamethasone sodium phosphate (0.25–1 mg/kg IV) or methylprednisolone sodium succinate (30 mg/kg IV).
4. Administer diphenhydramine (1 mg/kg IV or 2 mg/kg IM).
5. Administer crystalloid fluids (0.9% sodium chloride, Normosol, lactated Ringer's solution) at 90 mL/kg/hr in dogs and 44 mL/kg/hr in cats if hypotension occurs.
6. If anaphylactic shock occurs, administer epinephrine (0.01 mL/kg 1:1000 epinephrine IV or IO; 0.2–0.5 mL/kg IM). Administer epinephrine every 15–20 minutes if clinical signs are not resolving.

TABLE 13-1   EXPECTED NEUTROPHIL NADIR IN DOGS AND CATS FOR COMMONLY USED CYTOTOXIC AGENTS

Drug	Expected Nadir
Cyclophosphamide	7–10 days
Lomustine	21 days (dogs); 28 days (cats) (can vary significantly)
Doxorubicin	7–10 days
Mitoxantrone	7–10 days
Vincristine	5–7 days
Vinblastine	5–7 days
Cisplatin	7–14 days (double nadir reported in dogs)
Carboplatin	10–14 days

and/or dexamethasone 15 to 20 minutes before the chemotherapy infusion is warranted.

Hematologic Complications

Neutropenia

Neutropenia is the dose-limiting toxicity of most chemotherapy drugs. The neutrophil nadir (low point in the neutrophil count following chemotherapy administration) is species, patient, and drug specific. For many commonly used drugs, the nadir occurs between 7 and 10 days after treatment. See Table 13-1 for commonly used chemotherapy agents and their expected nadirs. Vincristine (VCR) and l-asparaginase (L-ASP) as single agents are not typically myelosuppressive at standard dosages. However, one study demonstrated that VCR/L-ASP in combination were more likely to result in neutropenia than when the drugs were used individually.[14] A grading scheme of hematopoietic toxicity adopted by the Veterinary Cooperative Oncology Group is outlined in Table 13-2.[15]

Animals with an absolute neutrophil count of <1000 cells/μl are at risk for developing a secondary infection; however, they will remain asymptomatic unless an infection should develop. Generalized malaise and fever are the two most common clinical signs associated with a secondary infection. The organisms causing infections in cancer patients often come from environmental reservoirs or the host's own flora and, therefore, are not typically mutated, resistant bacteria. Potential sources of bacterial entry include the GI tract, cutaneous lesions, pre-existing urinary tract infections, and intravenous catheter sites. Unfortunately, neutropenia and GI toxicity frequently occur at similar times, resulting in an increased potential for bacterial translocation across the GI tract wall. Broad-spectrum antibiotics can be chosen based on the presumed origin of the organisms. Generally, cutaneous sources of infection are gram positive, whereas GI tract, urinary tract, and respiratory infections are commonly gram negative in origin.

Because of the risk for neutropenia following chemotherapy administration, a complete blood count (CBC) should be performed the day of treatment (or within 24 hours before the treatment) to ensure an adequate neutrophil count at the time of dosing. In general, treatment should be delayed if the absolute neutrophil count is <3000 cells/μl. The exception to this rule is if the tumor is causing the neutropenia and treatment is necessary for the bone marrow to repopulate. This can occur in stage V lymphoma patients exhibiting myelophthisis (displacement of the bone marrow cells by neoplastic cells). A CBC is also recommended 1 week after treatment, or at the time of the expected neutrophil nadir. If the neutrophil count is <1500 cells/μl on the post-treatment CBC evaluation and the animal is feeling well, broad-spectrum oral antibiotics (e.g., amoxicillin/clavulanic acid or trimethoprim-sulfa) should be initiated to prevent a secondary infection from developing. If the animal is not well or is febrile as well as neutropenic, septicemia should be presumed. This animal should be hospitalized and treated with IV fluid therapy as well as IV

TABLE 13-2 HEMATOLOGIC AND GASTROINTESTINAL TOXICITY GRADING FROM THE VETERINARY COOPERATIVE ONCOLOGY GROUP (VCOG)[15]

Adverse Event	1	2	3	4	5
Blood/Bone Marrow					
Bone marrow cellularity	Mildly hypocellular; <25% reduction from normal cellularity for age	Moderately hypocellular; >25 to <50% reduction from normal cellularity for age	Severely hypocellular; >50% reduction of cellularity from normal for age	—	—
Hemoglobin	Dog: 10 g/dl – <LLN Cat: 8.0 g/dl – <LLN	Dog: <10–8.0 g/dl Cat: <8.0–6.5 g/dl	Dog: <8.0–6.5 g/dl Cat: <6.5–5.0	Dog: <6.5 g/dl Cat: <5.0	—
Neutropenia	1500/µl – <LLN	1000-1499/µl	500-999/µl	<500/µl	—
Thrombocytopenia	100,000/µl – <LLN	50,000–99,000/µl	25,000–49,000/µl	<25,000	—
Other (Specify, ___)	Mild	Moderate	Severe	Life-threatening; disabling	Death
Gastrointestinal					
Anorexia	Coaxing or dietary change required to maintain appetite	Oral intake altered (<3 days) without significant weight loss; oral nutritional supplements indicated	Of 3–5 days duration; associated with significant weight loss or malnutrition; IV fluids, tube feeding or TPN indicated	Life-threatening consequences; >5 days duration	Death
Colitis	Asymptomatic, pathologic, or radiographic findings only	Abdominal cramping/pain; mucus or blood in stool	Abdominal pain, fever, change in bowel habits, ileus, peritoneal signs	Life-threatening consequences (e.g., perforation, bleeding, ischemia, necrosis)	Death
Constipation	Occasional or intermittent symptoms; occasional use of stool softeners, laxatives, dietary modification or enema	Persistent symptoms with regular use of laxatives or enemas indicated	Symptoms interfering with ADL; obstipation with manual evacuation indicated	Life-threatening consequences (e.g., obstruction, megacolon)	Death
Dehydration	Increased oral fluids indicated; dry mucous membranes; <skin turgor	Parenteral (IV or SC) fluids indicated <24 hr	IV fluids indicated >24 hr	Life-threatening (e.g., hemodynamic collapse)	Death
Diarrhea	Increase of >2 stools per day over baseline	Increase of 2–6 stools per day over baseline; Parenteral (IV or SC) fluids indicated <24 hr; not interfering with ADL	Increase of >6 stools per day over baseline; incontinence; IV fluids >24 hr; hospitalization; interfering with ADL	Life-threatening (e.g., hemodynamic collapse)	Death

(Continued)

TABLE 13-2 HEMATOLOGIC AND GASTROINTESTINAL TOXICITY GRADING FROM THE VETERINARY COOPERATIVE ONCOLOGY GROUP (VCOG)[15] —CONT'D

Adverse Event	GRADE				
	1	2	3	4	5
Gastrointestinal					
Dysphagia	Symptomatic but able to eat regular diet	Symptomatic and altered eating/swallowing (e.g., altered dietary habits, food consistency); Parenteral (IV or SC) fluids indicated <24 hr	Symptomatic and severely altered eating/swallowing (e.g., inadequate oral caloric or fluid intake); IV fluids >24 hr, tube feeding or PPN/TPN indicated	Life-threatening (e.g., obstruction, perforation)	Death
Enteritis (inflammation of the small bowel)	Asymptomatic, pathologic, or radiographic findings only	Abdominal pain/cramping; mucus or blood in stool	Abdominal pain/cramping, fever, change in bowel habits with ileus; peritoneal signs	Life-threatening (e.g., perforation, bleeding, ischemia, necrosis)	Death
Flatulence	Mild	Moderate	—		
Ileus, GI (functional obstruction of bowel, i.e., neuro-constipation)	Asymptomatic, radiographic finding only	Symptomatic; altered GI function (e.g., altered dietary habits); parenteral (IV or SC) fluids indicated <24 hr	Symptomatic and severely altered GI function; IV fluids, tube feedings, or PPN/TPN indicated >24 hr	Life-threatening consequences	Death
Incontinence, anal	Occasional	Daily	Interfering with ADL; operative intervention indicated	Permanent	Death
Mucositis/stomatitis	Erythema of the mucosa	Patchy ulcerations or pseudomembranes	Confluent ulcerations or pseudomembranes; bleeding with minor trauma	Tissue necrosis; significant spontaneous bleeding; life-threatening	Death
Nausea	Loss of appetite without alteration in eating habits	Salivation or "smacking of lips" <12 hr	Salivation or "smacking of lips" >12–24 hr	Salivation or "smacking of lips" >24 hr	—
Vomiting	<3 episodes in 24 hr	3–5 episodes in 24 hr; <3 episodes/day for >2 days but <5 days; parenteral (IV or SC) fluids indicated <24 hr	>5 episodes in 24 hr; vomiting >4 days; IV fluids or PPN/TPN indicated >24 hr	Life-threatening (e.g., hemodynamic collapse)	Vomiting
Other (Specify, ___)	Mild	Moderate	Severe	Life-threatening	Other (Specify, ___)

ADL, Activities of daily life; *LLN,* lower limit of normal.

broad-spectrum antibiotics (enrofloxacin and ampicillin or cefazolin, ampicillin/sulbactam, or ticarcillin/clavulanic acid). Once the fever has resolved and the animal is feeling well, oral antibiotics can be dispensed if the animal remains neutropenic. Future doses of the specific chemotherapeutic agent resulting in a neutropenia of <500 cells/μl should be decreased by 20% in an attempt to prevent severe neutropenia with subsequent doses. In severely neutropenic patients or patients experiencing a prolonged neutropenia, recombinant human granulocyte colony-stimulating factor (rh-GCSF; Filgrastim; 5 μg/kg SQ daily)[16,17] can be administered to help stimulate granulopoiesis and ameliorate the myelosuppression.[18] It should be noted that evidence of a left shift or degenerative left shift is expected following rh-GCSF administration because of the release of immature granulocytes into the circulation. In addition, this is a human origin product, and antibodies may develop after repeated dosing (usually >20 doses) that can result in prolonged neutropenia. Although septicemia leading to death as a result of chemotherapy is rare, any animal that is not feeling well after chemotherapy should be evaluated immediately with a CBC so that appropriate therapy can be instituted. A few hours delay in treatment may be the difference in survival for septic, neutropenic patients.

Thrombocytopenia

Thrombocytopenia may occur following treatment with chemotherapy drugs but is rarely severe enough to necessitate treatment. Cumulative thrombocytopenia occurs in dogs receiving prolonged CCNU (lomustine) treatment,[19] and thrombocytopenia has also been reported as a common toxicity associated with use of the rescue lymphoma protocol, DMAC (dexamethasone, melphalan, actinomycin D, and cytosine arabinoside).[20]

Anemia

Anemia is a common hematologic finding with cancer patients; however, chemotherapy-induced anemia is a rare entity in our experience.

Gastrointestinal Toxicity

Anorexia, vomiting, and diarrhea are the most commonly reported GI toxicities resulting from chemotherapy.[21,22] Box 13-2 shows the relative emetogenic potential of some of the most common chemotherapy drugs used in veterinary oncology. Further information regarding the mechanisms and management of chemotherapy-induced nausea and vomiting can be found in Chapter 18, Section A. Chemotherapy-induced enterocolitis resulting in diarrhea most often occurs with doxorubicin

---

BOX 13-2   EMETOGENIC POTENTIAL OF COMMONLY USED CHEMOTHERAPEUTIC AGENTS

Highly Emetogenic
Cisplatin
Dacarbazine
Doxorubicin
Dactinomycin
Streptozocin

Moderately Emetogenic
Carboplatin
Cyclophosphamide
Procarbazine
Vinorelbine
Mitoxantrone

Mildly Emetogenic
L-Asparaginase
Chlorambucil
Cytarabine
Vincristine
Vinblastine
Melphalan
Fluorouracil
Hydroxyurea

---

administration, but it can potentially occur with any chemotherapeutic agent. It is generally self-limiting; however, symptomatic treatment may be necessary if diarrhea is severe. Fluid therapy and medications such as loperamide[16] (0.08 mg/kg PO TID; Collie-related breeds may be overly sensitive) or medications containing bismuth subsalicylate[23] (Pepto-Bismol 3–15 ml q8–12 hr; should be used in dogs only) can be used if necessary.

Greater rates of high grade GI toxicity have been reported with 25 mg/m^2 of doxorubicin, when given in combination with cisplatin at 60 mg/m^2, as adjuvant treatment for canine osteosarcoma.[24] Moore et al.[25] also reported a higher incidence of toxicity with the combination of doxorubicin and vincristine. It appears that small dogs with a mean body weight of 9.9 kg are more likely to have adverse GI effects as a result of carboplatin therapy.[26]

Hepatotoxicity

Approximately 6% of dogs developed hepatic toxicity after treatment with oral CCNU in one study.[27] The same study concluded that CCNU could cause delayed, cumulative, dose-related, chronic hepatotoxicity that is irreversible and can be fatal. Serum ALT should be monitored in patients receiving CCNU and the drug discontinued if a four-fold increase above baseline is noted.

Pancreatitis

Pancreatitis is a rare complication of chemotherapy. The drugs commonly associated with pancreatitis include L-asparaginase, azathioprine, and glucocorticoids.[28-30] The mechanism of drug-induced pancreatitis is not known, and the treatment is symptomatic.

Cardiotoxicity

Cardiotoxicity is a well-described adverse effect of doxorubicin in dogs, but it has not been reported in cats.[31-33] It is dose dependent and related to peak plasma concentrations of the drug. Arrhythmias are common during drug administration. The cumulative adverse effects of doxorubicin mimic dilated cardiomyopathy, eventually leading to heart failure.[34] Doxorubicin-associated cardiotoxicity has been reported to occur at cumulative doses as little as 90 mg/m^2 in dogs[35] but is of greater risk in normal dogs at cumulative doses >200 mg/m^2.[36] Recommendations for total cumulative dose in dogs is between 150 and 240 mg/m^2. Because of the toxicity also being related to peak plasma concentrations, doxorubicin should be diluted and infused over 30 minutes or longer. Obtaining a baseline echocardiogram to evaluate fractional shortening before beginning doxorubicin treatment and periodically during the treatment protocol should be considered, especially in animals with a predisposition to dilated cardiomyopathy.

Dexrazoxane (Zinecard), an iron-chelating agent, has been shown to reduce the cumulative cardiotoxicity in people and dogs when administered concurrently with doxorubicin.[37,38] In people it is recommended to be given at a ratio of 10:1 (dexrazoxane:doxorubicin) 30 minutes before doxorubicin administration.[39] The dexrazoxane package insert recommends a total elapsed time of 30 minutes from the start of the dexrazoxane infusion to the completion of doxorubicin infusion. A pegylated-liposomal formulation of doxorubicin (Doxil) has been shown to have a reduced risk of causing cardiotoxicity in dogs.[40] The dose-limiting toxicity of Doxil in dogs is palmar-plantar erythrodyesthesia.[41] Unfortunately, the cost of Doxil prohibits its use for many veterinary patients.

Uroepithelial Toxicity

Sterile hemorrhagic cystitis (SHC) can occur after administration of the alkylating agents cyclophosphamide and ifosfamide. Acrolein, a metabolite of cyclophosphamide and ifosfamide, is toxic to the urinary mucosa and responsible for SHC.[42-44] Clinical signs include hematuria, dysuria, and pollakiuria. The most effective therapy is immediate discontinuation of the drug. Intravesicular administration of 1% formalin or 25% to 50% of dimethyl sulfoxide has been used to treat persistent SHC.[45,46] Concurrent administration of furosemide when cyclophosphamide is given intravenously may reduce the likelihood of developing SHC.[42] Saline diuresis and the thiol compound, mesna, are used to prevent urothelial toxicity caused by ifosfamide.[43]

Pulmonary Toxicity

Cisplatin causes fatal pulmonary toxicity in cats that is clinically manifested as severe hydrothorax with pulmonary and mediastinal edema.[47] Because of this toxicity, cisplatin is contraindicated for use in cats.

Neurotoxicity

Neurotoxicity is a side effect of 5-fluorouracil (5-FU) in all species but is fatal in cats.[48-51] The use of any formulation of 5-FU in cats is contraindicated. The vinca alkaloids, particularly vincristine, can also cause neurotoxicity. Constipation in cats and peripheral neuropathy with licking and chewing at the digits has been reported in dogs receiving vincristine.[52]

Nephrotoxicity

Cisplatin and carboplatin are both nephrotoxic and can induce, to a different degree, impairment in glomerular function. Nephrotoxicity is the most important dose-limiting toxicity of cisplatin.[53,54] To prevent renal toxicity with cisplatin treatment, diuresis with 0.9% sodium chloride at a rate of 20 ml/kg/hour for 4 hours before and 2 hours following cisplatin administration is recommended. Dose-limiting renal toxicity has also been noted with the combination of the cyclooxygenase-2 inhibitor, piroxicam, and cisplatin in dogs with transitional cell carcinoma of the urinary bladder.[55,56] Nephrotoxicity appears to be the dose-limiting toxicity of doxorubicin in cats.[57,58]

Acute Tumor Lysis Syndrome

Acute tumor lysis syndrome (ATLS) refers to the constellation of metabolic disturbances that may be seen after tumor response to the initiation of cytotoxic therapy. It is classically noted with bulky, rapidly proliferating, treatment-responsive tumors such as lymphoma and leukemia.[59,60] Following chemotherapy, a large number of neoplastic cells are killed rapidly, leading to release of intracellular ions and metabolic by-products into the systemic circulation. The syndrome is characterized by rapid development of hyperuricemia, hyperkalemia, hyperphosphatemia, hypocalcemia, and acute renal failure and may manifest clinically as collapse, muscle fasciculations, and cardiorespiratory compromise within 48 hours of treatment initiation.[59,60] Treatment for ATLS includes supportive care with fluid diuresis and medical management of hyperkalemia and metabolic acidosis. The main principle of prevention of ATLS is identification of high-risk patients and ensuring they are adequately hydrated and monitored closely.

TUMOR-RELATED COMPLICATIONS

Tumor-related complications or emergencies are most often associated with a paraneoplastic condition associated with the tumor (e.g., hypercalcemia or hypoglycemia), which are discussed in detail in Chapter 11. A functional obstruction of an organ (GI obstruction or urinary obstruction) may also be an emergent situation and is discussed in Chapter 14. In addition to paraneoplastic and obstructive complications, animals with hematopoietic neoplasia, such as lymphoma or leukemia, may be presented for bone marrow suppression as a result of myelophthisis. Treatment of lymphoma is discussed in Chapter 25.

Selected References*

Charney SC, Bergman PJ, Hohenhaus AE, et al: Risk factors for sterile hemorrhagic cystitis in dogs with lymphoma receiving cyclophosphamide with or without concurrent administration of furosemide: 216 cases (1990-1996), *J Am Vet Med Assoc* 222:1388, 2003.

This retrospective study supports the administration of furosemide with cyclophosphamide, resulting in a decreased incidence of cyclophosphamide-associated sterile hemorrhagic cystitis in this study.

Kristal O, Rassnick KM, Gliatto JM, et al: Hepatotoxicity associated with CCNU (lomustine) chemotherapy in dogs, *J Vet Intern Med* 18:75, 2004.

A retrospective study suggesting that CCNU can cause drug-specific hepatotoxicity. The hepatotoxicity in this study was cumulative and dose related.

Poirier VJ, Hershey AE, Burgess KE, et al: Efficacy and toxicity of paclitaxel (Taxol) for the treatment of canine malignant tumors, *J Vet Intern Med* 18:219, 2004.

An overall unacceptable toxicity of paclitaxel with 64% of dogs experiencing allergic reactions. A lower starting dose is suggested for future evaluations of paclitaxel in dogs.

Sorenmo KU, Baez JL, Clifford CA, et al: Efficacy and toxicity of a dose-intensified doxorubicin protocol in canine hemangiosarcoma, *J Vet Intern Med* 18:209, 2004.

This study indicated that dose-intense regimens can be performed with tolerable clinical toxicity. However, this study failed to show an association between dose intensity and clinical outcome.

Veterinary Cooperative Oncology Group: Common terminology criteria for adverse events (VCOG CTCAE) following chemotherapy or biological antineoplastic therapy in dogs and cats v1.0, *Vet Comp Oncol* 2:95, 2004.

This reference describes the grading schemes for chemotherapy toxicity.

■ *For a complete list of the references cited in this chapter, please go to www.smallanimaloncology.com.

SECTION B: Treatment of Chemotherapy Extravasations

Valerie J. Wiebe and Eric Simonson

KEY POINTS

• The treatment of chemotherapy extravasations depends on the vesicant properties of the specific agent that is extravasated.

• A vesicant is an agent that is capable of causing tissue damage and/or necrosis.

• Sites of extravasation of agents that are high in potential vesicant properties should be treated aggressively before symptoms develop.

Extravasation is the leakage of a vesicant drug into the subcutaneous tissue, which is capable of causing pain, necrosis, or sloughing of tissues. Most chemotherapy agents are not vesicants and rarely cause ulceration of tissue if inadvertently extravasated. The incidence of accidental extravasations in human medicine is reported to be between 0.5% and 6% of chemotherapeutic administrations.[1] The incidence in veterinary medicine is unknown but most likely exceeds that found in

BOX 13-3 CLASSIFICATION OF CHEMO- THERAPY VESICANT PROPERTIES

High Vesicant Potential
Dactinomycin
Daunorubicin
Doxorubicin
Epirubicin
Mechlorethamine
Mitomycin-C
Vinblastine
Vincristine

Low Vesicant Potential
Cisplatin
Dacarbazine
Etoposide
5-Fluorouracil
Liposomal doxorubicin
Mitoxantrone

Irritant
Bleomycin
Carboplatin
Cyclophosphamide
Carmustine
Gemcitabine
Melphalan
Streptozocin

released from dying cells and further exposing adjacent cells to cytotoxic drug.[4] Surgery using wide excision technique or even amputation may be indicated to remove residual drug and non-viable tissues. Agents that are considered low in vesicant potential or that are irritants typically cause pain at the site of injection with or without an inflammatory reaction. In general, these extravasations are treated conservatively. However, these agents may also be considered vesicants if large amounts or high concentrations of drug are extravasated.

Because few antidotes are available that effectively inhibit the debilitating complications of inadvertent chemotherapy extravasations (Box 13-4), prevention of extravasations is critical. Many guidelines for the prevention of chemotherapy extravasations have been published,[3] and are covered elsewhere (see Chapter 12). Despite attempts to prevent extravasations, inadvertent extravasations may still occur and the veterinarian should be prepared in advance. Effective anecdotes and protocols for management of high vesicant extravasations should always be immediately available prior to the administration of these agents. The clinician may want to keep on hand an extravasation kit containing both supplies and management protocols (Boxes 13-5 and 13-6).

humans. Extravasation should be presumed if any of the following occur during chemotherapy administration:
- Inability to obtain blood return from an IV site
- Swelling at the injection site
- Patient appears painful at the injection site

The treatment of chemotherapy extravasations is not always required and is dependent on the vesicant properties of the specific agent (Box 13-3 and Table 13-3).[2] A vesicant is an agent that is capable of causing tissue damage and/or necrosis. Agents that are high in potential vesicant properties should be treated aggressively before symptoms develop. Symptoms may range from local inflammation to extensive necrosis, ulceration, and sloughing of the skin and underlying structures (Figure 13-1).[3] Tissue damage from anthracyclines is often very severe. Binding of drug to the DNA causes cell death with subsequent lysis, allowing the drug to be

Selected References*

Bertelli G, Dini D, Forno GB, et al: Hyaluronidase as an antidote to extravasation of Vinca alkaloids, *J Cancer Res Clin Oncol* 120:505, 1994.
The first clinical report confirming the efficacy of hyaluronidase for local treatment of vinca alkaloid extravasation in people.
Ener RA, Meglathery SB, Styler M: Extravasation of systemic hemato-oncological therapies, *Ann Oncol* 15:858, 2004.
This is a thorough review from the human literature discussing prevention and management of cytotoxic drug extravasations.
Langer SW, Thougaard AV, Sehested M, et al: Treatment of anthracycline extravasation in mice with dexrazoxane with or without DMSO and hydrocortisone, *Cancer Chemother Pharmacol* 57:125, 2006.
This study compares the efficacy of topical DMSO, intralesional hydrocortisone, and systemic dexrazoxane for the treatment of anthracycline extravasation and shows the use of dexrazoxane to be efficacious and superior to DMSO and hydrocortisone.

■ *For a complete list of the references cited in this chapter, please go to www.smallanimaloncology.com.

TABLE 13-3   SPECIFIC TREATMENT OF VESICANT CHEMOTHERAPEUTICS

Drug/Reference	Antidote	Local Care	Comments
Cisplatin (Platinol)	Isotonic sodium thiosulfate; use 2 ml antidote per each 100 mg cisplatin extravasated[2]	None proven effective	Treat if cisplatin concentration is >0.5 mg/ml × 20 ml; irritant below that[2]
Dactinomycin (Cosmegen)	None proven effective	Cold pack	Heat will increase damage; NaCl, hydrocortisone, Na thiosulfate not effective.
Daunorubicin (Cerubidine)	Dexrazoxane[5]—administer as a separate IV infusion within 3 hr. (See Box 13-4)	Wide surgical resection and debridement may be required	DMSO, cold, hydrocortisone shown not effective.[6] Immediate pain, followed by erythema, edema within hours; ulceration, necrosis within 1-3 weeks.
Doxorubicin (Adriamycin)	Dexrazoxane[5]—administer as a separate IV infusion within 6 hr. (See Box 13-4)	Wide surgical resection and debridement may be required	DMSO, cold, hydrocortisone shown not effective.[6] Immediate pain, followed by erythema, edema within hours; ulceration, necrosis within 1-3 weeks.
Epirubicin (Ellence)	Dexrazoxane[5]—administer as a separate IV infusion within 6 hr. (See Box 13-4)	Wide surgical resection and debridement may be required	DMSO, cold, hydrocortisone shown not effective.[6] Immediate pain, followed by erythema, edema within hours; ulceration, necrosis within 1-3 weeks.
Mechlorethamine (Mustargen)	Isotonic sodium thiosulfate[2]; Immediately! (See Box 13-4)	Heat/cold not effective	Immediate pain/phlebitis Use 2 ml antidote for every 1 mg drug extravasated.
Mitomycin-C (Mutamycin)	DMSO[2]	Cold pack	May get delayed reactions at distant sites.
Vinblastine (Velban)	Hyaluronidase[2] or if not available NaCl plus dex. 4 mg (See Box 13-4)	Apply dry heat compresses	Immediate pain, slow-healing ulcers
Vincristine (Oncovin)	Hyaluronidase[2] or if not available NaCl plus dex. 4 mg (See Box 13-4)	Apply dry heat compresses	Immediate pain, slow-healing ulcers
Vinorelbine (Navelbine)	Hyaluronidase[2] or if not available NaCl plus dex. 4 mg (See Box 13-4)	Apply dry heat compresses	Immediate pain, slow-healing ulcers

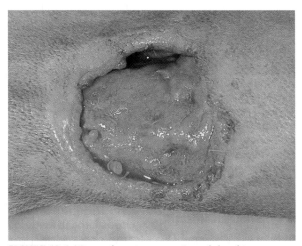

FIGURE 13-1 Tissue ulceration, necrosis, and sloughing occurred as a result of extravasation of vinblastine in the lateral rear limb of this patient.

BOX 13-4   ANTIDOTES

1. Hyaluronidase (Wydase)
   a. Indications: Vinca alkaloids, epipodophyllotoxin extravasations (if Wydase not available, see dexamethasone/saline alternative below).[7,8]
   b. Mechanism: Breaks down subcutaneous tissue bonds promoting drug diffusion through the interstitial space. Enhances absorption of injected substances.
   c. Contraindications: Anthracycline extravasation, infected or cancerous sites.[7,8]
   d. Admix: Use 10% sodium thiosulfate; mix 150 units (1 vial) of hyaluronidase with 1 ml of sterile saline.
   e. Administration: Attempt to remove by aspiration as much extravasated drug as possible; then inject 1 ml for each 1 ml of drug; infiltrate directly into existing IV line or subcutaneously within 1 hour of extravasation. Change needle between subcutaneous injections. Inject approximately 5 x 30 units (0.2 ml) of the 150 unit/ml hyaluronidase around the edge of the extravasation site.
2. Dexrazoxane (Zinecard)
   a. Indications: Anthracyclines (doxorubicin, daunorubicin, epirubicin, idarubicin)[5,6]
   b. Mechanism: Unknown; may be due to topo II interactions, not due to free radical scavenging; lesions reduced by > 70%.
   c. Contraindications: aclarubicin, merbarone
   d. Admix: Dilute according to the manufacturer's instructions (i.e., add either 25 or 50 ml of the manufacturer's diluent to a 250- or 500-mg vial to make a 10 mg/ml solution). This is then further diluted to a 1.3–5.0 mg/ml solution in either 0.9% sodium chloride or 5% dextrose injection. The solution is stable for up to 6 hours.
   e. Administration: IV only! This product is a vesicant alone. Administer first dose as a separate infusion within 6 hours of extravasation, ideally within 2–5 hours if possible.[5] Dose is 1:10 of vesicant:dexrazoxane; infuse IV (approximately 300 mg/m^2 BID on day 1), then daily for 2 days. Triple doses have been shown to be more effective than a single dose.[5]
3. Sodium thiosulfate
   a. Indications: Mechlorethamine (nitrogen mustard), cisplatin extravasations[9,10]
   b. Mechanism: Neutralizes vesicant effect of mechlorethamine by providing an alternative target for alkylation to form non-toxic thioesters, which can be excreted into urine.
   c. Contraindications: Dactinomycin
   d. Admix: If 10% sodium thiosulfate solution: Mix 4 ml with 6 ml preservative-free sterile water for injection. If 25% sodium thiosulfate solution: Mix 1.6 ml with 8.4 ml of preservative-free sterile water for injection. This results in a 1:6 Molar ratio.
   e. Administration: This is time sensitive and should be administered immediately. Inject 1 ml for each 1 ml of vesicant extravasated through the existing line. Then consider injecting 1 ml subcutaneously in 0.1-ml doses clockwise around the site. This may be repeated several times over the next 3–4 hours.
4. DMSO
   a. Indications: Mitomycin-C[11]
   b. Mechanism: Enhances skin permeability that may facilitate absorption of extravascular drug. Also has free radical scavenging/antioxidant properties that may speed up removal of drugs.
   c. Contraindications: Shown to reduce the efficacy of dexrazoxane.[6]
   d. Administration: Apply topical gel or 1–2 ml of a 1 mM 50%–90% (w/v) DMSO using a cotton swab, over the skin of the extravasation site. Apply topically, allow to dry, and do not cover. Repeat every 6–8 hours for 1–2 weeks.
5. Local Cooling
   a. Indications: Dactinomycin, Mitomycin-C[2]
   b. Mechanism: Causes vasoconstriction and tends to restrict spread of drug
   c. Contraindications: Nitrogen mustard, dacarbazine, vinca alkaloids
   d. Administration: Cooling may be achieved with ice packs, cooling pad, or cryogel packs. This should be done four times daily for 15–30 minutes for 48 hours after the extravasation.

(Continued)

BOX 13-4 ANTIDOTES—CONT'D

6. Local heating (dry heat only)
    a. Indications: Vinblastine, vincristine, vinorelbine[2]
    b. Mechanism: Produces local vasodilation and increased blood flow in area
    c. Contraindications: Nitrogen mustard, dactinomycin, anthracyclines
    d. Administration: Heating can be accomplished with a heating pad. Moist heat should not be used. This should be done four times daily for 15–30 minutes for 48 hours after the extravasation.
7. Dexamethasone/hydrocortisone with saline
    a. Indications: Venous flare reactions caused by doxorubicin or for vinca alkaloid extravasations when Wygase is not available.[2]
    b. Mechanism: May reduce ulcer size or reduce inflammation in flare reactions.
    c. Contraindications: May worsen symptoms of extravasation if high or multiple doses are used.
    d. Administration: Administer 10 ml of preservative-free 0.9% saline with 4 mg of dexamethasone sodium phosphate subcutaneously proximal to the extravasation site. Alternatively, hydrocortisone can be used in low doses (<50 mg).[12]

BOX 13-5 EXTRAVASATION KIT: SUPPLY LIST

Preservative-free 0.9% NaCl (10-ml vial)	25- to 27-gauge needles × 5
Sodium thiosulfate 10% (10-ml vial)	Instant cold pack
Preservative-free sterile water for injection (10-ml vial)	Instant hot pack (dry)
Alcohol pads	Hyaluronidase (refrigerated item)
6-ml syringe × 2	DMSO gel
12-ml syringe × 2	Cotton swabs
18-gauge needle	Dexrazoxane (Zinecard)
½-inch needle × 3	Sterile dressing

BOX 13-6 MANAGEMENT OF ACUTE EXTRAVASATIONS

1. Stop drug flow immediately.
2. Do not remove the needle or catheter.
3. Withdraw any remaining fluid and drug from the IV line with a syringe.
4. Using a syringe, attempt to withdraw as much infiltrated drug as possible through the needle (3–5 ml of blood).
5. If known antidote (see Table 13-3), prepare as described in Box 13-4.
6. Administer at least 5 ml directly through the existing line if still in place and/or subcutaneously (dexrazoxane-IV only!) if the line is no longer in place.
7. Antidotes may also be administered subcutaneously with a 25- to 27-gauge needle in a series of one to four injections clockwise around the extravasation site.
8. Note: Not all vesicants have antidotes (see Table 13-3).
9. Remove the needle or catheter and apply a sterile dressing.
10. Apply appropriate hot or cold compresses, if applicable (see Table 13-3).
11. Animal should have cage rest for 48 hours.
12. Avoid any pressure or friction to the skin that may aggravate the injury.
13. Cover area with a light dressing.
14. Document the extravasation (amount of drug extravasated, area, size, treatment).
15. Provide analgesics and/or local pain medication and home instruction sheet to client (see website for sample sheet).
16. If skin blisters or small ulcers form, silver sulfadiazine (Silvadene) can be applied every 12 hours until healing occurs. Surgery may be indicated for larger areas.

SECTION C: Transfusion Considerations

Ann E. Hohenhaus

KEY POINTS

- Red blood cell transfusions should be given only to patients with a symptomatic anemia or serious hemorrhage anticipated to result in symptomatic anemia.
- Fresh frozen plasma may be transfused to correct coagulation factor deficiencies resulting from hepatic neoplasia or tumor-induced disseminated intravascular coagulation.
- Platelet transfusions using cryopreserved platelets can be performed in dogs with cancer-associated thrombocytopenia.
- Neutropenia results from tumor infiltration into the bone marrow, chemotherapy, and radiation toxicity. Granulocyte transfusions are impractical in dogs and cats.

RED BLOOD CELL TRANSFUSIONS

Both solid tumors and hematologic malignancies can be associated with anemia and a need for transfusion of red blood cells (RBCs) (Tables 13-4 and 13-5). Studies of RBC transfusions in dogs indicate that 16% to 28% of transfused dogs had cancer as their underlying disease.[1,2] Cats with a diagnosis of cancer appear to have a similar frequency of RBC transfusion as dogs, with 7% to 21% of transfused cats reported to have cancer.[3,4] Tumors commonly associated with a need for RBC transfusion are hemangiosarcoma, acute and chronic leukemia, lymphoma, and nasal and GI tumors.[5-7]

The principles of RBC transfusion are the same in cancer patients as any other patient with anemia. RBC transfusions should be given only to patients with a symptomatic anemia or serious hemorrhage anticipated to result in symptomatic anemia. The amount of blood transfused should be adequate to alleviate the clinical signs, but restoration of hematocrit to normal is not required for successful transfusion. The most commonly used blood product in the treatment of anemia in dogs is packed RBCs. Although the product insert should be the source of dosing information, a general guideline is 6 to 10 ml/kg. Because dogs have a low incidence of naturally occurring alloantibodies, a crossmatch is not typically performed before a first transfusion.[8] Because of the small volume of blood collected and transfused in cats, whole blood is the product most frequently transfused to anemic cats. The recommended dosage for whole blood is 10 to 20 ml/kg. The cat is a species with naturally occurring alloantibodies, and blood typing is required before the first transfusion. If blood typing is not available, crossmatching blood of the recipient to a type A donor will infer the type of the recipient. An incompatible major crossmatch implies the cat is type B,

TABLE 13-5   TUMORS ASSOCIATED WITH NEED FOR TRANSFUSION IN DOGS AND CATS

Blood Product		
Red Blood Cells	Fresh Frozen Plasma	Platelets
Hematologic malignancy	Lymphoma	Multiple myeloma
Lymphoma	Mast cell tumor	Lymphoma
Leukemia, acute and chronic	Hemangiosarcoma	Leukemia
Multiple myeloma		Malignant histiocytosis
Mast cell tumor		Sertoli cell tumor
Hemangiosarcoma		Hemangiosarcoma
Nasal tumors		
Gastrointestinal leiomyosarcoma		
Adenocarcinoma		
Sertoli cell tumor		

TABLE 13-4   CAUSES OF ANEMIA IN CANCER PATIENTS

Hemolysis	Blood Loss	Bone Marrow Failure
Paraneoplastic immune-mediated	Tumor-associated hemorrhage	Myelophthisis
Microangiopathy	Thrombocytopenia	Myelodysplasia
Sepsis	Paraneoplastic immune-mediated	Myelofibrosis
Hemophagocytic syndrome	Bone marrow failure	Chemotherapy
	Surgical hemorrhage	Radiation therapy
	Coagulopathy	Anemia of chronic disease
	Disseminated intravascular coagulation	Megaloblastic anemia
	Paraneoplastic gastric ulceration	

and a compatible major crossmatch indicates the cat is type A. Because each transfusion can induce the production of new antibodies, resulting in serologic incompatibility, crossmatching should be performed if more than 4 days elapse between transfusions in both dogs and cats.

FRESH FROZEN PLASMA TRANSFUSIONS

Although coagulopathies resulting from feline hepatic lymphoma and canine hemangiosarcoma have been reported, the true incidence of cancer-associated coagulopathy is unknown.[9,10] Treatment of disseminated intravascular coagulation (DIC) is a common indication for fresh frozen plasma (FFP) transfusion in cancer patients.[11,12] Correction of the coagulation abnormality with FFP transfusion may facilitate surgery, chemotherapy, or radiation in patients with a wide variety of tumor types (see Table 13-5). FFP is not a good source of albumin or nutritional support in hypoalbuminemic cancer patients suffering from malnutrition, since a large volume is required to increase serum albumin concentration.[13] When it is removed from the freezer, the FFP bag is extremely fragile and prone to cracking. To prevent this, the bag should not be removed from its protective box until it has been allowed to warm for 15 minutes. Then the bag may be placed in a plastic zipper bag and immersed in water <37°C if rapid thawing is necessary. *Microwave ovens are not recommended for plasma thawing.* The initial dosage of FFP for the treatment of coagulopathy is 6 to 10 ml/kg one to three times daily depending on the condition being treated and the response to therapy. Response should be assessed by serial coagulation profiles. Crossmatching is unnecessary before transfusion of FFP, although feline FFP should be the same blood type as that of the recipient cat.

PLATELET TRANSFUSIONS

Thrombocytopenia is a common occurrence in dogs and cats with cancer. In one study, thrombocytopenia was reported in 10% of 2059 dogs with cancer.[14]

As many as 75% of dogs with hemangiosarcoma have thrombocytopenia.[10] In one retrospective study of cats with thrombocytopenia, 20% had an underlying neoplasia.[15] Despite the frequency with which thrombocytopenia occurs in cancer patients, platelet transfusions are not commonly performed (Table 13-5). One reason for the limited number of platelet transfusions reported is that the degree of thrombocytopenia in approximately half of the patients is not severe enough (<50,000/μl) to result in hemorrhage.[14,15] Another reason for the lack of platelet transfusions is the difficulty associated with producing components containing functional platelets. Stored whole blood, stored packed RBCs, and FFP do not contain functional platelets, and special equipment is required to produce platelets for transfusion.[16] Frozen canine platelets are commercially available. They are collected through plateletpheresis and preserved in DMSO. Because the product contains DMSO, it should not be infused rapidly or bradycardia will result. The platelet transfusion should be given over 1 to 2 hours at a dosage of 1 unit of platelets per 10 kg of body weight. This should increase the platelet count at 1 to 2 hours after transfusion by 20,000/μl.

GRANULOCYTE TRANSFUSIONS

Depression of granulopoiesis can occur in cancer patients as a result of chemotherapy and radiation therapy or as a result of bone marrow infiltration by tumor cells. The severity of hematological toxicity varies with the drug and protocol used, but virtually any chemotherapy drug can result in severe neutropenia. If the neutrophil count is below 1000/μl, the risk for developing an opportunistic infection or sepsis is significant. Prophylactic antibiotics are frequently administered when the neutrophil count is below 1000/μl and the patient is afebrile. Febrile neutropenia should be addressed as an emergency and is covered in Section A. Although neutropenia is a common and serious problem in cancer patients, granulocyte transfusion

TABLE 13-6 GUIDELINES FOR ADMINISTERING TRANSFUSIONS

Blood Product	Recommended Dosage	Transfusion Rate	Cross-match Needed
Whole blood	10–20 ml/kg	4-hr infusion	Yes*
Packed red blood cells	6–10 ml/kg	4-hr infusion	Yes*
Fresh frozen plasma	6–10 ml/kg	4–6 ml/minute	No
Platelets	1 U/10 kg	1- to 2-hr infusion	No

*Crossmatch needed before first transfusion in cats because of naturally occurring alloantibodies; in dogs, crossmatch is recommended for second and subsequent transfusions.

requires highly specialized equipment and is not currently practical in clinical veterinary oncology.

GENERAL TRANSFUSION PRINCIPLES

All blood and components should be administered through an administration set with an integral filter designed to remove clots and debris formed during collection and storage. Typically, a 170-μ filter is used; however, for a small volume transfusion given from a syringe, the use of an 18-μ filter attached to the syringe is recommended. Patient evaluation prior to transfusion should include body weight, temperature, heart rate, and respiratory rate. These parameters should be reassessed intermittently during and after the transfusion to identify potential transfusion reactions.[17] Table 13-6 shows general transfusion administration guidelines. RBC-containing products should be administered slowly, over a period of less than 4 hours. Plasma may be administered more rapidly (4–6 ml/min) than products containing RBCs.

Selected References*

Abrams-Ogg A: British Practical blood transfusion, In Day MJ, Mackin A, Littlewood JD, editors: *BSAVA manual of canine and feline haematology and transfusion medicine,* Quedgeley, Glouchester, 2000, Small Animal Veterinary Association

Contains an excellent step-by-step description of crossmatching, including color photographs of incompatible crossmatches.

Hohenhaus AE: Transfusion reactions, In Feldman BF, Zinkl JG, Jain NC, editors: *Schalm's veterinary hematology,* ed 5, Philadelphia, 2000, Lippincott, William & Wilkins

A comprehensive review of transfusion reactions, including monitoring recommendations, and therapeutic interventions.

Schneider A: Blood components: collection, processing and storage, *Vet Clin North Am Small Anim Pract* 25:1245, 1995.

A thorough description of the equipment, supplies, and skills required for collection and processing of blood for transfusion.

■ *For a complete list of the references cited in this chapter, please go to www.smallanimaloncology.com.

14 Surgical Interventions in Cancer

Eric R. Pope

KEY POINTS

- Whenever possible, a diagnosis should be established before definitive surgical therapy.
- Surgical procedures for oncology patients should be planned thoroughly; the first surgery is more likely to achieve a cure than subsequent procedures.
- *Always* submit excised tissues for histopathological examination.
- Surgical margins should be marked to aid assessment of completeness of excision.

Surgery is an integral part of comprehensive cancer treatment. Surgery can be used to establish a diagnosis, achieve a cure, palliate clinical signs, aid patient support, or reduce tumor burden in order to maximize the efficacy of other treatment modalities Thorough preoperative assessment is important to avoid over-treating or, more commonly, under-treating a patient. Two of the most important questions that should be considered prior to any surgery are: (1) What is the most appropriate surgical procedure, if any, for this patient? and (2) Do I have the skills and expertise to perform this surgery? A poorly planned or executed surgery can have profound negative effects on a patient with a potentially curable tumor. It is better to perform staged procedures (e.g., biopsy followed by definitive surgery) if knowing the type or grade of tumor could influence the aggressiveness of the definitive surgery. Performing a less-aggressive surgery because of lack of familiarity with a procedure or concerns about ability to close a wound is generally not in the patient's best interest. See Box 14-1 on p.144 for common mistakes related to surgical oncology.

BIOPSY (see Chapter 6 for detailed descriptions)

In most instances, the diagnosis should be established before the definitive surgery.[1-4] If that is not possible because of the location of the tumor or inability to obtain a diagnostic sample, intraoperative evaluation can be performed. Fine-needle aspirates (FNAs), impression smears, and/or frozen sections can provide valuable information for intraoperative decision-making. The results of these tests may be helpful in avoiding over- or under-treating patients and in helping pet owners decide whether or not to continue treatment. The ability to use these techniques obviously depends upon the availability of a cytopathologist to process the samples in a timely manner.

Surgical biopsies can be either incisional or excisional. Incisional biopsy is indicated when the diagnosis cannot be established by less invasive methods, and knowing the diagnosis might influence the aggressiveness of the surgical procedure.[5,6] Incisional biopsy is most commonly used for lesions on or near the skin surface. Deeper lesions can usually be adequately sampled by needle core biopsy, especially when image guidance is used.[7,8] Incisional biopsies should include normal tissue at the edge of the lesion as long as new tissue planes will not be invaded.[3,5,9] Removing a deep, narrow wedge of tissue facilitates closure of the biopsy site. Inflamed, ulcerated, and necrotic areas should be avoided because they often interfere with obtaining an accurate diagnosis. Incisional biopsies—all biopsies, for that matter—should be performed so that the biopsy tract can be excised during the definitive surgery without altering the surgical plan[1,3,5] (Figure 14-1). Failure to remove the entire biopsy tract increases the risk of recurrence because of potential seeding of the tract with tumor.

Excisional biopsy is indicated when the type of surgery would not be influenced by establishing a definitive diagnosis preoperatively,[3,5] such as a primary lung tumor or a dermal mass located in an area where additional surgery, if needed because of dirty margins, would not result in significantly increased morbidity. Excisional biopsy should not be performed as a convenience to the owner or to avoid multiple procedures (diagnostic and then therapeutic) because an incomplete excision can have a negative impact on treatment options and the ability to achieve a cure if the mass is malignant. Excisional biopsy should be performed adhering to the guidelines

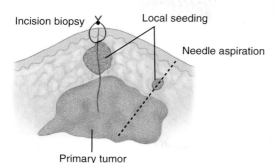

Incision biopsy   Local seeding

Needle aspiration

Primary tumor

FIGURE 14-1 Incisional biopsy. The biopsy should be planned so that new tissue planes are not opened. The biopsy site can be sutured closed while awaiting results, and the biopsy tracts will be removed when the definitive surgery is performed.

shown in the section "Surgery for Local Control" later in this chapter.

CYTOREDUCTION (DEBULKING)

The concept of cytoreductive surgery is often misunderstood and misused. The goal is to reduce the tumor burden to enhance the efficacy and/or reduce the morbidity associated with other treatments. It should not be considered a primary treatment modality. Simply removing easily accessible parts of a large mass is unlikely to improve the final outcome and may result in significant patient morbidity, particularly if wound healing complications occur. One gram of tumor in a wound leaves approximately 1 billion tumor cells.[10] In many instances, the tumor left in the wound is from the most biologically active areas of tumor (capsule or pseudocapsule), and tumor regrowth is often rapid.

Ideally the tumor burden should be reduced to microscopic levels when performed prior to radiotherapy or chemotherapy.[11] Marginal excision of a mass meets this criterion (see subsequent discussion). Since radiation therapy and chemotherapy interfere with wound healing, these procedures are often delayed after surgery to allow the surgical wound to heal before initiating therapy. Unfortunately, the longer the delay, the greater the chance that significant regrowth will occur, particularly if gross tumor is left within the wound or it is an aggressive tumor. Radiation therapy should be delayed for at least 1 week after surgery, but a recent study showed that there was not a significant improvement in wound healing if radiation therapy was delayed longer (Henry CJ, personal communication, 2003).

Cytoreductive surgery may also be performed in conjunction with photodynamic therapy (see Chapter 17).

The goal in this instance is to reduce the depth (thickness) of the tumor to less than the depth of penetration of the light source used to activate the photosensitizer. A potential benefit of this approach is an improved ability to maintain cosmetic appearance and function, compared with traditional surgical methods. An example is the use of photodynamic therapy to treat oral squamous cell carcinoma.[12] Superficial tumors with limited bone involvement may be effectively treated without having to perform a segmental mandibulectomy (Figure 14-2).

SURGERY FOR LOCAL CONTROL

Complete surgical excision of many benign and malignant tumors can be curative or provide long-term remission. The adage that *the first chance is the best chance* should guide preoperative planning.[1,2] Surgery for recurrent tumors is typically more complicated because differentiating scar tissue from tumor can be difficult and potential seeding of tissue planes opened during the prior surgery necessitates a more extensive resection.[1,2]

Preoperative Management

Complete staging to determine the local and distant extent of disease is essential for preoperative planning.[2] Routine use of the TNM (tumor, node, metastasis) system to document the extent of disease is recommended.[13,14] Recording the location(s) and size(s) of all masses and presence or absence of regional lymph node or distant metastasis is also important for assessing response to treatment during follow-up evaluations. The regional lymph nodes should be assessed preoperatively by palpation and/or imaging techniques. FNA or needle biopsy should be performed preoperatively. If the results are questionable, the lymph node(s) can be removed for biopsy during the definitive surgery. Advanced imaging techniques such as CT and MRI (see Chapter 10, Section B) are also useful for planning, particularly for cases where there is concern about the ability to completely excise a mass because of invasion into important structures. This is especially true with soft-tissue sarcomas, for which tumor margins may be difficult to discern at the time of surgery.

Preoperative blood work should be consistent with the suspected tumor type, physical examination findings, and American Society of Anesthesia classification. The minimum data base for most cancer patients includes CBC, biochemical profile, and urinalysis. Consult the chapters on specific tumor types for more detailed recommendations concerning preoperative assessment.

Infection rates after oncologic surgery have been shown to be significantly higher than for other surgical

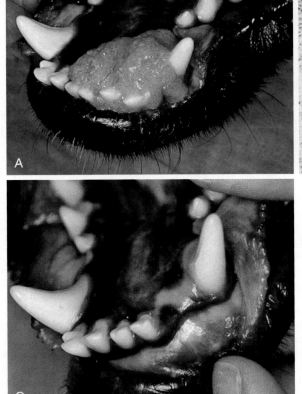

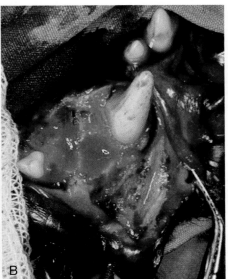

FIGURE 14-2 A, Oral squamous cell carcinoma. **B**, Tumor has been surgically debulked to a thickness <1 cm prior to photodynamic therapy. **C**, Healed site. Excellent cosmetic appearance and function have been maintained. (Courtesy of Dr. Dudley McCaw, Kansas State University.)

procedures.[4] The decision to administer perioperative antimicrobials should be based on anticipated length of the anesthesia/surgical period, whether or not the use of implants is anticipated or are pre-existing (e.g., pacemaker or total hip replacement implants) and if infection would have a catastrophic effect on the outcome of the procedure. Prophylactic perioperative antimicrobials are generally not continued for longer than 24 hours after surgery unless there is a demonstrated therapeutic need.

Operative Planning

Preoperative planning is essential in surgical oncology. Knowledge of the tumor type and its likely biological activity is useful for deciding what type of surgery is most likely to achieve local tumor control while minimizing morbidity.[2] Rarely should the aggressiveness of the surgery be tempered by concerns about the ability to close a wound.[1] The presence of metastatic disease may influence the aggressiveness of the procedure or the decision as to whether or not surgery is even indicated.

When considering all options, it is important to remember that the treatment should never be worse than the disease.

Surgery on previously irradiated tissues presents additional challenges.[2] Gentle tissue handling and preservation of blood supply are always important but may be even more so in previously irradiated tissues. In humans, major wound complications occurred in 30% to 44% of patients following preoperative radiation of soft-tissue sarcomas.[15] Major wound complications included those requiring an additional surgical procedure or prolonged wound care. In one veterinary study evaluating the tolerance of skin and mucosal flaps to radiation therapy performed either preoperatively or postoperatively, 77% of the dogs had at least one complication postoperatively.[16] Flap complications included necrosis, dehiscence, infection, and ulceration of the flap. The severity of complications was greater in patients irradiated preoperatively.

Excision Classifications (Table 14-1)

Complete tumor removal may be accomplished by marginal, wide, or radical excision. Intracapsular removal is rarely indicated because the capsule or pseudocapsule left behind is usually composed of viable tumor cells.[2,4] Incision into the tumor also increases the risk of seeding adjacent areas with tumor. *Marginal excision* removes the macroscopic tumor but follows closely around the edge of the tumor and, in most instances, leaves microscopic disease if the lesion is malignant or no normal tissue around the tumor is also removed. Differentiating wide and radical excisions can be difficult because there is not a standard definition. A *wide excision* removes enough normal tissue surrounding the mass so that all macroscopic and microscopic disease is removed. *Radical excision* typically means removal of all affected or potentially affected tissue (e.g., an entire organ or limb or an entire compartment such as a portion of the abdominal or thoracic wall) (Figure 14-3).

Marginal excision is appropriate for many benign tumors such as lipomas (Figure 14-4) because the risk of recurrence is low; even if they do recur, they can usually be managed by repeated marginal excision. Excising a rim of "normal" tissue along with mass, particularly with undiagnosed masses, affords the pathologist the opportunity to assess whether or not vascular or lymphatic invasion has occurred if the mass turns out to be a malignant tumor.

Most malignant tumors are best treated by wide excision. Wide excision implies removal of the tumor with sufficient surrounding normal tissue to achieve durable local control (Figure 14-5). The goal is to remove the tumor without ever directly observing it during the surgery. How wide the margins should be is determined by the tumor type and its biological activity rather than using specific measurements.[2] For those tumors with established grading criteria, determining the grade preoperatively may provide important information in guiding the aggressiveness of the surgery. For example, grade 1 mast cell tumors may be excised with a 1-cm margin, whereas grade 2 tumors should have at least 2-cm margins.[17] The biological activity may also be influenced by the size and location of the tumor. Melanoma in the oral cavity or nail bed is usually malignant while melanomas in haired skin are typically benign.[18] The recommendations for margin size vary and have not been clearly established for all tumors. The reader should consult the chapters on individual tumor types for current recommendations.

Margins of 1 to 3 cm are sufficient for most malignant tumors.[2] Since tumors extend out easily through fat and along vessels and nerves, it is essential to maintain the margins three-dimensionally around the tumor. The tendency to creep the dissection closer to the tumor as the wound depth increases must be avoided. For most tumors, an intact fascial layer to which the tumor is not attached is used as the deep margin. Fascia is considered a good barrier to tumor extension as long as the tumor is not attached (fixed) to it. If the tumor is attached, the fascia should be considered invaded and the excision should extend down to the next intact fascial layer.

It is helpful to mark the planned lateral margins preoperatively with a skin marker or other method so that primary contraction of skin as it is incised does not

TABLE 14-1	EXCISION TECHNIQUES
Classification	Comments
Intracapsular	Rarely indicated and performed in veterinary surgery
Marginal	Removes all macroscopic disease; an attempt should be made to include a rim of normal tissue completely around the mass
Wide	En bloc removal of the tumor with sufficient surrounding tissue to achieve durable local control
Radical	En bloc removal of the tumor including the entire tissue compartment involved or removal of an affected organ

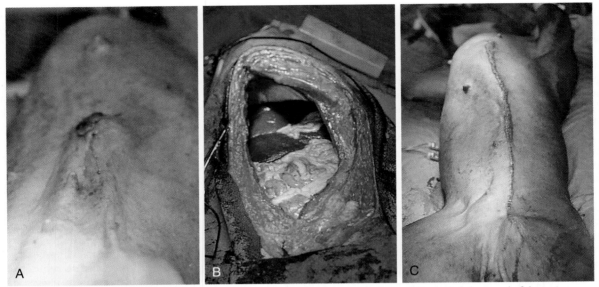

FIGURE 14-3 A, Recurrent squamous cell carcinoma on the ventral abdomen. **B**, Radical excision included removal of the entire thickness of the body wall (since the initial surgery included the external fascia) in addition to taking wider lateral (5 cm) margins. **C**, The wound was closed by direct apposition of tissues despite the large size of the wound.

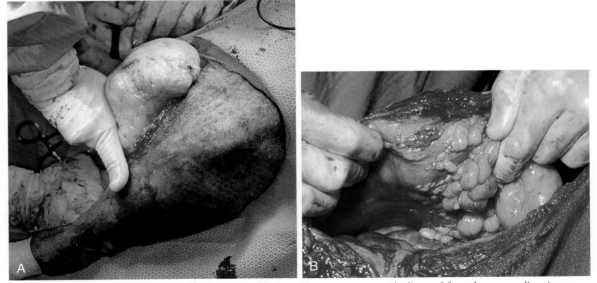

FIGURE 14-4 A, Marginal excision of a well-circumscribed lipoma. These tumors are easily dissected from the surrounding tissues. **B**, Infiltrative lipomas invade the surrounding tissues as evidenced by the extensive involvement of the body wall. Complete excision of infiltrative lipomas is often difficult because the margins are indistinct and complete excision may not be possible without interfering with normal function.

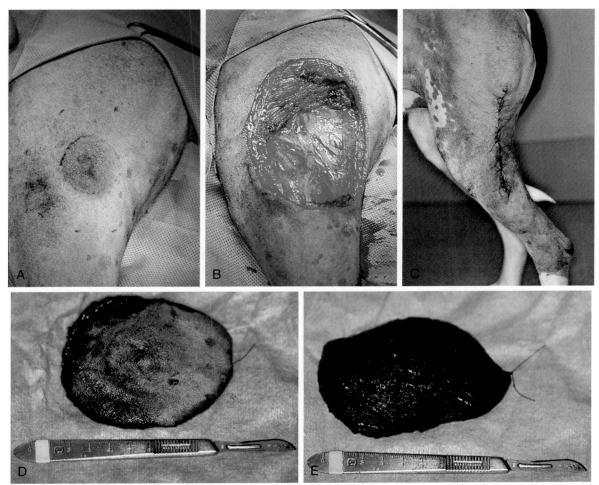

FIGURE 14-5 Wide excision of a mast cell tumor on the caudal thigh. **A**, Grade 2 dermal mast cell tumor with indistinct margins *(solid line)*. Dotted lines indicate 2-cm lateral margins around tumor. **B**, Wound bed after excision including one intact fascial layer below tumor. The popliteal lymph node was removed through the same incision for staging purposes. **C**, Postoperative appearance. There was no interference with normal function. **D**, Excised mass. **E**, The underside of the mass has been painted with India ink to mark surgical margins before fixing the tissue. The suture was placed to indicate the distal margin.

result in removal of a greater or lesser amount of tissue than desired. Gentle tissue handling is important in reducing postoperative complications. Direct manipulation of the tumor should be minimized to reduce the risk of embolizing clumps of tumor cells into the blood stream.[1] Maintaining hemostasis improves visualization during surgery and minimizes the risk of hematoma formation after surgery. Early ligation of the blood supply is ideal but not often possible.[1,4] The use of stay sutures in unaffected tissue surrounding the tumor is a good

way of minimizing tumor manipulation.[4] Use of clamps or other retractors that could potentially penetrate the tumor and exfoliate tumor cells into the wound bed should be avoided.[2,4]

Lymph node removal at the time of definitive surgery is controversial, especially if nodal metastasis has not been documented prior to surgery and they are not enlarged or abnormal in appearance.[1,4] Assessment of sentinel lymph nodes is commonly performed in human medicine to guide recommendations for adjunctive therapy.[19] The sentinel lymph node is the first lymph node receiving drainage from a specific area of the body. In humans, the sentinel lymph node has been shown to be a highly sensitive and specific indicator for a patient's true metastatic status. Unfortunately, the sentinel lymph nodes have not been defined for many anatomic regions in dogs and cats, and sentinel lymph node evaluation is not routinely performed. If the lymph nodes are biopsied or removed intraoperatively and they are not in the same area as the primary tumor, fresh gloves and instruments should be used if the lymph node is approached after excision of the primary tumor. This will reduce the risk of seeding tumor cells into the lymph node bed. Regional nodes should be biopsied when the primary tumor is located in an area that would be difficult to access at a later time. Examples include hilar lymph nodes with lung tumors and abdominal lymph nodes. The benefits of the information gained offset the potential drawbacks in these instances.

The value of wound lavage in removing tumor cells from the wound bed is controversial.[2] Although exfoliated cells may be removed, there is also a possibility they could be disseminated in the wound bed if removal of the lavage solution is not complete. Wound lavage is effective in removing tissue debris and blood and maintains tissue hydration. Gloves and instruments should be changed before beginning wound closure. If postoperative radiation therapy is anticipated, metallic clips can be placed in the wound bed to delineate the extent of the surgical wound.[20,21] This can provide the radiation oncologist with important radiation therapy planning information.

Although controlled studies are lacking, biological implants should be used with caution, particularly if there is concern about residual disease. Since many biological implants contain growth factors that promote angiogenesis and could increase the risk of local recurrence, it seems prudent to limit their use until more information is available. The use of other implant materials, such as polypropylene mesh, should also be minimized to reduce the risk of postoperative seroma formation and infection, particularly if radiation therapy or chemotherapy is planned.[2] The use of drains should be avoided if possible. If drains are used, they should be placed so that the opening of new fascial planes is minimized.[21] They should also be exited in a location that will enlarge the treatment field as little as possible if postoperative radiation therapy is anticipated.

The selection of suture material is an important consideration in cancer surgery. Many cancer patients are older and may heal slower. Cancer cachexia,

chemotherapy, and radiation therapy also delay wound healing. Long-lasting monofilament absorbable suture materials are sufficient in most instances, but if the need for wound support beyond 60 days is anticipated, the use of monofilament nonabsorbable suture materials may be indicated. Braided suture materials are associated with increased tumor recurrence and should be avoided if there is any concern about completeness of excision.[2,22,23] Skin sutures are generally left in place for at least 14 days after surgery to account for potentially delayed wound healing.

Primary wound closure is preferred, but if there is any doubt about completeness of the excision, it is better to leave the wound open until the surgical margins have been evaluated.[2] This is especially important if wound closure would entail the use of skin flaps or other reconstructive procedures. If extensive reconstruction is performed at the initial surgery and the margins are incomplete, further surgery with the intent to achieve a cure may not be possible since both the original wound bed and the skin flap donor site should be considered contaminated. Similar recommendations to treat all tissues manipulated during surgery have been made for patients undergoing radiation therapy,[21,24] but in one recent study, no dogs developed recurrence at the donor site when this protocol was followed even though the donor site was not included in the radiation field.[16]

All excised masses should be submitted for histopathologic evaluation. The surgical margins should be marked before fixing the tissue. Marking the surgical margins with an indelible dye facilitates differentiation of surgical margins from sectioning margins created during tissue processing.[25] If the tumor is visible at or near the dyed margin, the excision is considered incomplete.

Postoperative Care

The immediate postoperative management centers on patient support and pain control. The amount of support necessary varies significantly depending on the preoperative condition of the patient, the type of surgery performed, and potential metabolic disturbances associated with the tumor. Intravenous fluid therapy is indicated until the patient is sufficiently recovered to take in adequate fluids and food orally.

Pain management protocols should be established preoperatively. Pre-emptive multimodal techniques incorporating local anesthetics, epidurals, and/or systemic drugs can be used depending on the type of surgery performed. Combinations of nonsteroidal inflammatory drugs (NSAIDs) and opioids are commonly used because they usually provide excellent analgesia for moderate to

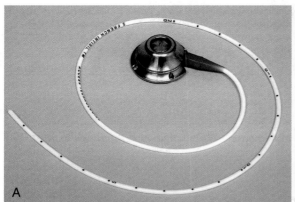
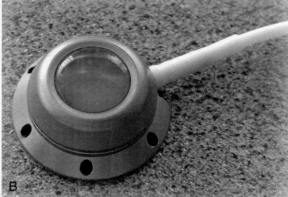

FIGURE 14-6 **A,** Vascular access ports such as the one shown here are implanted in the subcutaneous tissue and can be used for blood draws or fluid and drug administration. **B,** Close-up view of the port demonstrating suture holes that are used for securing the port in place. The port is made of titanium, with a silicone diaphragm for access with a Huber needle. (Courtesy of Norfolk Vet, a division of Access Technologies.)

severe pain, possibly because of synergistic interaction.[26] Sedatives are often used in the immediate postoperative period for patients that exhibit excitement or anxiety during recovery. The duration of therapy is variable but is generally most intense during the first 24 to 48 hours after surgery. See Chapter 18, Section C for additional information regarding pain management.

PATIENT SUPPORT AND ADJUNCTIVE THERAPY

Surgery may play a role in facilitating delivery of adjunctive therapy. Surgery may be necessary to provide vascular access for interventional procedures such as regional chemotherapy administration. Intraoperative radiation therapy allows delivery of a large dose of radiation to the tumor while reducing damage to surrounding normal structures.

Vascular Access Ports

Patients that require frequent vascular access may benefit from implantation of a vascular access port as shown in Figure 14-6 (e.g., The Companion Port, Norfolk Vet Products, Skokie, Illinois [www.Norfolkvetproducts. com]). Examples include patients undergoing chemotherapy that need regular blood draws and chemotherapy administration and patients undergoing radiation therapy necessitating access for administration of anesthetic agents. The port can also be used for intermittent intravenous fluid administration. The ports are implanted in the subcutaneous tissues and are accessed by use of a specially designed needle known as a Huber needle (Figure 14-7). In most instances, the catheter is inserted into

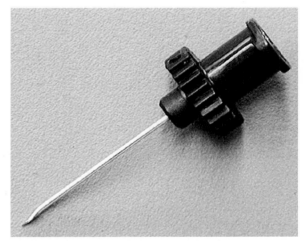

FIGURE 14-7 Huber needle designed to provide port access without coring the silicone diaphragm, as would occur with use of standard needles. (Courtesy of Norfolk Vet, a division of Access Technologies.)

the jugular vein and the port secured subcutaneously in the cervical area. The catheter can also be placed in the femoral vein and the port secured in the dorsal flank area. Strict aseptic technique must be followed during implantation and each time the port is accessed to minimize the risk of infection. Infected ports can rarely be salvaged and should be removed. The peripheral vein used for inserting the catheter can be preserved by using a "tear-away" introducer. Alternatively, the vein can be ligated distally prior to inserting the catheter through a venotomy incision. The catheter tip should be in a large central vein that has good flow to minimize the risk of catheter occlusion.

The most common causes of catheter obstruction are fibrin flap formation at the tip of the catheter, a clot within the catheter or port, or complete encasement of the catheter tip by a fibrous connective tissue sheath.[27] The latter is typically a late complication and associated with the catheter chronically "rubbing" against the vessel wall. These catheters cannot be salvaged. Catheters with a clot at the tip can often still be used for infusion, but attempts to withdraw samples fail because the clot acts like a one-way valve. Clots within the catheter or port can rarely be managed effectively; therefore, prevention is the key. The port and catheter should be flushed thoroughly with 5 to 10 ml of saline after each use, depending on the size of the catheter. The catheter and port should then be "locked" with anticoagulant. Although many solutions have been used, taurolidine citrate solution (Norfolk Vet Products, Skokie, Illinois) is available as a premixed solution. Taurolidine citrate also has antibacterial properties because of its ability to inhibit biofilm overgrowth on the catheter.[28] The typical recommendation is to lock the catheter with 1.5 to 2 times the volume of the catheter to insure complete flushing. It is also important to still be injecting the lock solution as the Huber needle is being withdrawn. If the needle is removed after the injection is completed, negative pressure can be generated in the system that will pull blood into the catheter, enhancing clot formation. With proper care, venous access ports can be maintained for months to years.

Feeding Tubes

Nutritional support is an important aspect of patient management. Cachexia is a relatively common complication of cancer in companion animals. Some chemotherapy protocols may also affect appetite. The placement of a feeding tube enhances the clinician's ability to maintain adequate nutritional support. Use the most minimally invasive technique that will adequately meet the patient's needs. Since many of these patients are also immunocompromised and heal at a slower rate, the decision to place a feeding tube must be weighed against the risk of potential complications.

PREVENTION

The efficacy of ovariohysterectomy in reducing the risk of mammary tumors in dogs is well documented.[1,2] Similarly, castration is effective in the control of perianal adenomas and eliminates the risk of tumors developing in cryptorchid testicles.[1] Other examples of preventive surgeries include excision of actinic lesions, which may transform into squamous cell carcinoma, and the removal of rectal polyps that could progress to carcinomas.

PALLIATION

The goal of palliative surgery is to improve or maintain quality of life but not necessarily prolong life.[1,2] Primary bone tumors such as osteosarcoma are often very painful and are predisposed to pathologic fracture as bone destruction progresses. Amputation of the limb removes the primary source of pain and is an example of a palliative surgery.

Splenectomy for a bleeding hemangiosarcoma reduces the immediate risk of a life-threatening hemorrhage but has little impact on the final outcome. Pericardectomy for pericardial effusion as a result of hemangiosarcoma or other cardiac tumors is another example.

BOX 14-1   COMMON MISTAKES RELATED TO SURGICAL ONCOLOGY

1. "Wait and see"—Few masses resolve spontaneously. Waiting only provides time for further growth and metastasis. There are few contraindications to FNA or needle core biopsy to obtain a diagnosis.
2. "It shelled out nicely" —Except for lipomas and a few other benign masses, close marginal excision invariably leaves tumor in the wound bed. Additional surgeries typically must be more aggressive because of altered tissue planes.
3. "It looks benign" —Although some tumors have a characteristic appearance, it is not possible to accurately diagnose or rule out cancer based on gross appearance of a mass alone. If surgical excision is warranted, so too is histopathological examination of the excised tissue.
4. "I only submitted the masses that looked suspicious" —If multiple masses are removed, *all* should be submitted for histopathology. This is especially true for canine mammary masses, since benign and malignant lesions are often present concurrently.
5. "It's an old dog (cat)" —Age is not a disease. Treatment options should be offered and the decision left to the owner.

Palliative therapy is discussed in more detail in Chapter 18, Section D.

SUMMARY

Surgical oncology is a vital component of comprehensive cancer care. When discussing surgery as an option with clients, practitioners must address the potential for morbidity and mortality and provide pet owners with the information necessary to make an informed decision. If patient referral to a specialty oncology practice is being considered, one should identify those practices that adopt a team approach including medical, radiation, and surgical oncology. Whether surgical intervention is intended to provide a diagnosis or facilitate a cure, it is vital to apply the basic principles of surgical oncology discussed herein and to make treatment decisions using an evidence-based approach.

Selected References*

Ehrhart N: Principles of tumor biopsy, *Clin Tech Small Anim Pract* 13:10, 1998.
An in-depth review of biopsy principles, biopsy techniques, and sample handling.
Lascelles D, White D: Principles of oncological surgery, *In Practice* 21:163, 1999.
This article contains very practical information that should be of interest to general practitioners performing oncologic surgery.
Soderstrom MJ, Gilson SD: Principles of surgical oncology, *Vet Clin North Am Small Anim Pract* 25:97, 1995.
A very good review of oncological surgical principles including a thorough discussion of preoperative assessment, surgical technique, and potential complications.

*For a complete list of the references cited in this chapter, please go to www.smallanimaloncology.com.

15 Radiation Therapy

SECTION A: External Beam Radiation Therapy (Teletherapy) and Brachytherapy

Jimmy C. Lattimer and David A. Bommarito

KEY POINTS

- Radiation therapy should be considered a localized therapy and is most effective against microscopic disease.
- Computerized treatment planning permits the radiation oncologist to maximize the dose to the tumor and minimize the dose to critical normal tissues.
- Splitting the total radiation dose into many small "fractions" is necessary to minimize the impact on normal highly differentiated tissues such as the brain.
- The use of electron beam therapy allows treatment of superficial tumors while minimizing radiation dose to underlying organs.
- Administration of a few large fractions of radiation to a tumor is only acceptable for palliation of pain and should not be considered as treatment with curative intent.

HISTORICAL PERSPECTIVE

Radiation in the form of an external beam has been used for many years in the management of solid cancers. Beginning in the 1930s, orthovoltage x-ray machines, which have an energy range of 150 to 500 kVp, were used for therapy. These units were largely replaced with higher energy Cobalt 60 and Cesium 137 machines following the development of the nuclear reactor in the late 1940s and 1950s. These sources have energies of 1.25 Mev and 0.662 Mev, respectively, based on the radioactive core contained within the machine. They became popular replacements to orthovoltage units because of their simplicity, stability, and, most importantly, ability to penetrate deeper tissues because of their higher energies. Today, Cobalt 60 and Cesium 137 units are falling out of favor because of concerns and liability related to replacement of the radioactive source, as well as modern-day issues of security and public safety. For these reasons, linear accelerator machines, which produce 4 to 15 megavolt x-ray beams, have largely replaced isotope machines.

LINEAR ACCELERATORS

Linear accelerators (LINAC) used in radiation therapy today are compact and highly reliable machines that, when integrated with computer control systems, can deliver radiation therapy (photon) beams at a constant dose rate and with a high degree of precision and repeatability. These factors are increasingly important in veterinary oncology with the advent of more complex approaches to radiation therapy planning for pets with cancer. In addition, many linear accelerators are configured to also deliver electron beams that are used to treat skin and superficial tumors. When considering patient referral for radiation therapy, practitioners should seek treatment sites with equipment best suited to provide the needs for each individual patient. While electron capabilities may not be important for the treatment of many deep-seated tumors, they provide an advantage when treating superficial or cutaneous lesions.

TELETHERAPY

Teletherapy refers to the use of an external beam for radiation treatment, as is done with linear accelerators and Cobalt 60 or Cesium 137 machines. Typical tumors treated this way include, but are not limited to, nasal carcinomas and sarcomas, brain tumors, oral neoplasms, isolated lymphoma, adenocarcinoma of the salivary gland and thyroid, mediastinal tumors, spinal column tumors, and malignancies of the pelvic canal. External beam radiation is also used to treat skin, subcutaneous tissue, and muscle after incomplete surgical resection of a tumor. Radiation therapy may be used to treat tumors in sites such as the distal limb, where surgical removal would require amputation or severely disfiguring surgery and for which there is a reasonable probability of controlling the neoplasm using radiation therapy alone or in combination with chemotherapy. Mast cell tumors and solitary cutaneous lymphoma are examples. External beam radiation therapy is also used for palliative treatment of tumors such as osteosarcoma of the limb to control pain when amputation is not a viable option.

External beam radiation therapy protocols are developed such that the total dose of radiation is given in a number of treatments referred to as fractions. This is done to maximize the killing effect on the tumor, while minimizing deleterious effects on the normal tissues. This is particularly important for normal tissues that do not have a large degree of cell turnover, such as muscle and bone.[1] The slow turnover of some normal tissues is protective against radiation damage if fractionation is used, because tissues are less sensitive to radiation damage if they are not actively dividing. This protective effect is negated, however, if radiation is delivered as a single large fraction, because large doses are damaging to both replicating and non-replicating tissues. Fractionation of the treatment over time allows for reassortment of tumor cells within the cell cycle, which improves the likelihood that each cell will be irradiated during the more sensitive phase of the cell cycle. Fractionation also allows for the return of hypoxic cells in the tumor population to a more oxic state as the radiation kills the more sensitive oxic cells between the hypoxic cells and the blood supply. This allows these cells to be irradiated in a more sensitive oxic state. Fractionation also allows time for normal cells killed by radiation to be repopulated from surviving cells. This also happpens in tumors but to a lesser degree. Normal cells are also more efficient at repairing radiation injury to the DNA when it is delivered in multiple small doses rather than in a single large dose. Tumor cells are generally not as good at this as normal cells in the dose range for most fractionation protocols. Taken together, these principles are referred to as the 4R's of radiation therapy—reassortment, reoxygenation, repopulation, repair—and form the foundation for modern radiation therapy protocols. Modern, definitive (intent to cure) veterinary radiation therapy protocols typically call for the administration of the total radiation dose over 10 to 20 daily fractions in 2 to 4 weeks, although many variations exist to meet individual circumstances. Veterinary radiation therapy requires anesthesia of the patient, not because there is any pain associated with the treatment, but in order to ensure they are immobilized and radiation is delivered accurately to the tumor site. This requirement for anesthesia is the major obstacle to using protocols similar to those used in human radiation oncology, where the total

dose of radiation is typically divided into 30 to 40 fractions. Therefore, the total dose of radiation delivered to veterinary patients is often somewhat lower and in larger fractions than that administered to people for tumors of similar types. Typical fraction sizes used in veterinary radiation therapy are in the 2.5 to 4 Gray (1 Gy = 100 rads) range when treating with curative intent. This represents a trade-off between using ideal radiobiological principles and the practicality related to the requirement for anesthesia, protracted hospitalization, cost, and owner acceptance.

STEREOTACTIC RADIOSURGERY/"GAMMA KNIFE" THERAPY

Stereotactic radiosurgery is an advanced form of radiation therapy used to treat small lesions (<2 cm) that are not surgically treatable (e.g., brain stem tumors). Between one and a few large doses are used, so extremely fine control is needed to avoid lethally damaging normal structures. Experience, computerized planning, and special positioning and beam limiting devices are required. Very few veterinary facilities have the expertise required to perform this technique.

THERAPY PLANNING

Within the last 10 years, computers have markedly changed many of the concepts related to radiation therapy planning. Previously, simple plans used one or two beams of radiation, and planning and dosimetry calculations were done by hand. Now it is common practice to use sophisticated computer plans that use data derived from computed tomography (CT) and the therapy machine's dosimetry tables to provide a 3D map of the radiation dose delivery to the tumor and the surrounding tissues (Figure 15-1). These programs allow prescription of radiation therapy plans that use more beams than were typically used in the past. By doing this, the radiation oncologist is able to conform the region of high radiation dose to the shape of the tumor and to shape the treatment field in ways that prevent a high radiation dose from being delivered to critical normal structures such as the optic nerve or spinal cord. This approach permits the delivery of higher radiation doses to tumors while minimizing acute local reactions such as moist desquamation or mucositis, and chronic effects such as bone necrosis or strictures, all of which are discussed in Section C.[2,3]

PATIENT SET-UP AND POSITIONING

When planning a course of radiation therapy, the radiotherapist must first define the location of the tumor to be treated. Tumor margins and the location of associated

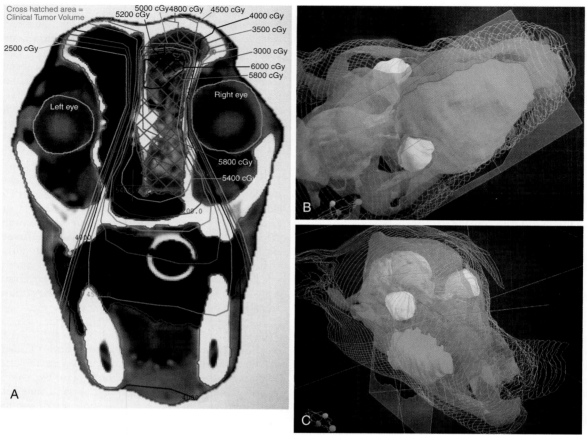

FIGURE 15-1 Computer-aided treatment plans used in many veterinary radiation treatment facilities today facilitate the use of CT images (**A**) to create treatment plans that maximize the dose to tumor tissues while sparing normal tissues. Here, plans for a dog with nasal carcinoma (**B**) and a dog with a maxillary mass (**C**) are shown. Tumor tissue, shown in red, receives the maximum dose, whereas eyes and normal surrounding tissues receive a smaller dose.

vital structures are typically determined using contrast CT scans or MRI. When treatment plans are based on CT images, it is vitally important to reproduce the positioning from the CT scan to the treatment table as accurately as possible. Many different positioning systems have been used, with the simplest such systems using various rigid or semi-rigid foam pads of various shapes as well as sandbags and tape to position the animal. Using vacuum cradles or custom cast foam cradles can improve the accuracy of positioning, especially for the head. The addition of a mouth block incorporating a dental mold has been shown to further improve the positioning accuracy to ±0.1 cm under optimum conditions.[4] In general, accurate positioning of the head is easier than for other anatomic sites because of the more prominent bony landmarks and rigid nature

of the skull. Consequently, larger volumes of normal tissue are often incorporated into the treatment volume in other parts of the body to ensure the inclusion of the entire tumor.[5] This inherently increases the likelihood of damage to normal surrounding tissues. Minimizing patient positioning errors is of paramount importance in not only maximizing tumor control, but in preventing post-irradiation complications.

SKIN-SPARING EFFECTS

Linear accelerators produce beams that are highly penetrating. Although the physics of high-energy x-rays is complex, once the effective energy of the beam exceeds approximately 500 keV, the maximum dose of radiation delivered by the beam (also called Dmax) to the tissue no longer occurs at the surface of the skin. This effect increases with energy to the point that for a 10-MeV beam, the Dmax is approximately 3 cm below the skin surface and the dose to the skin is approximately 30% of the dose at Dmax. This marked "skin sparing" effect is advantageous for treatment of deep tumors within the body. Once the dose maximum is reached, the intensity of the beam decreases relatively slowly beyond that point. Because of this, the dose to the skin on the side where the beam exits is substantially higher than that on the side of entry. This may be counterintuitive to clients, and they may question why skin effects would occur on the side opposite a treated lesion. Thus, pretreatment client consultation to explain potential side effects is vitally important.

Many beam-modifying devices can be used to conform the radiation dose to specific anatomical variations noted in small animal oncology patients. These include blocks, cutouts, filters, and wedges that are beyond the scope of this discussion but are shown in Figure 15-2.

As mentioned previously, electron beams may be used instead of photons for superficial and cutaneous tumors. Electrons, because of their charge and mass, lose energy very quickly once they enter the body. Consequently, the rate of dose fall-off after Dmax is much greater for electrons than for x-ray (photon) beams. In practical terms, this means that a therapeutic dose is delivered to the superficial tissues, while underlying

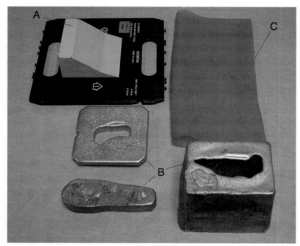

FIGURE 15-2 Treatment aids used in megavoltage radiation therapy. Wedges *(A)* help to provide uniform depth dose when the field is incident on an angled field. Custom blocks *(B)* shield vital normal structures. Bolus *(C)* brings the Dmax closer to the surface of the skin.

tissues are spared. Thus, electron beam therapy is ideal for treatment of many cutaneous and superficial masses, especially those that are overlying critical structures.

PALLIATIVE EXTERNAL BEAM RADIATION

Some neoplasms, because of their biology and other factors, such as the presence or likelihood of distant metastasis, are unlikely to be cured by radiation therapy. Osteosarcoma is a prime example of such a tumor.[6] In these instances, treatment with "palliative intent" may be the best choice. Palliative intent treatments typically involve treatment with one to five large fractions of 6 to 10 Gray administered at weekly or longer intervals. Palliative intent treatments are given in order to slow tumor progression and, most importantly, decrease pain associated with the tumor. Radiation oncologists vary widely in their approach to palliative treatments, and there is no uniform recommendation with regard to the number or size of fractions for any given tumor. When recommending palliative treatment, it is important to be cognizant of the type of normal tissue complications that can arise, since large fractions are more likely to have severe late effects on normal tissue, such as bone necrosis, than are small fractions. The total dose of radiation that can be given is also less than would be the case for smaller fractions given over the same period. As a result, ultimate control of the tumor is less likely. Treatment with a larger number of smaller fractions will typically result in fewer complications and more durable tumor control and should be recommended when all other factors are equal. However, many mitigating factors including client preference and patient life expectancy may make palliative treatment the better choice in some cases.

BRACHYTHERAPY

Brachytherapy (from the Greek *brachy,* meaning short distance) consists of placing radioactive sources in or near the target tissue. The dose rate from these sources falls exponentially with distance, allowing for the delivery of very high doses to the tumor and much lower doses to the normal surrounding tissues. Brachytherapy has been limited in veterinary medicine by concerns about radioactive exposure to clinicians and hospital staff, the potential for lost or ingested radioactive material, and the lack of appropriate radiation isolation facilities. Despite these issues, various animal malignancies have been successfully treated using brachytherapy. Brachytherapy can be delivered through several different methods, each having distinct advantages and disadvantages. The choice of brachytherapy method depends on shape, size, and location of the target tissue. Examples of brachytherapy techniques used in veterinary medicine include the following:

1. ***Interstitial brachytherapy*** refers to the surgical placement of radioactive implants directly inside the target tissue. An example is interstitial iridium 192, which has been used with some success after surgical removal of canine mast cell tumors.[7]

2. ***Intracavitary brachytherapy*** refers to the placement of radioactive implants inside a body cavity in close proximity to the target tissue. Intranasal iridium implants have been used to treat dogs after surgical debulking of nasal cavity malignancies.[8]

Plesiotherapy involves direct application of a radioactive source onto the target tissue. Strontium 90 probes (Figure 15-3) are the most common application of this type of therapy in veterinary medicine and have been used with great success to treat very superficial lesions. Strontium is a beta emitter, and almost the entire radiation dose is deposited superficially, with only about 5% going beyond 4 mm. Cats with superficial nasal planum squamous cell carcinoma treated with a single dose of strontium plesiotherapy had a 98% response rate, with 88% of these having complete resolution of their lesions.[9] Feline mast cell tumors have also been successfully treated with strontium. One report cited a 98% local control rate after single or multiple applications.[10]

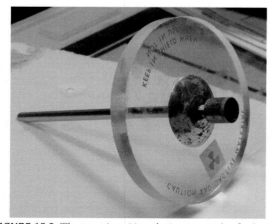

FIGURE 15-3 The strontium 90 probe is an example of a device used for plesiotherapy, where a radioactive source is directly applied to the target tissue. The shield *(red arrow)* protects the user's hand from the radioactive source located at the end of the probe *(yellow arrow)*.

EXPECTATIONS

Although radiation therapy is usually administered with "curative intent," there are many instances in which the treatment is more likely to result in delay of disease advancement and/or palliation of pain and clinical signs. Regardless, the patient's quality of life is improved, and the owner is afforded the opportunity to enjoy his or her companion for a longer time than would have otherwise been the case. Even when the likelihood for cure is low, one need not necessarily exclude radiation therapy as an option, as long as the owners have been properly counseled regarding the probable outcome and other treatment options. When referral for radiation therapy is desired, practitioners are encouraged to personally contact the radiation oncologist in order to gather information regarding prognosis, anticipated side effects, and the appropriate timing of radiation therapy in relation to other treatments such as surgery and chemotherapy. General information regarding side effects of radiation therapy and their management is provided in Section C, and a listing of sites offering teletherapy and brachytherapy can be found at: http://www.vetcancersociety.org/index.php?c-6, using the tab radiation facilities. A listing of board-certified veterinary radiation therapists can be found at www.acvr.org.

Selected References*

McEntee MC: Veterinary radiation therapy: review and current state of the art, *J Am Anim Hosp Assoc* 42:94, 2006.
This review paper provides a good basis for understanding the fundamentals of veterinary radiation therapy, including which cancers can be effectively treated with external beam therapy and what side effects should be expected.
Thames HD Jr, Withers WR, Peters LJ, et al: Changes in early and late radiation responses with altered dose fractionation: implications for dose-survival relationships, *Int J Radiat Oncol Biol Phys* 8:219, 1982.
This is a basic reference that provides an overview of the radiobiological basis of fractionated radiation therapy.
Walker M, Durrer R, Weir V, et al: A study to evaluate single port, central axis dosimetry and verification techniques for veterinary radiotherapy, using the canine nasal cavity as a model target, *Vet Radiol* 35:210, 1994.
This reference provides an overview of the problems encountered in and some of the techniques for determining the actual radiation dose delivered to complex anatomic areas.

*For a complete list of the references cited in this chapter, please go to www.smallanimaloncology.com.

SECTION B: Radioisotopes in Cancer Therapy

Jimmy C. Lattimer and Jeffrey N. Bryan

KEY POINTS

- Radioiodine therapy effectively manages canine and feline thyroid carcinoma that is unresectable.
- Samarium-153-EDTMP can effectively palliate bone pain, but causes myelosuppression, which may delay chemotherapy.
- One dose of Phosphorus-32 is generally sufficient to control polycythemia vera and essential thrombocythemia in dogs.

Therapeutic use of radioisotopes in veterinary oncology may be divided into two categories: (1) the administration of a radioisotope solution by oral, subcutaneous, intramuscular, or intravenous routes for the treatment of a neoplastic disease and, less commonly, (2) the implantation of high-activity sealed sources directly into the tumor. Both methods have been used for many years in both veterinary and human oncology. Radioisotopes that localize within, or are implanted into, tumors have the advantage that they provide continuous treatment and, in many cases, require far less hospitalization than external beam radiation therapy. In addition to continuous irradiation of the tumor, which takes full advantage of the benefits of the four Rs of radiobiology (see Section A), there is the added advantage that the radiation dose to adjacent normal tissues is often markedly reduced and the dose to the tumor can often be increased. However, there are significant concerns with regard to the safe use and administration of radioisotope treatments and prevention of significant radiation exposure to those in contact with treated pets. Administration of this therapy is restricted to individuals who have had specific training in the safe use and handling of radioisotopes and are licensed by the Nuclear Regulatory Commission. The most common veterinary applications for radioisotopes are summarized below, and current availability is outlined in Table 15-1.

RADIOISOTOPES: PARENTERAL ADMINISTRATION

Samarium-153-EDTMP

This bone-seeking radiopharmaceutical has been used to treat primary tumors of bone, including osteosarcoma, multilobular osteochondrosarcoma, and chondrosarcoma, as well as metastatic-to-bone cancer.[1-3] The intent of therapy in appendicular osteosarcoma is to preserve limb function in dogs for which amputation is not an acceptable option.[4] In metastatic-to-bone cancer, the intent of therapy is purely palliative to restore comfort and function.[2] Documented rates of complete response to ^{153}Sm-EDTMP as a primary therapy range from 1 of 9 dogs with osteosarcoma to 7 of 40 dogs with a variety of tumors including osteosarcoma.[2,3] In the larger study, 25 of 42 dogs exhibited a partial response with good palliation of signs of pain.[2] A recent study observed palliation of clinical signs in 63% of 32 dogs.[5] Palliation of the clinical signs of osteosarcoma allowed the dogs to live a median of 93 days, not dissimilar to amputation alone.[5] The currently practiced whole-body dose of ^{153}Sm-EDTMP of 1 mCi/kg is calculated to deliver from 20 to 160 Gy to an active bone lesion.[6] Patients must be pre-screened with ^{99m}Tc-MDP bone scans to identify a tumor to normal bone ratio of at least 4:1 before a significant therapeutic effect can be expected.[2] Myelosuppression is common and lasts up to 4 weeks after administration.[2] This can be expected to delay chemotherapy. Henry and others reported a synergistic myelosuppression when ^{153}SM-EDTMP was administered intercurrently with external beam radiation therapy (Henry CJ, personal communication, 2001).

Iodine-131

This radiopharmaceutical is ideal for treating thyroid neoplasia, since it is an element that is selectively accumulated by the thyroid tissue without modification. As a result, thyroid tissue at the primary tumor location as well as metastatic sites may be targeted with intravenously administered sodium iodide ^{131}I.[7] Thyroid hyperplasia and neoplasia in cats is routinely treated with ^{131}I with excellent results.[8,9] Unresectable thyroid carcinoma of dogs has been reported to be responsive to ^{131}I therapy with a median survival of 839 days for dogs with Stage II or III disease and 366 days for dogs with stage IV disease (see Chapter 26, Section B).[7]

Phosphorus-32

Accumulating in the bone, this radiopharmaceutical has been used to treat chronic diseases of the bone marrow. In a review of 11 cases, five of eight dogs with polycythemia vera and two of three dogs with essential thrombocythemia required only a single treatment to cause beneficial clinical response.[10] This is potentially preferable to many owners over administering oral chemotherapy on a regular basis chronically.

TABLE 15-1   VETERINARY RADIOISOTOPE AND IMPLANTABLE BRACHYTHERAPY AVAILABILITY IN THE UNITED STATES

Source	Indication	Site	Contact Information
Implantable brachytherapy			
Iridium-192	Various	Auburn University	334-844-4690 www.vetmed.auburn.edu
Cesium-137	Various	University of Missouri-Columbia	573-882-7821 www.cvm.missouri.edu/ oncology/index.htm
Radioisotope			
I-131 (cats)	Thyroid hyperplasia and carcinoma	Many	See listings at: www.vetcancersociety.org
I-131 (dogs)	Thyroid carcinoma	Arizona Veterinary Specialists	480-635-1110 www.azvs.com
		Veterinary Specialty Center, Buffalo Grove, IL	847-459-7535 www.vetspecialty.com
		University of Missouri-Columbia	573-882-7821 www.cvm.missouri.edu/ oncology/index.html
		Southeast Veterinary Oncology	904-278-3870 www.petcancercare.com
		SouthPaws Veterinary Specialists and Emergency Center	703-752-9100 www.southpaws.com
		University of Tennessee	865-974-8387 www.vet.utk.edu
		Colorado State University	970-297-4195 www.csuanimalcancercenter.org
P-32	Polycythemia vera	Arizona Veterinary Specialists	480-635-1110 www.azvs.com
		Southwest Veterinary Oncology	520-888-3177 www.southernazvets.com
		Southeast Veterinary Oncology	904-278-3870 www.petcancercare.com
Sm-153	Primary or metastatic bone lesions	Veterinary Specialty Center, Buffalo Grove, IL	847-459-7535 www.vetspecialty.com
		University of Missouri-Columbia	573-882-7821 www.cvm.missouri.edu/ oncology/index.htm
		Colorado State University	970-297-4195 www.csuanimalcancercenter.org

GENERAL PATIENT CONSIDERATIONS

When a radioisotope is administered parenterally, it is distributed throughout the body and all tissues receive some radiation dose. Most of the tissues that do not concentrate the isotope will receive minimal dose, representing an acceptable risk, provided the dose to the target (tumor) is therapeutic. However, dose to the organs in the excretion pathway can be quite significant. If the kidneys are the organs excreting the unused isotope, they will receive more dose than other non-target organs. If the animal does not urinate promptly, the urinary bladder may receive a very large dose of radiation that could cause substantial local tissue damage. Animals that are to have radioisotope administered should have normal kidney function and be encouraged to urinate frequently for the first 24 hours after the isotope is given, since this is the time of major excretion for unused isotopes.

RADIOISOTOPES: BRACHYTHERAPY

Implantation of sealed radioisotope sources into a tumor for local irradiation is known as *brachytherapy* (see Section A). Brachytherapy is particularly suited for treatment of small tumors that are accessible but adjacent to sensitive normal structures or for treatment of patients for which repeated anesthesia is not advisable, such as horses. Current availability of brachytherapy in the United States is outlined in Table 15-1.

Selected References*

Lattimer JC, Corwin LA Jr, Stapleton J, et al: Clinical and clinicopathologic response of canine bone tumors patients to treatment with Samarium-153-EDTMP, *J Nucl Med* 31:1316, 1990.

This paper described the therapeutic effect of Samarium-153-EDTMP and has been the basis for further study of this agent in canine osteosarcoma.
Smith M, Turrel JM: Radiophosphorus (32P) treatment of bone marrow disorders in dogs: 11 cases (1970-1987), *J Am Vet Med Assoc* 194:98, 1989.
This paper describes the use of radioactive phosphorous in managing bone marrow disorders in dogs.
Turrel JM, McEntee MC, Burke BP, et al: Sodium iodide I 131 treatment of dogs with nonresectable thyroid tumors: 39 cases (1990-2003), *J Am Vet Med Assoc* 229:542, 2006.
This paper demonstrated the utility of treating canine thyroid carcinoma with radioactive iodine in the largest population yet examined.

*For a complete list of the references cited in this chapter, please go to www.smallanimaloncology.com.

SECTION C: Management of Radiation Toxicity and Complications

William R. Brawner and Gregory T. Almond

KEY POINTS

- Radiation therapy is not specific for tumor cells; it will also affect normal cells located within the treatment field. This is the basis for side effects noted with radiation therapy.
- Effects of radiation therapy are limited to those cells, normal or abnormal, located within the treatment field.
- Acute radiation side effects occur in radiosensitive tissues, develop during the radiation treatment or shortly thereafter, and resolve or heal within weeks after completion of the therapy.
- Late radiation side effects occur in the relatively radio-resistant tissues. Little therapy exists for most late effects and in some tissues can be life limiting.

THE BASIS OF RADIATION TOXICITY

When ionizing radiation is delivered to tissues, DNA is damaged. Some of the damage is repaired, but some is irreparable and leads to cell death. Unfortunately, radiation damages DNA in both normal and neoplastic cells. The goal of radiation therapy is to maximize damage to neoplastic tissue while minimizing damage to normal tissues. However, there is minimal difference between the sensitivity of tumors and normal tissues to radiation therapy. If a high enough dose of radiation is given to ensure eradication of the tumor, there is often a high probability of damage to surrounding normal tissues. As a result, *the limiting factor in the ability to completely eradicate tumors with radiation therapy is the response of associated normal tissues.*

Despite advanced imaging techniques and sophisticated 3D computerized planning software, normal tissues are irradiated in even the best radiation therapy plans. There are several reasons why this occurs. First, inclusion of normal tissues may be unavoidable based on the location of the tumor. This can occur when the beam traverses normal tissue to reach a deep-seated mass. Second, radiation delivery to normal tissues is often by design. To effectively treat microscopic disease beyond the grossly visible tumor, margins around the tumor are intentionally included in the treatment plan. Factors used to determine margin width include the biologic behavior of the particular tumor being treated, regional lymphatic drainage, and clinical uncertainty of the extent of microscopic disease.

SECONDARY EFFECTS ON NORMAL TISSUES

Secondary effects of radiation therapy to normal tissues are categorized as early (acute) or late (delayed) effects. Dose of radiation per fraction, number of fractions, overall treatment time, and total radiation dose affect the likelihood of adverse reactions in normal tissues. It is important to note that within a group of patients, considerable variation in normal tissue reactions can occur, even with the same treatment protocol.[1] Secondary effects occur only in tissues in the radiation beam. Radiation sickness with vomiting, diarrhea, and other systemic signs reported in humans occurs with irradiation of internal organs. Since tumors of internal organs are infrequently irradiated in veterinary medicine, these symptoms are rarely seen. The Veterinary Radiation Therapy Oncology Group has devised an internationally accepted radiation toxicity scoring system, which can be found on the website (http://www.acvr.org/members/radiation_oncology/vrtog/scoring_scheme.pdf).[2] This system is referred to when evaluating radiation toxicity among veterinary patients.

Acute effects of radiation therapy usually begin in the second or third week of definitive, intent-to-cure, fractionated protocols. Acute effects occur in tissues that are characterized by rapid cell turnover such as the epidermis of the skin, mucous membranes, and gastrointestinal epithelium. Early effects are directly associated with fraction size, total dose, and overall treatment time.[3] See Table 15-2 for common acute responses encountered in veterinary medicine.

Late effects occur months to years after irradiation in slowly proliferating tissues such as cells of the liver, kidney, lung, nervous system, and bone. They can also develop as a result of severe acute effects such as in the skin. Late effects result in fibrosis or necrosis of skin or mucosa (caused by loss of germinal cells), bone necrosis, radiation encephalitis, myelitis, pulmonary fibrosis, cataracts, and radiation-induced tumors at previously treated sites.[4] Late effects are directly associated with radiation dose per fraction.[3] Higher dose per fraction regimens, such as palliative therapy protocols, are at risk for the development of late effects. However, when recommending palliative protocols, the radiation oncologist often presumes that the life expectancy of the patient will be shorter than the time necessary for the development of late effects and, therefore, the benefit to the patient outweighs the risk of the toxicity.

TABLE 15-2   ACUTELY RESPONDING TISSUES AND POTENTIAL TOXICITIES

Location	Toxicity
Skin	Erythema, epilation, dry desquamation, moist desquamation, ulceration, alopecia
Mouth	Mucositis, ulceration, foul odor
Eyes	Conjunctivitis, blepharitis, keratitis, corneal ulceration, keratoconjunctivitis sicca
Foot pads	Ulceration, sloughing
Perineal region	Proctitis, cystitis, colitis

TREATMENT OF ACUTE EFFECTS

The vast majority of acute effects will begin to heal within 2 to 3 weeks after treatment is completed. When radiation-induced acute effects are severe enough to require medical treatment, a frequent concern is the choice of appropriate therapeutic agents. Treatment of radiation-induced injury does not require unique medications; those appropriately used to treat acute inflammation can be used safely to treat radiation acute effects. These medications often will not speed healing, but rather make the patient more comfortable while healing occurs.

Skin

One of the most common acute effects observed with radiation therapy is radiation dermatitis. Clinical experience suggests that animals with allergic skin conditions are more likely to experience adverse secondary skin reactions. Initially this may appear as erythema of skin in the radiation field during the course of radiation therapy or a few days after the end of therapy. Mild cases of radiation dermatitis heal spontaneously as long as self trauma by the patient is prevented with the use of bandages or Elizabethan collars. Prevention of scratching, licking, chewing, or rubbing the treated site is critical for successful healing. Management is symptomatic with particular attention to hygiene and prevention of self trauma. Patients with dry desquamation (Figure 15-4) can be treated with topical products such as Zn7 (Addison Biological Laboratory, Inc., Fayette, MO) or Carra Vet Wound Gel (Carrington Laboratories, Inc., Irving, TX). Patients with moist desquamation (Figure 15-5) require clipping of hair in the affected areas and gentle lavage or warm compresses with normal saline or water. Applying a warm compress of Domeboro (Bayer,

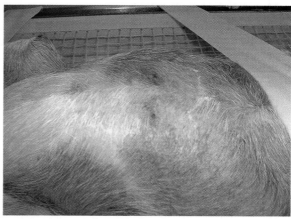

FIGURE 15-4 Dry desquamation.

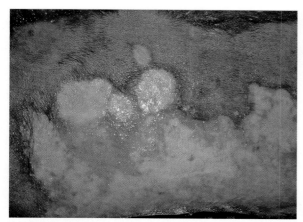

FIGURE 15-5 Moist desquamation.

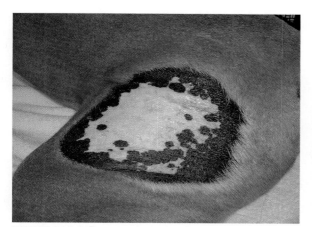

FIGURE 15-6 Pigmentary changes on the lateral thigh of a boxer after electron therapy.

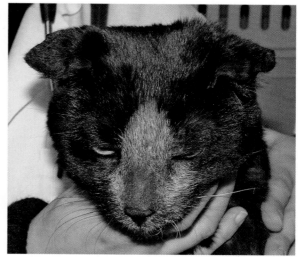

FIGURE 15-7 Grey hairs in the radiation field resulting from nasal lymphoma irradiation. (Courtesy of Dr. Dudley McCaw.)

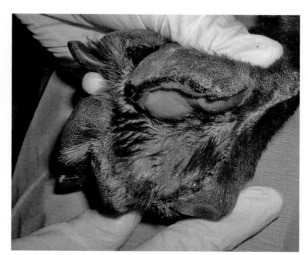

FIGURE 15-8 Sloughing metacarpal pad.

Morristown, NJ) solution to the site or soaking an appendage in the solution for 15 to 20 minutes twice daily is helpful to dry the area and provides relief to the patient. Other topical products that can be used include aloe-based topical gels, silver sulfadiazine cream, Zn7, CarraVet Wound Gel, colloidal oatmeal, and non-petroleum-based topical products. Topical application of extracts of black or green tea three times daily can be beneficial.[5] Systemic pain medications (NSAIDs, tramadol, etc.) may also help with the discomfort. Although moist desquamation can appear relatively severe, it usually heals within 2 to 3 weeks. Hair will usually regrow within the treatment field, albeit months before a normal amount of hair is present. In addition, clients should be advised that permanent pigmentary and hair color changes within the radiation field will likely occur (Figures 15-6 and 15-7). When the distal extremity

is included in the radiation field, sloughing of the pads can occur (Figure 15-8). With conservative care as described for moist desquamation, re-epithelialization can occur with satisfactory results (Figure 15-9). However, complete recovery will take an extended period of time.

Eyes

When the eyes or adjacent tissues are within the radiation field, as frequently occurs with treatment of nasal tumors, there is a risk of acute damage to the lacrimal glands. This can result in keratoconjunctivitis sicca, which can be treated with

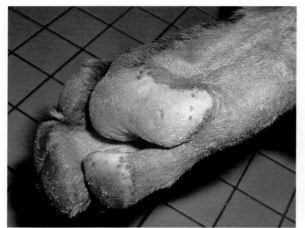

FIGURE 15-9 Healed pad. Notice that the healed tissue is smoother than normal and lacks the typical heavily keratinized conical papillae.

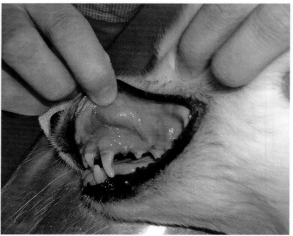

FIGURE 15-10 Mild mucositis.

artificial tears and/or cyclosporine ophthalmic ointment. Corneal ulceration may also occur. This can be treated with topical ophthalmic antibiotics and ophthalmic atropine for pain. As with any corneal ulcer, ophthalmic medications containing steroids should be avoided in these patients.

Mucositis

Inflammation within the oral cavity, pharynx, or esophagus can occur with irradiation of the head or neck. Mucositis within the oral cavity is frequently seen with irradiation of nasal tumors. Most commonly, the patient will exhibit signs of oral tenderness (Figure 15-10), have thick ropy saliva, and a foul odor to the breath. Mild mucositis can be treated with twice-daily oral flushes of decaffeinated tea, or if the animal will drink the tea, it can be provided in its bowl. The tannic acid in tea is an astringent and is helpful in drying the mouth and soothing the oral discomfort. A "radiation mouthwash" of equal parts liquid diphenhydramine, viscous lidocaine, and aluminum hydroxide/magnesium hydroxide (such as Maalox) may also be helpful.[6] If the mouth is flushed with this mouthwash solution shortly before eating, discomfort may be alleviated enough that the animal is willing to eat. Systemic pain relief agents (NSAIDs, tramadol, etc.) may also be beneficial. If oral mucositis is severe, supportive care such as subcutaneous fluids and placement of an esophagostomy or gastrostomy tube may be necessary. For perianal discomfort, radiation-induced proctitis, Proctofoam HC (Duchesnay, Inc., Blainville, QC, Canada) (combination of hydrocortisone and the topical anesthetic pramoxine) may be helpful.

TREATMENT OF LATE EFFECTS

Late effects are difficult and discouraging to treat. They are the limiting factor of radiotherapy success because they limit the radiation dose that normal tissues can tolerate and remain functional. Higher doses would completely eradicate more tumors but would result in unacceptable rates of severe normal tissue complications. Some late effects such as cataracts, and bone necrosis can be treated with surgery. Strictures in hollow organs such as the rectum can be treated with surgery or bougienage for stricture breakdown. However, since most late effects are not well treated or reversed, they must be avoided by using low dose per fraction (i.e., more small fractions rather than fewer large fractions) and limiting total dose to known tolerance levels.

Selected References*

LaDue T, Klein MK: Toxicity criteria of the veterinary radiation therapy oncology group, *Vet Rad Ultrasound* 42(5):475, 2001.
Explanation of the grading scheme for radiation toxicoses seen in veterinary medicine.
McEntee MC: Veterinary radiation therapy: review and current state of the art, *J Am Anim Hosp Assoc* 42:94, 2006.
A thorough and up-to-date review of radiation therapy in veterinary medicine. Includes discussion of the mechanisms of action of radiation therapy, responses of various tumor types, and commonly encountered toxicities.

█ *For a complete list of the references cited in this chapter, please go to www.smallanimaloncology.com.

16 Immunotherapy

Philip J. Bergman

KEY POINTS

- The immune system is generally divided into two primary components: the *innate immune response*, and the highly specific, but more slowly developing *adaptive or acquired immune response*.
- Immune responses can be further separated by whether they are induced by exposure to a foreign antigen (an "active" response) or if they are transferred through serum or lymphocytes from an immunized individual (a "passive" response).
- The ideal cancer immunotherapy agent would be able to discriminate between cancer and normal cells (i.e., specificity), be potent enough to kill small or large numbers of tumor cells (i.e., sensitivity), and lastly be able to prevent recurrence of the tumor (i.e., durability).
- Tumor immunology and immunotherapy is one of the most exciting and rapidly expanding fields at present.
- The veterinary oncology profession is uniquely able to greatly contribute to the many advances to come in the cancer immunotherapy field.

The term *immunity* is derived from the Latin word *immunitas*, which refers to the legal protection afforded to Roman senators holding office. Although the immune system is normally thought of as providing protection against infectious disease, the immune system's ability to recognize and eliminate cancer is the fundamental rationale for the immunotherapy of cancer. Multiple lines of evidence support a role for the immune system in managing cancer, including: (1) spontaneous remissions in cancer patients without treatment, (2) the presence of tumor-specific cytotoxic T-cells within tumor or draining lymph nodes, (3) the presence of monocytic, lymphocytic, and plasmacytic cellular infiltrates in tumors,

(4) the increased incidence of some types of cancer in immunosuppressed patients, and (5) documentation of cancer remissions with the use of immunomodulators.[1] With the tools of molecular biology and a greater understanding of mechanisms to harness the immune system, effective tumor immunotherapy is becoming a reality. This new class of therapeutics offers a more targeted and therefore precise approach to the treatment of cancer. It is extremely likely that immunotherapy will have a place alongside the classic cancer treatment triad components of surgery, radiation therapy, and chemotherapy within the next 5 to 10 years.

TUMOR IMMUNOLOGY

Cellular Components

The immune system is generally divided into two primary components: the *innate immune response*, and the highly specific, but more slowly developing *adaptive or acquired immune response* (Figure 16-1, *A*). Innate immunity is rapidly acting but typically not very specific and includes physico-chemical barriers (e.g., skin and mucosa); blood proteins such as complement, phagocytic cells (macrophages, neutrophils, dendritic cells [DCs], and natural killer [NK] cells); and cytokines that coordinate and regulate the cells involved in innate immunity. Adaptive immunity is thought of as the acquired arm of immunity that allows for exquisite specificity, an ability to remember the previous existence of the pathogen and differentiate self from non-self, and importantly the ability to respond more vigorously upon repeat exposure to the pathogen. Adaptive immunity consists of T and B cells. The T cells are further divided into CD8 (cluster of differentiation) and MHC (major histocompatibility complex) Class I cytotoxic T lymphocytes (CTL) and helper T cells (CD4 and MHC class II), NK cells, and regulatory T cells. B cells produce antibodies (humoral system) that may activate complement, enhance phagocytosis of opsonized target cells, and induce antibody dependent cellular cytotoxicity (ADCC). B-cell responses to tumors are thought by many investigators to be less important than the development of T-cell mediated immunity, but there is little evidence to fully support this notion.[2] The innate and adaptive arms of immunity are not mutually exclusive; they are linked by (1) the innate response's ability to stimulate and influence the nature of the adaptive response, and (2) the sharing of effector mechanisms between innate and adaptive immune responses.

Immune responses can be further separated by whether they are induced by exposure to a foreign antigen (an "active" response) or if they are transferred through serum or lymphocytes from an immunized individual (a "passive" response). Although both approaches have the ability to be extremely specific for an antigen of interest, one important difference is the inability of passive approaches to confer memory. The principal components of the active/adaptive immune system are lymphocytes, antigen-presenting cells, and effector cells. Furthermore, responses can be subdivided by whether they are specific for a certain antigen, or a non-specific response whereby immunity is attempted to be conferred by up-regulating the immune system without a specific target. These definitions are helpful because they allow methodologies to be more completely characterized, such as active-specific, active-nonspecific, passive-nonspecific, etc.

Immune Surveillance

The idea that the immune system may actively prevent the development of neoplasia is termed *cancer immunosurveillance*. Sound scientific evidence supports some aspects of this hypothesis,[3,4] including: (1) IFN-γ protects mice against the growth of tumors, (2) mice lacking IFN-γ receptor were more sensitive to chemically induced sarcomas than normal mice and were more likely to spontaneously develop tumors, (3) mice lacking major components of the adaptive immune response (T and B cells) have a high rate of spontaneous tumors, and (4) mice that lack IFN-γ and B or T cells develop tumors, especially at a young age.

Immune Evasion by Tumors

There are significant barriers to the generation of effective anti-tumor immunity by the host. Many tumors evade surveillance mechanisms and grow in immunocompetent hosts as is easily illustrated by the overwhelming numbers of people and animals succumbing to cancer. There are multiple ways in which tumors evade the immune response including those noted in Box 16-1.

NON-SPECIFIC TUMOR IMMUNOTHERAPY

Dr. William Coley, a New York surgeon in the early 1900s, noted that some cancer patients developing incidental bacterial infections survived longer than those without infection.[9] Coley developed a bacterial "vaccine" (killed cultures of *Serratia marcescens* and *Streptococcus Pyogenes*, or "Coley's toxins") to treat people with sarcomas, which provided complete response rates of approximately 15%. Unfortunately, high failure rates and significant side effects led to discontinuation of this approach. His seminal work laid the foundation for nonspecific modulation of the immune response in the treatment of cancer. Non-specific tumor immunotherapy approaches are numerous, and relevant examples are listed in Table 16-1.[10-42]

BOX 16-1   METHODS BY WHICH TUMORS MAY EVADE THE IMMUNE RESPONSE

1. Immunosuppressive cytokine production
   - Examples: TGF-β and IL-10[5,6]
2. Impaired DC function
   - Via inactivation ("anergy")
   - Via poor DC maturation through changes in IL-6/IL-10/VEGF/GM-CSF[7]
3. Induction of cells called regulatory T cells (Treg)
   - Treg cells were initially called suppressor T cells and are CD4/CD25/CTLA-4/GITR/Foxp3-positive cells that can suppress tumor-specific CD4/CD8+ T cells[8]
4. MHC I loss
   - Structural defect in MHC I
   - Changes in B2-microglobulin synthesis
   - Defects in transporter-associated antigen processing
   - Actual MHC I gene loss (i.e., allelic or locus loss)
5. MHC I antigen presentation loss through B7-1 attenuation
   - B7-1 is an important co-stimulatory molecule for CD28-mediated T-cell receptor and MHC engagement when the MHC system in no. 4 remains intact.

TABLE 16-1   EXAMPLES OF NON-SPECIFIC IMMUNOTHERAPY APPROACHES

Immunotherapy Approach	Agent(s)	Tumor Types Investigated with this Approach in Veterinary Medicine	Reference
Biological response modifiers	BCG	Canine mammary carcinoma, mast cell tumors, and transmissible venereal tumor	10-14
		Equine sarcoids	
		Bovine ocular squamous cell carcinoma	
	Corynebacterium parvum	Canine melanoma and mammary carcinoma	10, 16
	Mycobacterial cell wall-DNA complexes	Canine osteosarcoma and transitional cell carcinoma	Abstract only[*,†]
	Attenuated Salmonella (VNP20009)	Various	17
	Bacterial superantigens	Various, including canine melanoma	18, 19
	Oncolytic viruses (Newcastle disease virus, reovirus, vesicular stomatitis virus, Vaccinia, adenovirus, herpes simplex virus, canine distemper virus)	Various, including canine lymphoma	20-22
	Liposome-encapsulated muramyl tripeptide-phosphatidylethanolamine (L-MTP-PE)	Canine mammary carcinoma, melanoma, osteosarcoma	23-28
	Recombinant canine and human granulocyte macrophage colony-stimulating factor (rcGM-CSF and rhGM-CSF)	Melanoma	26, 29
	Imiquimod (Aldara)	Feline Bowen's disease	30
	Liposome-DNA complexes	Canine osteosarcoma, soft tissue sarcoma	31, 32
Recombinant cytokines	IL-2	Canine melanoma; feline fibrosarcoma	33-36
	Liposomal IL-2	Pre-clinical	37
	IL-12	Pre-clinical	38
	IL-15	Pre-clinical	39, 40
	Interferons	Pre-clinical	41, 42

*Filion MC, Filion B, Phillips NC: Effects of mycobacterial cell wall-DN complex (MCC), alendronate, and pamidronate on canine osteosarcoma cell lines, *2004 Veterinary Cancer Society Annual Conference Proceedings*, p 54.

†Knapp DW, Filion B, Filion MC, et al: Antitumor activity of mycobacterial cell wall-DNA complex (MCC) against canine urinary bladder transitional cell carcinoma cells, *2004 Veterinary Cancer Society Annual Conference Proceedings*, p 39.

‡Canine Melanoma DNA Vaccine, Merial, Inc, Duluth, GA.

CANCER VACCINES

The ultimate goal for a cancer vaccine is elicitation of an anti-tumor immune response that results in clinical regression of a tumor and/or its metastases. Responses to cancer vaccines may take several months or more to appear because of the slower speed of induction of the adaptive arm of the immune system, as outlined in Table 16-2.

There are numerous types of tumor vaccines in phase I-III trials across a wide range of tumor types. The immune system detects tumors through specific tumor-associated antigens (TAAs) that are recognized by both CTLs and antibodies. TAAs may be common to a particular tumor type, may be unique to an individual tumor, or may arise from mutated gene products such as ras,

TABLE 16-2   COMPARISON OF CHEMOTHERAPY AND ANTI-TUMOR VACCINES

Treatment Type	Mechanism of Action	Specificity	Sensitivity	Response Time	Durability of Response
Chemotherapy	Cytotoxicity	Poor	Variable	Hours to days	Variable
Anti-tumor vaccine	Immune response	Good	Good	Weeks to months	Variable to long

p53, p21, and/or others. Although unique TAAs may be more immunogenic than the other aforementioned shared tumor antigens, they are not practical targets because of their narrow specificity. Most shared tumor antigens are normal cellular antigens that are overexpressed in tumors. The first group to be identified was termed cancer testes antigens because of expression in normal testes, but they are also found in melanoma and various other solid tumors such as the MAGE/BAGE gene family. This chapter highlights those tumor vaccine approaches that appear to hold particular promise in human clinical trials and some that have been tested to date in veterinary medicine. A variety of approaches have been taken to date to focus the immune system on the aforementioned targets, including the following:

1. Whole cell or tumor cell lysate vaccines (autologous, or made from a patient's own tumor tissue; allogeneic, or made from individuals within a species bearing the same type of cancer; or whole cell vaccines from γ-irradiated tumor cell lines with or without immunostimulatory cytokines)[29,35,43]
2. DNA vaccines that immunize with syngeneic and/or xenogeneic (different species than recipient) plasmid DNA designed to elicit antigen-specific humoral and cellular immunity (to be discussed in more detail later in this chapter)
3. Viral vector-based methodologies designed to deliver genes encoding TAAs and/or immunostimulatory cytokines[36]
4. DC vaccines that are commonly loaded or transfected with TAAs, DNA, or RNA from TAAs, or tumor lysates[44]
5. Adoptive cell transfer (the "transfer" of specific populations of immune effector cells in order to generate a more powerful and focused antitumor immune response)
6. Antibody approaches such as monoclonal antibodies,[45] anti-idiotype antibodies (an idiotype is an immunoglobulin sequence unique to each B cell, and therefore antibodies directed against

these idiotypes are referred to as anti-idiotype) or conjugated antibodies

The ideal cancer immunotherapy agent would be able to discriminate between cancer and normal cells (i.e., specificity), be potent enough to kill small or large numbers of tumor cells (i.e., sensitivity), and lastly be able to prevent recurrence of the tumor (i.e., durability).

This author has developed a xenogeneic DNA vaccine program for melanoma in collaboration with human investigators from Memorial Sloan-Kettering Cancer Center.[46,47] Preclinical and clinical studies by our laboratory and others have shown that xenogeneic DNA vaccination with tyrosinase family members (e.g., tyrosinase, GP100, GP75) can produce immune responses resulting in tumor rejection or protection and prolongation of survival, while syngeneic vaccination with orthologous DNA does not induce immune responses. These studies provided the impetus for development of a xenogeneic DNA vaccine program in canine malignant melanoma (CMM). Cohorts of dogs received increasing doses of xenogeneic plasmid DNA encoding human tyrosinase (huTyr), murine GP75 (muGP75), murine tyrosinase (muTyr), muTyr ± HuGM-CSF (both administered as plasmid DNA) or MuTyr "off-study" intramuscularly biweekly for a total of four vaccinations. Minimal to mild pain was noted on vaccination, and one dog experienced vitiligo (Figure 16-1, *B*). We have recently investigated antibody responses in dogs vaccinated with HuTyr and found two- to five-fold increases in circulating antibodies to huTyr, which can cross-react to canine tyrosinase, suggesting the breaking of tolerance.[48] The clinical results with prolongation in survival have been reported previously.[46,47] The results of these trials demonstrate that xenogeneic DNA vaccination in CMM: (1) is safe, (2) leads to the development of anti-tyrosinase antibodies, (3) is potentially therapeutic, and (4) is an attractive candidate for further evaluation in an adjuvant, minimal residual disease Phase II setting for CMM. A USDA licensure study of huTyr in dogs with advanced malignant melanoma was initiated in April, 2006 in addition to a Phase I trial of murine CD20 for dogs and cats with

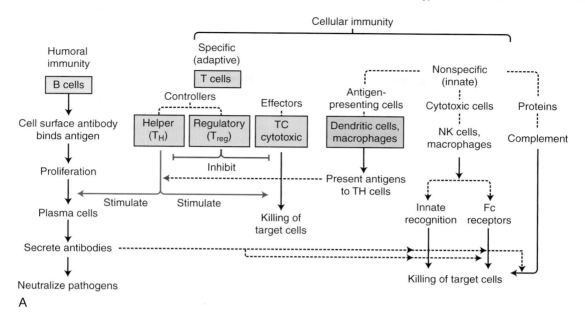

Cellular immunity

Humoral immunity — B cells

Specific (adaptive) — T cells

Controllers — Helper (T$_H$), Regulatory (T$_{reg}$)

Effectors — TC cytotoxic

Antigen-presenting cells — Dendritic cells, macrophages

Nonspecific (innate)

Cytotoxic cells — NK cells, macrophages

Proteins — Complement

Cell surface antibody binds antigen → Proliferation → Plasma cells → Secrete antibodies → Neutralize pathogens

Inhibit

Stimulate

Present antigens to TH cells

Killing of target cells

Innate recognition

Fc receptors

Killing of target cells

A

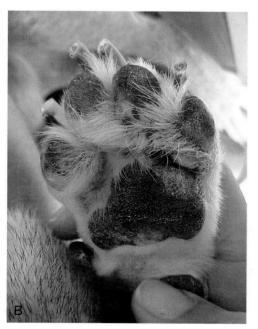

FIGURE 16-1 A, Diagram of the primary components of the immune system. Innate immunity is nonspecific, and physicochemical barriers, blood proteins, phagocytic cells, NK cells, and cytokines compose this arm of the immune system. Adaptive immunity is acquired, allowing for specificity and memory. It is composed of B and T cells. The innate and adaptive immune responses are not mutually exclusive, as evidenced by their interactions in this diagram. **B,** Presumed footpad autoimmune depigmentation (vitiligo) in a dog with stage III oral melanoma that began receiving murine tyrosinase DNA vaccination approximately 5 months before this photograph was taken. (**A** From Weinberg RA: *The biology of cancer,* New York, 2007, Garland Science [Taylor Francis].)

B cell lymphoma. The USDA granted conditional licensure for the use of HuTyr in dogs with locally controlled stage II or III oral malignant melanoma in March, 2007. This represents the first U.S. government–approved vaccine for the treatment of cancer across species.

Tumor immunology and immunotherapy is one of the most exciting and rapidly expanding fields at present. Significant resources are focused on mechanisms to simultaneously maximally stimulate an anti-tumor immune response while minimizing the immunosuppressive aspects of the tumor microenvironment. The recent elucidation and blockade of immunosuppressive cytokines (e.g., TGF-β, IL-10, and IL-13) and/or the negative costimulatory molecule CTLA-4[49] may dramatically improve cell-mediated immunity to tumors. As investigators more easily generate specific anti-tumor immune responses in patients, we will need to remain vigilant to not push the immune system too far into pathologic autoimmunity. In addition, immunotherapy is unlikely to become a sole modality in the treatment of cancer, since the traditional modalities of surgery, radiation, and/or chemotherapy are extremely likely to be used in combination with immunotherapy in the future. Like any form of anticancer treatment, immunotherapy appears to work best in a minimal residual disease setting, suggesting its most appropriate use will be in an adjuvant setting with local tumor therapies such as surgery and/or radiation. Similarly, the long-held belief that chemotherapy attenuates immune responses from cancer vaccines is beginning to be disproved through investigations on a variety of levels.[50,51]

In summary, the future looks extremely bright for immunotherapy. Similarly, the veterinary oncology profession is uniquely able to greatly contribute to the many advances to come in this field. Unfortunately, what works in a mouse will often not reflect the outcome in human cancer patients. Therefore, comparative immunotherapy studies using veterinary patients may be able to better "bridge" murine and human studies. To this end, a large number of cancers in dogs and cats appear to be remarkably stronger models for counterpart human tumors than presently available murine model systems. This is likely due to a variety of reasons including, but not limited to, extreme similarities in the biology of the tumors (e.g., chemoresistance, radioresistance, sharing metastatic phenotypes and site selectivity); spontaneous syngeneic cancer (vs. typically an induced and/or xenogeneic cancer in murine models); and finally the fact that the dogs and cats that are spontaneously developing these tumors are outbred,

immune-competent, and live in the same environment that humans do.

Selected References*

Bergman PJ, Camps-Palau MA, McKnight JA, et al: Development of a xenogeneic DNA vaccine program for canine malignant melanoma at the Animal Medical Center, *Vaccine* 24(21):4582, 2006.
Concise review of the development of a cancer immunotherapy program between the Animal Medical Center and Memorial Sloan-Kettering Cancer Center using xenogeneic DNA cancer vaccines.
Emens LA, Jaffee EM: Leveraging the activity of tumor vaccines with cytotoxic chemotherapy, *Cancer Res* 65(18):8059, 2005.
Excellent review of the status and possible breakdown of the long-held paradigm of cytotoxic chemotherapy attenuating immune responses to cancer vaccines.
MacEwen EG, Kurzman ID, Vail DM, et al: Adjuvant therapy for melanoma in dogs: results of randomized clinical trials using surgery, liposome-encapsulated muramyl tripeptide, and granulocyte macrophage colony-stimulating factor, *Clin Cancer Res* 5(12):4249, 1999.
This paper is another seminal work by the MacEwen group using a number of agents in randomized clinical trials for canine melanoma.
Reilly RT, Emens LA, Jaffee EM: Humoral and cellular immune responses: independent forces or collaborators in the fight against cancer? *Curr Opin Investig Drugs* 2(1):133, 2001.
This is a great review of both arms of the immune system and how they may interact within the context of cancer immunotherapy.
Smyth MJ, Godfrey DI, Trapani JA: A fresh look at tumor immunosurveillance and immunotherapy, *Nat Immunol* 2(4):293, 2001.
Excellent review of the immunosurveillance theory and its impact on cancer immunotherapy strategies.

*For a complete list of the references cited in this chapter, please go to www.smallanimaloncology.com.

17 Photodynamic Therapy

Dudley L. McCaw and Jeffrey N. Bryan

KEY POINTS

- Photodynamic therapy (PDT) kills tumor cells by activating a photosensitizing agent with light of a specific wavelength.
- Efficacy of PDT for the treatment of canine oral squamous cell carcinomas (SCCs) and feline cutaneous SCC has been reported.
- Mast cell tumors can also be successfully treated with PDT.
- Animals treated with photodynamic therapy must avoid direct sunlight for a few weeks after treatment.

Photodynamic therapy (PDT) is a relatively new therapy that has advantages over other therapies (Box 17-1), but also has its own complications (Box 17-2). Three components are necessary for successful PDT: a photosensitizer, a light source, and oxygen. The process involves the injection of a photosensitizer, then activating that agent with light of the appropriate wavelength (Figure 17-1). The activation of the sensitizer in the presence of oxygen results in the production of oxygen radicals causing cell death. This technique is used for dermatologic, ocular, and esophageal disease as well as cancer therapy in people. In veterinary medicine, the primary use is for cancer treatment.

PHOTOSENSITIZERS

Most photosensitizers are activated in the red spectrum of light from 630 to 700 nm. Penetration of tissue by the light is increased as the wavelength of the light increases. Greater penetration of light allows for larger tumors to be treated, but it also means that more normal tissue will be irradiated (Box 17-3). For dermatologic use, the photosensitizer is activated by a blue light so that only the superficial tissues are treated. The currently approved agents are listed in Table 17-1.

LIGHT AND LIGHT SOURCES

Any light of the proper wavelength can be used for PDT. In fact, the first light sources were slide projectors with the proper filters to allow only the desired wavelength to reach the patient. The activation of the sensitizer is a function of the total light exposure, so these low power sources resulted in unacceptably long treatment times. The advent of lasers has made PDT more clinically appealing, since they are a source of high power light of only one wavelength. This has decreased treatment times and eliminated the need for filters. Another significant advantage of laser light is the ability to couple fiberoptic cables to the laser to improve the delivery of light to the tissue. Initially, lasers were very large and could not be moved. However, diode lasers that are portable are now available, making this therapy more feasible in a practice setting.

MECHANISMS OF CELL KILLING

Cells are killed by PDT by one of three mechanisms: (1) directly from the production of oxygen radicals, (2) indirectly from resulting inflammation, and (3) by immunologic mechanisms. The direct killing occurs when tumor cells or vascular endothelial cells contain the photosensitizer.[1] The tissue location of the sensitizer depends upon its properties, but the result is the same regardless of whether the tumor cells are directly killed or whether blood vessels are damaged and the tumor cells die from lack of blood supply. In the process of killing cells, PDT creates acute inflammation that attracts neutrophils, causing more cell killing.[2] Dendritic cells that process antigens to present to antibody-producing cells are also attracted to the dying tumor. Antibodies produced against tumor antigens have the potential to kill tumors distant to the original tumor as well as the primary tumor.[3] In mouse and rat models, PDT treatment

BOX 17-1   ADVANTAGES OF PHOTODYNAMIC THERAPY

- Although normal tissue is not totally spared, the damage to normal tissue does appear to be less than that of neoplastic tissue.
- With the use of a fiberoptic cable, the light can be delivered in areas not readily accessible by surgery.
  - In the treatment of gingival squamous cell carcinomas, dogs with caudal mandibular lesions were successfully treated.[10]
  - If the same lesions were treated with surgery, a partial mandibulectomy with disarticulation of the temporomandibular joint would have been necessary.
- Passage of the fiberoptic cable through an endoscope allows for non-invasive treatment of esophageal inflammatory lesions (Barrett's esophagus) and bronchial neoplasms in people.
- Even though a single treatment is usually sufficient, it can be repeated. Unlike radiation therapy, there is no cumulative effect on normal tissue.
- In contrast to chemotherapy, no tumor resistance occurs.
- Healing is very cosmetic with less scarring than surgery.

BOX 17-2   POTENTIAL SIDE EFFECTS OF PHOTODYNAMIC THERAPY

- Swelling: There is considerable swelling beginning immediately after treatment. Resolution takes about 4 days.
  - If treating the oropharynx, a tracheostomy tube must be placed until swelling subsides.
- Necrosis, draining, and odor: The tumor dies over a short period, but necrotic tissue must be removed by macrophages. Healing takes about 4 weeks, and during this time there can be significant odor.
  - This problem can be reduced by flushing the affected area two to three times daily with water or a mild antiseptic solution.
- Infection: Because the treated area is, in effect, an open wound with necrotic tissue, infection is common during the healing phase. This can be successfully treated with antibiotics.
- Photosensitization: The sensitizer may be retained in skin, causing a severe reaction if the animal is exposed to sunlight. This was a significant problem with the early sensitizers, but this is of lesser concern with the newer generation sensitizers.
- Pulmonary edema: Some cats treated for squamous cell carcinoma developed pulmonary edema. No fatalities occurred.

of tumors resulted in development of a systemic immune response that produced rejection of tumor upon rechallenge.[3]

VETERINARY EXPERIENCE

Most veterinary reports of cancer therapy using PDT include data from early stage trials in which a variety of tumors were treated in dogs, cats, birds, and snakes.[4-7] Among the common tumor types that were successfully treated were canine mast cell tumors (Figure 17-2) and SCC in multiple species. Four studies in dogs and cats have looked at single tumor types. Two studies have shown successful treatment of feline SCCs of the head and nose.[8,9] Success of PDT for dogs with gingival SCCs was equal to surgical treatment. The major advantage was a better cosmetic effect because surgery would have involved mandibulectomy or maxillectomy.[10] The treatment of canine hemangiopericytomas (HPCs) with PDT has not been shown to be clinically advantageous over surgery alone.[11] In one prospective study, HPCs

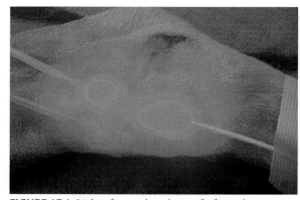

FIGURE 17-1 Light of a wavelength specific for each photosensitizing agent is used to activate the compound at the tumor site. Shown here is the use of an intratumoral catheter to permit activation of photosensitizer within a canine mast cell tumor.

BOX 17-3   MYTHS REGARDING PHOTODYNAMIC THERAPY

1. The sensitizer is present only in tumor tissue, and normal tissue will not be killed by PDT.
In the experience of the authors, normal tissue that receives a sufficient amount of light will be killed. Protection of normal tissue can be achieved by limiting the size of the treated area and by covering normal tissue with drapes or moistened gauze sponges.
2. Photodynamic therapy is a painless procedure.
During the procedure the animals will have increased heart rates in spite of being anesthetized. The authors have attributed this to pain. We routinely administer narcotic analgesics for 18 hours after treatment.

TABLE 17-1   PHOTOSENSITIZERS APPROVED IN ONE OR MORE COUNTRIES AND THEIR USE[1]

Trade Name	Generic Name	Indications
Photofrin	Hematoporphyrin derivative	*Neoplasia:* Gastric, cervical, endobronchial, and esophageal carcinomas
		Inflammatory: Barrett's esophagus
Visudyne	Benzoporphyrin	*Ocular:* Age-related macular degeneration
Foscan	Meta-tetrahydroxyphenyl-chlorin	*Neoplasia:* Head and neck tumors
Levulan	5-aminolevulinic acid	*Dermatologic:* Actinic keratosis
Metvix	5-aminolevulinic acid-methylesther	*Neoplasia:* Basal cell carcinoma

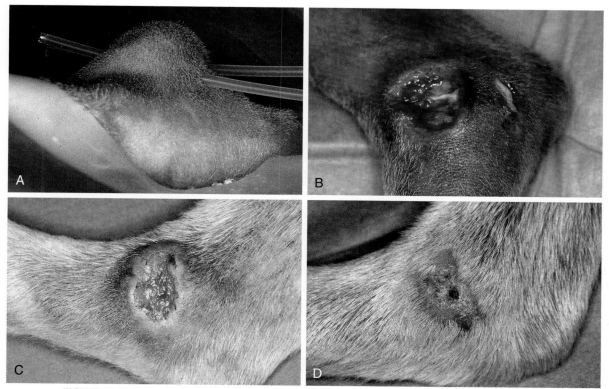

FIGURE 17-2 A, Placement of catheters in a mast cell tumor. A fiberoptic fiber equipped with a lens that diffuses the light laterally is inserted into each catheter. **B,** Treated tumor 1 week after photodynamic therapy (PDT) treatment. Tumor necrosis appears complete. **C,** Four weeks after PDT treatment. The lesion is healing and a good bed of granulation tissue is present. **D,** Eight weeks after PDT treatment. There is near complete epithelialization of the treated area.

were surgically debulked prior to PDT treatment. Sixteen dogs were treated and nine had recurrence within 29 months (median 9 months). Smaller tumors had a better response than large tumors. Slow wound healing, infections, and tumor recurrences before healing were problems.

Prospective clinical trials to evaluate the use of PDT in more tumor types are warranted. Previous experience indicates that the canine tumors amenable to treatment with PDT include mast cell tumor and oral SCCs. In cats, aural and facial SCCs respond to PDT. As with any therapy, small tumors (<3 cm) are more successfully treated than larger tumors.

Selected References*

Castano AP, Mroz P, Hamblin MR: Photodynamic therapy and anti-tumour immunity, *Nature Rev Cancer* 6:535-545, 2006.
This paper reviews the immunological processes that occur with PDT.
Magne ML, Rodriguez CA, Autry SA, et al: Photodynamic therapy of facial squamous cell carcinoma in cats using a new photosensitizer, *Lasers Surg Med* 20:202-209, 1997.
This manuscript reports the outcome of 51 cats with facial SCC treated with PDT. The complete response rate was 49%. Tumors staged as T1a (<1.5 cm and noninvasive) had a 100% complete response (15 cats).
McCaw DL, Pope ER, Payne JT, et al: Treatment of canine oral squamous cell carcinomas with photodynamic therapy, *Br J Cancer* 82(7):1297-1299, 2000.
This is a report of 11 dogs with gingival squamous cell carcinoma that were treated with PDT. Eight of the dogs were tumor-free for at least 17 months and were considered cured.

▌ *For a complete list of the references cited in this chapter, please go to www.smallanimaloncology.com.

18 Supportive Care of the Cancer Patient

SECTION A: Prevention and Management of Nausea and Vomiting

Mary Lynn Higginbotham

KEY POINTS

- Mechanisms of vomiting for chemotherapeutic agents are drug and dose dependent.
- Prevention of chemotherapy-associated nausea and vomiting is more effective than treatment.
- Multi-agent therapy may be necessary to most effectively control chemotherapy-associated nausea and vomiting.

INCIDENCE OF CHEMOTHERAPY-ASSOCIATED NAUSEA AND VOMITING

The management of chemotherapy-associated nausea and vomiting is an important aspect in the treatment of animals with cancer. Quality of life (QOL) is of utmost importance to owners and practitioners alike and therefore pre-emptive treatment of chemotherapy side effects is necessary. A 1983 survey of human oncology patients found that nausea and vomiting are the most feared side effects of chemotherapy,[1] and, in the author's experience, this is true for pet owners as well. When nausea and vomiting occur, the practitioner is not only faced with the sick patient, but also with poor compliance of the recommended therapy and/or decreased dose and dose intensity, resulting in an inferior long-term outcome for the patient. In addition, chemotherapy-associated nausea and vomiting (CANV) is easier to prevent than it is to treat. Few studies have been performed in veterinary medicine evaluating the incidence or treatment of CANV; therefore, most information on this subject has been derived from the human literature and clinical experience.

CLASSIFICATION OF CHEMOTHERAPY-ASSOCIATED NAUSEA AND VOMITING

CANV can be classified into three categories: acute, delayed, and anticipatory.[2-4] *Acute* vomiting is described as vomiting within 24 hours of receiving chemotherapy; *delayed* is vomiting after the first 24 hours of receiving chemotherapy; and *anticipatory* is a conditioned response to previous vomiting, either acute or delayed, in response to chemotherapy.[2-4] Chemotherapy-associated vomiting is drug and patient dependent. Whereas anticipatory vomiting is rarely encountered, delayed vomiting is most common in veterinary patients.

MECHANISMS OF CHEMOTHERAPY-ASSOCIATED NAUSEA AND VOMITING

Vomiting is mediated through the vomiting center located in the reticular formation of the medulla oblongata. The vomiting center receives stimulatory input from various afferent pathways, including the cerebral cortex, the chemoreceptor trigger zone (CRTZ), the vestibular apparatus, and vagal or sympathetic stimulation from peripheral sensory receptors such as those located within the abdominal viscera, including the GI tract.[5,6] The CRTZ is located in the area postrema of the medulla, where the blood–brain barrier is less effective and is thus able to detect toxins in the blood and CSF.[5,7] The CRTZ stimulates the vomiting center by releasing neurotransmitters. Neurotransmitters involved in emesis include serotonin ($5\text{-}HT_3$), substance P, dopamine, histamine, and enkephalins, among others. In addition to stimulation of the CRTZ, chemotherapeutic agents may stimulate the vomiting center via vagal afferents caused by release of serotonin from the enterochromaffin cells within the GI tract wall.[3] Serotonin has been implicated as a primary mediator of acute phase CANV but does not appear to be as important in the delayed phase of CANV,[8] whereas substance P may play more of a role in delayed CANV.[4,8]

PHARMACOLOGY OF CHEMOTHERAPY-ASSOCIATED NAUSEA AND VOMITING

Serotonin Receptor Antagonists

Although there are several generations of 5-HT$_3$ receptor antagonists, those most commonly used in veterinary medicine include dolasetron (Anzemet) and ondansetron (Zofran). These agents bind to both the 5-HT$_3$ receptors located peripherally on the afferent vagal neurons of the GI tract as well as those located in the CRTZ. Metoclopramide has also been shown to be a weak antagonist of peripheral 5-HT$_3$ receptors at high doses.[3]

Neurokinin-1 Receptor Antagonists

Neurokinin-1 (NK-1) receptor antagonists inhibit the binding of substance P to NK-1 receptors in the vomiting center, perhaps inhibiting both peripherally and centrally mediated vomiting. An NK-1 receptor antagonist, maropitant (Cerenia, Pfizer Animal Health, New York), was approved in 2007 for use in dogs as a general antiemetic. A recent study has shown maropitant to be more effective than metoclopramide when treating vomiting of various causes.[9] Maropitant was also found to be effective at preventing and controlling emesis associated with cisplatin administration when compared with placebo.[10,11]

Dopamine Receptor Antagonists

Dopamine receptor antagonists also have some anti-emetic activity by inhibiting stimulation of the emetic center by the CRTZ. Metoclopramide is the most frequently used antidopaminergic agent. Another class of frequently used antidopaminergic agents is the phenothiazines, including prochlorperazine (Compazine) and chlorpromazine (Thorazine). These agents may also have antihistaminic and weak anticholinergic effects that also contribute to their function as anti-emetics. The efficacy of dopamine receptor antagonists in treating CANV is limited at best.

Opiates

Opiate receptors are found in abundance in the CRTZ; although some narcotic agents can induce emesis, others have anti-emetic properties. Butorphanol significantly reduces the emetogenesis associated with cisplatin[12] and streptozocin[13] administration in dogs. One side effect to note with butorphanol is the sedative effect associated with its use.

Histamine Receptor Antagonists

Histamine receptors are also found in abundance within the CRTZ; however, the H$_2$ receptor antagonists such as cimetidine, ranitidine, and famotidine are not effective as anti-emetic agents. Diphenhydramine and other H$_1$ receptor antagonists also have not been shown to be helpful for CANV.[3]

USE OF ANTI-EMETIC AGENTS IN THE ONCOLOGY PATIENT

For those agents that are highly emetogenic and likely to cause acute CANV (cisplatin and streptozocin) pretreatment anti-emetic agents such as butorphanol or maropitant, are a necessity. Butorphanol has been effective when given subcutaneously 20 minutes before cisplatin administration,[12] as has maropitant when given subcutaneously 1 hour before cisplatin administration.[10] No standard protocols exist for treatment of delayed CANV; however, using agents such as ondansetron or maropitant as necessary for symptomatic care is reasonable. In addition, for patients that have experienced delayed CANV with previous chemotherapy doses, pre-treatment with an antiemetic as well as dispensing an oral formulation (available for ondansetron and maropitant) for at-home use to control CANV is recommended (see Table 18-1 for anti-emetic agents used in veterinary medicine).

SPECIES VARIATIONS

Species variations important to the management of veterinary patients should be noted. Rather than vomiting, cats tend to have more nausea and anorexia associated with treatment. Although metoclopramide may be used in felines, it can cause excitement. More often, steroids or cyproheptadine (an antiserotonergic agent) may be used as appetite stimulants and a transdermal formulation of cyproheptadine is available to avoid the added stress of pilling cats.

SUMMARY

Because of the multifactorial nature of CANV and inter-patient and species variations, it is important to consider anti-emetic agents associated with each individual situation. Pre-emptive attempts at controlling nausea and vomiting will help decrease both acute and delayed CANV and help improve the QOL of our patients while undergoing treatment. It will also prevent undesirable delays and dose reductions, ultimately decreasing the efficacy of our chemotherapy protocols.

TABLE 18-1   ANTI-EMETIC AGENTS USED IN VETERINARY MEDICINE

Drug	Trade Name	Mechanism of Action	Dose	Route	Frequency
Metoclopramide	Reglan	Dopamine antagonist	K9: 0.1–0.4 mg/kg	PO, SQ, IM	q6–8h
		Weak peripheral 5-HT$_3$ antagonist	1–2 mg/kg/day	IV CRI	
			Fe: 0.2–0.4 mg/kg	PO, SQ	q6–8h
			1–2 mg/kg/day	IV CRI	
Dolasetron	Anzemet	5-HT$_3$ antagonist	K9: 0.5–0.6 mg/kg	PO, SQ, IV	q24h
			Fe: 0.6 mg/kg	IV	q24h
Ondansetron	Zofran	5-HT$_3$ antagonist	K9: 0.1–1.0 mg/kg	PO, IM	q12–24h
			0.11–0.22 mg/kg	IV	
			Fe: 0.1–0.15 mg/kg	IV	q6–12h
Maropitant	Cerenia	NK-1 receptor antagonist	K9: 1.0. mg/kg	SQ	q24h (max 5 d) or 1 hr before cisplatin administration
			2 mg/kg	PO	q24h (max 5 d)
Prochlorperazine	Compazine	Dopamine antagonist	K9: 0.1–0.5 mg/kg	IM, SQ	q8h
		Histamine antagonist Anticholinergic	Fe: 0.1–0.5 mg/kg	IM, SQ	q8h
Chlorpromazine	Thorazine	Dopamine antagonist	K9: 0.1–0.5 mg/kg	IM, SQ	q6–8h
		Histamine antagonist Anticholinergic	Fe: 0.22–0.5 mg/kg	IM, SQ	q6–8h
Butorphanol	Torbugesic	Opiate antagonist	K9: 0.4 mg/kg	IM, SQ	20 min before cisplatin or immediately after streptozotocin administration

5-HT$_3$, 5-hydroxytryptamine (serotonin); K9, canine; PO, per os; SQ, subcutaneous; IM, intramuscular; IV, intravenous; CRI, continuous rate infusion; Fe, feline; NK-1, neurokinin-1.

Selected References*

Puente-Redondo VA, Siedek EM, Benchaoui HA, et al: The antiemetic efficacy of maropitant (Cerenia™) in the treatment of ongoing emesis caused by a wide range of underlying clinical aetiologies in canine patients in Europe, *J Small Anim Pract* 48(2):93, 2007.
Prospective study evaluating the efficacy of the NK-1 receptor antagonist, maropitant, for vomiting induced by multiple causes.
Vail DM, Rodabaugh HS, Conder GA, et al: Efficacy of injectable maropitant (Cerenia) in a randomized clinical trial for prevention and treatment of cisplatin-induced emesis in dogs presented as veterinary patients, *Vet Comp Oncol* 5(1):38, 2007.

Prospective study evaluating the efficacy of maropitant as an antiemetic in cisplatin-treated dogs.
Washabau RJ, Elie MS: Antiemetic therapy, In Bonagura JD (ed): *Kirk's current veterinary therapy XII: small animal practice*, Philadelphia, 1995, WB Saunders, p 679.
In-depth review of the physiology of vomiting and pharmacology of anti-emetic agents available in 1995.

■ *For a complete list of the references cited in this chapter, please go to www.smallanimaloncology.com.

SECTION B: Nutritional Management of the Cancer Patient

S. Dru Forrester, Philip Roudebush, and Deborah J. Davenport

KEY POINTS

- Nutritional management is an important component of cancer care that may affect quality of life and survival time.
- One therapeutic food containing increased amounts of omega-3 fatty acids and the amino acid arginine has been shown to improve survival and quality of life in dogs with cancer.
- To lessen the likelihood of side effects (e.g., diarrhea), it is critical to gradually (over 10–14 days) transition to therapeutic foods formulated for cancer patients.
- If feeding a therapeutic food is not possible, it is important to facilitate caloric intake and maintain body condition by feeding a complete and balanced food that the patient will eat.
- Nutritional recommendations for overweight or obese cancer patients may need to be adjusted, especially if there are concomitant conditions (e.g., increased risk for pancreatitis, arthritis).
- Many supplements have been suggested for cancer patients; however, most have not been critically evaluated in dogs or cats.

Nutritional management can improve quality and quantity of life for cancer patients. Many owners understand the importance of nutrition in cancer patients and are willing to implement nutritional recommendations that can potentially increase the quality of their pet's life. This chapter reviews metabolic consequences of cancer, evidence supporting nutritional intervention in dogs and cats with cancer, and guidelines for implementing nutritional management.

NUTRITIONAL CONSEQUENCES OF CANCER AND CANCER TREATMENT

Weight loss and decreased body condition may occur in cancer patients as a result of tumor location (e.g., oral masses), cancer cachexia, or complications of cancer treatment (e.g., decreased appetite caused by chemotherapy). Cancer cachexia is a paraneoplastic syndrome characterized by progressive weight loss and decreased body condition, despite adequate nutritional intake. It is not known how many dogs and cats with cancer suffer from cachexia. In a study of dogs presented to a veterinary oncology service, only 4% exhibited cachexia, defined as thin body condition, whereas 29% were markedly overweight.[1] However, 15% had clinically relevant muscle wasting, and 68% had lost weight compared with their body weight before cancer was diagnosed. In the same study, dogs with hematopoietic neoplasia (e.g., lymphoma) were significantly more likely to lose more weight compared with dogs with solid tumors. Human patients with cancer cachexia respond less favorably to treatment and have decreased survival time compared with patients that have not lost weight.[2-6] Cachexia also has negative effects on quality of life in human cancer patients.[2,3] It seems reasonable that similar consequences occur in veterinary cancer patients; however, this has not been critically evaluated.

METABOLIC ALTERATIONS IN CANCER PATIENTS

Dogs with lymphoma and other malignant diseases have significant alterations in carbohydrate metabolism; these alterations occur because tumors preferentially metabolize glucose (carbohydrates) for energy, forming lactate as an end product.[7-12] Dogs with cancer must then expend energy to convert lactate back to glucose, resulting in a net energy gain by the tumor and net energy loss by the patient. Following intravenous administration of glucose, dogs with cancer have increased blood lactate and insulin concentrations, which persists after successful treatment with chemotherapy or surgery.[10,13] In addition, administration of lactate-containing fluids increases blood lactate concentrations in dogs with lymphoma; these findings are the basis for recommending avoidance of glucose- or lactate-containing fluids in dogs with cancer.[11]

In addition to altered carbohydrate metabolism, cancer patients have altered protein and fat metabolism. In one study, cancer-bearing dogs had significantly lower plasma concentrations of several amino acids (e.g., arginine); these alterations in plasma amino acid profiles did not normalize after tumors were removed surgically.[14] Altered lipid profiles have also been reported in dogs with lymphoma.[9] Decreased fat synthesis or increased lipolysis can deplete fat stores and contribute to cachexia; several cytokines (e.g., tumor necrosis factor alpha) produced in cancer patients appear responsible for altered lipid metabolism and may contribute to cachexia.

THE IDEAL NUTRITIONAL PROFILE FOR PATIENTS WITH CANCER

Nutritional management is an important component of multi-modality therapy of dogs and cats with cancer and should be given equal consideration when planning treatment (chemotherapy, radiotherapy, surgery, and pain management). Providing appropriate nutrition may improve QOL, enhance effectiveness of cancer treatment, and increase survival time. Pending further studies in cats, therapeutic principles for feline patients with cancer should follow those for people and dogs with cancer. Key nutritional factors in dogs and cats with cancer include soluble carbohydrate, fiber, protein, arginine, fat, and omega-3 fatty acids (Table 18-2). It is also critical to supply the pet's energy needs (i.e., calories) to maintain ideal body condition.

Soluble Carbohydrate and Fiber

Most adult, non-producing dogs and cats do not require soluble carbohydrates; however, pet food manufacturers include ingredients with soluble carbohydrates because they are good energy sources and their unique properties aid in manufacturing processes. Soluble carbohydrates may be poorly used by pets with cancer and can contribute to increased lactate production. For this reason, it is recommended that soluble carbohydrates comprise <25% of food on a dry matter basis (Table 18-2). Soluble (fermentable) and insoluble (poorly fermentable) fiber sources may help maintain intestinal health, especially in pets undergoing cancer treatment. Increased dietary fiber may help manage abnormal stool quality or diarrhea, which may occur when changing from high-carbohydrate, dry foods to high-fat commercial or homemade foods.

Protein and Arginine

Dietary protein should be highly digestible and exceed maintenance levels for adult dogs and cats because patients with cancer have altered protein metabolism and may suffer loss of lean muscle mass (Table 18-2). Arginine is an essential amino acid that may have specific therapeutic value in pets with cancer. Adding arginine to parenteral solutions decreased tumor growth and metastatic rates in rodent cancer models.[15,16] Increased dietary arginine in conjunction with increased dietary omega-3 fatty acid intake improved clinical signs, QOL, and survival time in dogs treated for cancer.[17,18] The minimal effective level of dietary arginine for pets with cancer is

unknown; however, the positive correlation between plasma arginine concentrations and survival in dogs with lymphoma suggests it should be >2.5% arginine on a dry matter basis.

Fat and Omega-3 Fatty Acids

Some tumor cells have difficulty using lipids as a fuel source, whereas host tissues can use lipids for energy. This finding led to the hypothesis that foods relatively high in fat may benefit pets with cancer compared with foods relatively high in carbohydrates. In North America, pets receive most of their nutrient intake from commercial dry pet foods; these foods are usually high in soluble carbohydrate (25%–60%) and relatively low in fat (7%–25%). These characteristics make most of these foods inappropriate for nutritional management of dogs with cancer; this may also be true for cats, although it has not been evaluated (see Table 18-2).

Omega-3 fatty acids, especially those found in certain types of fish and fish oil (eicosapentaenoic acid [EPA], docosahexaenoic acid [DHA]), are probably the most important to consider for pets with cancer. Fish oil and EPA/DHA supplementation have many beneficial effects, including inhibition of lipolysis and muscle protein degradation associated with cachexia. Several human epidemiologic studies have suggested that consumption of fish or higher levels of omega-3 fatty acids protect against certain types of cancer. The recommendation for feeding high levels of omega-3 fatty acids such as EPA and DHA to pets with cancer is based on *in vitro* cell culture studies, extensive studies in rodent cancer models, clinical trials in human patients with severe forms of cancer, and clinical trials in dogs treated for lymphoma and nasal tumors.[19]

Antioxidants

Use of antioxidants in cancer patients is somewhat controversial. Some believe that supplementation with high-dose dietary antioxidants such as vitamin E may improve effectiveness of cancer therapy by enhancing immune function, increasing tumor response to radiation or chemotherapy, decreasing toxicity to normal cells, and helping reverse metabolic changes contributing to cachexia. Others believe that dietary antioxidants may protect cancer cells against damage by chemotherapy or radiation therapy. At present, megadose vitamin therapy does not appear indicated if pets are fed a complete and balanced commercial food. Instead, levels of vitamin E and other antioxidant nutrients should be appropriate for the level of polyunsaturated fatty acids, trace minerals, and oxidants in the food.

TABLE 18-2   KEY NUTRITIONAL FACTORS FOR DOGS AND CATS WITH CANCER AND LEVELS IN SELECTED COMMERCIAL FOODS*

	Protein	Soluble Carbohydrate	Fat	Omega-3 Fatty Acids	Arginine	Crude Fiber
Recommended levels for dogs with cancer	30–45	<25	25–40	>5	>2.5	>2.5
Recommended levels for cats with cancer	40–50	<25	25–40	2-3	>2.5	>2.5
Products						
Hill's Prescription Diet n/d Canine, moist	38	20	33.2	7.3	2.95	2.7
Hill's Prescription Diet a/d Canine/Feline, moist	44.2	15.4	30.4	2.6	2.4	1.3
Hill's Prescription Diet p/d Feline, moist (Canada)	49	16.2	24	1	2.3	2.8
Hill's Prescription Diet p/d Feline, dry (Canada)	39	24	29	1.1	2.2	1.3
Hill's Science Diet Puppy Healthy Development Savory Chicken Entrée	28.2	39.2	23.6	0.4	1.8	1.3
Hill's Science Diet Kitten Healthy Development Liver & Chicken Entrée	49	16	24	1	2.3	2.8
Hill's Prescription Diet m/d Feline, dry	52	14.7	22	0.23	2.64	5.9
Hill's Prescription Diet m/d Feline, moist	53	15.7	19.4	0.3	3.2	6.0
Iams Eukanuba Maximum Calorie/Canine & Feline, moist	42	12	37	0.22 (minimum)	NA	0.5
Purina CV Feline Formula, moist	42.5	23	27	NA	NA	1
Purina DM Feline Formula, dry	58	15	18	0.39	3.57	1.3
Purina DM Feline Formula, moist	57	8.1	24	0.88	NA	3.7
Royal Canin Veterinary Diet Canine and Feline Recovery RS	53.4	2.3	33.4	NA	5.9 g/1000 kcal	3.4
Dry grocery brand dog foods (average)[†]	25.3	52.2	12.3	<1	<2	3.1
Dry specialty brand dog foods (average) [†]	28.1	45.1	16.3	<1	<2	3.3
Moist grocery brand dog foods (average) [†]	41.2	19.9	27.1	<1	<2	1.8
Dry grocery brand cat foods (average) [†]	34.8	43.9	12.3	<1	<2	2.2
Dry specialty brand cat foods (average) [†]	35.3	37.4	18.5	<1	<2	2.4
Moist grocery brand cat foods (average) [†]	51.2	9.7	26.6	<1	<2	1.5

NA, Information not available from manufacturer

*Nutrients expressed on a percent dry matter basis unless otherwise indicated. Values obtained from manufacturers' published information.

[†]Data from Debraekeleer J: Nutrient profiles of commercial dog and cat foods (Appendix L). In Hand MS, Thatcher CD, Remillard RL. et al (eds): *Small animal clinical nutrition,* ed 4, Topeka, 2000, Mark Morris Institute, pp 1073-1083.

EVIDENCE SUPPORTING NUTRITIONAL MANAGEMENT OF CANCER PATIENTS

Several well-controlled clinical trials have evaluated a high-fat, low-carbohydrate, arginine- and fish oil–supplemented therapeutic food (Prescription Diet n/d Canine, Hill's Pet Nutrition, Inc.) in dogs undergoing single-agent chemotherapy for lymphoma with doxorubicin or radiation therapy for nasal tumors.[17,18,20] Dogs fed the therapeutic food had higher serum concentrations of omega-3 fatty acids and arginine compared with dogs fed the unsupplemented control food. Higher concentrations of EPA and DHA were associated with lower plasma lactic acid responses and longer disease-free interval and median survival time in dogs with Stage III lymphoma.[18] In one study, improved QOL was noted in dogs with lymphoma fed the fish oil and arginine supplemented food.[20] Additional beneficial effects (i.e., lower tissue concentrations of inflammatory mediators, improved performance scores, and less histologic damage to normal tissues from radiation therapy) were observed in dogs undergoing radiation therapy for nasal tumors when fed the fish oil and arginine–supplemented food.[17] It is expected that similar clinical responses would occur in patients with a wide range of cancer types; however, this has not been reported.

FORMULATING A NUTRITIONAL PLAN FOR CANCER PATIENTS

The goals of nutritional management of cancer patients are to provide adequate nutrients to facilitate recovery, minimize metabolic consequences of cancer, and maintain lean body mass. Before establishing and implementing a nutritional plan for cancer patients, it is helpful to remember these goals, which help guide patient assessment and monitoring, nutritional recommendations, and education of pet owners.

Patient Assessment

A thorough dietary history should be obtained prior to initial management of cancer patients. This should include detailed information about current foods (brands, quantity, and frequency) and any over-the-counter supplements. Physical examination should include weighing the patient and determining body condition. Body condition can be assessed by assigning a score ranging from 1 to 5 (1 = very thin, 3 = ideal body condition, 5 = grossly obese).[21] This is a more objective method for determining fat stores and body composition. A body condition score should be determined and recorded in the patient's medical record along with body weight as a routine part of the physical examination at each visit. This allows for detecting changes in body condition over time, which is important in cancer patients.

Selecting a Food

Selecting the appropriate food for management of cancer patients should include consideration of owner/pet preferences, body condition, and presence of concurrent diseases. Foods prepared by a reputable manufacturer and tested in feeding trials are preferred over homemade foods because they are more likely to provide complete and balanced nutrition, are more readily available, and are convenient to use. When owners are interested in preparing homemade foods, veterinarians should consult a clinical nutritionist or additional resources to assist with creating a nutritionally balanced food.[22] Based on current evidence, the authors believe that bones and raw food (BARF) diets should not be fed because cancer patients are immunocompromised and are at risk for septicemia as a result of bacterial contamination.[23,24] Body condition and presence of concurrent disorders must also be considered when selecting a food. Foods formulated for cancer patients are relatively high in fat, which is appropriate for dogs and cats that are underweight or in good body condition. However, they may not be ideal for overweight or obese patients, particularly if there are concomitant conditions such as pancreatitis, hyperlipidemia, osteoarthritis, or anticipated need for amputation of a limb (e.g., osteosarcoma). When managing patients with multiple problems, it may be helpful to consult with a clinical nutritionist for advice.

Several commercially available foods provide key nutrients in appropriate levels for cancer patients (Table 18-2). One food (Prescription Diet n/d Canine) has been shown to improve lifespan and QOL in selected canine patients with cancer.[18,25] Similar foods are recommended in cats with cancer, although no studies have been done to evaluate their effects. When changing to a food with increased fat, it is critical to gradually transition (over a period of 10–14 days) to the new food in order to avoid complications. Sudden introduction of a food containing relatively higher amounts of fat may cause unacceptable side effects (e.g., refusal to eat the new food, loose stools or severe diarrhea), causing pet owners to abandon a potentially beneficial treatment. It may also be helpful to divide the daily food amount and give three to six small meals per day during the initial feeding of the new food. In patients that will not eat a recommended therapeutic food, it is reasonable to try a different food. When owners are not willing or able to purchase a therapeutic food formulated for cancer patients, it is important to maintain caloric intake and body condition by offering a complete and balanced food that the patient will eat.

Using Supplements

Some owners may ask about adding supplements to their pet's regular food in an attempt to improve effectiveness of treatment or save money. Although many supplements and nutraceuticals have been suggested for cancer patients, only the combination of fish oil and arginine in a therapeutic food has been shown to have a significant effect in dogs.[19] In general, use of therapeutic foods formulated to aid in nutritional management of dogs with cancer is preferable to supplementing typical pet foods (e.g., with fish oil and arginine). To achieve levels of omega-3 fatty acids shown to be effective, typical pet foods need to be supplemented with 12 to 20 fish oil capsules per day for a 10-kg dog; this is not practical for most pet owners and is more expensive than using a therapeutic food.

Determining Amount to Feed

Most commercial foods are formulated to be nutritionally complete and balanced when fed to meet a pet's caloric needs (please see the form at www.smallanimaloncology. com. to determine caloric needs). Feeding instructions provided by the manufacturer can be used as an initial guide; these instructions usually give a recommended range for amount to feed. It is important to keep in mind that this is a starting point only and that some pets may need more or less food to maintain ideal body condition.

Feeding Methods

For most cancer patients, voluntary oral intake is appropriate if the amount of food consumed maintains ideal body condition. Pet owners should carefully monitor amount of food offered and amount consumed so that adjustments can be made as needed. If patients are not consuming adequate amounts of food, additional strategies (e.g., using highly palatable and caloric dense foods, hand-feeding, warming the food, giving multiple smaller meals per day, syringe-feeding) should be implemented. Appetite stimulants such as cyproheptadine (2–4 mg/cat PO q12–24h, 5–20 mg/dog PO q12–24h), diazepam (1 mg/cat PO q24h, 0.1–0.2 mg/kg PO q12–24h in dogs), and oxazepam (1.25–2.5 mg/cat PO q12–24h, 0.3–0.4 mg/kg PO q12–24h in dogs) can be attempted, although there is little evidence to support their effectiveness. Mirtazapine (0.6 mg/kg PO once daily, with a daily maximum of 30 mg for dogs; 3–4 mg/cat PO q3days) is a newer drug that shows promise for the treatment of anorexia in dogs and cats.[26]

TABLE 18-3   FEEDING GUIDELINES FOR AVAILABLE LIQUID DIETS—HILL'S PRESCRIPTION DIET A/D CANINE/FELINE

Body Weight (LB)	Guideline (ML/DAY)
5	140
8	200
10	236
20	397
30	538
40	668
50	789
60	905
70	1016
80	1123
90	1227
100	1327

This food intended for intermittent or supplemental feeding only. The above daily intakes are intended as a guide and should be adjusted as needed to achieve or maintain body weight. Divide a 5.5-oz can into three to six equal daily feedings to minimize gastrointestinal side effects (1 can = 150 ml).

For patients in whom normal gastrointestinal function has been compromised by anorexia, a 3-day transitional feeding strategy may be necessary:

Day One: 1/3 of daily caloric intake with 2/3 water dilution.
Day Two: 2/3 of daily caloric intake with 1/3 water dilution.
Day Three: Entire daily caloric intake.
Consult the company product guide or website for additional information.

Assisted feeding is indicated if inadequate nutritional intake persists for more than 3 to 5 days or if patients have lost 10% of their body weight in a 1- to 2-week period.[27,28] Enteral feeding is preferred because it provides adequate nutrition in a simple and cost-effective manner; it also supports enterocyte health and helps maintain intestinal immune function. Parenteral-assisted feeding is indicated for patients with intractable vomiting or severe gastrointestinal disease (e.g., intestinal lymphoma). Consult additional resources for information on use of feeding tubes and formulating a nutritional plan for enteral and parenteral feeding.[27-30] Tables 18-3 and 18-4 provide information regarding the amount of commercially available liquid diet to feed.

Side Effects Associated with Foods for Cancer Patients

It has been noted by one of the authors (DJD) that approximately 10% of dogs with cancer develop soft stools or diarrhea when initially fed a high-fat canned food in conjunction with other cancer therapy. Of

TABLE 18-4   FEEDING GUIDELINES FOR AVAILABLE LIQUID DIETS—IAMS VETERINARY FORMULA MAXIMUM-CALORIE/CANINE & FELINE

	Weight (LB)	Maintenance (CANS/DAY)	Weight Gain (CANS/DAY)
Dogs	3–10	⅓–¾	¾–1⅔
	10–20	¾–1¼	1⅔–2½
	20–30	1¼–1⅔	2½–3⅓
	30–40	1⅔–2	3⅓–4
	40–60	2–2⅔	4–5⅓
	60–80	2⅔–3¼	5⅓–6½
	80–100	3¼–3¾	6½–7⅔
Cats	4	¼–⅓	½
	8	½–¾	¾–1
	12	¾–1¼	1⅓–1⅔
	16	1–1½	1¾–2¼
	22	1½–2	2⅓–3

These guideline amounts are a starting point, and individual patients may need more food depending upon age, activity, and temperament. In order to reach an optimal body condition, you may need to adjust food intake. The chart represents the total recommended volume of food per day. You should divide the total recommended volume by the number of times the patient will be fed per day to get the actual portion size per feeding. Consult the company product guide or website for additional information.

TABLE 18-5   USING INCREASED FIBER TO IMPROVE STOOL QUALITY IN CANCER PATIENTS EATING HIGH-FAT FOODS

Substance	Instructions/Dose
Psyllium (Metamucil, Procter & Gamble)	1 tsp/5–10 kg body weight with each meal
High-Fiber Cereals Post 100% Bran (28% fiber) Kellogg's All-Bran (50% fiber) General Mills Fiber One (43% fiber)	Mix ½–1 cup of cereal/can of food
High-Fiber Foods Hill's Prescription Diet, Canine r/d, dry Hill's Prescription Diet, Canine w/d, dry Royal Canin Veterinary Diet Calorie Control CC 29 High Fiber, dry	Replace 10% of total daily calories with the high-fiber food and mix the dry kibble with the canned food at each meal

these dogs, about half will adjust to the dietary change and develop normal stool consistency, and the other half (about 5% of total cases) continue to have stool consistency issues that pet owners find unacceptable. Abnormal stool quality can be minimized by gradually changing from commercial dry foods to higher fat moist foods over 10 to 14 days. Increasing dietary fiber may also be very helpful (Table 18-5).

Other potential adverse effects of fish oil supplementation include platelet dysfunction, pancreatitis, fishy breath odor, and nutrient interactions (e.g., need for additional vitamin E in the food). Although high levels of dietary omega-3 fatty acids can alter platelet function, studies in normal dogs and dogs with cancer have not shown this.[31,32] One study failed to detect significant changes in platelet aggregation or mucosal bleeding time in normal cats supplemented with EPA and DHA; however, two other studies revealed decreased platelet aggregation and increased toenail or mucosal bleeding time in normal cats fed omega-3 fatty acid–enriched foods.[33-35] Because of potential for bleeding problems, cats with cancer should be given foods with lower levels of fish oil or omega-3 fatty acids than dogs (Table 18-2).

Reassessment

After implementing nutritional management, cancer patients should be reassessed periodically for changes in nutritional status, which may impact quality and quantity of life and dictate need for changes in the nutritional plan. This can be accomplished during routine visits for evaluation of response to other cancer treatments (e.g., monitoring complete blood counts during chemotherapy) or more frequently as needed. Pet owners should again be asked about food and supplements offered and amounts consumed. Body weight and body condition score should be determined at each visit so trends can be detected over time and adjustments made as needed.

Selected References*

Marks SL: Nasoesophageal, esophagostomy, and gastrostomy tube placement techniques, In Ettinger SJ, Feldman EC, (eds): *Textbook of veterinary internal medicine*, ed 6, St Louis, 2005, Saunders/Elsevier, pp 329-336.
Brief description of common techniques for placement of enteral feeding tubes in dogs and cats.
Mauldin GE: Nutritional support of the cancer patient. In Bonagura JD (ed): *Kirk's current veterinary therapy (small animal practice) XIII*, Philadelphia, 2000, WB Saunders, pp 458-462.

Techniques for meeting nutritional needs of small animal patients with cancer.

Ogilvie GK: Alterations in metabolism and nutritional support for veterinary cancer patients: recent advances, *Compend Contin Educ Pract Vet* 15:925, 1993.
Review of metabolic abnormalities in cancer patients and effect on nutritional recommendations.

Ogilvie GK, Marks SL: Cancer. In Hand MS, Thatcher CD, Remillard RL, et al(eds): *Small animal clinical nutrition*, Topeka, 2000, Mark Morris Institute, pp 887-905.
Review of nutritional effects of cancer and key nutritional factors for cancer patients.

Remillard RL, Armstrong PJ, Davenport DJ: Assisted feeding in hospitalized patients: enteral and parenteral nutrition. In Hand MS, Thatcher CD, Remillard RL, et al(eds): *Small animal clinical nutrition*, Topeka, 2000, Mark Morris Institute, pp 351-399.
Recommendations for assisted feeding of dogs and cats.

Remillard RL, Paragon BM, Crane SW, et al: Making pet foods at home. In Hand MS, Thatcher CD, Remillard RL, et al (eds): *Small animal clinical nutrition*, Topeka, 2000, Mark Morris Institute, pp 163-181.
Recommendations for formulating homemade foods for dogs and cats.

Roudebush P, Davenport DJ, Novotny BJ: The use of nutraceuticals in cancer therapy, *Vet Clin North Am (Sm Anim Pract)* 34:249, 2004.
Review of metabolic alterations in cancer patients and effects of using functional foods for nutritional management.

Thatcher CD, Hand MS, Remillard RL: Small animal clinical nutrition: an interactive process, In Hand MS, Thatcher CD, Remillard RL, et al (ed): *Small animal clinical nutrition*, Topeka, 2000, Mark Morris Institute, pp 1-19.
Basic review of evaluating nutrient content of pet foods and making appropriate nutritional recommendations for patients.

■ *For a complete list of the references cited in this chapter, please go to www.smallanimaloncology.com.

SECTION C: Assessment and Management of Pain in the Cancer Patient

Louis-Philippe de Lorimier and Timothy M. Fan

KEY POINTS

- Pain is common in cancer-bearing pets and may be associated with the tumor, paraneoplastic syndromes, diagnostic or therapeutic procedures, or concurrent conditions.
- Chronic pain negatively impacts quality of life and important physiologic functions, and treating it is mandatory.
- Cancer pain is best treated by addressing the underlying tumor when possible, and by using a multimodal approach when moderate to severe.

Pain commonly accompanies cancer in humans, with an incidence of 30% to 90%, and more advanced disease correlates with increased frequency and intensity of pain.[1,2] Pain control should be a priority for clinicians, since pain negatively affects quality of life (QOL) and key physiologic functions. Over 70% of human patients with cancer pain are relieved with opiate-based regimens.[1,2] Such data do not currently exist for pets, but estimates suggest that over 50% of cancer-bearing dogs and cats may experience some degree of pain.

ASSESSING CANCER PAIN

Pain can be classified using various criteria such as the temporal aspect (acute, chronic, breakthrough), intensity (mild to excruciating), type (somatic, visceral, neuropathic), or cause (primary tumor, metastases, paraneoplastic syndrome, diagnostic or therapeutic procedures, concurrent conditions).[1,2] Arguably, the best way to classify pain may be to differentiate between physiologic pain (generally acute) and maladaptive pain (generally chronic). Early recognition and frequent reassessments are essential for adequate cancer pain management. Barriers preventing appropriate management of cancer pain are numerous and include poor recognition with many tumor types, difficulty assessing pain in pets, improper reassessment once therapy is implemented, fear of using or lack of knowledge regarding certain analgesic drugs, and suboptimal communication with owners.[3-6]

Owners know their pet the best and can identify abnormal behaviors as reliable signs that something is wrong. Believing owners who think their pet may be in pain and getting them involved in regular reassessment are important first steps in pain recognition.[3,4,6] As a general rule, if an animal seems to be in pain, it most likely is, and treating for pain and observing the improvement is a clinically useful way to confirm it.[7] Many physiologic parameters (pupil size, blood pressure, etc.) have been used as surrogate measures of pain in veterinary patients but are influenced by other factors and stressors in a clinical setting.[6] Close observation of behavior alterations (movement, posture, grooming, etc.) may provide a better estimate of the degree of pain experienced.[3,4,6] Objective methods of pain measurement exist and are useful in controlled studies, but their clinical application and usefulness in evaluating a patient with a given painful condition is debatable.[7] Various observer pain scales exist, but more crucial than the type of scale used is to have a system that is understood by all observers, easy to use, and repeatable.[3,4] The score must be noted for all patients initially and regularly reassessed during therapy.

Veterinary Cancers Causing Pain

Any tumor type can lead to pain (Table 18-6).[7] It may result from invasion and destruction of surrounding tissues by the primary tumor, including nerves and bones; from regional or distant metastasis to sites such as bone, body cavity, or meninges; from stretching the capsule of certain visceral organs or by causing flow obstruction.[7] Inflammation or secondary infection may also lead to pain at the tumor site, and certain paraneoplastic syndromes can be quite painful.

Pain from Diagnostic and Therapeutic Procedures

Invasive diagnostic or therapeutic procedures can result in pain. The spectrum of painful surgical procedures extends from incisional biopsies to aggressive *en bloc* excisional surgeries.[7] Appropriate preemptive multimodal analgesic protocols must be in place, in addition to standard, rather than "as needed," post-operative pain management.

Cytotoxic chemotherapy may lead to painful side effects such as constipation from vincristine (cats) and sterile hemorrhagic cystitis with cyclophosphamide.[7] Perivenous extravasation of vesicant drugs, including vincristine and doxorubicin, will result in painful tissue destruction sometimes severe enough to necessitate surgical debridement. Prevention is best, and clean-stick catheters should be placed in intact veins just prior to administering these vesicants.

Pain may result from the early side effects of radiation therapy, such as mucositis (mouth, intestine) and moist dermatitis observed with curative protocols (daily fractions for 3–4 weeks).[1,2,7] Preventing further self-trauma is critical. Oral rinse solutions can be used for stomatitis, a corticosteroid enema often will help for proctitis, and topical application of colloidal oatmeal, wheat extracts, and aloe gel may benefit pets with acute moist dermatitis.[7] Petroleum-based products must be avoided. Broad-spectrum antibiotics may benefit the patient with opportunistic infection. Pain may also accompany late side effects of radiation therapy,

months after completion. Computerized planning and dose distribution analysis help prevent side effects to normal tissues.

TREATING THE UNDERLYING CAUSE

The best way to alleviate cancer pain, when possible, is to treat the tumor. Occasionally, with resistant, refractory, recurring, or terminal cancers, only standard analgesic therapy can truly benefit the patient. Purely palliative therapy does not intend to alter the course of the disease. The goal is rather to control pain and improve the patient's overall QOL, through the use of traditional anticancer therapeutic modalities, various analgesic therapies, and supportive care. Surgical, chemotherapeutic, and radiation approaches to pain management are covered in chapters specific to those treatment modalities. The reader is also referred to Section D for more information on palliative care.

TRADITIONAL ANALGESIC THERAPY

A three-step analgesic ladder for treating cancer pain has been proposed by the World Health Organization (WHO).[1,2,3-6,8] Mild pain is treated initially with non-opiate drugs, generally non-steroidal anti-inflammatory drugs (NSAIDs). When pain persists, or with moderate pain, a "weak opiate" can be added. If still not controlled, or with severe pain, stronger opiates, preferably full mu agonists, are added on the final rung. Adjuvant analgesic drugs can be incorporated at any step. Further steps are added for human patients with painful advanced cancer with intrathecal administration of opiates, neurostimulation, or peripheral neuroablation as a fourth step, and central neuroablative procedures as a fifth step.[8] An inverted pyramid is used by others when chronic pain with central sensitization is suspected.[6] This refers to use of a multimodal approach first to reverse such changes, before gradually eliminating one drug at a time, as proper pain control is achieved.

Non-Steroidal Anti-Inflammatory Drugs (Table 18-7)

By far, NSAIDs are the drugs most often used to control various types of pain in pets. By inhibiting cyclooxygenases (COX), COX-2 being the main target with coxibs, NSAIDs are very helpful in the treatment of cancer pain. Prostaglandins play a key role in peripheral sensitization of nociceptors and may also lead to central sensitization and institution of a chronic pain state.[2,4] In humans, NSAIDs are effective for moderate to severe pain from bone metastases, compression of muscles and tendons, and carcinomatosis.[2] Anecdotally, cancer pain in pets also appears to respond to NSAIDs,

TABLE 18-6 VARIOUS TUMOR TYPES AND THE TYPE OF PAIN THAT MAY ACCOMPANY THEM

Tumor	Pain Severity	Comments
Bone sarcomas (primary)	Moderate to severe	Osteosarcoma is most common (80%), followed by other sarcomas. The vast majority are painful, from lytic and proliferative bone remodeling.
Joint tumors	Moderate to severe	Capsular stretching and bone invasion by primary joint tumors (synovial cell sarcoma, histiocytic sarcoma, etc.) or tumors invading joints (e.g., oral tumor invading TMJ) can be very painful.
Metastatic bone tumors	Moderate to severe	Primary carcinomas from mammary gland, prostate, anal sacs (apocrine glands), lungs, and bladder TCC. Spine (esp. lumbar) and long bones can be affected. Most are painful and typically are lytic, although metastasis from prostate is often proliferative. In cats, digit metastasis from pulmonary carcinoma is well reported.
Multiple myeloma	Moderate to severe	Common feature is purely osteolytic lesions (spine, long bones), with risk for pathologic fractures. Soft-tissue component or pathologic fracture can compress spinal cord and cause neuropathic pain.
Oral tumors	Mild to severe	Many cause bone destruction and soft-tissue inflammation. Most common in dogs are melanoma, SCC, and fibrosarcoma. In cats, SCC is most common (70%).
Nasal tumors	Mild to severe	Can cause considerable destruction and invasion of surrounding tissues leading to pain. See orbital and CNS pain.
Urinary tumors	Mild to severe	Pain can be from invasion of tissues and inflammation, spasms, urinary obstruction, or renal capsule stretching. Secondary infection common.
Prostate tumors	Mild to severe	Pain from similar causes as urinary tumors.
Vaginal tumors	Moderate to severe	Pain from similar causes as urinary tumors.
Mammary gland tumors	None to severe	Inflammatory carcinoma is very painful, causing pain in nearly 100% of cases. Lymphatic obstruction can be painful. Recently described in 3 cats, was extremely painful in all 3.
Carcinomatosis (pleural or peritoneal)	Moderate to severe	From various tumors (carcinomas, mesothelioma, sarcomas), diffuse body cavity pain from serosal involvement. Pleural pain can be very severe.
Mast cell tumors and other skin tumors	None to severe	Mast cell tumors especially painful when degranulation and peritumoral inflammation is present. Ulcerated and inflamed carcinomas can be painful.
Pancreatic carcinoma	Moderate to severe	Extremely painful in humans (invasion around nerves); pain likely an important component in veterinary equivalent.
Liver and splenic tumors	None to moderate	Capsular stretching, from primary or metastatic neoplasia, can lead to considerable visceral pain.
Orbital tumors	Moderate to severe	Can be primary orbital, or secondary from invasion by oral or sinonasal tumors. Can also cause pain upon opening the mouth.
Central nervous system	Moderate to severe	Can be primary CNS tumor, or involvement of the meninges and nerves by disseminated neoplasia (lymphoma, carcinomas, melanoma, sarcomas), or of cranial vault by sinonasal tumors. In humans with brain tumors, headaches are common.
Ear tumors	Mild to severe	Ear canal tumors can be painful, especially when secondary infection is present. Middle ear tumor, although uncommon, can be very painful with bone destruction and pain upon opening the mouth.
Brachial plexus tumor	Moderate to severe	Uncommon, but most often very painful from direct neuropathic and neurogenic pain.

CNS, Central nervous system; *SCC,* squamous cell carcinoma; *TCC,* transitional cell carcinoma; *TMJ,* temporomandibular joint.

TABLE 18-7   NSAIDS AND COX INHIBITORS USED IN DOGS AND CATS IN NORTH AMERICA

NSAID	Veterinary Product	Dosage Dog*	Dosage Cat†
Acetaminophen‡	No¶	10–15 mg/kg PO q8–12h	Toxic!
Aspirin	No¶	10 mg/kg PO q12h	10 mg/kg PO q48–72h
Carprofen	Rimadyl (Pfizer)	2.2 mg/kg PO bid *or* 4.0 mg/kg PO qd	1-2 mg/kg PO q3d
Deracoxib	Deramaxx (Novartis)	1–2 mg/kg PO qd	Not used
Etodolac	EtoGesic (Fort Dodge)	10-15 mg/kg PO qd	Not used
Firocoxib	Previcox (Merial)	5 mg/kg PO qd	Not used
Ketoprofen	Anafen (Merial)	1 mg/kg qd × 4–5 days	1 mg/kg PO qd × 3–5 days
Meloxicam	Metacam (Merial)	0.1 mg/kg PO qd; when chronic, use lowest effective dosage	0.025–0.1 mg/kg PO qd—not approved for chronic use; use lowest effective dosage
Piroxicam	No‡	0.3 mg/kg PO qd *or* q2d	0.3 mg/kg PO qd *or* q2d
Robenacoxib	Onsior§ (Novartis)	1–2 mg/kg PO qd; when chronic, use lowest effective dosage	1–2.4 mg/kg PO qd for up to 6 days
Tepoxalin	Zubrin (Schering-Plough)	10 mg/kg PO qd	5 mg/kg PO q12h × 3 days, then 4 days off
Tolfenamic acid	Tolfédine (Vétoquinol)	4 mg/kg PO qd × 4 days, 3 days off	4 mg/kg PO qd × 4 days, 3 days off

*Use the chronic dosage for cancer pain treatment; none is specifically approved for this use.

†Carprofen and tepoxalin are not approved for use in cats in North America, but their safe use has been described in that species.

‡No anti-inflammatory effect in humans; certain studies have demonstrated an anti-inflammatory effect in dogs.

¶Many manufacturers and generic drugs. The dosage listed here is what is considered "safe."

§Not yet available in North America as of this writing.

alone or in combination with opiates and adjuvant analgesics when pain is more severe. Veterinary approved NSAIDs appear equianalgesic for cancer pain. The clinical responses and toxicity profiles vary between patients for a given drug and are usually not predictable. If a patient fails to benefit from a given NSAID or suffers side effects, it is reasonable to try another drug, after a washout period of 4 to 7 days, although there are no established guidelines.[9]

Another motive to use NSAIDs, in addition to their analgesic effects, is their potential anticancer and chemopreventive effects in humans and pets. Overexpression of COX-2 is known to occur in many human and canine tumors, including many carcinomas, osteosarcoma, and malignant melanoma.[9] This permits immune evasion, decreased apoptosis, increased angiogenesis, and increased proliferation, all benefiting the cancer cells. Canine studies showed tumor responses with NSAIDs alone and additive effects when combined with chemotherapy.[9]

The past decade saw the approval of many veterinary NSAIDs (Table 18-7), to the benefit of our patients. In North America, these include deracoxib, firocoxib, carprofen, meloxicam, etodolac, tepoxalin, tolfenamic acid, and ketoprofen. Other NSAIDs occasionally used in pets include aspirin (mostly dogs), acetaminophen (dogs only), piroxicam, and ketorolac (IV, post-op only). Blood work and urinalysis to evaluate renal and liver function must be performed before chronic dosing with NSAIDs. Baseline values should be established, rechecked after 2 to 4 weeks, and then reassessed every 2 to 4 months thereafter. Owners should monitor for melena, vomiting, lethargy, altered water intake, and urine output. The most common side effects with NSAIDs and coxibs are gastrointestinal irritation, renal or liver toxicity, and antithrombotic effects (aspirin mainly).

The use of NSAIDs in cats is delicate, since species differences in the glucuronoconjugation pathways account for their longer half-life in cats when compared with dogs. Meloxicam, tolfenamic acid, ketoprofen, carprofen, and piroxicam have all been used in cats, and robenacoxib was recently approved for use in cats in Europe. A practical guideline for safe NSAID dosing in cats is to use the lowest effective dosage and to avoid their use when altered renal function is present. *Acetaminophen is extremely toxic to cats and should never be used in that species.*

Opiates (Table 18-8)

Opiates are the basis of effective cancer pain therapy in humans, and it should be no different in veterinary oncology.[1,2] Because there is no ceiling effect, dosages can be gradually and safely increased to offer the desired level of analgesia. Side effects are more frequent at higher dosages but are fairly predictable and tolerable, with the exception of the sporadic occurrence of dysphoria. Other side effects may include sedation, constipation, bradycardia, respiratory depression, panting, mydriasis (cats), cough suppression, altered laryngeal reflexes, vomiting, and histamine release (IV bolus of morphine).[1,2,4] Opiates are used for moderate to

TABLE 18-8   MAJOR OPIOIDS USED IN THE TREATMENT OF CANCER PAIN IN COMPANION ANIMALS

Opioid	Dosage Dog	Dosage Cat	Comments
Buprenorphine	0.01–0.03 mg/kg SC, IM, IV q4–8h	0.01–0.03 mg/kg SC, IM, IV q6–8h 0.02–0.05 mg/kg sublingual q6–12h *or* as needed for breakthrough pain	Moderate pain. Useful in cats (transmucosal) to control breakthrough pain.
Butorphanol	0.5–2.0 mg/kg PO q6–8h 0.2–0.8 mg/kg SC, IM, IV q2–4h		Kappa agonist, mu antagonist. For *mild pain only*. Sedation at high dose. Short duration of analgesia.
Codeine	0.5–2 mg/kg PO q6–8h	0.5–1.0 mg/kg PO q6–8h	Mild to moderate pain. Do not use the combination with acetaminophen in cats!
Fentanyl	Constant IV infusion: 0.002–0.01 mg/kg/h Transdermal: 25, 50, 75, or 100 µg/h Dosage: 2–5 µg/kg/h (cover part of 25 µg/h patch in small cats and very small dogs)		Moderate to severe pain. Sedation, nausea, respiratory depression, and bradycardia are possible. Transdermal absorption varies with patients. Change patch q3–4d.
Hydromorphone	0.05–0.2 mg/kg SC, IM, IV q2–4h		Moderate to severe pain. Less histamine release than with morphine. May cause emesis and dysphoria.
Methadone	0.5–2.0 mg/kg SC, IM q3–6h; 0.1 mg/kg IV	0.1–0.5 mg/kg SC, IM q–6h; 0.05–0.1 mg/kg IV	Mu receptor agonist. Also has noncompetitive antagonistic effect on NMDA receptors. Used more commonly in UK and Australia.
Morphine	0.2–2.0 mg/kg SC, IM; 0.05–0.4 mg/kg IV Slow-release tablets: 0.5–1.5 mg/kg PO q8h. Lower dosage at first, titrate up to effect.	0.05–0.2 mg/kg SC, IM Liquid: 0.2–0.5 mg/kg PO q6–8h	Moderate to severe pain. Sedation, respiratory depression, bradycardia, nausea, hypothermia, constipation, dysphoria at high dose in non-painful cats. Administer IV slowly to avoid histamine release.
Oxycodone	0.1–0.3 mg/kg q8–12h	Not used.	Moderate to severe pain. Mu receptor agonist. Risk of abuse in humans.
Tramadol	3–5 mg/kg PO q8–12h (starting dosage, can be titrated up)	2–5 mg/kg PO q12–24h	Mild to severe pain. Has mu receptor agonistic effect. Also serotonin and norepinephrine reuptake inhibition.

The analgesic effect of opiates is improved when combined with other agents (NSAID, alpha-2 agonists, sodium channel blockers, etc.).

severe pain and are potentiated when combined with NSAIDs.

The standard opiate is morphine, a pure mu receptor agonist. This inexpensive drug, with predictable and tolerable side effects, can be administered via various routes. Other pure mu agonists include fentanyl, hydromorphone, oxymorphone, and oxycodone, and they are equally useful for cancer pain. Buprenorphine, a longer-acting partial agonist, is very effective for breakthrough pain in cats via the transmucosal (oral) route.[10] Butorphanol, a mixed agonist/antagonist (kappa/mu), is inadequate for moderate to severe cancer pain.[2,8] With lower analgesic potency and short-lived analgesia (20–90 min) compared with that of sedation (hours), it may lead to a false sense of pain relief.[4,11] Methadone, a mu agonist also acting via antagonism of the *N*-methyl-D-aspartate (NMDA) receptors, is increasingly used to treat chronic cancer pain in humans.[1,2] Its use for the treatment of pain in companion animals is presently more common in Europe and Australia.

Weaker opiates are helpful for moderate cancer pain. In recent years, tramadol has become common use for chronic pain in humans and pets. A good analgesic for moderate cancer pain in humans, it has fewer side effects than equipotent true opiates.[2,10,12] Few reports exist on the efficacy of tramadol for treating pain in dogs or cats, but studies are ongoing. Recent PK/PD studies in dogs, along with growing anecdotal support of efficacy, suggest tramadol is safe and effective for many painful conditions in dogs.[13] Tramadol is a mu receptor agonist that also inhibits serotonin and norepinephrine reuptake. Combination with NSAIDs provides better analgesia.

Alpha-2 Agonists

Alpha-2 agonists are good analgesics, especially when combined with other analgesics such as opiates, ketamine, and lidocaine.[4] Medetomidine is commonly used to provide analgesia for moderately to severely painful procedures because of its well-known opiate-sparing effect. Alpha-2 agonists may cause bradycardia from increased vagal tone and are contraindicated in patients with a decreased cardiac output and increased afterload.[4] They may also cause transient hypertension. The use of medetomidine is generally safe in otherwise healthy geriatric cancer-bearing pets.[8]

Adjuvant Analgesic Drugs (Table 18-9)

Local anesthetics are very valuable and often used for local or regional blocks.[4] The oral, intravenous, or transdermal route can also be helpful in certain conditions. The use of sodium channel blockers (lidocaine, bupivacaine, mexiletine) helps provide good pain control and potentiates other analgesics, and it is becoming increasingly popular for the treatment of cancer pain in pets and humans.

NMDA antagonists are drugs such as ketamine, tiletamine, amantadine, and dextromethorphan. The NMDA receptor antagonistic effect of ketamine plays a key role in its central analgesic effect.[4] Ketamine has a sparing effect on opiates and is effective at a microdose in a continuous rate infusion, for intraoperative and postoperative analgesia, combined with fentanyl or morphine. Amantadine is an oral NMDA receptor antagonist first developed for its antiviral properties against human influenza. It is now often used for chronic cancer pain.[2,10] A placebo-controlled study on dogs with degenerative joint disease showed improved physical activity in dogs receiving an NSAID combined with oral amantadine when compared with those receiving the same NSAID and placebo.[14]

Anticonvulsants help in the treatment of neuropathic pain or chronic pain with central sensitization. Best described is gabapentin, a structural analogue of gamma-aminobutyric acid (GABA), providing analgesia through its effect on certain calcium channels in the CNS.[2,4,15] Well-tolerated, highly bioavailable, and rapidly metabolized in dogs, gabapentin works best with other analgesic agents, such as NSAIDs. Further studies with dogs and cats await.

Tricyclic antidepressants (TCAs), including amitriptyline and clomipramine, may provide pain relief for malignant and non-malignant chronic pain states.[16] Working best when combined with other classes of analgesics, TCAs act on endogenous monoaminergic pain modulating systems involving norepinephrine and serotonin.[1,2,4,6] Their use is still poorly described in dogs and cats.

Bisphosphonates are analogues of inorganic pyrophosphate. By concentrating at sites of active bone turnover and inhibiting osteoclasts, they are mostly used in the management of malignant bone pain.[1,2,17,18] Potent intravenous aminobisphosphonates such as pamidronate and zoledronate are preferred for osteolytic bone pain from metastatic carcinoma and multiple myeloma in humans, and studies evaluated their use in dogs and cats with primary and metastatic bone cancer.[17-21]

Corticosteroids have mild analgesic effects and are occasionally useful for cancer pain, especially if inflammation contributes to the ongoing nociceptive stimuli.[9] *They should never be used concurrently with NSAIDs.*

TABLE 18-9   ADJUVANT ANALGESIC DRUGS

Drug	Dosage Dog	Dosage Cat	Comments
Amantadine	3–5 mg/kg PO q24h		NMDA receptor antagonist. Most effective in combination with NSAID. GI side effects occasionally. Do not use with MAO inhibitor. Chronic pain.
Amitriptyline	1.0–1.5 mg/kg PO q12–24h	2.0–3.0 mg/kg PO q24h	Tricyclic antidepressants (TCAs). Potentiate analgesia. For mild to moderate chronic or neuropathic pain. Work best with an NSAID. Do not use with tramadol or SSRIs.
Clomipramine	1–3 mg/kg PO q24h	1–5 mg/kg PO q24h	
Dexamethasone	0.10–0.20 mg/kg SC, PO q24–48h		Corticosteroid. Occasionally useful for mild to moderate pain, especially if caused by inflammation or when CNS is involved.
Gabapentin	5–10 mg/kg PO q8–12h starting dosage (Note: some start with q24h at bedtime for 5–7 days, then increase frequency and dosage gradually)		Structural GABA agonist. Low dose initially, titrate up to effect. For chronic pain with central sensitization, or neuropathic pain. Most effective with an NSAID.
Imipramine	0.5–1.0 mg/kg PO q8h	2.5–5.0 mg/kg PO q12h	Tricyclic antidepressant (TCA). Potentiate analgesia. For mild to moderate chronic or neuropathic pain. Works best with an NSAID. Do not use with tramadol or SSRIs.
Ketamine	IV bolus of 0.5 mg/kg, then CRI at 0.3–1.0 mg/kg/h		NMDA receptor antagonist. Microdose infusion helps attenuate dysphoric effect of opioids post-operatively.
Lidocaine	IV bolus 2–4 mg/kg, followed by infusion at 0.02–0.05 mg/kg/min	IV bolus 1–2 mg/kg, followed by infusion at 0.01–0.04 mg/kg/min	Sodium channel blocker. Markedly decreases anesthetic and post-operative analgesic requirements. Lidocaine may be used transdermally (e.g., gel, EMLA).
Methocarbamol	10–40 mg/kg PO q8–12h		Muscle relaxant. Sedation is a side effect at higher dosages.
Mexiletine	4–10 mg/kg PO q12h	Not used	Sodium channel blocker. To potentiate analgesic effect of other drugs. Adjuvant use for neuropathic pain.
Pamidronate	1–2 mg/kg IV over 2 hr, in 250mL 0.9% sodium chloride, q21–28d (100mL of 0.9% sodium chloride for dogs <10kg)	1–1.5 mg/kg IV over 2 hr, in 50mL 0.9% sodium chloride, q21–28d	Aminobisphosphonate. For osteolytic bone pain. Monitor renal function before each dose.
Prednisone	0.25–1.0 mg/kg PO q24h	0.5–1.5 mg/kg PO q24h	Corticosteroid. Occasionally useful for mild to moderate pain, especially if caused by inflammation or with CNS involvement.
Zoledronate	0.15–0.25 mg/kg IV over 15 minutes, in 50mL 0.9% sodium chloride, q28d (25 mL 0.9% sodium chloride for dogs <10kg)	0.15–0.20 mg/kg IV over 15 min, in 25mL 0.9% sodium chloride, q28d	Aminobisphosphonate. For osteolytic bone pain. Monitor renal function before each dose.

Complementary Therapies and Rehabilitation Medicine

Complementary therapies are increasingly used in management of human cancer pain.[1,2,22] These include acupuncture, massage, stretch and manipulation, hydrotherapy, superficial heat and cold, percutaneous electrical stimulation, transcutaneous electrical nerve stimulation, laser therapy, ultrasound, and pulsed magnetic field therapy.[1,2,4,22] Although their use for veterinary cancer pain is not well described in the literature, their growing availability, anecdotal-reported efficacy, and good tolerability profile make them an attractive addition to other therapeutic options in that setting.

Combination Therapies and Drug Interactions

A multimodal approach is best suited for the treatment and alleviation of cancer pain, often combining two or more analgesics for moderate to severe pain. Caution should be applied with geriatric patients, and new drugs should ideally be introduced one at a time, in a sequential manner. When side effects are encountered or once a drug is used at its maximum safe dosage without benefit to the patient, it should be discontinued.

The possibility of pharmacokinetic or pharmacodynamic drug interactions should be carefully evaluated whenever multiple drugs are used concomitantly.

Selected References*

Bruera ED, Portenoy RK (eds): *Cancer pain: assessment and management*, Cambridge, 2003, Cambridge University Press.
This thorough textbook focuses on human cancer pain, with most information applicable to veterinary oncology.
Gaynor JS, Muir WW: *Handbook of veterinary pain management*, ed 2, St Louis, 2009, Mosby/Elsevier.
This handbook covers veterinary pain management in detail. Excellent chapters on analgesic drug classes and management of various conditions associated with pain.
Lascelles BD: Management of chronic cancer pain. In Withrow SJ, Vail DM, (eds): *Withrow and MacEwen`s small animal clinical oncology*, ed 4, St Louis, 2007, Saunders/Elsevier.
This chapter is a good resource on cancer pain management in small animals, and specifically focuses on chronic pain assessment and management.

■ *For a complete list of the references cited in this chapter, please go to www.smallanimaloncology.com.

SECTION D: Palliative Care for the Cancer Patient

J. Paul Woods

KEY POINTS

- The goal of palliative care is to control clinical signs of disease as best as possible to provide a desirable quality of life to the veterinary patient while providing emotional support to their owners or family.
- A team of veterinary health care professionals is necessary to provide comprehensive palliative care to cancer patients.
- Palliative care is not limited to any particular therapy; rather, it is any therapy that will improve the patient's quality of life regardless of the prognosis of the primary disease.

The World Health Organization (WHO) has defined palliative care as follows:

> "…an approach that improves the quality of life of patients and their families facing the problems associated with life-threatening illness, through the prevention and relief of suffering by means of early identification and impeccable assessment and treatment of pain and other problems, physical, psychosocial and spiritual."[1]

Pet owners and veterinarians are strong advocates for the quality of life (QOL) of pets during cancer therapy. Although there are cancers for which there are no cures, there are few pets with cancer for which we cannot improve the QOL. Improving the pet's QOL may be done through the amelioration of signs of disease via palliative care such as analgesics, anti-emetics, and nutritional support, as well as radiation therapy or surgical procedures. The resultant enhancement in QOL may lead to an increase in quantity of life for the pet with cancer. The goals of palliative care are listed in Box 18-1.

THE PALLIATIVE CARE TEAM

A partnership between the pet owners and the professional team (veterinarians, technicians, staff, and counselors if available) is necessary to achieve the goals of palliative care. A closely knit, skillfully integrated, and interdependent team is required to provide complete care to the patient and the family. A mutually supportive team is required to share the responsibility and the emotional strain of palliative care. Similar to all of veterinary medicine, good communication is at the heart of good care. Many problems can stem from poor communication, which is not unique to palliative care; however, palliative care often focuses on loss and death, which requires skilled empathetic communication. Palliative care is planned care, not crisis intervention, and many of the problems encountered by the team are not unique to cancer (e.g., chronic pain). Although unexpected emergencies and crises do occur, many can be avoided by team-sharing and planning. With greater knowledge of each condition and its management, it is easier to reassure the client that their pet is receiving the best care possible.

QUALITY OF LIFE

Although each person may carry a strong intuitive feeling about QOL, it is a poorly defined term with different meanings to different people. In addition to the various opinions about what constitutes QOL, the issue is confounded in veterinary medicine because QOL is assessed by proxy by pet owners and the palliative care team. Often subjective measures such as general health, physical functioning (performance status), clinical signs, cognitive function, and activity level are used to assess QOL.[2,3]

Palliative care involves the amelioration of clinical signs emanating from the pet's cancer or cancer treatment. It is a difficult transition to change the team's goal of cancer therapy from cure to care. However, if signs such as pain, dyspnea, or obstruction can be improved by removing or shrinking the tumor, QOL may be greatly improved even if life is not prolonged.

PRINCIPLES OF PALLIATIVE CARE

1. Control clinical signs. Each clinical sign should be addressed, although priority should be given to those most significantly affecting the patient's QOL.

2. Maintain a problem-solving diagnostic approach throughout the illness. Pets with advanced cancer may become acutely ill and are in a changing situation with new problems arising such as metastases or pathologic fractures. However, pets with cancer can develop medical conditions unrelated to their cancer, and one should not assume that every condition is due to their cancer. These conditions may be treatable with routine medical care.

3. Regularly evaluate the patient as the cancer evolves to adjust therapies in order to maintain the best QOL possible for the pet.

4. Combine medications if needed to control a clinical sign (e.g., the use of different anti-emetics that act on different receptors for nausea and vomiting). However, beware of the complexity created by many drugs so that new signs are not created because of inappropriate drug use (e.g., lethargy).

5. Do not rule out invasive or specialized procedures for specific situations in which drugs are ineffective. An example is the use of radiation therapy to control pain in patients with bone tumors.[4]

6. Anticipate events such as pain and nausea and treat prophylactically to avoid them rather than initiating therapy after symptoms occur and subsequently affect QOL. Many of the problems experienced by pets with advanced cancer are predictable and can either be avoided or deferred.

TYPES OF PALLIATIVE CARE

Pain Control

A three-step "ladder" for cancer pain relief has been developed by the WHO Cancer Programme. If pain develops, the prompt administration of oral drugs should begin (1) non-opioids such as aspirin, (2) mild opioids, and (3) strong opioids as necessary until the patient is free of pain. Adjuvant methods, such as bisphosphonate therapy or radiation therapy, may be included in any of these three steps to improve pain control as necessary. It is also recommended that drugs be given "by the clock" rather than as needed to maintain pain control.[5] Further discussion of the management of pain in the cancer patient can be found in Section C.

Gastrointestinal Signs

Anorexia, nausea, vomiting, and diarrhea are all possibilities resulting from either the cancer itself or the treatment of cancer. Treatment of nausea and vomiting are discussed in Section A. Diarrhea is often self limiting; however, it can be severe, so treatment with loperamide at standard doses may be helpful. Constipation can also be a clinical sign noted with cancer, such as with perianal tumors or tumors that have metastasized to the lumbar lymph nodes. Softening the stools with lactulose may be particularly helpful in these instances. Begin at the low end of the recommended dose and escalate to a dose and frequency that is most helpful to the patient without causing fecal incontinence.

Nutrition

Nutritional supplementation may be necessary in the cancer patient, and an in-depth discussion of this topic can be found in Section B. Anorexia may require correction of mechanical problems (e.g., pyloric outflow obstruction, intestinal obstruction, etc.) or treatment of metabolic causes (e.g., hypercalcemia). It may also be treated with anti-emetics or appetite-stimulating drugs, depending upon the cause. Cyproheptadine is more effective in cats than dogs to stimulate the appetite and can be formulated as a topical medication to be placed on the inner aspect of the pinnae for easy administration in cats.

Anemia

Supportive blood products may be necessary to correct anemia resulting from hemorrhage or coagulopathies or caused by decreased RBC production (in the case of myelophthisis). See Chapter 13, Section C.

Malignant Effusions

Malignant effusions, most often caused by mesotheliomas or carcinomas, may necessitate periodic abdominocentesis, thoracocentesis, or both. Intracavitary chemotherapy has been used with some success for the treatment of malignant effusions caused by these tumors, and further description of the procedure can be found in Chapter 12, Section E.

Mechanical Obstructions

Mechanical obstructions can occur directly from tumors of the gastrointestinal or urinary tracts, or indirectly from lymphadenopathy associated with metastatic disease or primary lymphoid neoplasia (i.e., lymphoma). Treatment may entail stents for urethral obstruction by transitional cell carcinoma[4] or debulking/removing the tumor in the case of gastrointestinal or urinary tract tumors. In the case of perianal tumors with lymph node metastasis, obstruction of the rectum may be noted and either surgical extirpation of the nodes/tumor or stool softening agents may be helpful. In the case of dyspnea caused by mediastinal lymph node enlargement, radiation therapy may be helpful in shrinking the nodes to alleviate dyspnea.

SUMMARY

Palliative care is the active care of the pet focusing on enhancement of QOL by a team of professionals when the pet's cancer is no longer responsive to traditional treatment or the owners do not wish to pursue standard therapy. Support is provided in a patient-centered (rather than pathology-centered) manner to allow for optimal QOL regardless of the length of life. The principles of pain and clinical sign control, support and empathy, and team-caring used in palliative care are vital and should not be limited to cancer care, but should also be the norm for the practice of veterinary medicine in other fields beyond cancer care.

Selected References*

Mayer MN, Grier CK: Palliative radiation therapy for canine osteosarcoma, *Can Vet J* 47:707, 2006.
This review discusses the pathophysiology of bone cancer pain and the use of radiation therapy as a palliative treatment to improve quality of life in dogs suffering from bone tumors.
Mellanby RJ, Herrtage ME, Dobson JM: Owners' assessment of their dog's quality of life during palliative chemotherapy for lymphoma, *J Small Anim Pract* 44:100, 2003.
This study evaluates owners' perception of their dog's quality of life while undergoing treatment for lymphoma.
Weisse C, Berent A, Todd K, et al: Evaluation of palliative stenting for management of malignant urethral obstructions in dogs, *J Am Vet Med Assoc* 229:226, 2006.
This is a prospective study evaluating the efficacy and outcome of urethral stenting in dogs with urethral obstructions resulting from malignant disease.
Wojciechowska JI, Hewson CJ: Quality-of-life assessment in pet dogs, *J Am Vet Med Assoc* 226:722, 2005.
This review article discusses the philosophy and assessment of quality of life in pet dogs.

*For a complete list of the references cited in this chapter, please go to www.smallanimaloncology.com.

19   Nervous System Neoplasia

Joan R. Coates and Gayle C. Johnson

KEY POINTS

- Meningioma is the most common primary brain tumor in dogs and cats.
- Glioma is the most common primary brain tumor in brachycephalic breeds.
- Prognosis for meningioma is favorable with surgical resection and radiation therapy.
- Seizure is the most common clinical sign of brain tumors in dogs, whereas nonspecific behavior changes are common in cats.
- Lymphoma is the most common spinal cord tumor in cats, whereas meningioma is most common in dogs.
- Dogs with peripheral nerve sheath tumors commonly present with chronic lameness and severe muscle atrophy.

PRIMARY BRAIN TUMORS

Incidence

Brain tumors develop with a frequency of 14.5 in 100,000 dogs[1] and 2.2 to 3.5 in 100,000 cats.[1,2] The tumor classification system most widely used is from the World Health Organization Classification System and can be found in Table 19-1. Meningioma is the most common brain tumor in dogs and cats[3-5] and accounts for approximately 45% of primary intracranial neoplasms in dogs[4,5] and 59% in cats.[3] Glial cell tumors are the second most common primary brain tumor in dogs[3,5] and the fourth most common in cats.[3] Brain tumors typically affect older dogs with a median age of 9 years (range, 4–13 years) and 95% are older than 5 years of age.[4] Golden Retrievers and Boxer dogs are at increased risk for intracranial neoplasia.[5] Dolichocephalic breeds may be at increased risk for meningiomas, whereas brachycephalic breeds may have increased risk for gliomas.[5] Cats with brain tumors are older with a mean age of 11.3 ± 3.8 years (range, 0.5–21.5 years).[3] Male cats are affected slightly more than female cats (male:female ratio of 1.5:1).[3] The domestic shorthair cat is the most common breed identified.[3]

Etiology and Risk Factors

Definitive risk factors for development of brain tumors are unknown for dogs and cats. Inheritance may have a role in some breeds of dogs. Hormones such as estrogen and progesterone can influence tumor genesis.[7,8] Young cats with mucopolysaccharidosis type I have a high incidence of meningiomas, providing suspicion for a genetic basis.[9]

Clinical Features

Clinical signs of brain tumors develop as a result of damage to surrounding normal neural tissue from tumor expansion and associated edema.[10] Brain edema is a prominent feature of intracranial neoplasms. Brain edema may initially cause few or no clinical signs. As the edema worsens, a mass effect occurs with distortion and displacement of brain tissue, subsequently causing a rise in intracranial pressure[11] and shift of brain tissue to areas of lower pressure. Neurologic deficits produced by these displacements are additive to the clinical signs caused by the tumor itself.[12] Table 19-2 summarizes clinical signs associated with herniation. Hydrocephalus may also occur, either as a result of altered cerebrospinal fluid (CSF) resorption or ventricular obstruction.[13,14]

Diagnosis and Staging

Common neurologic signs observed in animals with brain tumors include altered mentation (obtundation, stupor, coma), seizures, ataxia, circling, and behavioral changes. Seizures (45%) are the most common clinical sign in dogs, but circling (23%), ataxia (21%), and head

TABLE 19-1　HISTOLOGIC CLASSIFICATION OF TUMORS OF THE NERVOUS SYSTEM

Tissue/Region	Cell Origin	Subtype
Tumors of neuroepithelial tissue	Astrocytic tumors	Fibrillary
		Protoplasmic
		Gemistocytic
		Anaplastic
		Glioblastoma
	Oligodendroglial tumors	Oligodendroglioma
		Anaplastic
	Other gliomas	Mixed glioma
		Gliosarcoma
		Gliomatosis cerebri
		Spongioblastoma
	Ependymal tumors	Ependymoma
		Anaplastic
	Choroid plexus tumors	Choroid plexus papilloma
		Choroid plexus carcinoma
	Neuronal tumors	Gangliocytoma
		Ganglioglioma
		Neuroblastoma
		Ganglioneuroma
		Paraganglioma
	Embryonal tumors	Primitive neuroectodermal tumors
		Neuroblastoma
		Ependymoblastoma
		Epithelioneuroblastoma
	Pineal parenchymal tumors	Pineocytoma
		Pineoblastoma
Meningeal tumors	Meningioma	Meningotheliomatous
		Fibrous
		Transitional
		Psammomatous
		Angiomatous
		Papillary
		Granular cell
		Myxoid
		Anaplastic
	Mesenchymal tumors	Fibrosarcoma
		Diffuse meningeal sarcomatosis
Hematopoietic tumors	Lymphoma	Primary
		Secondary
	Neoplastic reticulosis	
	Microgliomatosis	
	Malignant histiocytosis	
Tumors of sellar region	Suprasellar germ cell tumor	
	Pituitary tumors	Pituitary adenoma
		Pituitary carcinoma
	Craniopharyngioma	
Other primary tumors/cysts	Hamartoma	
	Cysts	Epidermoid
		Pituitary
		Other
Tumors of peripheral nervous tissue	Peripheral nerve sheath tumor	Schwannoma
		Neurofibroma
		Malignant schwannoma
		Neurofibrosarcoma
Metastatic tumors	Local extension	
	Hematogenous	

(Adapted and modified from Koestner A, Bilzer T, Fatzer R, et al: Histological classification of tumors of the nervous system of domestic animals [WHO international classification of tumors of domestic animals], Washington DC, 1999, Armed Forces Institute of Pathology.)

TABLE 19-2   CLINICAL SIGNS OF BRAIN HERNIATION SYNDROME

Herniation Type	Anatomic Displacement	Clinical Signs
Foramen magnum	Caudal displacement of cerebellum and compression of medulla and cerebellum	Tetraplegia (flaccid) Pupils midposition to dilated Loss of brainstem reflexes Apnea Coma Opisthotonus
Caudal transtentorial	Herniation of temporal cortex and compression of midbrain and traction of oculomotor nerve	Pupils dilated (asymmetric) Loss of brainstem reflexes Tetraplegia Apnea Coma Opisthotonus
Rostral transtentorial	Compression of rostral cerebellum against the tentorium	Possible cerebellar dysfunction Decerebellate posture
Cingulate gyrus (falcine)	Movement of the cingulated gyrus beneath the falx and compression of opposite cingulated gyrus	Possible forebrain dysfunction Circling Head pressing Seizures Abnormal mentation

tilt (13%) also occur.[15] Brain neoplasia should be considered as a differential diagnosis when a dog has its first seizure after 4 years of age.[4] Clinical signs in cats are similar but often are vague or nonspecific, with anorexia and lethargy being most common. Reported neurologic signs in cats include altered mentation (26%), circling (23%), seizures (23%), ataxia (16.9%), and behavioral changes (15.6%).[3] A sudden onset of aggression is the most common behavioral change reported in cats.[3]

A minimum database including a complete blood count, serum biochemical analysis, and urinalysis should be performed to evaluate for metabolic abnormalities in animals suspected of having a brain tumor. Radiographs of the thorax and abdomen as well as abdominal ultrasound are recommended to rule out metastatic and concurrent disease prior to advanced diagnostics and surgery.[5] Neuroanatomic localization of the central nervous system (CNS) lesion will vary based on location of the tumor and amount of mass effect caused by the edema and tumor.[16,17] Table 19-3 summarizes clinical signs associated with specific lesion localization within the brain.

Magnetic resonance imaging (MRI) is the diagnostic imaging modality of choice for diagnosis of brain tumors. See Chapter 10, Section B, for discussion and comparisons of MRI and CT. A normal contrast-enhanced MRI most likely rules out the possibility of a brain tumor. Analysis of CSF can aid in diagnosis and ruling out overt inflammatory diseases. Increased protein concentration

(normal, <25 mg/dl) and a normal to mild increase in total nucleated cell count (normal, <5 cells/μL)are typical for a brain tumor.[18] Rarely, neoplastic cells may be identified in CSF.[19] Collection of CSF should be avoided when increased intracranial pressure is suspected based on clinical signs and imaging studies (deviation of falx cerebri, ventricular compression, hydrocephalus).

Electroencephalography and auditory brainstem evoked potential have been used to further confirm lesion extent and physiologic function but lack specificity and sensitivity for detecting brain masses.[20] Regardless of diagnostic findings, definitive diagnosis of brain tumors is made by histopathologic examination and can be helpful in prognostication of some tumor types. A summary of brain tumor types is provided in Table 19-4.

Metastasis

Rarely, primary CNS tumors will spread systemically. Tumors with potential for extraneural spread include meningiomas, primitive neuroectodermal tumors (PNETs), malignant gliomas, malignant histiocytic tumors, and choroid plexus tumors. Very rarely a meningioma may metastasize outside the CNS with lung and pancreas as reported sites.[21,22] Nasal meningiomas of dogs are more aggressive and may invade the brain through the cribriform plate.[23] Glial tumors rarely metastasize unless there is ventricular involvement. Choroid plexus tumors implant along CSF pathways and may localize within the spinal

TABLE 19-3   CLINICAL SIGNS ASSOCIATED WITH INTRACRANIAL LOCALIZATIONS

Intracranial Division	Brain Region	Clinical Signs
Supratentorial (rostral to the osseous tentorium)	Cerebral cortex	Seizures Obtundation/stupor or normal mentation Behavioral abnormalities Ipsilateral circling with normal gait Contralateral menace response deficit Contralateral loss of touch and pain recognition Contralateral postural reaction deficits Cervical spinal pain
	Diencephalon	Obtundation/stupor Normal gait (compulsive) or circling Cranial nerve (CN) II deficits Loss of thermoregulation Abnormal eating or drinking Endocrine dysfunction Cervical spinal pain
Infratentorial (caudal to the osseous tentorium)	Brainstem	Obtundation/stupor Vestibular dysfunction (central) Ipsilateral cranial nerve deficits Asymmetric tetraparesis/plegia
	Cerebellum	Dysmetria and ataxia Intention tremor Absent menace response but visual Vestibular dysfunction (central)
Cavernous Sinus	CN III, IV, V, VI sympathetic nerve	External and internal ophthalmoparesis, Ptosis Horner's syndrome Sensory deficits—corneal, facial

cord.[24-27] Choroid plexus carcinomas tend to invade locally into surrounding brain parenchyma.[28] Ependymomas have potential to implant along CSF pathways and seed to distant spinal cord tissue. Primary CNS lymphoma is uncommon in dogs and cats, whereas secondary CNS lymphoma is more common and part of a multicentric process.[3,5] Primary renal lymphoma in cats is likely to relapse in the CNS.[29] The meninges are also a site for metastatic lymphoma.[30,31] With progression to the spinal cord, lymphoma often appears as an extradural compressive mass.[32-35]

Treatment Modalities

The goals for treatment of brain tumors are size reduction or complete tumor removal and control of secondary effects (edema, increased intracranial pressure [ICP]).[18] Guidelines for treatment of specific types of brain tumors are lacking in veterinary medicine. Treatment options depend upon tumor type and location, onset of clinical signs, costs, and associated morbidity/mortality.[18] Often a combination of surgery, chemotherapy, and radiation is used in the treatment regimen. Surgery alone can be curative for selective tumor types when complete resection is achieved but is often limited by anatomy and extent of disease.[36,37] Surgery also allows for a histologic diagnosis and control of clinical signs. Ultrasonographic, stereotactic, and endoscopic techniques have increased access to tumors located deep within the brain parenchyma.[38,39] Aspiration pneumonia is the most common complication associated with intracranial surgery.[40] Stereotactic radiosurgery for brain tumors is used to administer a single-fraction, high-dose radiation treatment[39] and is promising in the treatment of brain tumors.[41] The use of chemotherapy for treatment of brain tumors in veterinary medicine is primarily anecdotal. Several reports exist for use of nitrosurea compounds in dogs.[42-45] The blood–brain barrier (BBB) has been considered a major hindrance to the use of chemotherapy for brain tumors. Lipophilic agents more readily cross the BBB. The BBB can be iatrogenically disrupted with mannitol administration before administration of agents.[46] Intrathecal administration may also bypass the BBB.

Glucocorticoids and anti-epileptic drugs (AEDs) provide beneficial effects in controlling clinical signs of edema

TABLE 19-4   SUMMARY OF BRAIN TUMOR TYPES, FEATURES, AND ANTICIPATED CLINICAL OUTCOME FOR THE MOST COMMON BRAIN TUMORS OF DOGS AND CATS

Tumor Type	Histologies	Cell of Origin	Incidence	Diagnostic Findings	Behavior	Treatment	Survival
Meningioma	Cystic areas common in cats[102]	Arachnoid layer of the meninges	• 45% canine intracranial tumors[4,5] • 59% feline intracranial tumors[3]	• Solitary mass • Multiple masses in cats common[2,103,104] • Broad-based mass extra-axial to brain tissue[105,106] • Dural tail sign on MRI	• Infiltrative in dogs, encapsulated in cats[107] • Usually histologically benign • Rare metastasis to lung and pancreas reported[21,22]	• Glucocorticoids • Surgery • Radiation therapy • Surgery and radiation	• 2–4 mo[49,108] • 6–7 mo[52,53] • 8 mo[50,54,108] • 16.5 mo[7,53,108]
Glial tumors	Astrocytoma Oligodendroglioma Glioblastoma multiforme	Astrocytes Oligodendrocytes Mixed cell origin	• 20%–37% canine intracranial tumors[4,5,105] • 10% all canine CNS tumors[93] • 12% feline intracranial tumors[3]	• Ring enhancement pattern common on MRI[105,109]	• Rarely metastasize unless there is ventricular involvement	• Radiation therapy • Chemotherapy o Lomustine • Glucocorticoids	• 6–10 months[108] • 7–11 months[42,43,45] • 52 days in cats[3,111]
Choroid plexus tumors	Papilloma Carcinoma	Choroid plexus	• 6% canine intracranial tumors[4,5,105] • 0.6% feline intracranial tumors[3]	• Secondary obstructive hydrocephalus common • >100 mg/dl protein on CSF often found with choroid plexus carcinomas[112]	• Implant along CSF pathways	Not reported	Poor
Ependymoma		Ependymal cells that line the ventricles of the brain and spinal cord	Rare in both dogs and cats	• Hydrocephalus if mass is obstructing CSF flow[113]	• Usually benign • Malignant ependymomas reported in cats[114] • Implant along CSF pathways and seed to distant spinal cord	• Surgery • Glucocorticoids	Dependent upon response to therapy
Lymphoma	T-cell lymphoma common[101]		• 4%–7% primary canine intracranial tumors[5,101] • 3% feline intracranial neoplasms[3]	• Multifocal neurologic signs and seizures[19,34]	• Secondary CNS lymphoma more common than primary lymphoma in dogs and cats[3,5] • Primary feline renal lymphoma often relapses in CNS[29]	See Chapter 25, Section A	See Chapter 25

and seizures.[47] Prednisone (0.25–0.5 mg/kg PO BID) or dexamethasone (0.25–2.0 mg/kg PO SID) may be used with the dosage adjusted based on clinical response.

Osmotherapy such as mannitol is useful to control acute increases in ICP associated with herniation syndrome.[11] Mannitol is most widely used at a 25% solution administered as an intravenous bolus at a dosage of 0.5 to 1.0 g/kg. Hypertonic saline solutions (3%) at 0.5 to 1.0 ml/kg IV may also be effective. Furosemide 0.7 mg/kg IV may also have synergistic effects of rapid reduction of vasogenic edema.[48] Single administrations of these agents usually only have a short-term effect and may need to be repeated. AED therapy is indicated for tumor-associated seizures.[16,18,47] For acute seizure control, AEDs (e.g., valium) that rapidly permeate the BBB are indicated. Maintenance AED therapy (e.g., phenobarbital or potassium bromide) is often indicated for long-term control.

Prognosis and Survival

In general, prognosis for brain tumors in dogs and cats treated only with palliative therapy is poor. Except for feline and canine meningiomas, the prognosis for brain tumor types is quite variable. Dogs that receive only glucocorticoids or AEDs had mean survival times ranging from 2 to 4 months.[49-51] Median survival times for all tumor types reported in dogs and cats after surgery alone vary around 2 to 7 months.[6,52,53] Reported median survival times in dogs with intracranial tumors that receive radiation therapy alone vary from 4.9 to 14.4 months.[6,54,55] Survival rates of 1 and 2 years for dogs with intracranial neoplasia undergoing radiation therapy are 37% and 5%, respectively.[54] Median survival times of 16 months have been reported in dogs with intracranial meningiomas that received a combination of tumor resection and radiation therapy.[53] Median survival time for cats with meningiomas not treated with surgery is <1 month compared with up to 27 months for cats treated with surgery.[3,56,57] Well-designed controlled case studies with large patient numbers are lacking in veterinary medicine as well as understanding of the biologic behavior of these tumors.

BRAIN METASTASES
Incidence

Common locations for CNS metastases of extra-neural tumors in dogs and cats are the cerebrum with caudal fossa and spinal cord metastases occurring less commonly.[58] Routes for CNS metastases are through local extension or hematogenous spread. Brain metastases may be single or multiple. Tumors of primary CNS origin rarely metastasize by spread within CSF pathways (drop metastases) to other parts of the nervous system. However, PNETs, ependymomas, pineal region tumors, and malignant gliomas have been reported to do so. Although rare, meningeal carcinomatosis describes a diffuse or multi-focal infiltration of leptomeninges with carcinoma cells.[25,27,59] Prevalence of secondary brain neoplasms is unknown in dogs and reported as 22% (excluding pituitary tumors) in cats.[3]

Etiology and Risk Factors

Most secondary brain tumors in dogs are local extensions of nasal tumors, which account for 30% of tumors with CNS metastasis.[18,58] Other tumors that can extend into the brain include squamous cell carcinoma, pituitary tumors, and osteochondrosarcomas. Metastatic tumor types in dogs that have been reported to undergo hematogenous spread to the CNS include transitional cell carcinoma, hemangiosarcoma (HSA),[35,60] mammary carcinoma, adenocarcinoma, melanoma, lymphoma, and undifferentiated sarcoma.[58] A recent retrospective study evaluated common secondary brain tumors in dogs to include HSAs (51%), pituitary tumors (25%), lymphosarcoma (12%), and metastatic carcinoma (12%).[61] Pulmonary metastases were found in 80% of animals with hematogenous spread of tumors to the CNS.[58] Brain metastasis has been reported to occur in 14% of dogs with HSAs, and dogs having pulmonary metastases are at greater risk.[60] In cats, the most common secondary brain tumors are lymphoma and pituitary tumors.[3] Hematogenous spread of neoplasia to the brain in cats is rare (<6%), with pulmonary adenocarcinoma being the most likely to spread by this route.[3] Other metastatic neoplasms in cats include adenocarcinoma, squamous cell carcinoma, fibrosarcoma, malignant fibrous histiocytoma, sarcoma, and HSA.[3]

Clinical Features

Onset and progression of clinical signs of metastatic neoplasms are more rapid than with primary CNS neoplasms. Clinical signs are determined by tumor location and are multifactorial. Since most tumors are located in the cerebrum, a mentation change is the most common presenting clinical sign.[61] Secondary manifestations of increased ICP, obstruction of CSF flow, and herniation syndrome become more apparent as metastases increase in size.

Diagnosis/Staging

To obtain a presumptive diagnosis of CNS metastasis, advanced brain imaging is performed. Biopsy will provide a definitive diagnosis. However, it is important to perform a thorough systemic work-up in any animal suspected of having intracranial neoplasia prior to advanced imaging or surgery.[5]

Treatment Modalities

Metastatic neoplasia is treated with palliative-based medical therapies to alleviate subsequent clinical signs associated with increased ICP. Radiation therapy and chemotherapy may provide temporary improvement of clinical signs. Complete surgical resection may be feasible for solitary tumors of superficial location.

Prognosis and Survival

In general, prognosis for metastatic CNS neoplasia is poor. Factors contributing to a poor prognosis are inability to obtain an early diagnosis and presence of disseminated disease.[35]

SPINAL CORD NEOPLASIA

Tumors affecting the spinal cord are classified as extradural, intradural-extramedullary, or intramedullary.[62,63] Extradural tumors are primary bone tumors, metastatic tumors, and lymphoma. Intradural-extramedullary tumors are meningioma, nephroblastoma, lipoma, metastatic carcinoma, and nerve sheath tumor. Intramedullary spinal cord tumors include astrocytomas,[64,65] ependymomas,[66-69] and oligodendrogliomas.[70] Metastatic spinal tumors that have intramedullary involvement include lymphoma and HSA.[35] The cervical spinal cord is most commonly affected, with the majority being extradural tumors.[62,71,72] Meningiomas[24,73] and nerve sheath tumors[74] commonly occur in the cervical region, whereas lymphoma in cats[32,75] and neuroepitheliomas[76] occur in the thoracolumbar region.

Incidence/Etiology/Risk Factors

Meningiomas are the most common spinal cord tumor in dogs followed by metastatic choroid plexus tumors, astrocytoma, and ependymoma.[24] Meningiomas are the most common primary spinal cord tumor in cats older than 8 years of age, and lymphoma is among the most common spinal cord diseases in cats older than 2 years.[75] Canine neuroepithelioma or nephroblastoma is an intradural extramedullary neoplasm in young dogs between 6 months and 3 years of age.[76] Many breeds have been reported to be affected, but German Shepherd dogs may be predisposed.[77]

Clinical Features

Clinical signs are due to the space-occupying effects of the tumor. Neurologic localization depends on presence of upper or lower motor neurons in the pelvic and/or thoracic limbs. Initial neurologic deficits are often asymmetric and unilateral with monoparesis or hemiparesis but progress to bilateral involvement of the spinal cord. Micturition dysfunction and urinary retention occur with more severe involvement of spinal cord tissue and loss of voluntary motor function. Paraspinal hyperesthesia is a clinical feature of extradural and intradural-extramedullary tumors. Intramedullary tumors usually lack paraspinal hyperesthesia. Onset of neurologic signs is often insidious and progressive. Intramedullary tumors can have acute onset of clinical signs.[62] Neurologic deficits may progress rapidly if malacia or hemorrhage occurs. As for nephroblastomas, abdominal radiography and ultrasound can assess for primary renal involvement.

Diagnosis and Staging

Survey radiography can detect vertebral tumors that are osteolytic or chondromic, as well as enlarged intervertebral foramina that result from osteonecrosis secondary to slowly expansile tumors within the spinal canal. Myelography or CT/myelography is useful for delineating extradural, intradural-extramedullary, and intramedullary involvement. Meningiomas are usually intradural extramedullary lesions, and a "dural tail" sign has been reported to be associated with canine spinal meningiomas on MRI.[78] Analysis of CSF for spinal cord tumors often is nonspecific.[79]

Metastasis

Extraspinal metastasis has not been reported for spinal meningiomas. Rarely will renal nephroblastoma secondarily metastasize to the spinal cord and other extraneural tissues.[80] Intraspinal metastasis from a primary spinal nephroblastoma has been reported in a dog.[81]

Treatment Modalities

A decompressive laminectomy procedure by itself will provide improvement of neurologic deficits.[73,82] Surgical resection is a viable option for extradural and intradural-extramedullary tumors. Some intramedullary tumors can also be resected using a rhizotomy procedure.[68,83] In comparison to intracranial meningiomas, complete surgical resection of spinal meningiomas is more difficult because of meningeal adhesion and more intimate association with the spinal cord tissue.[73] Radiation may be used for tumors not surgically accessible or as an adjunct to partial surgical resection.[82] Chemotherapy has been mainly used for hematopoietic tumor types. Glucocorticoid treatment is used as palliative therapy to reduce peritumoral edema. If nephroblastomas are detected early, limited morbidity is associated with surgical resection.[77,84,85] Adjuvant radiation is considered when complete surgical resection is not possible.[86,87] Chemotherapy has only limited success.[88]

Prognosis and Survival

Median survival time tends to be longer in dogs with benign spinal cord tumors versus malignant.[71] Average survival time of dogs treated for spinal meningiomas was greater than 1 year, whereas untreated dogs had an average survival time of 15 days after diagnosis.[24] Other studies report good long-term outcome of up to 3 years.[71,73] Poor surgical results are associated with intumescence involvement and tumors with ventral location and invasion of the neural parenchema.[71,73,82] Survival may be enhanced with radiation.[82] The prognosis for nephroblastomas is considered guarded because spinal cord involvement is often extensive by the time of diagnosis. Tumor recurrence is likely.[77]

PERIPHERAL NERVE SHEATH TUMORS

Incidence

In dogs, peripheral nerve sheath tumors (PNSTs) have been reported in various anatomic sites but spinal nerves in the lower cervical and upper thoracic region as well as cranial nerves are affected with greatest frequency.[74,89,90] The trigeminal nerve is the most commonly involved cranial nerve.[91] Peripheral nerve sheath tumors are rare in cats.[71,92]

Etiology and Risk Factors

Peripheral nerve sheath tumors arise from Schwann cells, perineural fibroblasts, or both.[93] These tumors can differentiate into schwannomas, neurofibromas, and neurofibrosarcomas. Benign tumors are classified as schwannoma (neurilemoma) or neurofibroma. The malignant counterparts, malignant schwannoma and neurofibrosarcoma, are more generally termed malignant PNST. Malignancy is determined by mitotic index and degree of anaplasia.

Clinical Features

Severe asymmetric muscle atrophy is a key finding on clinical examination.[74] Dogs with spinal nerve involvement commonly have lameness and muscle atrophy in the affected limb.[74,90] Findings of pain and a palpable mass are less frequent. Average time from development of signs to diagnosis ranges from 4 to 6 months.[90] Masses associated with the brachial plexus often extend proximally into the spinal canal and eventually cause deficits in the pelvic limbs. Unilateral atrophy of the muscles of mastication is the most common clinical sign in dogs with trigeminal nerve sheath tumors.[91]

Diagnosis and Staging

Survey radiography rules out orthopedic-related diseases, causing lameness. Slow intradural expansion may cause resorption and enlargement of the adjacent intervertebral foramina. An intradural-extramedullary filling pattern is evident with myelography[63] if there is spinal canal involvement.[74] CT, MRI,[94] and ultrasonography have been used to identify PNSTs.[95] Thoracic radiography is recommended to evaluate for metastatic disease. Analysis of CSF is usually normal.[74]

Metastasis

Metastasis is rare, but pulmonary metastasis has been reported.[89,96]

Treatment

Successful treatment of PNSTs depends on early surgical intervention.[74,97] Local resection, limb amputation, laminectomy, or combinations are recommended surgical procedures. Tumors within the brachial plexus are treated with local resection[98] and/or limb amputation. Tumors involving the spinal canal are explored with a laminectomy. Repeated surgeries may have little benefit in treatment outcome.[74] Local surgical resection is the preferred treatment for trigeminal NSTs.[91,99] Efficacy of radiation therapy is unknown.

Prognosis

Malignant PNSTs have a high rate of recurrence (82%), and overall long-term prognosis is considered poor.[74] Median survival time of dogs with root and peripheral nerve involvement is 5 and 12 months, respectively.[74] The median relapse-free interval of plexus associated tumors was 7.5 months.[74] Early and aggressive surgical management may extend survival.[97,100] Dogs with peripherally located tumors had longer median survival times compared with those with more proximal tumors.[74] Survival times for trigeminal nerve sheath tumor in dogs that were not treated range from 5 to 21 months.[91]

Selected References*

Marioni-Henry K, Van Winkle TJ, Smith SH, et al: Tumors affecting the spinal cord of cats: 85 cases (1980-2005), *J Am Vet Med Assoc* 232:237, 2008.
　This article represents a retrospective study to determine prevalence of spinal tumors in cats. Data documented signalment, clinical history, neurologic examination, diagnostic imaging, and tumor location. Lymphosarcoma was the most common tumor in cats. Paraspinal hyperesthesia and asymmetry were common clinical signs.
Snyder JM, Lipitz L, Skorupski KA, et al: Secondary intracranial neoplasia in the dog: 177 cases (1986-2003), *J Vet Int Med* 22:172, 2008.

A summary of prevalence of secondary intracranial neoplasia in dogs. Common metastatic neoplasms and clinical signs are discussed. Post-mortem findings are also highlighted.

Snyder JM, Shofer FS, Van Winkle TJ, et al: Canine intracranial primary neoplasia: 173 cases (1986-2003), *J Vet Intern Med* 20:669, 2006.

This article describes pathologic and clinical findings of canine brain tumors. Meningiomas were most common. Tumors were most commonly located in the forebrain with seizures as the common presenting clinical sign. Thoracic radiography and abdominal ultrasonography are indicated to evaluate for extracranial neoplasia prior to imaging.

Troxel MT, Vite CH, Massicotte C, et al: Magnetic resonance imaging features of feline intracranial neoplasia: retrospective analysis of 46 cats, *J Vet Intern Med* 18:176, 2004.

This article describes a retrospective study evaluating MRI characteristics of feline brain tumors to document these characteristics to respective tumor types.

Troxel MT, Vite CH, Van Winkle TJ, et al: Feline intracranial neoplasia: retrospective review of 160 cases (1985-2001), *J Vet Intern Med* 17:850, 2003.

This article describes a retrospective study that determined the frequency of brain tumors in cats. Signalment, clinical signs, tumor type and location, imaging results and treatments were reviewed. Meningioma was the most common tumor type. Common neurologic signs of brain tumors were altered consciousness, seizures, and circling.

■ *For a complete list of the references cited in this chapter, please go to www.smallanimaloncology.com.

SECTION A: Oral and Salivary Gland Tumors

Carolyn J. Henry and Mary Lynn Higginbotham

KEY POINTS

Oral Tumors

- Melanoma, squamous cell carcinoma (SCC), and fibrosarcoma are the most common malignant oral tumors in dogs; SCC is the most common feline oral malignancy, by far.
- Approximately 5% of oral tumors in dogs are benign dental tumors (epulides), which do not metastasize and warrant an excellent prognosis.
- Lymph node palpation alone does not accurately predict nodal metastasis.
- The presence of loose teeth in a patient with otherwise good dentition warrants a search for oral neoplasia.
- Obtain incisional biopsies from sites that can be easily excised at the time of definitive surgery (i.e., lesions should be approached from within the oral cavity, such that any regions that may be needed later for wound closure using tissue flaps are not contaminated with tumor cells).

Salivary Gland Tumors

- The majority of canine and feline salivary tumors are malignant, with adenocarcinoma the most frequent diagnosis.
- Metastasis at the time of diagnosis is more common in cats than dogs and may develop in the regional lymph nodes and other distant locations late in the course of disease.
- Local recurrence is common with surgical excision alone.

ORAL TUMORS

Incidence—Morbidity and Mortality

Oral tumors account for 3% to 10% of all feline neoplastic diseases and are the fourth most common neoplasm in dogs.[1-3] The most common oral malignancies in dogs are malignant melanoma (MM), squamous cell carcinoma (SCC), and fibrosarcoma (FSA). In cats, SCC predominates, with FSA seen less frequently. The most common tongue tumor diagnosed in cats is SCC, whereas lingual melanomas occur more often in dogs, followed by SCC (Figure 20-1; Boxes 20-1 and 20-2).[1-14] Benign neoplastic and inflammatory lesions (viral papillomatosis, epulides/ameloblastomas, odontomas, and eosinophilic granulomas) are differential diagnoses to consider for patients presenting with an oral mass.

Etiology/Risk Factors

Unlike oral cancer in people, which is largely attributable to the use of smokeless tobacco products, the underlying etiology for most oral malignancies in companion animals is unknown. Three notable exceptions are: (1) viral papillomatosis occurs subsequent to horizontal transmission of papovavirus from dog to dog (see Chapter 3, Section B); (2) radiation-induced oral sarcomas and carcinomas may occur years after radiation therapy for benign oral tumors such as epulides[15,16]; and (3) an association between exposure to environmental tobacco smoke and development of some feline oral SCC is supported by both epidemiologic and molecular evidence.[17]

Clinical Features

Animals with tumors located in the rostral oral cavity are usually presented for evaluation of a visible mass. Rostral tumors are detected earlier and therefore are usually smaller. This means there is a greater likelihood for complete excision; and such tumors often have a good prognosis, especially canine SCC.[3,5,18] Tumors in other sites may go undetected since they are difficult to see or may be ignored because of their benign outward appearance. Oftentimes, suspicion of oral cancer develops during routine dental prophylaxis. One such

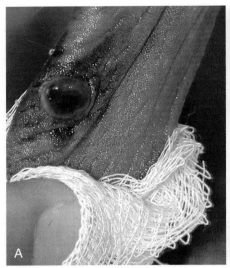 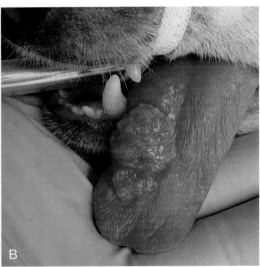

FIGURE 20-1 A, Melanoma and, **B,** squamous cell carcinoma are the most common lingual tumors in dogs.

BOX 20-1 REPORTED ORAL MALIGNANCIES IN DOGS AND CATS[1-14]

- Melanoma (most common oral malignancy in dogs)
- Squamous cell carcinoma (most common oral malignancy in cats)
- Fibrosarcoma
- Osteosarcoma
- Mast cell tumor
- Extramedullary plasmacytoma
- Lymphoma
- Chondrosarcoma
- Hemangiosarcoma
- Anaplastic sarcoma
- Multilobular osteochondrosarcoma/Multilobular tumor of bone
- Myxosarcoma
- Neurofibrosarcoma
- Rhabdomyosarcoma
- Transmissible venereal tumor
- Ectopic thyroid carcinoma (tongue)

BOX 20-2 TONGUE TUMORS REPORTED IN DOGS AND CATS[7,9-13]

Malignant
Squamous cell carcinoma (most common in cats)
Malignant melanoma (most common in dogs)
Fibrosarcoma
Mast cell tumor
Adenocarcinoma
Leiomyosarcoma
Neurofibrosarcoma
Rhabdomyosarcoma
Hemangiosarcoma
Ectopic thyroid carcinoma
Benign
Plasmacytoma
Granular cell myoblastoma
Papilloma
Rhabdomyoma
Lipoma
Hemangioma
Myxoma

---

hallmark of oral neoplasia is the presence of loose teeth in a patient with otherwise good dentition. This presentation warrants tissue biopsy at the time of tooth extraction. FSAs of the maxilla are often associated with considerable facial deformity (Figure 20-2) and may be biologically aggressive, despite a low-grade appearance on histopathology. Other typical clinical signs that should prompt a thorough oral examination are listed in Box 20-3. The presence of multiple concurrent oral lesions is most consistent with benign conditions,

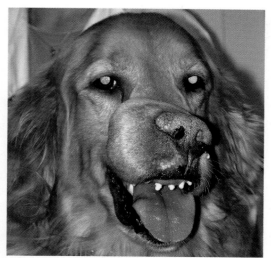

FIGURE 20-2 Maxillary fibrosarcoma (FSA) is locally aggressive and can create considerable facial deformity. Golden retrievers in particular may have histologically low-grade, yet biologically aggressive FSA.

BOX 20-3   CLINICAL SIGNS ASSOCIATED WITH ORAL TUMORS

- Ptyalism
- Halitosis
- Dysphagia
- Weight loss and/or decreased oral intake
- Mandibular or retropharyngeal lymph node enlargement
- Disinterest in chew toys
- Blood-stained food, water bowls, and bedding
- Exophthalmos
- Facial asymmetry
- Sneezing
- Nasal discharge
- Pawing at mouth

---

including papillomas and epulides, but does not rule out malignancy.

Diagnosis and Staging

Diagnostic methods and staging procedures depend upon tumor location and ease of sampling. Friable and rostrally located masses may be easily sampled under light sedation, whereas general anesthesia is suggested for biopsy of more caudal masses or those that are likely to bleed excessively. Before anesthesia, full physical examination, complete blood count, serum chemistries, and urinalysis are warranted. If malignancy is suspected, three-view thoracic radiographs are advised before other testing because detection of pulmonary metastatic disease warrants a poor prognosis and may influence case management decisions. Although the overall rate of pulmonary metastasis at the time of diagnosis is relatively low (14% or less for all oral malignancies), this finding means that local surgery is unlikely to be curative, and may therefore contraindicate aggressive surgery.[19] Radiographic or CT imaging of the affected site aids in determining tumor extent and in planning therapy. Over 50% of oral tumors arising from or near the gingiva have bone lysis demonstrable on radiographs.[19] Visual assessment may greatly underestimate the extent of the cancer, particularly feline oral SCC. In some cases, imaging may reveal the diagnosis, as was the case for the dog in Figure 20-3. However,

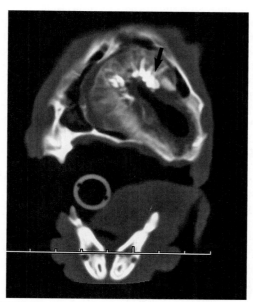

FIGURE 20-3 Computed tomography scan of a dog with an odontoma reveals teeth *(arrow)* within the mass. In this case, imaging provided a diagnosis and surgery was curative.

in most cases a biopsy is essential because inflammatory lesions and benign masses can look outwardly similar to malignant tumors. When lesions are small and superficial, excisional biopsy with curative intent is encouraged. Incisional biopsy is recommended for larger or invasive lesions, since treatment planning will vary depending on tumor histology and stage. Biopsy samples should

TABLE 20-1   IMMUNOHISTOCHEMICAL (IHC) STAINS USEFUL FOR DIFFERENTIATING ORAL MALIGNANCIES

IHC Stain	TUMOR TYPE		
	SCC	Melanoma	FSA
Vimentin	−	+/−	+
Cytokeratin	+	−	−
S-100	−	+	−
Melan A	−	+	−
HMB-45 and MEL-1	−	+	−
Neuron-specific enolase	−	+	−

FSA, Fibrosarcoma; *SCC,* squamous cell carcinoma.

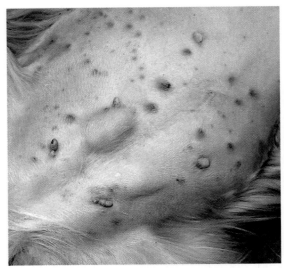

FIGURE 20-4 Cutaneous metastasis on the ventral abdomen of a dog with oral malignant melanoma.

be large and representative of the mass, with care taken not to sample too superficially or in necrotic areas. The biopsy site should be planned so that it can be excised at the time of definitive surgery. Lesions should be sampled via an oral approach, such that skin that may be needed later for wound closure using tissue flaps is not contaminated with tumor cells.[20] Use electrocautery only after biopsy specimens are obtained because cautery distorts the histologic appearance of the tissue.[15] A veterinary pathologist with immunohistochemistry (IHC) expertise should evaluate biopsy specimens. Useful IHC stains for poorly differentiated oral tumors are listed in Table 20-1.[21,22] Melanomas may be difficult to differentiate from other malignancies because their cells can be round (like lymphoma and plasmacytoma), ovoid (like carcinomas), or spindle shaped (like sarcomas). Melanomas may also be amelanotic, thus lacking the granules that aid in diagnosis. For this reason, it is advisable to make impression smears of biopsy tissues before placing them in formalin so that cytologic evaluation can be compared with the histologic appearance.

Tumor staging should include fine-needle aspiration (FNA) of the regional lymph nodes (particularly those ipsilateral to the mass) even if they are not enlarged. The procedure should be performed *after* CT imaging, since FNA immediately before CT will cause artifactual changes in the appearance of the node on CT. Physical examination alone is a poor predictor of lymph node metastasis.[23,24] In one report, 40% of dogs with MM had nodal metastasis despite having normal-sized lymph nodes.[24] When nodal metastasis is suspected, based on imaging results or node enlargement, excision should be considered. There is no evidence that node excision facilitates distant metastasis. Furthermore, nodal biopsy

may reveal metastasis that is not evident on cytology of an FNA sample.[25] It is important to remember that as well as mandibular nodes, the parotid and medial retropharyngeal nodes, although rarely palpable, also receive lymphatic drainage from the oral cavity. Imaging of all these regional nodes, in addition to the primary tumor, is warranted.[20,26]

Metastasis

Of the oral malignancies encountered in dogs, MM is the most likely to metastasize, with a reported metastatic rate exceeding 80% (Figure 20-4).[19] Feline oral MM is diagnosed infrequently, but has also been associated with pulmonary and other systemic sites of metastasis.[27] Regional lymph node metastasis is relatively uncommon with SCC, although canine tonsillar (Figure 20-5) and canine lingual SCC are exceptions.[4,6,28,29] In some dogs with tonsillar SCC, regional lymph node enlargement caused by metastasis may be the reason for initial presentation, with the primary tumor only clinically evident later in the disease course.[6,30,31] The overall metastatic rate for canine FSA is less than 25%, with the regional lymph nodes or lungs most often affected.[5,18,19,32-34] Osteosarcoma (OSA) within the oral cavity is less likely to metastasize than appendicular OSA.[5,35,36] Benign oral lesions including epulides, ameloblastomas, and odontomas do not metastasize. However, left untreated, they will become quite large and impede normal function (Figure 20-6).

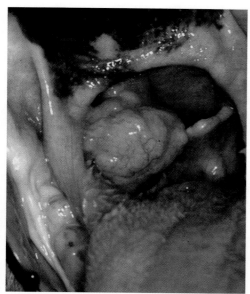

FIGURE 20-5 Tonsillar squamous cell carcinoma as shown here warrants a poor prognosis due to its high metastatic rate and tendency to be detected late in the course of disease.

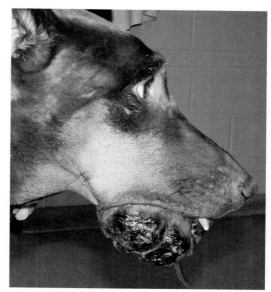

FIGURE 20-6 Epulides, while not malignant, may be life-threatening due to expansive growth that can affect food intake.

Treatment Modalities

Surgery

Complete surgical excision affords the best chance of a cure for most oral malignancies. Epulides do not metastasize and, if small, can be cured with excision alone. When multiple concurrent epulides occur in cats, they are more likely to recur after excision than in dogs; thus, wide excision is advised.[37] Rostrally located malignancies have the best prognosis; thus tumors in this location, including those on the tongue, should be excised with curative intent.[18] Even with excision of over half of the mobile portion of the tongue, dogs can maintain the ability to eat and drink.[6,28,38] Cats, on the other hand, may not tolerate extensive oral surgery as well and may have problems with prehension or compromised grooming ability after partial glossectomy. Results of surgery are summarized in Table 20-2.[5,5,39-47] As long as surgical margins exceed 2 cm, complete maxillectomy or mandibulectomy may not be necessary. In one study, case outcome was similar regardless of the extent of surgery (radical vs. limited) for dogs with MM.[46] Considerable shrinkage of the surgical margins occurs after excision, formalin fixation, and slide preparation of lesions from the tongue and labiobuccal tissue. In fact, surgical margins of 8 to 10 mm are necessary in order to obtain clean histologic margins of 5 mm.[48] This should be taken into account when evaluating histopathology reports after resection and may alter interpretation of literature citing necessary surgical margins at these sites. Owner satisfaction with partial maxillectomy or mandibulectomy in dogs was 85% in one report. Owners perceived that the surgery afforded pain relief and were most pleased with results of rostral mandibulectomy, as compared with partial maxillectomy.[49] Gastrostomy tube placement may be an important aspect of postoperative and palliative care. Dietary management with gastrostomy tube placement is reviewed in Chapter 18, Section B. Cryosurgery can provide good results for small (<2 cm diameter) lesions with minimal bone invasion.[5,6,50,51] Complications such as oronasal fistula or bone necrosis and fracture may occur when cryosurgery is attempted for larger tumors.

Radiation Therapy

Radiation therapy may be used with curative intent for small SCC and epulides, for localized tumors with microscopically incomplete surgical margins, and as a palliative option for unresectable masses, including those crossing the midline of the hard palate. Results with radiation are summarized in Table 20-2.[52-61] Response rates are generally best for SCC, although in one prospective clinical trial of megavoltage irradiation for 105 dogs with oral SCC, FSA, or MM, the only prognostic factor identified was tumor size regardless of tumor type.[52]

TABLE 20-2	REPORTED TREATMENT OUTCOME FOR COMMON ORAL TUMORS IN DOGS AND CATS		
Tumor Type	Outcome Measured	Surgery	Radiation Therapy	Chemotherapy
SCC	1 year survival	Dogs: 70%–91% with mandibulectomy 25% for lingual Cats: <10%	Cats: 30% with adjuvant mitoxantrone 57% with mandibulectomy	
	MST	Dogs: 18 mos	Dogs: 15–16 mos 34 mos when combined with surgery	Dogs: MST not reached with median follow-up of 534 days after piroxicam and carboplatin
		Cats: <6 mos with mandibulectomy 14 mos if surgery combined with radiation and gastrostomy tube placement	Cats: 60 days with hypofractionation 6 mos with adjuvant mitoxantrone 111.5 days with palliative fractionation and adjuvant gemcitabine	
	Response rate			Dogs: 17% with piroxicam 57% with carboplatin and piroxicam Cats: 44% (1 CR and 3 PR in 9 cats) with doxorubicin and cyclophosphamide
FSA	1-year survival	Dogs: 23%–50% with mandibulectomy	Dogs: 331 days with fine fractionation (52.5 Gy) 310 days with coarse fractionation (3 × 8 Gy or 5 × 6 Gy18–26 mos as adjuvant to surgery	
	MST	Dogs: 11 months		
MM	1-year survival	Dogs: 21%–35% with partial mandibulectomy 27% with maxillectomy		
	MST	Dogs: 8–9.9 mos overall 5–10 mos with maxillectomy 7–17 mos with mandibulectomy 511 days for lesions <2 cm and 164 days for lesions >2 cm222 days with lingual	Dogs: 7 months 363-days with hypofractionation and cisplatin or carboplatin chemotherapy Cats: 146 days with hypofractionation	Dogs: Carboplatin and surgery gave 57-day median DFI and 299-day mean DFI
Epulis	Response rate 1-year survival	Dogs: 90%–97%		Dogs: 28% to carboplatin Dogs: 75% with intralesional bleomycin
	MST	Dogs: 36–49 months		

CR, Complete response; *DFI*, disease-free interval; *MST*, median survival time; *PR*, partial response; *SCC*, squamous cell carcinoma.

Therefore, radiation therapy is most likely to be effective when used early in the course of treatment of oral tumors rather than for salvage therapy against large tumors late in their clinical progression. Although radiation response may be short-lived, it is sometimes possible to re-irradiate tumors that do respond, in hopes of achieving a second positive response.[53] Both coarse and fine fractionated radiation protocols (see Chapter 15, Section A for definitions) have been evaluated for treatment of oral tumors. Once-weekly fractionation provides similar clinical responses to standard fractionation for dogs with MM and those with non-resectable soft tissue sarcomas.[54,55] Accordingly, this option may be considered in an effort to prevent extended hospitalization. Coarse fractionation is not recommended for cats with oral cancer because of poor efficacy and unacceptable treatment complications.[56] Hyperthermia improves response to radiation therapy, but is labor-intensive and not readily available.[33]

Medical Therapy

Because local disease progression, rather than metastasis, is often the reason for deaths associated with oral malignancies such as SCC and FSA, systemic chemotherapy may be less important than localized therapy. Adjuvant chemotherapy with mitoxantrone, 5-FU, and cisplatin has improved responses of human head and neck cancers to radiation. These drugs may also prove useful as adjuvant therapy for small animal patients, but published veterinary reports are rare. Neither cisplatin nor 5-FU should be used in cats because of the potential for drug-related fatal toxicity. Improved response rates for non-resectable feline oral SCC may be achieved by combining radiation and mitoxantrone (median survival time = 6 months; 30% 1-year survival*) or gemcitabine chemotherapy.[60] Chemotherapy alone has traditionally offered little benefit in terms of clinical outcome for oral tumors in dogs and cats. Carboplatin has been used to treat oral MM and SCC in dogs with non-resectable tumors.[62,63] The non-steroidal anti-inflammatory drug (NSAID), piroxicam, has shown some promise as a palliative treatment for oral SCC, both as single-agent therapy and in combination with chemotherapy.[63,64] A dose of 0.3 mg/kg/day PO in dogs and q48h in cats may be used if renal function is adequate. Because gastric ulceration may result from the use of NSAIDs, some advocate concurrent administration of a prostaglandin analogue such as misoprostol. Reported

results with chemotherapy for oral malignancy are summarized in Table 20-2.[5,8,59,60,62-70] In an unpublished report, a protocol combining bleomycin (20 mg/m² SC on days 1–3, then weekly for a maximum of 20 doses) and methotrexate (15–20 mg/m² SC weekly on a 4 weeks on/4 weeks off cycle) resulted in an 87.5% overall response rate in 8 cats with SCC (5 CR and 2 PR).* Given this dramatic response rate and the reported lack of serious side effects, further evaluation of this protocol is warranted. Intralesional chemotherapy, usually with cisplatin, has been evaluated for treatment of oral tumors, including canine MM.[71,72] In one report, bleomycin (5 mg) was injected intralesionally once weekly to four dogs with recurrent acanthomatous epulis. All dogs responded, with complete responses in three dogs lasting over 1 year.[72] Intralesional chemotherapy is discussed in Chapter 12, Section E.

Photodynamic Therapy

Photodynamic therapy (PDT) (see Chapter 17 and Figure 14-2) shows promise in the treatment of oral SCC in dogs.[73,74] The treatment requires less hospitalization than radiation therapy and provides excellent cosmesis. In contrast, our experience with PDT for treatment of oral SCC in cats has been disappointing to date.

Immunotherapy/Gene Therapy

Immune enhancement techniques are the focus of active research and are covered in greater detail in Chapter 16. For the oral tumors that occur in veterinary patients, immunotherapy is most promising for MM.[75-78] In 2007, the U.S. Department of Agriculture granted conditional licensure for a canine melanoma vaccine that is intended for use in the minimal disease setting, after the primary tumor has been locally controlled via surgery or radiation therapy. The vaccine is initially being made available only to board-certified oncologists.

Prognosis

Prognosis for dogs and cats with oral tumors is highly dependent upon tumor type and location. Table 20-2 summarizes outcome for various tumor types and treatment modalities reported in the veterinary literature.

SALIVARY GLAND TUMORS

Incidence—Morbidity and Mortality

Tumors of the salivary gland are uncommon in both the dog and cat with a reported incidence of 0.09% in the dog and 0.6% in the cat.[79] In a study of 245

---

*LaRue SM, Vail DM, Ogilvie GK, et al. Shrinking-field radiation therapy in combination with mitoxantrone chemotherapy for the treatment of oral squamous cell carcinoma in the cat. *Proc 11th Ann Conf Vet Cancer Soc*, Minneapolis, Oct 27-29, 1991, p 99.

*Lowe R: *Proc Combined Eur Soc Vet Oncol/Vet Cancer Soc Conf* 2008:7.

BOX 20-4	LIST OF POTENTIAL DIFFERENTIAL DIAGNOSES FOR SALIVARY GLAND ENLARGEMENT[80,93]

Mucocele
Abscess
Salivary gland infarction
Sialadenitis
Sialolithiasis
Edema
Ductal ectasia
Primary neoplasia, malignant or benign
Metastatic neoplasia

BOX 20-5	WORLD HEALTH ORGANIZATION TNM STAGING FOR SALIVARY GLAND TUMORS [95]

T_1	< 2 cm largest dimension
T_2	2-4 cm largest dimension
T_3	> 4 cm largest dimension
N_0	No nodal involvement
N_1	Nodal involvement
M_0	No distant metastasis
M_1	Distant metastasis

Overall Tumor Stage

I	$T_1 N_0 M_0$
II	T_2 or T_3, $N_0 M_0$
III	Any T, $N_1 M_0$
IV	Any T, any N, M_1

salivary gland biopsy specimens, 42% of feline samples were neoplastic, whereas only 25% were neoplastic in dogs.[80] Benign tumors of the salivary gland are rare in both species.[79-82] A male sex predisposition may exist in cats[81]; however, none has been shown in dogs. Siamese cats[81] and spaniel dogs[83] may be predisposed; however, this has not been substantiated in all reports. Salivary tumors appear to occur in older animals with a median age of 10 years in dogs and 12 years in cats.[81]

Etiology and Risk Factors

Most salivary gland tumors in both dogs and cats are epithelial in origin with adenocarcinoma most common.[79-82,84] Other reported histologies include carcinoma,[79,80] acinic cell carcinoma,[81,82] SCC,[79,81,83] mucoepidermoid carcinoma,[82,83] cystadenocarcinoma,[3] mixed carcinoma,[79,82] basal cell adenocarcinoma,[85] sebaceous carcinoma,[86] salivary duct carcinoma,[87] pleomorphic adenoma,[79,80,88] FSA,[79,80] mast cell tumor,[79] lymphoma,[80,89] extraskeletal osteosarcoma,[90] and malignant fibrous histiocytoma (giant cell type).[91] No risk factors have been identified for the development of salivary gland tumors in dogs and cats.

Clinical Features

Most animals are presented for a non-painful swelling in the region of a salivary gland. Tumors can develop in either the major (mandibular, parotid, zygomatic, or sublingual) or minor salivary tissues throughout the oral cavity. The mandibular and parotid glands are most commonly affected in the dog and cat.[79-81,84] Bilateral salivary adenocarcinoma has been reported in a cat.[92] Other non-specific presenting complaints depending upon the salivary gland affected include halitosis, dysphagia, anorexia, weight loss, exophthalmos, the presence of Horner's syndrome, dysphonia, and sneezing.[92,93]

Diagnosis and Staging

FNA cytology is helpful in determining a diagnosis of salivary gland neoplasia.[92,94] Differential diagnoses to consider for salivary masses are included in Box 20-4.[80,93] Because of the potential aggressive biological behavior for salivary tumors, a thorough physical examination, regional lymph node aspiration cytology, and thoracic radiographs are warranted at initial presentation. Skull radiographs may show a soft tissue swelling with or without periosteal reaction of surrounding bone.[93] Computed tomography (CT) is useful to help determine the invasiveness of the neoplasm and to assist the surgeon in planning resection. The World Health Organization TNM staging scheme is shown in Box 20-5.[95]

Metastasis

Metastasis may develop with salivary tumors in both dogs and cats. Cats are more likely to have advanced disease at the time of diagnosis compared with dogs. Hammer et al. showed that at the time of diagnosis; 39% of cats and 17% of dogs had nodal metastasis, and 16% of cats and 8% of dogs had visceral metastasis.[81] The lung is the most frequently reported distant metastatic site.[79,83,92]

Treatment Modalities

When feasible, aggressive surgical resection is warranted. Unfortunately, many salivary neoplasms have extracapsular invasion and are locally extensive, making complete surgical excision unlikely.[82,93] Recurrence is common following surgical resection alone. Adjuvant radiation therapy has been reported and resulted in prolonged survival for three dogs with parotid salivary gland adenocarcinoma.[84] Because of the high potential for metastatic disease, chemotherapy is also warranted, particularly in cats. Drugs to consider should be based upon histologic diagnosis; either as single agents or alternating, doxorubicin and carboplatin are most often considered for salivary adenocarcinoma. Studies are lacking evaluating radiation and chemotherapy for the treatment of salivary neoplasms in companion animals; however, it is the authors' opinion that the best chance for long-term control of a salivary gland tumor is aggressive surgical excision followed by radiation therapy and possibly chemotherapy.

Prognosis and Survival

Incompletely excised salivary tumors consistently recur and adjuvant radiation therapy can be helpful in preventing recurrence.[81,84] Reported median survival times (MSTs) for 24 dogs and 30 cats with salivary gland neoplasms was 550 days and 516 days, respectively. Dogs with stage I or II disease had significantly longer survivals than dogs with stage III or IV disease. Stage of disease was not, however, prognostic in cats.[81]

Selected References*

Berg J: Principles of oncologic orofacial surgery, *Clin Techn Sm Anim Pract* 13:38, 1998.
This manuscript offers a thorough review of important considerations for orofacial surgery.
Carberry CA, Flanders JA, Harvey HJ, et al: Salivary gland tumors in dogs and cats: a literature and case review, *J Am Anim Hosp Assoc* 24:561, 1988.
This is a comprehensive review of salivary gland tumors in dogs and cats.

de Vos JP, Burm AGD, Focker AP, et al: Piroxicam and carboplatin as a combination treatment of canine oral non-tonsillar squamous cell carcinoma: a pilot study and a literature review of a canine model of human head and neck squamous cell carcinoma, *J Vet Comp Oncol* 3:16, 2005.
This pilot study provides the most encouraging results for chemotherapy of canine oral SCC to date.
Dhaliwal RS, Kitchell BE, Marretta SM: Oral tumors in dogs and cats. Part II. Prognosis and treatment, *Compendium* 20:1109, 1998.
This review paper provides useful recommendations for treatment of canine and feline oral tumors.
Evans SM, Thrall DE: Postoperative orthovoltage radiation therapy of parotid salivary gland adenocarcinoma in three dogs, *J Am Vet Med Assoc* 182:993, 1983.
This manuscript reports on response to radiation therapy of three dogs with parotid salivary gland adenocarcinoma.
Hammer A, Getzy D, Ogilvie G, et al: Salivary gland neoplasia in the dog and cat: survival times and prognostic factors, *J Am Anim Hosp Assoc* 37:478, 2001.
This is the largest and most recent clinical study of salivary gland tumors in dogs and cats and evaluates location, survival time, and prognostic factors.
Proulx DR, Ruslander DM, Dodge RK, et al: A retrospective analysis of 140 dogs with oral melanoma treated with external beam radiation, *Vet Radiol Ultrasound* 44:352, 2003.
This large retrospective study showed no difference in response rate of MM to radiation based on fractionation scheme and established rostral tumor location, lack of bone lysis, and smaller tumor volume as predictors of a better prognosis.
Syrcle JA, Bonczynski JJ, Monette S, et al: Retrospective evaluation of lingual tumors in 42 dogs: 1999-2005, *J Am Anim Hosp Assoc* 44:308, 2008.
This retrospective review highlights findings in dogs with tongue tumors and supports the previous report by Beck et al.[4] that lingual melanoma is more common than lingual SCC in dogs.

■ *For a complete list of the references cited in this chapter, please go to www.smallanimaloncology.com.

SECTION B: Nasal Tumors

Mary Lynn Higginbotham and Carolyn J. Henry

KEY POINTS

- Dogs with intranasal tumors are often presented for unilateral or bilateral nasal discharge that may be hemorrhagic and is often initially antibiotic responsive.
- Nasal discharge is less common in cats with intranasal tumors than dogs; epiphora and facial deformity are often associated with feline intranasal tumors.
- Radiation therapy is the primary treatment for canine intranasal tumors, with a median survival time of approximately 1 year.
- Lymphoma is a common intranasal feline tumor that has a good response to multi-modal therapy and median survival time in excess of 2 years.
- Nasal planum squamous cell carcinomas are locally invasive tumors of dogs and cats that carry a good long-term prognosis with early intervention and aggressive local therapy.

Incidence—Morbidity and Mortality

Nasal tumors may be *intranasal*—arising from the tissues inside the nasal cavity such as the epithelial lining, cartilage, bone, or lymphoid tissues— or they may be *extranasal*—arising from the nasal planum or other tissues covering the nose. The majority of canine and feline nasal tumors are malignant.[1] Common intranasal tumors include various carcinomas and sarcomas as well as lymphoma (Box 20-6). Adenocarcinoma is the most common intranasal tumor in the dog[1-3] whereas lymphoma is most common in the cat.[1,4,5] SCC is the most frequently encountered tumor of the nasal planum in both species.

Etiology and Risk Factors

Long-nosed dogs (dolichocephalic breeds) are suspected to be at increased risk for intranasal tumor development.[1] Exposure to environmental tobacco smoke, use of topical insecticides, and exposure to indoor coal or kerosene heaters have been associated with an increased risk of developing intranasal cancer.[6,7] Cyclooxygenase-2 (COX-2) expression has been found to be upregulated in canine intranasal carcinomas and may play a role in the pathogenesis of this disease.[8-10] Exposure to ultraviolet (UV) light is a risk factor for the development of nasal planum tumors in cats.[11]

Clinical Features of Canine Intranasal Tumors

Clinical signs associated with intranasal tumors are due to erosion of the mucosa, destruction of the turbinates, and invasion into the surrounding structures by the tumor (Box 20-7). The majority of animals with intranasal tumors are presented with nasal discharge that initially responds to antibiotics. Clinical signs often recur soon after the discontinuation of the antibiotic. Adenocarcinoma is the most frequently diagnosed intranasal tumor in the dog.[1-3] Metastasis at the time of diagnosis is rare,[12] but approaches 40% in dogs that succumb to the disease.[13] Lymph nodes and lungs are the most common metastatic sites, but other sites including skin[14] and bone[14,15] have been documented. Paraneoplastic hypercalcemia has been reported in dogs with nasal carcinoma.[16,17]

Chondrosarcoma (CSA) is the most common intranasal mesenchymal tumor in dogs.[1] Metastasis at the time of diagnosis of nasal sarcomas is uncommon. Paraneoplastic erythrocytosis has been documented in one dog with a nasal FSA.[18]

Clinical Features of Feline Intranasal Tumors

Lymphoma is the most frequently diagnosed feline intranasal tumor and often occurs in older cats.[5] It can cause significant erosion of the nasal or frontal sinus cavities, resulting in severe facial deformity. The majority of cats with nasal lymphoma do not have evidence of systemic disease at the time of diagnosis; however, up to 20% of cats will have disease progression outside of the nasal cavity with time.[19,20] Intranasal carcinomas also occur in cats. Metastasis at diagnosis is uncommon.

Clinical Features of Canine Extranasal Tumors

Extranasal SCC is most often associated with the nasal planum in dogs. Metastasis at the time of diagnosis is rare.[21,22]

When occurring within the extranasal tissue, lymphoma typically appears as a non-pigmented plaque associated with the mucocutaneous junction and nasal philtrum. Lymphoma in this site is often epitheliotrophic in nature, is of T-cell origin, and may be the only

---

BOX 20-6 MOST FREQUENTLY DIAGNOSED NASAL TUMORS IN DOGS AND CATS

Adenocarcinoma
Squamous cell carcinoma
Non-keratinizing squamous cell carcinoma (transitional carcinoma)
Undifferentiated carcinoma
Neuroendocrine carcinoma
Chondrosarcoma
Osteosarcoma
Fibrosarcoma
Hemangiosarcoma
Mast cell tumor
Lymphoma
Transmissible venereal tumor

BOX 20-7 CLINICAL SIGNS ASSOCIATED WITH INTRANASAL TUMORS

Unilateral or bilateral epistaxis
Unilateral or bilateral mucoid to mucopurulent nasal discharge
Sneezing
Reverse sneezing
Epiphora
Facial deformity
Neurologic signs

detectable disease at the time of diagnosis.[23] In general, however, lymphoma is considered a systemic disease, and thorough staging is recommended.

Clinical Features of Feline Extranasal Tumors

SCC is the most common feline extranasal tumor. Cats with nasal planum tumors are usually light skinned, white-haired cats that may also have lesions associated with their pinnae and conjunctiva resulting from chronic UV light exposure. These solar-induced lesions progress from what is described as actinic keratosis to non-invasive carcinoma *in situ* (where the tumor does not invade the epidermal basement membrane) to invasive SCCs.[11] These tumors are often confused with non-healing wounds early in the course of disease when they are ulcerated, scabbed lesions. Metastasis is uncommon and treatment is aimed at controlling local disease.[24]

Diagnosis and Staging

Physical Examination

For animals presenting with clinical signs associated with the upper airway, close attention should be paid to assessment of air flow through the nostrils, ocular examination, oral examination, and regional lymph node examination. Air flow may be assessed using either a glass slide or cotton ball and evaluating for condensation on the slide or

movement of the cotton as air flows from the nasal passage. The patient should be assessed for facial deformity (Figure 20-7) that indicates erosion of the nasal bone and infiltration into the extranasal soft tissues. Decreased retropulsion of either or both of the eyes suggests that the mass has eroded into the orbit. Ocular discharge may also be a sign of orbital compromise because of an invasive nasal tumor. An oral examination should be performed to assess for asymmetry of the hard and soft palates. Careful lymph node palpation should be performed, paying special attention to mandibular and prescapular nodes. Lymph node aspiration and cytology are recommended even if nodes are not considered palpably abnormal.

Bloodwork

A minimum database including a CBC, biochemical profile, and urinalysis should be performed in all patients suspected of having a nasal tumor. A coagulation profile and blood pressure measurement should be done for animals presenting with epistaxis in order to rule out etiologies other than primary nasal cancer.

Imaging Studies

Thoracic radiographs should be evaluated for the presence of pulmonary metastatic disease. Skull radiographs may be helpful in evaluating for a nasal mass, although

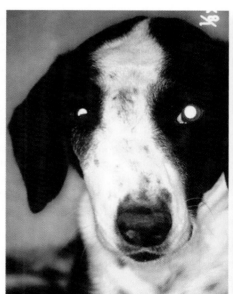
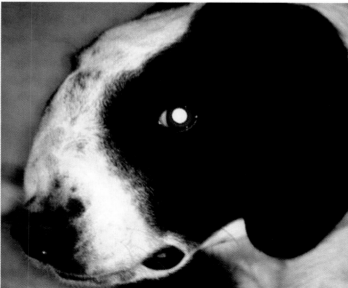

FIGURE 20-7 Facial deformity may be a feature of a nasal malignancy that has eroded through the nasal bone and infiltrated the extranasal soft tissues. (Photos courtesy of Dr. Eric Pope.)

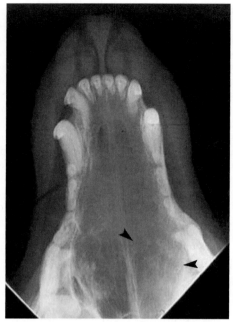

FIGURE 20-8 Intraoral radiograph of the nasal cavity in a dog with an intranasal adenocarcinoma. Note the increased soft tissue opacity in the caudal aspect of the right side of the nasal cavity. No radiographic evidence of lysis of the nasal septum or other structures is evident in this film. (Photo courtesy of the University of Missouri Veterinary Oncology Service.)

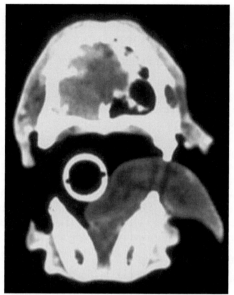

FIGURE 20-9 CT image of the dog in Figure 20-8. This nasal mass appears to originate in and consume the right nasal cavity. Note the erosion of the nasal septum and the extension of the mass into the left nasal cavity. (Photo courtesy of the University of Missouri Veterinary Oncology Service.)

lack of radiographic evidence of a nasal tumor does not rule out its presence. CT is superior to radiography when evaluating the nasal cavity and is recommended over radiographs when one has a high index of suspicion for a nasal malignancy.[25] Figures 20-8 and 20-9 offer comparison of radiography and CT for identification of a nasal mass in a dog. In addition to confirming the presence of a mass, a CT scan will enable assessment of the local disease and provide the images necessary for radiation treatment planning. Disease stage is prognostic for dogs who are treated with radiation therapy for intranasal tumors.[26,27] It is, however, important to remember that the CT scan should be performed before biopsy and aspiration of regional lymph nodes in order to prevent iatrogenic contrast enhancement that could be misinterpreted as neoplastic disease on the CT images.

Rhinoscopy

Rhinoscopy is useful for visualizing a mass before a transnasal biopsy, as well as for assessing for fungal plaques, nasal mites, or other non-neoplastic causes of

nasal disease. As with FNAs and biopsies, rhinoscopy may cause hemorrhage that leads to subsequent contrast enhancement on CT images. As such, rhinoscopy should follow, rather than precede, CT when both imaging modalities are used.

Biopsy and Histopathology

Histopathology is necessary to confirm a diagnosis and may be facilitated by transnasal biopsy. This technique is preferred over an approach through the skin, since it minimizes the possibility for creating a biopsy tract that will necessitate skin excision at a later date. Alligator forceps or forceps with a round cup biopsy tip are passed through the nares to the level of the mass, as indicated on CT scan or until resistance is met. The biopsy should be taken at this location. Before beginning the procedure, it is recommended to mark the biopsy instrument with tape or a marker at the depth of the medial canthus of the eye by aligning the instrument with the bridge of the nose to measure the distance from the nares to the caudal aspect of the nasal cavity (Figure 20-10). This will prevent inadvertently passing the biopsy instrument through the cribriform plate. A minimum of five tissue

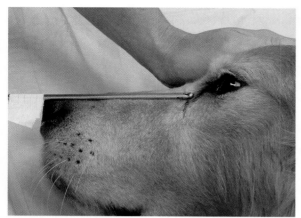

FIGURE 20-10 Before obtaining a transnasal biopsy sample, it is important to mark the biopsy instrument to indicate the length to the medial canthus. This will prevent inadvertent advancement of the biopsy instrument through the cribriform plate. (Photo courtesy of University of Missouri Veterinary Oncology Service.)

samples should be obtained in order to provide an adequate and representative sample for the pathologist to review. Aspiration[3] and hydropulsion* techniques have also been described to obtain nasal biopsies. The hydropulsion technique was successful in obtaining tissue in 92% of cases and provided clinical relief to the patient by non-invasive tumor debulking.*

Treatment Modalities

Canine Intranasal Tumors

Because of the relatively low metastatic rate, treatment recommendations for intranasal tumors are primarily aimed at controlling the local disease with either surgical resection or radiation therapy. Surgical resection results in an average survival time of 3 to 9 months[3,28] and has not been shown to be superior to radiation therapy in the treatment of canine intranasal tumors. Megavoltage radiation therapy (administered by a linear accelerator or Cobalt 60 machine) is the mainstay of treatment for intranasal tumors and appears to be superior to orthovoltage therapy.[14] (See Chapter 15, Section A, for a description of megavoltage and orthovoltage radiation therapy.) A significant survival benefit to combining surgery and radiation therapy over radiation therapy alone has yet to be demonstrated.[12,29] A survival benefit was noted, however,

---

*Ashbaugh EA, McKiernan BC, Miller CJ, et al: Hydropulsion to biopsy and debulk nasal tumors, abstract, 26th Annual American College of Veterinary Internal Medicine Forum, San Antonio, TX, June 4-7, 2008 (unpublished data).

when surgery was performed after radiation therapy to control residual or recurrent disease.[30] Toxicity and long-term side effects were also significantly higher in this small group of dogs treated with radiation therapy followed by surgery.[30] Few reports exist evaluating chemotherapy as sole treatment or as an adjuvant to radiation therapy. No survival benefit has been noted when chemotherapy has been used in a radiosensitizing role for the treatment of intranasal tumors.[31] Minimal response was noted to cisplatin alone,[32] but results were more promising with carboplatin-doxorubicin-piroxicam therapy.[33] COX-2 expression has been documented in intranasal carcinomas,[8-10] justifying the use of COX-2 inhibitors in the treatment of this disease, but studies evaluating response to this treatment are lacking at this time. See Table 20-3 for more information regarding treatment options and outcome for dogs with nasal tumors.

Feline Intranasal Tumors

Because of the potential for disease progression outside of the nasal cavity, multimodal therapy with multi-agent chemotherapy and radiation therapy is recommended for feline nasal lymphoma and has resulted in prolonged survival times in cats with this disease.[20] There are no reported prospective studies that compare outcome for cats with nasal lymphoma treated with chemotherapy or radiation therapy versus the combination of chemotherapy and radiation therapy. Radiation therapy is the recommended treatment for intranasal carcinomas in cats.

Canine Extranasal Tumors

Treatment of canine extranasal SCC often consists of surgery, with long-term survivals (>2 years) reported after nasal planum and premaxilla resection.[22,34,35] Figure 20-11 illustrates preoperative and postoperative images of dogs treated with surgery for nasal planum SCC. Reports of radiation therapy for canine nasal planum SCC have had less impressive results.[22] No consistent therapy recommendations exist for lymphoma associated with the nasal planum in the dog. Aggressive local therapy with surgery or radiation therapy followed by systemic chemotherapy or careful surveillance for disease recurrence after local therapy are reasonable treatment options. See Chapter 25, Section A, for further discussion of lymphoma.

Feline Extranasal Tumors

Surgery,[24] external beam radiation therapy,[36] and strontium 90 plesiotherapy[37,38] have all been shown to be effective treatments for SCC associated with the nasal planum in cats. If treated when the lesions are small and

TABLE 20-3   REPORTED SURVIVAL OF DOGS WITH INTRANASAL TUMORS FOLLOWING RADIATION THERAPY

Reference	No. of Patients	Histology	Type of Radiation	Total Dose	Median Survival (Mos)	Percentage Of 1- And 2-Year Survival
Thrall[42]	21	All types	O	26–55 Gy	23	57%, 48%
Adams[13]	67	All types	M and O	32–53 Gy	8.5	38%, 30%
McEntee[29]	27	All types	M	41.8–54 Gy	12.8	59%, 22%
Théon[26]	77	All types	M	48 Gy	12.6	60.3%, 25%
Adams[27]	21	All types	M	42 Gy	14.25	60%, 36%
Henry[12]	53	ACA	M	48 Gy	14.1	NR
Northrup[14]	42	All types	O	48 Gy	7.4	37%, 17%
Mellanby[44]	56	All types	M	36 Gy	7.0	45%, 15%
Correa[41]	6	Transitional carcinoma*	M	54–63 Gy	5.5	None
Lana[43]	51	All types	M	54 Gy	15.8	NR
Nadeau[31]	31	Carcinomas	M	48–50 Gy	14.4	NR
Adams[30]	53	All types	M	42 Gy	RT = 19.7 RT/sx = 47.7	RT = 68%, 44% RT/sx = 77%, 69%

ACA, Adenocarcinoma; *Gy*, gray; *M*, megavoltage radiation therapy; *NR*, not reported; *O*, orthovoltage radiation therapy; *RT*, radiation therapy; *sx*, surgery.

*Also known as non-keratinizing squamous cell carcinoma.

non-invasive, local control is likely. However, careful surveillance must follow, since new lesions often develop because of the diffuse UV light exposure.[38] Intralesional carboplatin therapy has also been described with reasonable response rates.[39]

Prognosis and Survival

Overall, the prognosis for nasal tumors is guarded. Most dogs with malignant nasal tumors eventually die from their tumor, usually due to progression of local disease.[40] Without treatment, the prognosis for dogs with nasal carcinomas is approximately 3 months.[3,40] Survival of dogs with intranasal tumors following radiation therapy is provided in Table 20-3. Prognostic information for intranasal tumors in dogs varies between studies. Factors evaluated—including tumor histology, local disease stage, patient age, and length of time clinical signs have been present—have not consistently been shown to have prognostic significance for dogs treated for intranasal tumors. However, regardless of treatment, SCC,[13] undifferentiated carcinoma[13] and non-keratinizing SCC (transitional carcinoma)[41] carry a more guarded prognosis than adenocarcinoma. No significant difference in prognosis has been demonstrated for intranasal sarcomas when compared with carcinomas in multiple studies[29,30,42-44] and

reported MSTs range from 7 to 23 months.[26,29,42-44] MST after radiation therapy for canine nasal CSA is approximately 12 months.[26] The presence of metastatic disease does appear to be a negative prognostic indicator in dogs with intranasal tumors.[12] In addition, facial deformity has been shown to be a negative prognostic indicator.[14]

An MST of 31 months has been reported for cats with nasal lymphoma treated with radiation therapy and chemotherapy,[20] compared with approximately 3 months for cats treated with chemotherapy alone.[5] See Chapter 25, Section A, for further discussion of lymphoma. MSTs for cats treated with radiation therapy for intranasal carcinomas range from 12 to 19 months[45,46] and 1-year survival rates from 44% to 63%.[46,47]

The prognosis for nasal planum SCCs in dogs and cats appears to be good with aggressive therapy and local disease control. Long-term survival of greater than 2 years has been reported after nasal planum and premaxilla resection in dogs with nasal planum SCC.[22,34,35] Without intervention, survival of 5 months is average for dogs with this disease.[21] Reported average survival times of 19 months[41] have been reported with surgery and 21 to 105 months with strontium 90 therapy for feline extranasal SCC.[37,38]

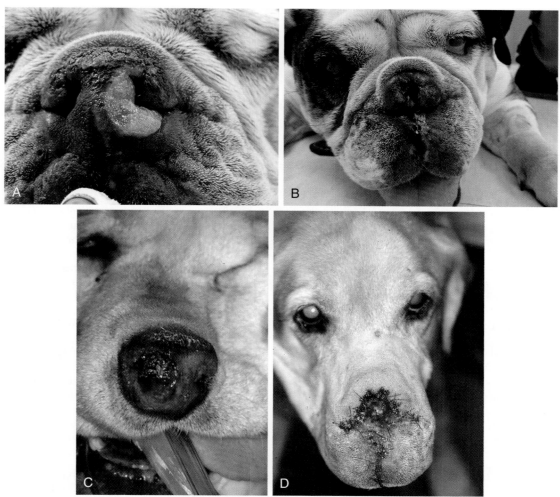

FIGURE 20-11 Preoperative and postoperative photos of two dogs treated for squamous cell carcinoma via partial nosectomy and bilateral alar fold plasty (**A, B**) or complete nasal planectomy (**C, D**). (Photos courtesy of University of Missouri Veterinary Oncology Service.)

Selected References*

Lana SE, Ogilvie GK, Withrow SJ, et al: Feline cutaneous squamous cell carcinoma of the nasal planum and the pinnae: 61 cases, *J Am Anim Hosp Assoc* 33:329, 1997.
This is the largest study evaluating the outcome for cutaneous squamous cell carcinoma associated with the ears and nasal planum in cats.
Lascelles BDX, Parry AT, Stidworthy MF, et al: Squamous cell carcinoma of the nasal planum in 17 dogs, *Vet Rec* 147:473, 2000.

This is the largest study evaluating the response to various treatment options for canine nasal planum squamous cell carcinoma.
Rassnick KM, Goldkamp CE, Erb HN, et al: Evaluation of factors associated with survival in dogs with untreated nasal carcinomas: 139 cases (1993-2003), *J Am Vet Med Assoc* 229:401, 2006.
This manuscript discusses prognosis for untreated nasal carcinomas in dogs.
Sfiligoi G, Théon AP, Kent MS: Response of nineteen cats with nasal lymphoma to radiation therapy and chemotherapy, *Vet Radiol Ultrasound* 48:388, 2007.

The response to treatment and prognosis associated with feline intranasal lymphoma are presented in this prospective study.

Théon AP, Madewell BR, Harb MF, et al: Megavoltage irradiation of neoplasms of the nasal and paranasal cavities in 77 dogs, *J Am Vet Med Assoc* 202:1469, 1993.
The response to radiation treatment, prognosis, and prognostic factors associated with outcome are evaluated in this paper.

Théon AP, Peaston AE, Madewell BR, et al: Irradiation of nonlymphoproliferative neoplasms of the nasal cavity and paranasal sinuses in 16 cats, *J Am Vet Med Assoc* 204:78, 1994.
Evaluation of response to treatment and prognosis of cats with non-lymphoma intranasal tumors are reported in this study.

■ *For a complete list of the references cited in this chapter, please go to www.smallanimaloncology.com.

SECTION C: Ocular and Periocular Tumors

Elizabeth A. Giuliano

KEY POINTS

- Exophthalmos and strabismus are the two most common presenting signs associated with orbital tumors.
- Typically, examination of the oral cavity in cases of retrobulbar neoplasia does not elicit the pain response seen in cases of retrobulbar abscessation.
- Whereas most eyelid tumors in dogs are benign and warrant an excellent prognosis, feline eyelid tumors are often malignant (squamous cell carcinoma and malignant melanoma).
- In contrast to intraocular melanocytoma in dogs, which is largely considered to be benign with a low metastatic potential, diffuse iris melanoma in cats can be an aggressive tumor with a potential of malignancy.
- Any eyelid or conjunctival mass, no matter how benign in clinical appearance, should be submitted for histopathologic examination.

OVERVIEW OF THE APPROACH TO OCULAR TUMORS

Patients with tumors affecting the orbit, eyelid, or globe may present with signs of ocular discomfort and/or vision loss.[1-5] Numerous primary and metastatic ocular and periocular tumors have been reported and classified histologically (Table 20-4).[6] Regardless of the underlying diagnosis, concern for the patient's vision and ocular comfort should guide the diagnostic and therapeutic plan. The patient should be examined first at a distance, and then at eye level. An examination room that can be completely darkened to permit accurate assessment of intraocular structures is essential. The "minimum ophthalmic data base" (Box 20-8) should be acquired during all ophthalmic examinations, almost without exception. Caution should be exercised when performing tonometry on any patient concurrently affected with a deep corneal ulcer to avoid globe perforation. Retropulsion and assessment of ocular motility is often helpful in cases of suspected orbital tumors or intraocular tumors with extrascleral extension. Additional diagnostic procedures that can be performed by the general practitioner include nasolacrimal flushing, conjunctival/corneal swabs for cytology and culture, and eyelid or conjunctival biopsy.

Once the ophthalmic examination is completed, more advanced diagnostic imaging such as ocular ultrasound, skull radiographs, and/or CT or magnetic resonance imaging (MRI) may be indicated. These additional diagnostics are especially helpful when evidence of extrascleral extension is likely to alter the diagnosis, prognosis, or surgical planning. Consultation with or referral to a veterinary ophthalmologist may be helpful. A list of board-certified ophthalmologists may be found at www.acvo.com.

Clinical Features and Biological Behavior of Common Ocular and Periocular Tumors

Orbital Tumors

The orbit is composed of bone, nerves, vessels, and soft tissue, any of which may give rise to neoplasia.[5,7] Specific histologic identification of some orbital tumors is problematic because the exact tissue of origin is frequently difficult to determine.[8] Resources in the literature reports are often limited to individual case reports, with diagnoses rarely confirmed by electron microscopy or IHC.[9-11] Both retrobulbar spindle cell tumors (e.g., rhabdomyosarcoma, hemangiosarcoma, liposarcoma, FSA, fibrous histiocytoma) and neural/neuroendocrine tumors may be difficult to identify histologically.[12-17]

When considering orbital tumors as a whole, signalment may vary. However, in general, the younger the animal is when diagnosed with a malignant neoplasm, the more guarded the prognosis.[7] Patients are

TABLE 20-4   HISTOLOGIC CLASSIFICATION SCHEME OF OCULAR TUMORS IN DOGS AND CATS DEMONSTRATING THE WIDE VARIETY OF POSSIBLE OPHTHALMIC TUMOR TYPES

Ocular Tumor	Possible Tumor Types

Orbital tumors	Retrobulbar spindle cell tumors
	  ○ Canine orbital meningioma
	Lacrimal gland tumors
	  ○ Lacrimal adenoma
	  ○ Lacrimal adenocarcinoma
	Bony tumors
	  ○ Multilobular osteoma
	  ○ Multilobular osteochondroma
	  ○ Multilobular osteochondrosarcoma
	  ○ Chondroma rodens

Eyelid and conjunctival tumors	Tumors of the haired eyelid
	  ○ Meibomian adenoma
	  ○ Melanocytoma and malignant melanoma
	  ○ Squamous cell carcinoma
	  ○ Squamous papilloma
	  ○ Chalazion
	Third eyelid and conjunctival tumors
	  ○ Squamous cell carcinoma
	  ○ Conjunctival malignant melanoma
	  ○ Hemangioma and hemangiosarcoma
	  ○ Angiokeratoma
	  ○ Adenocarcinoma
	  ○ Lymphosarcoma
	  ○ Nodular granulomatous episcleritis
	  ○ Mast cell tumor
	  ○ Conjunctival inclusion cyst

Intraocular tumors	Melanocytic tumors
	  ○ Canine anterior uveal melanocytoma
	  ○ Limbal melanocytoma
	  ○ Canine choroidal melanocytoma
	  ○ Canine diffuse uveal melanosis
	  ○ Feline diffuse iris melanoma
	  ○ Feline multifocal uveal melanocytoma
	Iridociliary epithelial tumors
	  ○ Iridociliary adenoma
	  ○ Iridociliary adenocarcinoma
	Medulloepithelioma
	Iridociliary cysts
	Feline primary ocular sarcoma (post-traumatic sarcoma)
	Iridal spindle cell tumor of blue-eyed dogs
	Optic nerve glioma
	Metastatic tumors

BOX 20-8   KEY COMPONENTS OF THE COMPLETE OPHTHALMIC EXAMINATION*

The Minimum Ophthalmic Database
1. Menace response
2. Pupillary light reflex (direct and consensual)
3. Palpebral reflex
4. Schirmer tear test
5. Fluorescein stain
6. Tonometry (note: exercise caution in those patients concurrently affected with a deep corneal ulcer)
7. Careful examination of the anterior and posterior segments. Indirect funduscopy is advocated over direct funduscopy whenever possible.
8. Globe retropulsion and assessment of ocular motility should be performed whenever an orbital tumor or intraocular tumor with extrascleral extension is suspected.

*To be performed, in the order listed, when working up or monitoring any patient affected with, or undergoing treatment for, an ocular or periocular tumor.

---

often not presented until the disease is quite advanced. Exophthalmos and strabismus are the two most common presenting signs. Globe deviation varies according to the position of the mass within the orbit. For example, a tumor arising from the superior-temporal quadrant of the orbit will more than likely result in a ventro-medial strabismus. Typically, examination of the oral cavity in cases of retrobulbar neoplasia does not elicit the pain response that is seen in cases of retrobulbar abscessation. If lagophthalmos (an inability to completely close the eyelids) occurs as a result of exophthalmos, exposure keratitis and corneal ulceration frequently result. Owners may first become aware of an orbital problem only after secondary corneal ulceration occurs and the dog or cat suddenly becomes painful. For this reason, any corneal ulcer should prompt careful comparison of globe position. By holding the patient's head horizontally and viewing from above, one can look for evidence of exophthalmos, which is distinguished from buphthalmos by comparing the limbus-to-limbus diameter between globes. In exophthalmos the limbus-to-limbus diameter should be symmetrical, whereas a buphthalmic globe will have an increased limbus-to-limbus diameter caused by globe stretching.

The most commonly reported and well-recognized orbital tumors include meningioma, lacrimal gland

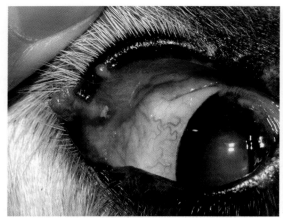

FIGURE 20-12 Two meibomian adenomas demonstrating typical fusiform shape along the margin of the upper eyelid in parallel with the meibomian glands. A proliferative, pedunculated, "cauliflower-type," squamous papilloma is seen overlying the temporal-most meibomian adenoma. These are the most common eyelid tumors in dogs.

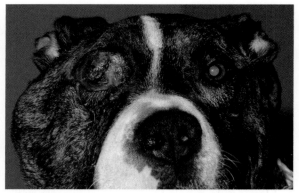

FIGURE 20-13 Superior right eyelid mast cell tumor in a 4-year-old, male, castrated Boxer. Note the extensive swelling along the right side of the face associated with this primary eyelid tumor.

tumors, and secondary tumors.[6,18-20] Orbital meningiomas arise from the meninges of the optic nerve and grow expansively within the periorbital region.[19] They may infiltrate retrograde through the sclera and into the choroid, eventually entering the subretinal space, or may travel normograde through the optic foramen into the calvarium.[21] Vision loss may occur. Lacrimal tumors may be benign (lacrimal adenoma) or malignant (lacrimal adenocarcinoma).[22] The latter may invade surrounding normal tissues even when the histologic appearance of the tumor cells suggests a less aggressive lesion (i.e., relatively mature appearing cells). Glandular orbital tumors may also arise from the zygomatic salivary gland, with the main clinical difference being tumor location (the zygomatic salivary gland is ventromedial, and tumors arising from the lacrimal gland originate superotemporally).[16,23,24] Secondary tumors affect the orbit either by direct extension from surrounding areas or by vascular metastasis from distant sites. Given the close proximity of the oral and nasal cavities, it is not uncommon for oral and nasal tumors to induce secondary ophthalmic manifestations including, but not limited to, exophthalmos, strabismus, and/or serosanguineous epiphora. Lymphoma may metastasize to the orbit in small animal patients, although this is most commonly recognized in cattle.[25] Finally, orbital invasion resulting from extrascleral extension of a primary intraocular neoplasm is most frequently seen in cases of feline ocular sarcoma (see intraocular tumors).[11,26]

Eyelid and Conjunctival Tumors

As a general rule, canine eyelid tumors are primary, are benign, do not metastasize, and carry a very favorable prognosis with low recurrence rates when treated appropriately.[27] The most common eyelid tumors in dogs include the meibomian adenoma and squamous papilloma.[28,29] Meibomian adenomas appear as irregular, fusiform, usually pigmented nodules along the eyelid margin and are prone to bleeding if irritated by the dog's rubbing. Squamous papillomas are proliferative, pedunculated lesions with a "cauliflower-type" appearance and variable pigmentation commonly seen overlying meibomian adenomas (Figure 20-12). A variety of other tumor types may arise from the eyelid, with mast cell tumors being some of the most impressive (Figure 20-13).[30] The eyelids can be the site of secondary, metastatic lymphoma (Figure 20-14) in addition to the more typical intraocular location of metastatic lymphoma.[31-33]

In contrast to dogs, eyelid tumors affecting cats are much more likely to be malignant.[34] SCC predominates, particularly in cats with little to no pigmentation.[35] UV light damage from sunlight is believed to be a predisposing factor in the development of this tumor type. Early, preneoplastic lesions are typically erythematous, scaly, slightly raised lesions along the eyelid margins that may be ulcerated. As the disease progresses, a firm intradermal or subcutaneous mass can be appreciated.

Melanocytic neoplasia affects the eyelids of dogs and cats and further illustrates the differences between these two species.[36] In dogs, melanocytic tumors arising from the haired skin are almost always behaviorally benign and, thus, more appropriately called melanocytomas.

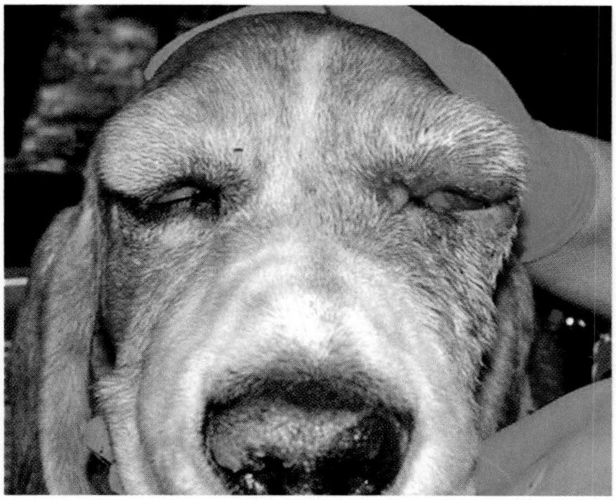

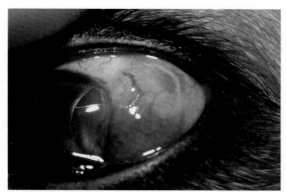

FIGURE 20-14 A 7-year-old, male, neutered Basset Hound presenting with marked bilateral eyelid swelling as the initial most significant finding after relapse from lymphoma. (Photograph courtesy of Dr. Kim Selting.)

FIGURE 20-15 Nodular granulomatous episcleritis in a dog. These nodular, pink to grey proliferative, subconjunctival lesions arise from the temporal limbus in young to middle-aged dogs and can be mistaken for neoplastic lesions. Etiology is thought to be autoimmune.

In contrast, in cats, more than half are malignant (i.e., MM), are often less pigmented than those seen in their canine counterparts, and show invasive growth.

Conjunctival MM occurs in both dogs and cats.[37] When arising from the conjunctiva, MM behaves much more aggressively than when it originates in the anterior uveal tract or haired skin of the eyelids. Conjunctival MM may or may not be pigmented, making diagnosis a challenge.[38,39] Canine conjunctival melanomas often arise from the bulbar surface of the third eyelid and are most common in dogs over 10 years of age.[40]

SCC and mast cell tumors also occur as primary conjunctival lesions, whereas conjunctival lymphoma may occur as a secondary lesion in a patient with generalized lymphoma.[41] A vascularized, raised lesion arising from the leading edge of the third eyelid or bulbar conjunctiva in the dog is most likely to be a tumor of vascular origin.[42] Differentials include hemangioma, angiokeratoma, or hemangiosarcoma.[43-46] As with any mass removal, all resected tissue should be submitted for histopathologic examination. Definitive diagnosis is largely based upon growth characteristics, rather than specific cytologic criteria. Adenocarcinoma arising from the third eyelid is occasionally reported in older-aged dogs and is rare in cats.[47] Nodular, pink to grey proliferative, subconjunctival lesions that arise from the temporal limbus in young to middle-aged dogs are most consistently termed nodular granulomatous episcleritis (NGE) (Figure 20-15). These lesions are not uncommon and collies and collie-crosses are

predisposed. Other terms for this condition include *nodular fasciitis, nodular granulomatous episclerokeratitis,* and *ocular fibrous histiocytoma.* Lesions are frequently bilateral, but not always symmetrical or identical in time of onset. NGE is composed of macrophages, lymphocytes, and plasma cells with no real features of malignancy. Most veterinary ophthalmologists consider the disease to be an immune-mediated phenomenon. Nevertheless, given its relatively common occurrence in dogs and its "cancer-like" appearance, NGE deserves consideration when examining nodular conjunctival ocular lesions.

Intraocular Tumors

The three primary intraocular tumors affecting dogs and cats that warrant discussion include melanocytic neoplasia, iridociliary epithelial tumors, and feline primary ocular sarcoma (post-traumatic sarcoma).[48-50] Melanocytic neoplasia is the most common intraocular tumor in both dogs and cats.[51,52] As discussed in the previous section, the biological behavior of this melanoma is highly species dependent.[53,54] In dogs, intraocular melanocytoma most commonly presents as a nodular mass arising from the anterior uveal tract (iris and/or ciliary body) (Figure 20-16).[55] The average age at diagnosis in dogs is 7 years, with no apparent gender predilection. Many different breeds are affected. In cats, the most common primary intraocular site is also the anterior uveal tract, but the lesion is more appropriately termed *diffuse iris melanoma (DIM)* because of its clinical appearance and

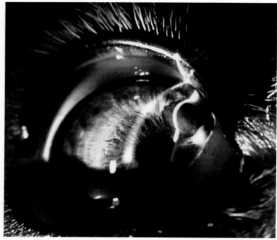

FIGURE 20-16 A 2-year-old, female, spayed Labrador Retriever with focal anterior uveal melanocytic neoplasia. Note the raised, hyperpigmented, nodular mass on the anterior iris surface as seen on slit-lamp biomicroscopy in this photograph. This patient responded very well to diode laser ablation and has been visual and comfortable for 5 years after surgery.

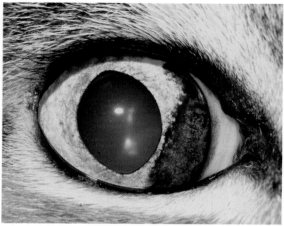

FIGURE 20-17 Fifteen-year-old female, spayed, domestic short-hair with a diffuse iris melanoma extending from the 1 o'clock to 6 o'clock position. Although the lesion was not raised on slit-lamp biomicroscopy, invasion into the iridocorneal angle was evident on gonioscopy.

biological behavior.[56] DIM is classically characterized by iridal golden to dark brown pigmented foci that begin to slowly (months to years) coalesce into larger pigmented areas that often involve most or all of the iris (Figure 20-17).[57] In contrast to intraocular melanocytoma in dogs where the condition is largely considered to be benign with a low metastatic potential, DIM in cats may be an aggressive tumor with the potential to metastasize, albeit often with long latency periods.[58,59] Metastasis, reported to be as high as 63% in cats in one study,[60] is usually first to regional lymph nodes and then to visceral organs and skeleton.

Iridociliary epithelial tumors arise from the neuroepithelium of the posterior surface of the iris and inner ciliary body.[61] Ciliary body epithelial tumors are the second most common primary intraocular tumor in dogs but are relatively rare in cats. They appear as unilateral pigmented to non-pigmented solid masses growing within the posterior chamber and affecting middle-aged to older dogs with no apparent breed or gender predisposition.[62] These tumors often displace the iris and lens and, as with extensive intraocular melanocytomas in dogs, the owner is often only first "alerted" to an ocular problem by recognizing secondary tumor effects such as uveitis, glaucoma, or hyphema. Iridociliary body tumors may be benign (iridociliary adenoma) or malignant (iridociliary adenocarcinoma), but there are no well-recognized

clinical features that help distinguish between the two (see next section for further discussion).

Feline ocular sarcoma is the second most common primary intraocular tumor in cats and is unique to this species.[49,63] This tumor type has also been called *post-traumatic sarcoma* because many affected cats have a history of trauma to the eye at some time, often many years, before oncogenesis.[26,64] Most affected cats appear with a change in the appearance of the globe as manifested by an alteration in size, shape, or color. As with many primary intraocular tumors, ocular pain is not usually noted until significant secondary complications arise (e.g., uveitis and/or glaucoma). Feline ocular sarcoma is highly malignant and may spread by direct invasion of the optic nerve and orbit, as well as by hematogenous metastasis to distant sites. Similar to the sarcomatous lesions that can develop at vaccination sites in this species, feline ocular sarcoma may develop in any eye affected by long-term inflammation. For this reason, cats with a history of ocular trauma should have regular evaluations to assess for changes in globe appearance, comfort, and vision that may indicate tumor development.

The globe is all too often ignored as part of a routine physical examination or necropsy; thus, estimates of the overall prevalence of metastatic disease within the eye is likely grossly underestimated. Lymphoma is the most common tumor metastatic to the eye, but hemangiosarcoma and carcinomas often manifest with ocular lesions as well.[65,66] In the author's experience, the lesions most consistently found with metastatic disease include bilateral uveitis with secondary glaucoma (lymphoma), hyphema (hemangiosarcoma), and characteristic "watershed zones" of wedge-shaped chorioretinitis radiating from the optic nerve head unique to metastatic feline bronchial adenocarcinoma.[67,68]

Diagnosis and Staging

The first step in the diagnosis of any ocular or periocular tumor is a complete ophthalmic examination (see Box 20-8). Early detection is key to ensuring a successful outcome with respect to vision, ocular comfort, and overall systemic health of the animal. In general, definitive histopathologic diagnosis of any orbital or adnexal tumor is obtained via biopsy. Additional diagnostics such as ultrasound, CT, or MRI may aid in identifying the optimal biopsy site, especially in orbital disease.[17,69-71] If a retrobulbar mass is present in a visual animal, the utmost care should be taken to avoid the optic nerve and globe during biopsy. Unfortunately, orbital neoplasia is often in an advanced stage at the time of presentation in many cases.[18] Adnexal tumors are, in contrast to orbital or intraocular lesions, easily biopsied, given their accessibility. For third eyelid or conjunctival tumors, it may be possible to obtain a snip biopsy of the affected tissue using only topical anesthesia in an awake patient.

With careful examination, early intraocular tumors can be detected on routine wellness examinations before the owner is even aware of an ophthalmic problem. However, a proliferative intraocular lesion in a visual, comfortable globe represents a significant diagnostic challenge.[72] Essentially, the clinician may opt to: (1) document any changes via drawings and/or photography with regular recheck examinations to assess for alterations in size, shape, or extent of the lesion, (2) attempt intraocular aspiration biopsy; however, the procedure may cause intraocular hemorrhage or damage to the lens and results are often inconclusive in terms of assessing malignancy, (3) refer the patient for intraocular surgery and excisional biopsy (e.g., cyclectomy or iridocyclectomy for anterior uveal tumors) in an attempt to save the globe and vision, or (4) enucleate and submit the globe for complete histopathologic examination. The latter is often an undesirable alternative in patients who are both visual and comfortable at the time of presentation. Recommendations for diagnostic tests depend on the species affected, the most likely tumor type involved, and whether or not the lesion is believed to be primary or metastatic. In the author's opinion, the greatest controversy involves the clinical approach to feline DIM. Despite its known metastatic potential, some veterinary

ophthalmologists do not advocate any additional diagnostics or therapy unless the patient has secondary chronic uveitis and glaucoma. Others routinely ablate early lesions of DIM using a diode laser. A third group of specialists typically recommend prompt globe removal through enucleation in an effort to prevent death resulting from metastasis. Gonioscopy enables the clinician to better examine the iridocorneal angle and to determine if tumor cells have invaded this region of the eye. If tumor cells have encroached into the iridocorneal angle, it is indicative of tumor invasiveness. However, this feature alone does not necessarily predict malignant potential. This is especially true for many canine anterior uveal melanocytomas. Another diagnostic tool to better evaluate extent of a lesion and monitor changes over time is high-resolution ultrasound or ultrasound biomicroscopy. In cases where the lesion is suspected to be metastatic, or in cases with known malignant potential (e.g., lymphoma, mast cell tumor, feline DIM, feline ocular sarcoma), a more complete systemic workup including organ function tests, thoracic radiographs, and abdominal radiographs is warranted.[73]

Therapy and Prognosis

Treatment of orbital tumors can be challenging for three principal reasons. First, tumors are usually quite advanced at the time of the initial diagnosis.[8,9,74] Second, surgical access to the orbit is limited and may require orthopedic surgical equipment (e.g., Hall air drill, Steinman pin).[75-78] Third, irradiation of an orbital tumor in a globe that is still visual will usually result in significant ocular side effects (keratoconjunctivitis sicca, cataract, and/or retinal degeneration). As a general rule, orbital tumors in small animal patients carry a guarded to poor prognosis. In cases demonstrating extensive invasion, an exenteration coupled with ancillary treatment (e.g., radiation therapy, chemotherapy) may be necessary.[79] The surgeon and oncologist benefit from combining their skills and expertise to best manage the patient. Canine orbital meningiomas frequently result in significant orbital remodeling. Metastasis of meningiomas and retrobulbar spindle tumors has been reported, but appears to be rare, with little published information on the latter tumor types especially.[21] In contrast, the unclassified non-lymphoid round cell tumors of neural or neuroendocrine origin are extremely aggressive, rapidly progressive tumors in young, large-breed dogs, and often invade the brain through the optic foramen.

The eyelids are the primary "windshield wipers" of the cornea and, as such, any irregularity in their shape or contour can result in chronic keratitis, ulceration, and discomfort. Preservation of eyelid function must be balanced with the need for adequate tumor resection. Appropriate surgical and ancillary treatment options for eyelid neoplasia depend on tumor type and eyelid conformation. Canine meibomian tumors are typically managed by surgical excision, cryoablation, or a combination thereof. They carry a favorable prognosis and seldom recur if treated appropriately. Tumors affecting greater than one fourth to one third of the eyelid margin cannot be removed by simple wedge resection in most cases because too much of the eyelid margin must be sacrificed. The reader is encouraged to refer to more detailed descriptions of ophthalmic surgical techniques (e.g., H-plasty, lip-to-lid, or bucket handle procedures) as needed.[80-84] Newer treatment modalities such as PDT (Chapter 17) show promise for the treatment of eyelid neoplasia.[85-87] Any eyelid or conjunctival mass, no matter how benign in appearance, should be submitted for histopathologic examination to ensure the most accurate diagnosis and to guide case management decisions.

Management of primary intraocular tumors varies depending on tumor type, species affected, and overall health of the eye at the time of diagnosis. The difficulties in obtaining a definitive histopathologic diagnosis in the non-extirpated globe have been discussed previously. Unfortunately, many intraocular tumors, unless associated with a significant color change in the iris, will go undetected until secondary complications such as uveitis or glaucoma have occurred and enucleation is frequently recommended to improve patient comfort. Additional diagnostics such as gonioscopy can help distinguish a canine anterior uveal melanocytoma with extrascleral extension necessitating enucleation from an epibulbar melanoma, which is typically managed with surgical resection and preservation of the globe.[88-91] Diode laser photocoagulation has been used to treat presumed iris melanoma in dogs.[92] Similarly, an ocular ultrasound may indicate whether extrascleral extension of an iridociliary body adenocarcinoma has occurred and helps the surgeon decide between an enucleation or

exenteration to best ensure complete tumor resection. In cases where an intraocular tumor is well circumscribed and demonstrates low risk for metastasis, surgery may be attempted to remove the intraocular tumor and still preserve vision (e.g., cyclectomy or iridocyclectomy).[93] The owner should be advised, however, that these resections can result in significant intraocular hemorrhage, cataract formation, or glaucoma.

Any patient affected with a secondary metastatic ocular or periocular tumor should undergo systemic workup and staging.[94-96] Consultation with an oncologist is recommended and the reader is referred to more detailed discussions of specific tumor types elsewhere in this book for further information.

Selected References*

Dubielzig RR: Ocular neoplasia in small animals, *Vet Clin North Am Sm Anim Pract* 20:837-848, 1990.
Primary canine and feline tumors of the globe with particular emphasis on morphologic features as a predictor for biological behavior are discussed. Melanoma and feline post-traumatic ocular sarcomas receive special attention in this review.
Giuliano E: Primary intraocular melanoma: a comparative approach, *Vet Cancer Soc Newsl* 24:5-6, 2000.
Clinical description and biological behavior of primary intraocular melanoma in dogs and cats, with significant comparisons to the disease in people, are reviewed.
Moore CP, Constantinescu GM: Surgery of the adnexa, *Vet Clin North Am Sm Anim Pract* 27:1011-1066, 1997.
A review of the functional anatomy of adnexal structures and presentation of surgical procedures involving the eyelid, conjunctiva, and third eyelid of small animals is provided. Illustrations of applied anatomy and various surgical techniques are included.

■ *For a complete list of the references cited in this chapter, please go to www.smallanimaloncology.com.

SECTION D: Aural Tumors

Mary Lynn Higginbotham

KEY POINTS

- Squamous cell carcinoma should be suspected in cats with non-healing wounds associated with the face (periaural, periocular, or nasal planum regions).

- Neoplasia should be suspected in dogs or cats with chronic otitis that is non-responsive or incompletely responsive to symptomatic therapy.

Aural tumors can develop in any of the protective and supporting structures of the ear including the

BOX 20-9 COMMON TUMORS OF THE PINNA

Canine	Feline
Squamous cell carcinoma	Squamous cell carcinoma
Mast cell tumor	Mast cell tumor
Histiocytoma	Melanoma
Sebaceous gland adenoma	Basal cell tumor
Sebaceous gland adenocarcinoma	Rhabdomyoma
	Hemangioma
	Hemangiosarcoma

TABLE 20-5 REPORTED TUMORS OF THE EAR CANAL[4]

Species	Benign	Malignant
Canine	Polyp	Ceruminous gland adenocarcinoma
	Papilloma	Carcinoma of undetermined origin
	Sebaceous gland adenoma	Squamous cell carcinoma
	Basal cell tumor	Round cell tumor
	Ceruminous gland adenoma	Sarcoma
	Histiocytoma	Malignant melanoma
	Plasmacytoma	Hemangiosarcoma
	Benign melanoma	
	Fibroma	
Feline	Polyp	Ceruminous gland adenocarcinoma
	Ceruminous gland adenoma	Squamous cell carcinoma
	Papilloma	Carcinoma of undetermined origin
		Sebaceous gland adenocarcinoma

pinna, external ear canal, middle ear, and inner ear. Compared with the incidence of cutaneous tumors in dogs and cats, aural tumors are relatively uncommon. Diagnosis of an aural tumor is often preceded by a chronic history of clinical signs such as otitis externa or progressive "scabs" associated with the pinna or periauricular region. Depending upon the type and severity of clinical signs, quality of life may be compromised as the disease progresses. SCC of the pinna is the most common ear tumor in cats, with a reported incidence of 26.9 in 100,000 cats.[1] Tumors of the external ear canal comprise 1% to 2% of all tumors in cats[2] and less than 3% of tumors in dogs presenting for surgery of aural disease.[3] Lists of reported pinnal and external ear canal tumors[4] are presented in Box 20-9 and Table 20-5.

Etiology and Risk Factors

Feline cutaneous SCC affecting the pinnae is associated with sunlight exposure. These solar-induced lesions often occur in non-pigmented areas, with white cats being 13.4 times more likely to develop SCC than colored cats.[1] Mutations of the tumor suppressor gene p53 have been identified in cases of feline pinnal SCC.[5] Although cats with cutaneous SCC have been reported to be FeLV and/or FIV positive, no correlation has been made to suggest that viral disease predisposes to the development of SCC. More than likely, they are concurrent diseases of outdoor cats.[6,7] The true etiology of external ear canal tumors is unknown; however, an association between chronic otitis externa and ear canal tumors has been proposed.[2,3] It is common for tumors of the ear canal to be associated with chronic inflammation and bacterial or yeast infections. Most ear canal tumors eventually become obstructive in nature, impairing drainage and leading to accumulation of cerumen and debris within the ear. In addition, chronic inflammation has been implicated in the development of tumors of the ear canal resulting in the progression of hyperplasia to dysplasia and eventually neoplasia.[2,8] It is unknown if the true order of etiological events is inflammation progressing to neoplasia or neoplasia with secondary chronic inflammation.

Clinical Features of Aural Tumors

Pinnal tumors in dogs usually are discrete masses. In cats, SCC frequently begins as cutaneous excoriations that progress over time to become invasive, ulcerative lesions. Multifocal lesions including the nasal planum, periocular region, and pinnae are common on the face of white cats.

Dogs and cats with external ear canal tumors often present because of chronic otitis externa with aural discomfort, purulent discharge that may also be hemorrhagic in nature, and possibly deafness or other neurologic signs such as head tilt, Horner's syndrome, or circling. Clinical signs are oftentimes prolonged, ranging from 0 to 96 months from onset to presentation in one retrospective study.[4] The appearance of the tumor will vary by histology and invasiveness, but may be pedunculated to broad-based, discrete to irregular, and potentially ulcerated.

Diagnosis and Staging

Neoplasia should be a differential for any animal presenting with chronic otitis, especially in those cases that are refractory or incompletely responsive to treatment. Thorough physical examination should be performed with close attention being paid to the regional lymph nodes, oral cavity and aural tissues. Bilateral tumors of the ear canal have been reported,[9] so evaluation of both ears is important. Extension into the oral cavity is possible with tumors involving the Eustachian tubes. Most malignant tumors of the aural region in dogs and cats are locally invasive, and if they metastasize, it is late in the course of disease. Metastasis is generally to the lymph nodes and lungs; thus, lymph node cytology and thoracic radiographs should be performed in animals suspected of having an aural malignancy. Skull radiographs, or preferably CT scan, will aid in the evaluation of disease extent. Cranial nerve evaluation is also important to assess for involvement of the inner ear. Diagnosis is generally via biopsy, although cytologic evaluation of FNA samples is adequate to distinguish inflammatory polyps from neoplastic lesions.[10]

Metastasis

Aural malignancies do not frequently metastasize. In one retrospective study of canine and feline ear canal tumors, 8% of dogs with malignant ear canal tumors had evidence of pulmonary metastasis at diagnosis. Only one dog had evidence of lymph node metastasis at the time of diagnosis. None of the cats with malignant tumors of the ear canal had evidence of pulmonary metastasis at the time of diagnosis, although 9% had lymph node metastasis.[4] In a separate retrospective series of ceruminous gland tumors in dogs and cats, no animals had evidence of pulmonary metastatic disease at the time of diagnosis.[11,12] Canine mast cell tumors of the pinnae tend to metastasize to the prescapular lymph nodes; thus cytological evaluation of lymph node aspirates is recommended before developing a treatment plan.*

Treatment Modalities

Aggressive surgical resection is the treatment of choice for ear tumors, regardless of their location. Feline superficial SCC of the pinna or periauricular region may be amenable to cryotherapy or strontium 90 plesiotherapy if appearance is of concern to the owners. Pinnectomy is recommended for tumors affecting the pinnae, since this will also prevent the development of de novo tumors, which is common with solar-induced neoplasia. Histologic evaluation should always be performed to confirm diagnosis and evaluate for completeness of surgical resection. PDT has also been reported as treatment for this tumor type and location.[13,14]

Ear canal ablation with lateral bulla osteotomy is recommended for dogs and cats with tumors of the external ear canal. Eleven dogs with ceruminous gland adenocarcinomas treated with this procedure had no recurrence with a median follow-up of 36 months, versus a 75% recurrence rate in four dogs treated with a lateral ear canal resection.[11] The same study was performed in cats with ceruminous gland adenocarcinomas showing a 25% recurrence rate in 16 cats treated with ear canal ablation and lateral bulla osteotomy with a median disease-free interval of 42 months, versus a 66.7% recurrence rate in 6 cats treated with a lateral ear canal resection with a median disease-free interval of 10 months.[12] Radiation has been evaluated as either primary therapy or adjuvant therapy for incompletely resected ceruminous gland adenocarcinomas in dogs and cats and is considered safe and effective for this tumor type.[15] Because of the low metastatic rate of these tumors in general, chemotherapy has not been evaluated adequately. Depending upon the histologic type and stage of disease, chemotherapy or immunotherapy may be indicated (such as with high-grade mast cell tumors or malignant melanomas).

Prognosis and Survival

In general, aural tumors warrant a fair prognosis if they are diagnosed and aggressively treated at an early stage of disease. Disease-free intervals and survival times of 681 and 799 days, respectively, have been reported with pinnal amputation for SCC in cats. Disease-free interval and survival time were significantly less for animals with concurrent SCC of the nasal planum and pinnae. Surgery provided the longest disease-free interval and survival times in this study when compared with cryotherapy or radiation therapy.[7] One must consider, however, that cases chosen for these therapies may have been more advanced and less amenable to complete resection. Early, aggressive treatment of this disease is essential to afford the best long-term prognosis.

Few reports exist describing the prognosis for dogs and cats with tumors of the ear canal. One retrospective study including all histologic types of ear canal tumors found an MST greater than 58 months for dogs with malignant ear canal tumors and 11.7 months for cats

---

*Higginbotham ML, Henry CJ, Watson Z, et al: Biological behavior of canine aural mast cell tumors. Twentieth Veterinary Cancer Society Annual Conference, Asilomar, CA, Oct 15-18, 2000, p 52 (unpublished data).

with malignant ear canal tumors. Dogs with tumors limited to the vertical or horizontal canal have an improved survival over those with bulla and ear canal involvement. Poor prognostic factors in cats include neurologic signs

TABLE 20-6   COMPARISON OF MEDIAN SURVIVAL TIMES FOR PROGNOSTIC FACTORS ASSOCIATED WITH EXTERNAL EAR CANAL TUMORS[4]

Species	Prognostic Factor	Median Survival Time
Canine	Involvement of bulla and ear canal	5.3 mo
	Tumor limited to vertical or horizontal ear canal	> 30 mo
Feline	Neurologic signs at diagnosis	1.5 mo
	No neurologic signs at diagnosis	15.5 mo
	SCC	3.8 mo
	Carcinoma of undetermined origin	5.7 mo
	Ceruminous gland adenocarcinoma	> 49 mo
	Tumor invasion of surrounding tissues	4 mo
	No tissue invasion	21.7 mo

at the time of diagnosis, histopathologic diagnosis of SCC or carcinoma of undetermined origin, and histologic evidence of tumor invasion of surrounding tissues.[4] A mitotic index (number of mitoses in 10 high-power fields) of 3 or more has also been associated with a negative prognosis in cats with ceruminous gland adenocarcinoma.[16] See Table 20-6 for survival times associated with various prognostic factors of ear canal tumors in dogs and cats. Although most malignant aural tumors are locally invasive, with early and aggressive local therapy, long-term survival is possible.

Selected References*

Fan TM, de Lorimier LP: Inflammatory polyps and aural neoplasia, *Vet Clin North Am Sm Anim Pract* 34:489, 2004.
This is a thorough review of aural neoplasms in dogs and cats.
London CA, Dubilzeig RR, Vail DM, et al: Evaluation of dogs and cats with tumors of the ear canal: 145 cases (1978-1992), *J Am Vet Med Assoc* 208(9):1413, 1996.
This retrospective study is the largest to date regarding ear canal tumors in dogs and cats.

■ *For a complete list of the references cited in this chapter, please go to www.smallanimaloncology.com.

SECTION E: Skull Tumors

Jarrod M. Vancil and Carolyn J. Henry

KEY POINTS

- The biological behavior of skull tumors can vary greatly in comparison with histologically similar tumors in other locations.
- CT is often necessary to accurately determine tumor borders and involvement of vital structures before making a plan for case management.
- Surgical excision is often an appropriate treatment option for tumors of the skull.

Incidence/Etiology and Risk Factors

Various tumor types have been reported to affect the canine skull, including multilobular tumor of bone (MLTB), which may also be referred to as multilobular osteochondrosarcoma (MLO), multilobular chondroma, or osteoma, chondroma rodens, calcifying aponeurotic fibroma, juvenile aponeurotic fibroma, or

cartilage analog of fibromatosis[1]; osteosarcoma (OSA); fibrosarcoma (FSA); and chondrosarcoma (CSA). Non-oral skull tumors in cats are extremely rare, with OSA and CSA being the histologies reported to date.[2-5] In one reported feline CSA case, the mass originated from within a multilobular chondroma of the skull.[3] Oral, nasal, and orbital neoplasms are reviewed in other sections; thus, tumors of the rest of the calvarium are the focus here.

Overall incidence and etiology of skull tumors is not well documented in the veterinary literature. Multilobular tumors of bone occur almost exclusively in the skull, but are relatively rare. OSA of the axial skeleton accounts for approximately one fourth of all canine OSAs and roughly one half of these occur on the head.[1,6] In cats, OSA of the skull is exceedingly rare, accounting for only 1 of 22 OSAs in one report.[5] Feline CSA is also rarely associated with the skull, accounting for only 2 of 46 CSAs in one study.[7]

Signalment

For many tumors of the calvarium, there are too few reported cases to determine breed or sex predilections. Multilobular tumors of bone occur primarily in middle-aged to older dogs (median = 8 years) of medium or large breed, but seldom in giant breed dogs.[1,8,9] This tumor type has also been reported in smaller dogs such as Chihuahua and Pekingese.[8-10] OSA generally affects middle-aged to older dogs and cats.[1,4] Boxers are reported to be the breed most commonly affected by OSA of the skull.[1] One study of 116 cases of axial skeletal OSA reported an overrepresentation among female dogs, although it was unclear if this was an actual female predominance found in dogs with axial OSA, or simply due to a female predominance in the general pet population of the area.[6] No sex predilection has been observed among the other skull tumor types.[8,9,11] In comparison to OSA, CSA occurs in a slightly younger population (average age, 6–7 years) and primarily affects medium and large breed dogs.[1,11] Small and giant breed dogs are rarely affected.[1,11] FSA of the skull (Figure 20-18) primarily affects medium and large breed dogs at a median age of 8 years (range = 3–13).[12]

Clinical Features

Multilobular tumors of bone are composed of bone or partially-to-completely calcified tissue that is surrounded by mesenchymal tissue and stroma. Multilobular tumors of bone arise from the flat bones of the canine skull, commonly involving the cranium, mandible, or maxilla, although other sites including the hard palate, orbit, tympanic bulla and zygomatic bone may be affected.[1,13] The typical appearance is a medium to large, lobulated, protruding mass or swelling, arising from the skull.[1,9] Clinical manifestations relate to the adjacent structures that are compressed by the mass rather than infiltrated by it (Figure 20-19). Neurologic signs, ocular pain, and pain with opening of the mouth are examples of these symptoms.[9,14]

OSA of the calvarium has a tendency to be purely osteoproductive.[15] As with other tumors of the calvarium, local invasion of vital structures determines the clinical symptoms.

CSA of the canine skull most commonly infiltrates the nasal cavity, frontal sinus, and frontal bones (Figure 20-20).[11,16] Clinical signs are determined by tumor location, with a palpable mass generally being the reason for presentation for non-nasal CSA of the skull.

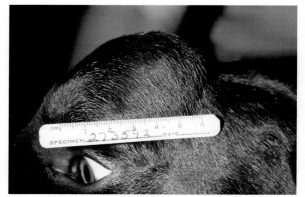

FIGURE 20-18 Fibrosarcoma of the calvarium is indistinguishable from osteoma and multilobular tumor of bone (MLTB) based on outward appearance. (Photo courtesy of University of Missouri VMTH.)

FSA is a tumor characterized by proliferation of fibrous connective tissue that often aggressively infiltrates adjacent normal tissue.[1,12] Although the mandible and maxilla are more common sites for skull FSA, these tumors can invade any regions of the skull and are often seen involving the zygomatic arch or temporal bone.[1] FSA presentation varies widely; however, dogs with skull FSA generally present with a firm swelling or mass. The severity of the clinical signs is related to the degree of tumor infiltration into the surrounding structures.

Diagnosis and Staging

Despite the varied biological behavior of skull tumors, one should approach each case with a similar process for staging and definitive diagnosis. A thorough physical examination and skull radiographs aid in the diagnosis of some tumors of the calvarium, particularly MLTB.[8] Radiographically, MLTBs appear as a mass with nodular or stippled mineralized opacities giving what has been referred to as a "popcorn ball" appearance (Figure 20-21).[9] CSA is usually characterized by varying degrees of osteolysis and proliferation that may make them difficult to differentiate from OSA.[1] With locally invasive proliferative tumors of the skull, the full size of the mass and extent of bone involvement can be difficult to determine with palpation and skull radiographs alone. CT or MRI should be performed in order to determine tumor borders and involvement of vital structures before making a plan for case management.[8,14,17] Biopsy is recommended in advance of definitive therapy when OSA or CSA of the skull is

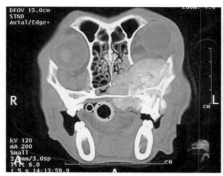
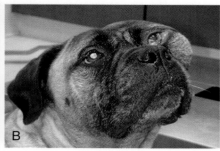

FIGURE 20-19 Tumor location determines clinical signs as in these two cases where local infiltration of a multilobular tumor of bone has caused deviation of the eye noted on CT (**A**) and apparently caused by facial deformity (**B**). (Photos courtesy of University of Missouri VMTH.)

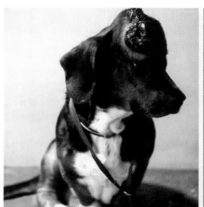
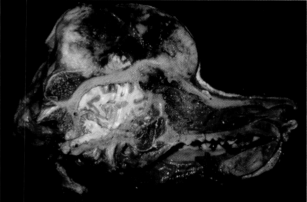

FIGURE 20-20 Chondrosarcoma with severe local infiltration of the calvarium and frontal sinus. (Photos courtesy of University of Missouri VMTH.)

suspected, or when results could change the owners' willingness to treat. Benign masses, such as osteoma, can be very similar in appearance (Figure 20-22), such that a biopsy is required to definitively differentiate them from malignant lesions. FNA of the mass and regional lymph nodes should be performed to aid in gaining a definitive diagnosis and to rule out local metastasis. With FSA and MLTB, histologic grade is important for determining overall prognosis and the development of a proper treatment plan.[9] However, FSA can appear histologically to be of low grade, but still have the biological behavior of a very high-grade tumor.[12] This should be carefully considered when treatment is chosen and overall prognosis is discussed. A complete diagnostic workup should include three-view thoracic radiographs, abdominal radiographs, and abdominal ultrasound to rule out any existing metastatic disease.

Biological Behavior/Metastasis

Multilobular Tumor of Bone

MLTBs are slow-growing, locally invasive tumors that often invade the cranial vault.[8-10,17] Although the metastatic rate exceeds 50%, metastases are slow to develop and are rarely the cause of significant clinical signs or the reason for death or euthanasia. Development of metastasis correlates significantly with incomplete surgical resection of the primary tumor.[8] In one report, 75% of dogs with completely excised tumors did not develop metastasis, whereas 86% of dogs with local recurrence developed metastasis.[8] The most common metastatic sites are

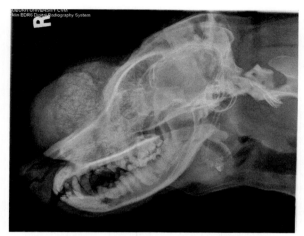

FIGURE 20-21 Skull radiograph of a dog with multilobular tumor of bone demonstrated the multilobular character of the lesion, sometimes described as a "popcorn ball" appearance. (Photo courtesy of Dr. John Hathcock Auburn University CVM.)

the lungs, mediastinum, ribs, long bones, kidney, pancreas, and cerebral cortex.[8,10]

Osteosarcoma

OSA is generally a locally invasive tumor with high metastatic potential. However, previous reports have indicated that OSA of the axial skeleton is associated with a better prognosis than OSA of the appendicular skeleton.[1,6,18] Whereas appendicular OSA carries a 90% potential for metastatic disease, 40% or fewer of dogs with axial skeletal OSA develop metastasis.[6] In a retrospective study of 116 dogs with axial skeletal OSA, pulmonary metastasis was evident on the initial thoracic radiographs in 11.1% of the dogs.[6] The overall metastatic potential of axial skeletal OSA varies with tumor location. Although in a report of 45 dogs with OSA arising from flat or irregular bones, only 13% had metastatic disease upon presentation, 35% of the dogs ultimately developed metastasis.[19]

Chondrosarcoma

According to reports of dogs with sinonasal tumors, the metastatic rate of CSA of the skull is less than that of OSA.[16] A metastatic frequency of 8.3% (1/12) was reported for dogs with sinonasal CSA, compared with 12.5% (1/8) for dogs with sinonasal OSA.[16] Both of these frequencies are lower than are noted with similar histologies at other more common anatomic locations. The metastatic rate for CSA of other sites in the canine

calvarium is poorly documented. In a retrospective study of 67 cases of feline CSA, none of the cats with follow-up information (n = 24) developed metastatic disease.[7] This included four cats with CSA of the oral or nasal cavity (one mandibular, two maxillary, and one nasal). Follow-up was not available for two cats with CSA of the skull (in sites other than the oral or nasal cavity).

Fibrosarcoma

The metastatic rate for non-oral FSA of the skull is poorly documented. Well-differentiated masses are unlikely to produce metastatic disease, whereas less well-differentiated or anaplastic FSA may metastasize hematogenously or via lymphatics. In a report of 25 dogs with histologically low-grade, but biologically high-grade, FSA of the mandible or maxilla, the metastatic rate was 20%; however, metastases were not present at the initial examination and none of the dogs with metastatic disease were euthanized or died because of these lesions.[12]

Therapy and Prognosis

Surgical options vary greatly depending on the location of the mass and the structures involved; however, surgical excision is often a viable and appropriate treatment option for dogs with tumors of the calvarium. Wide margins of excision should be the top priority when considering surgery as a treatment. With MLTB, significant correlation has been shown between incomplete excision and recurrence rate, as well as an increase in metastatic rate.[8-10] One study indicated an approximate 11-fold increased chance of significantly shorter time to local recurrence with incomplete surgical margins, when compared with dogs with complete surgical excision.[9] OSA of the skull is a locally invasive tumor, and treatment should be focused on preventing further local invasion into vital structures. Extrapolating from reports of treatment for oral OSA, surgical excision is considered the treatment of choice to remove the existing mass and prevent further invasion.[4,20,21] As with MLTB, studies have shown that prognosis worsens and recurrence rates increase with the inability to gain complete excisional margins with OSA.[20,21] Resection of at least 1 cm of normal tissue surrounding the excised skull tumor is recommended.[20,21] Acrylic cranioplasty, titanium mesh, axial pattern flaps, and other forms of craniectomy site repair have been used following extensive surgical resection of large tumors, or tumors in small patients.[10,14,22-24] However, because of the thick temporal muscles, these measures are often unnecessary.[10] With midline occipitotemporal tumors, resection is likely to disrupt the

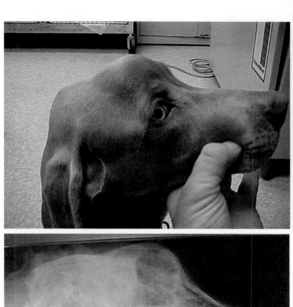

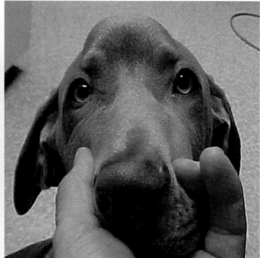

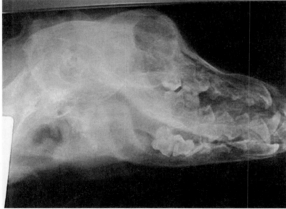

FIGURE 20-22 Benign osteoma of the skull in this Weimaraner has a smooth contour, lacking the multinodular densities on radiographs that are typical of multilobular tumor of bone. (Photos courtesy of University of Missouri VMTH.)

transverse venous sinuses and could result in significant morbidity and mortality. As such, preoperative planning and assessment of collateral circulation via MRI or CT is essential.[25]

Samarium-153 ethylenediaminetetramethylene phosphonic acid (Sm-153-EDTMP) is a bone-targeting radioisotope that is a treatment option for inoperable tumors of the skull. Although most reports in the veterinary literature address the treatment of appendicular tumors with this modality, initial evidence suggests that tumors of the calvarium may also be an appropriate target. In an unpublished report of 21 dogs with primary tumors of the skull including MLTB or osteoma

(n = 16) and OSA (n = 5), Sm-153-EDTMP was used as the primary treatment modality (Figure 20-23).* Tumor locations included occiput (n = 5), palate (n = 3), orbit (n = 3), frontal bone (n = 5), and zygomatic bone and/or maxilla (n = 5). Three dogs were still alive with survival times of greater than 48, 343, and 677 days, and four dogs were lost to follow-up, one of which had survived 757 days from the time of treatment. MST for all dogs was 180 days (range = 3 to >757 days). Although this

---

*McCoig AM, et al: Proceedings of the 24td Annual Conference of the Veterinary Cancer Society, 92, 2004 (unpublished data).

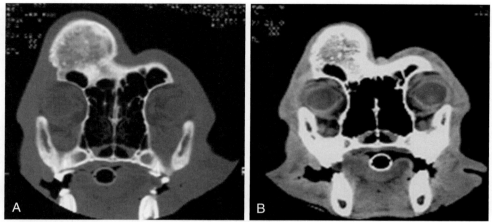

FIGURE 20-23 Multilobular tumor of bone in a juvenile mastiff before (**A**) and 2 years after (**B**) treatment with the radiopharmaceutical Sm-153-EDTMP. Although an obvious deformity remained, tumor growth had been rapid before treatment and ceased thereafter. (Photos courtesy of University of Missouri VMTH.)

treatment requires referral to a site licensed to administer the radioisotope, it may be a viable option for patients with unresectable tumors.

FSA and CSA of the skull can be difficult to completely excise because of location and involvement of vital structures. Radiation therapy following incomplete excision of CSA is often recommended. A wide variety of modalities have been attempted for treatment of FSA, including surgery, external beam radiation, chemotherapy, and combinations thereof. Aggressive and prompt treatment is necessary to significantly prolong survival of dogs with FSA.

The use of adjuvant therapy such as chemotherapeutic agents and radiation following surgical excision has not provided a significant overall increase in the survival time over surgery alone for dogs with skull tumors.[8-10,20,21] However, given the small number of reported cases, further investigation of adjuvant therapy is warranted.

Prognosis and Survival

The reported prognosis associated with skull tumors varies throughout the veterinary literature, but is generally favorable for MLTB. Although 47% of dogs undergoing treatment of MLTB had local tumor recurrence, and 56% had metastasis, the median time to recurrence, median time to metastasis, and MST were 797, 542, and 797 days, respectively, in one report.[9] Prognosis is affected by histologic grade (Grade I > Grade III), surgical margins, and tumor location (mandible > non-mandibular).[9]

The prognosis and survival for dogs with OSA of the skull is not well documented, except for mandibular and maxillary lesions. Dogs with mandibular OSA that are treated with complete surgical excision alone have a reported 1-year survival rate exceeding 70%,[20,21] whereas those with maxillary OSA have a reported MST of 4.6 months.[26] A study of 116 dogs with axial skeletal OSA indicated an MST of 22 weeks and a 1-year survival rate of 26.3%.[6] In an unpublished retrospective study of 60 dogs with OSA of the head, the metastatic rate was much lower than that of appendicular OSA (22% vs ~90%) and the MST for 10 dogs with clean surgical margins exceeded 1500 days.[†] Cats with axial skeletal OSA appear to have a shorter survival time and poorer quality of life when compared with cats undergoing amputation for appendicular OSA.[4] One study indicated a MST of 5.5 months for cats with axial skeletal OSA.[4]

With CSA, complete surgical excision of the mass is a key determinant of the overall prognosis. Recurrence is common with incompletely excised CSA, and is often the cause of euthanasia. FSAs typically grow slowly, but can invade many surrounding structures. Dogs often develop gross distortion of the face, loosening of teeth, and invasion of the nasal cavity, hard palate, and orbit.[12] Like the other skull tumors, incomplete excision and local recurrence is the usual reason for euthanasia in dogs affected with FSA.[12]

[†]Kazmierski KJ, et al: Proceedings of the 22nd Annual Conference of the Veterinary Cancer Society, 2002, p. 30 (unpublished data).

Selected References*

Dernell WS, Straw RC, Cooper MF, et al: Multilobular osteochondrosarcoma in 39 dogs: 1979-1993, *J Am Anim Hosp Assoc* 34:11, 1998.
This retrospective study examines a relatively large group of dogs presenting with multilobular osteochondrosarcoma (MLTB), and outlines the importance of histologic grade, surgical margins, and tumor location in relation to overall outcome.

Durham AC, Popovitch CA, Goldschmidt MH: Feline chondrosarcoma: a retrospective study of 67 cats (1987-2005), *J Am Anim Hosp Assoc* 44:124, 2008.
This retrospective study is one of the few reports to document outcome in cats with chondrosarcoma and includes six cases affecting the head, four mandibular/maxillary, and two of the skull.

Hathcock JT, Newton JC: Computed tomographic characteristics of multilobular tumor of bone involving the cranium in 7 dogs and zygomatic arch in 2 dogs, *Vet Radiol Ultrasound* 41:214, 2000.
Computed tomography findings are described and shown for canine multilobular tumor of bone, emphasizing the extent of local invasion that characterizes this disease and providing a compelling case for advanced imaging before treatment decisions.

█ *For a complete list of the references cited in this chapter, please go to www.smallanimaloncology.com.

SECTION F: Esophageal Tumors

Mary Lynn Higginbotham

KEY POINTS

- Primary esophageal tumors are rare and must be differentiated from non-esophageal primary tumors that can extend into the esophagus from surrounding tissues.
- Thorough diagnostic evaluation of esophageal masses should be performed to determine the potential for resection.
- Supportive care with an emphasis on adequate nutritional intake is necessary for animals with esophageal tumors.

Incidence—Morbidity and Mortality

Esophageal tumors are extremely rare in companion animals and consist of carcinomas[1] and sarcomas,[2-7] leiomyomas[1,8] and plasma cell tumors.[9] In a retrospective study reported by Ridgway and Suter, esophageal tumors were diagnosed in 8 of 49,229 cases over an 11-year period. Only two of the cases were primary esophageal neoplasms. The remainder were non-esophageal primary tumors that had invaded or metastasized to the esophagus.[1] Even fewer reports of esophageal tumors exist in the cat; predominantly squamous cell carcinomas have been reported,[10,11] but adenosquamous carcinoma[12] and neuroendocrine carcinoma[13] have also been reported. Because of the rarity of these tumors, there is a paucity of information in the literature regarding their behavior. What has been written suggests a relatively aggressive clinical course and guarded prognosis for malignant tumors of the esophagus.

Etiology and Risk Factors

Sarcomas, most notably OSA and FSA, are the most frequently reported esophageal tumors in the dog. *Spirocerca lupi*, the esophageal worm, is associated with canine esophageal sarcomas that develop in dogs living in areas endemic for the parasite. *S. lupi* can be found worldwide in tropical and subtropical climates.[2-6] Dogs at highest risk for *S. lupi* infection are free roaming, with access to the intermediate host, the dung beetle.[3]

The causes of other primary esophageal tumors are unknown. It does appear, however, that metastatic invasion of the esophagus is more common than are primary esophageal tumors. Tumors most frequently invading the esophagus include thyroid carcinomas, pulmonary neoplasms, and tumors of the stomach that extend beyond the cardia into the esophagus.[1]

Clinical Features

The clinical signs associated with esophageal tumors tend to be vague and progressive over time. These may include regurgitation, anorexia, salivation, weight loss,[1,14] dysphagia, hematemesis,[15] melena,[6] depression,[1] sneezing and nasal discharge,[7] and dyspnea.[1] Lameness may occur if hypertrophic osteopathy is present as a result of the intrathoracic mass.[16] Regurgitation is one of the most common clinical signs reported and is due not only to the obstructive nature of the mass, but also to the infiltration of tumor cells into the esophageal wall, resulting in altered motor activity of the musculature.[1] If the esophageal mass is an extension of a gastric mass, vomiting may be a presenting complaint.[15]

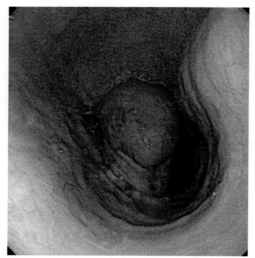

FIGURE 20-24 Endoscopic examination of a 9-year-old, female spayed, cocker spaniel presented with a 10-day history of hematemesis and regurgitation. A pedunculated esophageal mass was noted with esophagitis proximal to the mass. Biopsy confirmed a plasma cell tumor. No treatment was pursued, and the dog was euthanized at the owner's request.

Hematemesis or blood in the regurgitant is uncommon unless there is ulceration of the mucosal surface. Ulceration is relatively common in dogs with malignant lesions but was not reported in a series of dogs with esophageal leiomyoma.[8]

Diagnosis and Staging

Diagnosis of esophageal cancer relies on recognition of associated signs and an appropriate index of suspicion. Routine laboratory tests are often unrewarding, although in one report of dogs with *S. lupi*–associated esophageal cancer, microcytic hypochromic anemia was noted in 30% of dogs and leukocytosis occurred in 82%. Plain film thoracic radiographs may reveal a caudal esophageal mass or retention of gas within the esophageal lumen proximal to the lesion. Esophageal dilation may also occur proximal to the lesion.[14] Positive contrast radiography may prove to be more helpful for demonstrating either a stricture or filling defect within the esophageal lumen. Esophagoscopy affords the best visualization of an esophageal mass and allows for biopsy, which may aid in diagnosis (Figure 20-24). Multiple biopsies should be obtained, since malignant tumors are frequently ulcerated and contain secondary inflammation. A biopsy of the center of the mass

should be attempted, since the inflammatory reaction is typically superficial to the tumor. No fewer than three biopsy specimens are recommended. Thoracotomy and/or laparotomy may be necessary for visualization and appropriate biopsy sampling to be performed. In dogs with *S. lupi*–associated tumors, focal aortic mineralization, aortic dilation, and spondylitis of one or more vertebrae from T5–12 are common radiographic findings.[5] Fecal examination should be performed on initial presentation for dogs from endemic areas, since *S. lupi* ova are shed in the stool. Although this does not confirm a diagnosis, it is highly supportive in addition to the radiographic changes.

Biological Behavior/Metastasis

Metastasis of esophageal carcinomas and sarcomas is common and occurs by both hematogenous and lymphatic routes of dissemination. In the few reports of esophageal carcinomas (SCC and adenocarcinoma), metastasis was frequently present within regional lymph nodes on necropsy.[14,16] Metastases from esophageal sarcomas are most frequently pulmonary, but renal, gastric, adrenal, cardiac, and tongue metastases have been reported.[6,17] Metastasis of esophageal leiomyosarcomas or plasma cell tumors has not been reported.

Therapy and Prognosis

Treatment of esophageal tumors is difficult, in part because of their invasive nature at the time of diagnosis.[18,19] If no evidence of metastatic disease is present, surgical resection of the mass would be ideal. However, surgical complications are likely because of the nature and location of the esophagus, and they include poor exposure, wound tension, and compromised blood supply to the esophagus.[6,17,18] Recent retrospective reports have been published describing successful removal of *S. lupi*–associated sarcomas that are attached to the esophagus by a stalk.[6,17] Postoperative complications were minimal. Likewise, successful removal of a low-grade spindle cell sarcoma in a dog, with resultant resolution of regurgitation, was recently reported.[7] Carcinomas are much more difficult to resect because of their diffuse and invasive nature.

PDT has been described for the treatment of one dog with an esophageal SCC. A partial response was accomplished with three treatments. However, a new lesion was noted at a distal esophageal location and confirmed to be SCC 1 month after the third treatment. The dog survived with nutritional support for 278 days after the initial PDT treatment.[14]

The utility of chemotherapy and radiation therapy for the treatment of esophageal tumors is limited. Doxorubicin has been reported for treatment of dogs with *S. lupi*–associated sarcomas, although the true efficacy of the treatment could not be determined because of the small number of cases and variability in their treatment schedules.[6] Radiation therapy carries a substantial potential for morbidity because of the sensitivity of esophageal mucosal cells to radiation damage and because the proximity of the heart and lungs to the esophagus makes it likely that these normal surrounding tissues will receive considerable radiation dose.

Supportive measures to provide adequate nutrition are necessary in most patients with esophageal tumors. Enteral feeding tubes such as esophagostomy or gastrostomy tubes are useful if they can be placed such that they allow for the passage of food around the esophageal mass.

Based on the low likelihood of complete resection and potential for metastasis, malignant esophageal tumors are associated with a poor prognosis. The prognosis for leiomyomas, low-grade sarcomas, and plasma cell tumors is significantly better if resection is feasible.

Resection may be possible for the *S. lupi*–associated sarcomas if they are not broadly attached to the underlying mucosa; however, metastasis is common. Further evaluation is needed to determine the role of adjuvant chemotherapy in the treatment of dogs and cats with esophageal tumors. For five dogs with *S. lupi*–associated sarcomas that were treated with partial esophagectomy and adjuvant doxorubicin, the MST was 267 days.[6]

Selected Reference*

Ranen E, Shamir MH, Shahar R, et al: Partial esophagectomy with single layer closure for treatment of esophageal sarcomas in 6 dogs, *Vet Surg* 33:428, 2004.
Describes the surgical technique for esophagectomy.

■ *For a complete list of the references cited in this chapter, please go to www.smallanimaloncology.com.

SECTION G: Laryngeal and Tracheal Tumors

Jennifer E. Winter

KEY POINTS

- Laryngeal tumors encompass a wide variety of histologic types but nearly identical clinical signs of voice changes, dyspnea, and cough.
- Primary tracheal tumors most frequently lead to development of chronic cough, stridor, and wheezing.
- Advanced diagnostics, including laryngoscopy, bronchoscopy, and CT or MRI, are often necessary to definitively diagnose laryngeal and tracheal tumors.
- Aggressive local disease control is imperative to successful management of laryngeal and tracheal tumors, whereas adjunctive chemotherapy maintains an important role for treatment of round cell tumors of the larynx and trachea.

LARYNGEAL TUMORS

Incidence/Etiology and Risk Factors

Primary neoplasms of the larynx are rare in dogs and cats.[1-4] Various histologic types of laryngeal neoplasms have been described in canine patients, including rhabdomyomas (also called oncocytomas) and rhabdomyosarcomas, SCCs, osteosarcomas, mast cell tumors, and others.[2,3] In cats, lymphoma, SCC, and adenocarcinoma are the most commonly reported laryngeal tumors.[1]

In people, laryngeal tumors are associated with cigarette smoking; however, no risk factors have been identified in development of these tumors in companion animals.[5] Two of 15 cats with malignant laryngeal tumors in a recent report were positive for FIV on ELISA and Western blot, but the etiologic implication of this finding is uncertain.[1]

Clinical Features

Patients are usually older, with a median age of 8 years at diagnosis for dogs and 12 years for cats.[1,2] Benign rhabdomyomas are more common in younger dogs.[6] Canine laryngeal tumors may cause voice alteration, cough, and signs consistent with airway obstruction, such as choking and dyspnea.[2,3] Feline laryngeal tumors are often associated with similar signs, including voice change, dyspnea, cough, and weight loss.[1-4,7,8]

Diagnosis and Staging

A thorough oral and laryngeal examination, aided by sedation or general anesthesia, is imperative to determining the extent and etiology of laryngeal disorders.

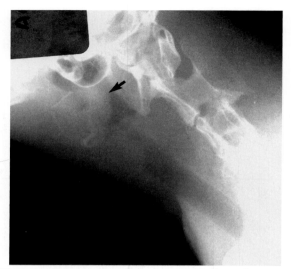

FIGURE 20-25 Lateral cervical radiograph of a dog with a space-occupying soft tissue mass within the laryngeal lumen *(arrow).* Biopsy of this mass revealed a rhabdomyosarcoma.

Where available, laryngoscopy may be a useful tool for obtaining cytologic or tissue samples of the lesion and for observing intraluminal changes that could suggest a non-neoplastic etiology for observed clinical signs. Non-neoplastic conditions that may mimic laryngeal tumors include foreign bodies, lymphoid hyperplasia, laryngeal paralysis, neurologic disorders, and other upper or lower airway obstructive diseases. In addition, the larynx may be invaded by neoplastic disease originating in adjacent tissues such as lymph nodes and thyroid tissue.

Lateral cervical radiographs may demonstrate intraluminal soft tissue masses within the laryngeal airways or laryngeal thickening in both dogs and cats (Figure 20-25).[1-3,7,8] In one study of feline laryngeal tumors, radiographic evidence of laryngeal opacity, decreased margination of laryngeal structures, or stenosis of the airways was noted in 16 of 19 cats.[1] Ultrasonographic examination of the larynx can be performed in order to evaluate laryngeal masses and obtain FNA samples for cytologic examination.[9] Thoracic radiographs should be obtained to evaluate for metastasis to the lungs, mediastinum, and thoracic lymph nodes. CT scan of the laryngeal region is beneficial to evaluate the extent of local disease and assist in surgical planning. This is especially important in cases in which the mass appears to have both intraluminal and extraluminal components. Cytologic and/or histopathologic examination of tissue samples is necessary to achieve a definitive diagnosis. In cases of lymphoma, additional systemic staging (see Chapter 25, Section A) is warranted.

Biological Behavior/Metastasis

Primary laryngeal tumors in dogs and cats may be either benign or malignant.[1,2] Benign rhabdomyomas in dogs can become quite large but are minimally invasive and do not metastasize. Malignant masses, however, tend to be quite locally invasive, with variable metastatic potential depending on histologic type. Oftentimes, obstructive disease becomes life threatening before metastatic disease occurs. Lymphoma, which is the most common laryngeal tumor in cats, may be characterized by systemic involvement affecting other lymphoid tissues.[1,7]

Therapy and Prognosis

Surgical resection of the primary tumor is the treatment of choice for control of local disease and to ensure proper airway and deglutitory function. For small, well-defined masses, complete surgical excision may be achieved. However, complete surgical resection of large or extensive laryngeal masses can be challenging because of the significant anatomic structures within this region. Furthermore, total laryngectomy must be accompanied by permanent tracheostomy.[2,6] For these reasons, radiation therapy may be a preferential treatment for radioresponsive tumors (such as lymphoma), to manage residual local disease and to sterilize margins from incomplete surgical excisions.

The role and efficacy of chemotherapy is variable based on histologic tumor type.[6,10] In one report, five cats with laryngeal masses (four with neoplasia and one with lymphoplasmacytic inflammation) that received chemotherapy as their sole treatment survived 59 to 370 days with an MST of 141 days. Chemotherapy protocols in the four cats with malignant laryngeal masses included a multi-drug protocol for the two cats with lymphoma and piroxicam for the two cats with SCC.[1]

Because many animals are euthanized at the time of diagnosis, large studies of treated patients are lacking in veterinary medicine, and the outcome for patients whose disease is allowed to run its natural course is largely under-reported. The prognosis for dogs and cats with benign laryngeal masses or radioresponsive reticuloendothelial tumors is favorable. Dogs with completely excised benign rhabdomyoma are reported to experience long-term disease control (1–4 years after complete excision).[2,6,11] Conversely, complete excision may be challenging in the majority of malignant laryngeal tumors and local recurrence is common; thus, prognosis for these patients is guarded.[1,2,6] In one study of cats with laryngeal and tracheal masses, four cats treated with multimodality therapy (various combinations of surgery, chemotherapy, and radiation) had a reported MST of 134.5 days, with a range of 80 to 183 days. However, one of these cats had tracheal, rather than laryngeal, disesase.[1]

TRACHEAL TUMORS

Incidence/Etiology and Risk Factors

Primary neoplasms of the trachea are rare in dogs and cats. In a multi-institutional retrospective study of cats with upper airway tumors, only five tracheal tumors were identified.[1] Likewise, only 16 canine tracheal tumors had been reported in the veterinary literature by 1991.[2] Canine tracheal neoplasms that have been reported include chondroma and CSA, adenocarcinomas, osteosarcomas, mast cell tumors, and extramedullary plasmacytomas. In cats, lymphoma appears to be the most common tracheal tumor, with various carcinomas (SCC, seromucinous carcinoma, and adenocarcinoma), leiomyosarcomas, and benign inflammatory polyps reported as well.[1,2,6,12-19]

Clinical Features

Primary tracheal neoplasia typically affects older patients, with median age between 9 and 11 years at diagnosis. The most common clinical signs associated with tracheal tumors in both dogs and cats include stridor, dyspnea, wheezing, and coughing. Clinical signs may be chronic in nature, as evidenced by the fact that patients in one report experienced clinical signs for 3 weeks to 6 months before diagnosis.[1,2,6,12-19]

Diagnosis and Staging

Primary tracheal tumors must be differentiated from non-neoplastic conditions including inflammatory or allergic processes, tracheal compression (from enlarged lymph nodes or pulmonary or mediastinal masses), laryngeal paralysis, or tracheal foreign bodies. As with laryngeal lesions, it is important to remember that tracheal masses may occur as primary tumors or as tumors of surrounding tissues that secondarily invade the trachea.

Cervical and thoracic radiographs may demonstrate intraluminal soft tissue masses within the tracheal lumen in both dogs and cats, and they should also be evaluated

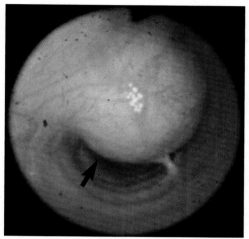

FIGURE 20-26 This bronchoscopic image from a dog demonstrates a large mass that extends from the wall of the trachea and nearly occludes the entire tracheal lumen.

for metastasis to the lungs, mediastinum, and thoracic lymph nodes. CT scan of the trachea is beneficial to evaluate the extent of local disease and assist in surgical planning. Bronchoscopy facilitates direct visualization of the mass (Figure 20-26), as well as sample collection for histopathologic examination, which is necessary to achieve a definitive diagnosis.[6]

Biological Behavior/Metastasis

Tracheal tumors in dogs and cats may be benign or malignant, although the factor of most clinical relevance initially relates to tumor size. Degree of local invasion varies with histology, as does metastatic risk.[2] As expected, local disease is an overwhelming concern, since airway capacity is usually significantly compromised at the time of diagnosis.

Therapy and Prognosis

Surgical resection is the treatment of choice for control of local disease and to ensure proper airway function.[1,6,12,13,20-24] Resection of up to three to four tracheal rings, with end-to-end anastomosis of residual normal tracheal tissue, can be achieved,[6] whereas complete surgical resection of infiltrative or diffuse tracheal masses is unlikely. Tube tracheostomy can provide palliative improvement in airway function; however, in one study, tube tracheostomy as sole therapy resulted in an MST of only 3 days in cats, with no cats surviving beyond 6 days.[1] Radiation therapy may be preferred over surgery for treatment of radiorespon-sive tumors (such as lymphoma and extramedullary plasmacytomas) and as adjunctive therapy to sterilize margins from incomplete surgical excisions. The role of chemotherapy is variable based on histologic tumor type, with lymphomas and extramedullary plasmacytomas demonstrating the most effective control with use of chemotherapy.[1,6,12,13,20,23,25]

The prognosis for dogs and cats with tracheal tumors ranges from good to poor. In one study of feline laryngeal and tracheal tumors, an MST of 5 days was reported; however, a majority of the cats in this study were euthanized at the time of diagnosis.[1] The prognosis for dogs and cats with benign tracheal masses or radioresponsive reticuloendothelial tumors is more favorable. One case series describes long-term control of feline tracheal lymphoma with use of systemic chemotherapy or radiation therapy. Three cats experienced local disease control of greater than 8, 17, and 19 months.[25]

Selected References*

Brown MR, Rogers KS, Mansell KJ, et al: Primary intratracheal lymphosarcoma in four cats, *J Am Anim Hosp Assoc* 39:468, 2003.
This article provides excellent descriptions of specific treatments and outcomes of four cats with primary tracheal lymphoma.
Jakubiak MJ, Siedlecki CT, Zenger E, et al: Laryngeal, laryngotracheal, and tracheal masses in cats: 27 cases (1998-2003), *J Am Anim Hosp Assoc* 41:310, 2005.
This paper provides a good description of the clinical picture and outcomes for feline upper airway tumors and inflammatory masses.
Venker-van Haagen AJ: Diseases of the larynx, *Vet Clin North Am Small Anim Pract* 22:1155, 1992.
This article provides an excellent overview of laryngeal diseases, including advanced diagnostics such as laryngoscopy and electromyography.

*For a complete list of the references cited in this chapter, please go to www.smallanimaloncology.com.

21 Tumors of the Thoracic Cavity

SECTION A: Primary Respiratory Tumors

Leslie E. Fox and Kerry C. Rissetto

KEY POINTS

- Identification of a solitary, well-circumscribed lung parenchymal mass with plain radiography in a middle-aged to older dog or cat should raise suspicion for a primary lung tumor.
- Since the majority of carcinomas affecting the feline digits are metastatic lesions from a primary lung tumor (rather than a primary digital carcinoma), thoracic radiographs are *always* indicated in cats with lytic lesions of P2/P3.
- At the time of thoracoscopy or thoracotomy, biopsy and histopathology of the tracheobronchial lymph nodes should be done if possible even if they are of normal size, since nodal metastasis has a marked negative effect on prognosis.
- Surgical excision is the treatment of choice for primary lung tumors. Those amenable to complete resection are associated with longer patient post-surgical survival time; average post-surgical survival is 1 year in dogs.

Incidence—Morbidity and Mortality

Primary lung tumors are uncommon in dogs and rare in cats but have been diagnosed more frequently in the past decade.[1] Although metastatic neoplasms are far more common than primary lung tumors, carcinomas/adenocarcinomas are the most common histology of tumors originating in the lungs of dogs and cats.[2] They are almost always malignant. Dogs and cats are typically older (average, 9–12 years), but these tumors may occur in young animals.[2]

Often dogs have no clinical signs suggesting the presence of a primary lung tumor.[1,2] If dogs are presented for signs referable to the respiratory tract, the most frequent abnormality, seen in 52% to 58% of primary lung tumor patients, is a chronic, nonproductive cough that fails to respond to antimicrobial and symptomatic therapies.[3-5]

Other clinical findings may include dyspnea, tachypnea, hemoptysis, and cyanosis, often with inappetence and subsequent weight loss. The original reason for presentation may be less obvious, including lameness caused by hypertrophic osteopathy (HO) (the most common paraneoplastic syndrome), dysphagia, fever, cranial vena cava obstruction leading to head and neck edema, ascites, pleural effusion, spontaneous pneumothorax, and diarrhea.[5] Cats are often symptomatic with dyspnea and/or tachypnea and coughing with or without lethargy, anorexia, and weight loss, but may be presented for only nonrespiratory signs like fever and decreased appetite.[2,6,7] Lameness in cats may be the only presenting clinical sign and is most likely due to lung-digit syndrome, in which metastasis from the primary lung tumor to one or more digits causes pain, swelling, paronychia, and pododermatitis unresponsive to antimicrobial and anti-inflammatory therapies.[8,9] In addition, cats often have serious concurrent illness, but usually do not have feline leukemia or feline immunodeficiency virus infections.[6]

Etiology and Risk Factors

Airborne carcinogens probably contribute to the development of lung cancer in cats and dogs, just as they do in people. An association between second-hand smoke and lung cancer has been made for both mesocephalic and brachycephalic breeds, with the hypothesis that a longer nose may confer a protective effect via additional turbinate filtration.[10] There may also be an association between urban environments and the development of these tumors.[3]

Diagnosis and Staging

Radiographic evidence of a solitary, well-circumscribed lung parenchymal mass in a middle-aged to older dog or cat raises the suspicion for primary or secondary neoplasms; however, lung tumors can present with almost any radiographic pattern in any age animal.[11,12] Because vascular, lymphatic, and alveolar tumor spread may be simultaneous, primary lung cancer is often observed radiographically as a solitary mass, but also as disseminated multifocal or diffuse parenchymal or interstitial patterns sometimes with lobar consolidation and/or pleural effusion. Abscesses, pneumonia, fungal granulomas, lymphomatoid or eosinophilic pulmonary granulomatosis, hematomas, pulmonary thromboembolism, cysts, bullae, and metastatic lung tumors are differential diagnoses for solitary or multifocal lung masses. Pneumonia, primary and metastatic lung neoplasms, granulomatous diseases and hemorrhage, edema, and fibrosis are differentials for disseminated pulmonary patterns. Multicentric neoplasms that may affect the lung parenchyma simultaneously with systemic abnormalities include lymphoma, malignant histiocytosis, metastatic histiocytic sarcoma (in dogs), and rarely, mast cell tumor (also in dogs).

Presurgical diagnosis of primary lung tumors involves ruling out non-neoplastic and metastatic cancer as causes for the observed radiographic findings with fine needle aspiration and cytology or histopathological examination of a biopsy specimen. A complete blood count including platelet count, serum biochemical panel, urinalysis, and coagulation panel or activating clotting time can be used to assess potential risks of hemorrhage and anesthetic complications and to assess for concurrent illness. Feline leukemia virus antigen, feline immunodeficiency virus antibody, and serum L-thyroxine assays are recommended for cats. Transthoracic fine-needle aspiration (25- or 27-gauge, 1.5-inch needle on a 6-ml syringe) or core biopsy (20-gauge Wescott needle) of peripherally located discrete nodules and tracheobronchial lymph nodes (TBLNs) can be effectively guided using ultrasound, fluoroscopy, or CT.[13,14] In fact, a recent study showed cytologic agreement with histopathology in an impressive 82% of cases.[14] Serious complications are infrequent and mainly include pneumothorax or hemothorax. A repeat thoracic radiograph taken 4 to 8 hours after the procedure or observation overnight is recommended after transthoracic aspiration/needle biopsy.

If a preliminary diagnosis cannot be determined from a cytologic or needle tissue biopsy sample and moderately invasive technique is desired, additional tissue obtained via thoracoscopy or limited thoracotomy will usually help distinguish neoplastic disease from non-neoplastic causes of parenchymal masses. Since surgical excision is the treatment of choice for resectable masses, confirmatory histologic specimens of suspected neoplasms are easily obtained during therapeutic thoracotomy via an intercostal or median sternotomy approach.

Clinical staging of primary lung tumors consists of thoracic radiographs or advanced imaging for tumor lung lobe localization and evidence of regional intra-thoracic spread, as well as histopathological evaluation of TBLNs. Even normal-sized lymph nodes should be examined histologically. In one study, CT evaluation of TBLN status agreed with histopathology in 93% of cases, versus only 57% for thoracic radiographs. Therefore, dogs without radiographic evidence of tracheobronchial lymphadenomegaly benefit from preoperative thoracic CT for a more complete assessment of regional metastasis, as well as a better indicator of prognosis.[15] If the preliminary cytologic examination suggests that the pulmonary disease is likely metastatic, a careful search of the abdomen with plain radiography and an ultrasonogram will complement a complete physical examination in identifying a tumor elsewhere in the body. The prostate, urinary bladder, and mammary glands are common extrathoracic sites.

Metastasis

Since the majority of primary lung tumors are carcinomas, there is reason to assume that most metastasis occurs through the lymphatics. However, metastasis can also be vascular, alveolar (by local cell migration in the airways), or through the pleura. Local metastasis to structures in the thorax is more common than systemic spread to bones and intra-abdominal organs. In greater than one third of all cases, multiple lobes are affected, and this will dramatically change surgical treatment options.[3] Regional lymph nodes (tracheobronchial and mediastinal) are the most common sites of intra-thoracic spread. The pattern of metastasis in cats is similar, but the metastatic rate is higher (>75%) at the time of diagnosis, likely due to a greater incidence of poorly differentiated carcinomas as well as the stoic nature of the feline patients, delaying outward clinical signs.[6,16] P2 and P3 are common sites of metastasis (i.e., lung-digit syndrome) for cats with primary pulmonary carcinomas and may be present in multiple toes and feet simultaneously. In fact, in a study examining cats with digital carcinomas, 87.5% were actually metastases from a primary lung carcinoma, with only 12.5% being primary digital tumors.[9] Thus, thoracic radiographs are always warranted prior to amputation for neoplastic digital lesions in feline patients.

Treatment

Whenever possible, lobectomy or partial lobectomy offers the best chance for the longest disease-free interval and survival (Figure 21-1). When treating canine

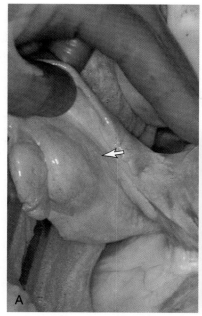
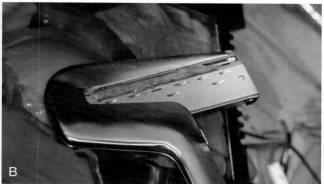

FIGURE 21-1 A, Intraoperative appearance of a primary pulmonary adenocarcinoma in a 12-year-old dog. **B,** The mass was completely excised via partial lobectomy.

patients, in which over half of all lung cancers affect only one lobe, immediate surgical excision is advised since small tumor size (<5 cm diameter) and completeness of tumor excision are associated with better outcomes.[2,4] Radiation and chemotherapies are largely untried. Inhalation chemotherapy has provided measurable responses in approximately 25% of treated dogs.[17] Improved targeting and safer methods of inhalant drug delivery are currently under investigation. Systemic chemotherapy is indicated for dogs and cats with pulmonary lymphoma, lymphomatoid granulomatosis, malignant histiocytic diseases, and mast cell neoplasms. Additional information regarding diagnostics, clinical staging, and multi-drug protocols for these diseases are found in the corresponding chapters. Systemic chemotherapy may also be warranted as adjuvant treatment for patients after surgical removal of the primary lung tumor. A partial response was observed in two dogs with gross evidence of bronchoalveolar carcinoma using vinorelbine, a mitotic inhibitor (given at 15 mg/m^2, IV infusion over 5 minutes, every 7 days), and may be helpful for dogs with residual microscopic disease.[18] The benefit of vinorelbine is its ability to achieve 13.8 times greater concentrations in lung tissue than other vinca alkaloids.[1,19] The

dose-limiting toxicity is typically neutropenia. Piroxicam is a nonsteroidal anti-inflammatory drug that indirectly decreases tumor proliferation, angiogenesis, and resistance to apoptosis and may be useful in the treatment of either primary or secondary lung carcinomas (0.3 mg/ kg PO, once a day).[20]Intracavitary chemotherapy (carboplatin or mitoxantrone) has also shown some success in treating dogs with thoracic or abdominal carcinomatosis, sarcomatosis, or mesothelioma, with one study achieving a median survival time of 332 days in treated patients versus 25 days in the control group.[21]

Although radiation therapy might improve control of incompletely resected tumors, radiation damage to intrathoracic structures with conventional radiation therapy is frequent and problematic.[22] However, newer methods for more precise delivery of local therapy can minimize normal tissue cell kill. One such treatment modality is intensity-modulated radiation therapy (IMRT), which uses multiple collimator beams to three-dimensionally conform to the tumor and minimize radiation doses to normal tissue surrounding it.[23] Another potential method of local treatment is called radiofrequency ablation (RFA) in which an electrode is percutaneously placed in the tumor and uses electrical currents to induce tumor cell necrosis.[24] Treatment of paraneoplastic HO, a periosteal proliferation of long bones, includes complete excision of the lung tumor that provides pain relief within 3 to 6 weeks and resolution of bone lesions only months later. Pain management with NSAIDs or corticosteroids is also helpful.[25]

Prognosis and Survival

The overall post-surgical median survival times for dogs is more favorable than for cats (11 months vs. 4 months, respectively) possibly because in cats, lung tumors are less well differentiated than in their canine counterparts, and the disease is usually more advanced at the time of detection.[3-7,26] However, the survival times for both species are longer when favorable prognostic factors are present (up to 26 months for dogs and 22 months for cats). Prognostic factors associated with longer survival times for dogs are reported as lack of clinical signs referable to their tumor (i.e., no coughing), normal-sized TBLN assessed intra-operatively and/or radiographically, histologic absence of tumor cells in the TBLN, lower histologic grade tumor, well-differentiated adenocarcinomas, low-grade papillary carcinoma, peripherally located tumors amenable to complete surgical excision, small tumors (<5 cm diameter), solitary tumors without metastatic disease, lack of pleural effusion, and complete surgical resection of the primary disease.[1-5,26] Post-surgical survival for cats is longer when pleural effusion, lymphatic or vascular invasion, and embolic, intrapulmonary, or TBLN metastasis are absent. A greater prognosis is also afforded to patients with moderately to well-differentiated tumors that are completely resected without evidence of metastasis.[6,7]

Selected References*

DeBerry JD, Norris CR, Samii VF, et al: Correlation between fine-needle aspiration cytopathology and histopathology of the lung in dogs and cats, *J Am Anim Hosp Assoc* 38:327, 2002.
A retrospective study of patients with spontaneous pulmonary disease found fine-needle aspiration cytology to accurately reflect histopathology in >82% of cases.
Hahn KA, McEntee MF, Paterson MM, et al: Prognosis factors for survival in cats after removal of a primary lung tumor: 21 cases (1979-1994), *Vet Surg* 27:307, 1998.
A retrospective study demonstrating prognostic factors for survival after attempted complete excision.
Jacobs TM, Tomlinson MJ: The lung-digit syndrome in a cat, *Feline Pract* 25:31, 1997.
Veterinary and human literature is reviewed in light of the case presentation, which demonstrates typical features of lung-digit syndrome resulting from a pulmonary carcinoma.
McNeil EA, Ogilvie GK, Powers BE, et al: Evaluation of prognostic factors for dogs with primary lung tumors: 67 cases (1985-1992), *J Am Vet Med Assoc* 211:1422, 1997.
Associations between clinical and histologic factors and outcome for dogs with primary lung tumors are made and a histologic grading system is suggested in this retrospective study.
Poirier VJ, Burgess KE, Adams WM, et al: Toxicity, dosage, and efficacy of vinorelbine (Navelbine) in dogs with spontaneous neoplasia, *J Vet Intern Med* 18:536, 2004.
The first evaluation of vinorelbine (a mitotic inhibitor) for use in dogs with cancer.
Rissetto KC, Lucas P, Fan TM: An update on diagnosing and treating primary lung tumors, *Vet Med* 103(3):154, 2008.
A review article summarizing diagnostic and treatment options for small animal patients with lung cancer.

█ *For a complete list of the references cited in this chapter, please go to www.smallanimaloncology.com.

SECTION B: Mediastinal Tumors

Annette N. Smith

KEY POINTS

- Thymoma and lymphoma are the most common tumors of the cranial mediastinum.
- Cytology may aid in differentiation of lymphoma from thymoma if lymphoblasts are present on review of a mediastinal mass aspirate.
- Surgery is the treatment of choice for non-invasive thymomas.
- Radiation is useful in the palliation of non-resectable thymomas and mediastinal lymphoma.

Incidence—Morbidity and Mortality

Lymphoma and thymoma are the most common cranial mediastinal masses diagnosed in companion animals.[1] Lymphoma is the most frequently diagnosed mediastinal malignancy in both the dog and cat, whereas thymomas are uncommon in the dog and rare in the cat.[2] The cranial mediastinum is the primary site of lymphoma in approximately 5% of canine lymphoma patients[3] and a common site of disease for feline leukemia positive (FeLV+) cats. A list of

---

BOX 21-1   LIST OF DIFFERENTIAL DIAGNOSES FOR MEDIASTINAL MASSES[1,2,4,5]

Lymphoma
Thymoma
Ectopic thyroid tissue
Ectopic thyroid carcinoma (follicular or medullary)
Branchial cyst
Chemodectoma
Neuroendocrine carcinoma
Expansile chest wall mass
Lymphangiosarcoma
Osteosarcoma
Liposarcoma
Soft tissue sarcoma
Fibroma
Undifferentiated sarcoma
Tracheal or esophageal tumor
Metastatic tumor
Lymphadenopathy (infectious or inflammatory)
Bacterial granulomas
Fluid (transudate, exudate, or hemorrhage)
Fat

BOX 21-2   LIST OF REPORTED PARANEOPLASTIC SYNDROMES ASSOCIATED WITH THYMOMA

Myasthenia gravis[12-14,23-28]
Hypercalcemia[13,22]
Polymyositis[23,29]
Skin disease[29-31]
Hypogammaglobulinemia[29]
Non-thymic tumors[12]
Arrhythmias[13,25]

---

differential diagnoses for mediastinal masses[1-5] can be found in Box 21-1.

Etiology and Risk Factors

Lymphoma is typically a disease of middle-aged to older animals with the exception of the FeLV-associated form, which primarily occurs in young cats.[1,6-10] Siamese and Oriental breeds are over-represented in some reports.[1,6,7,9,11] Thymomas are most common in older animals, and medium- to large-breed dogs may be over-represented.[12-14] The median age reported for nine dogs with mediastinal carcinoma was 10 years, with no breed or gender predisposition noted.[5]

Clinical Features

Dyspnea, coughing, and exercise intolerance can all be associated with a space-occupying mediastinal mass. On physical examination, lung sounds are often muffled, heart sounds are muffled or displaced, and, in cats or small dogs, chest compliance may be decreased. Regurgitation/vomiting or gagging can occur as a result of esophageal compression or megaesophagus associated with thymoma-associated paraneoplastic myasthenia gravis. Aspiration pneumonia and recurrent weakness or collapse can be associated with generalized myasthenia gravis.

Invasion or compression of the cranial vena cava by the mediastinal mass can result in swelling of the head, neck, and/or thoracic limbs, known as precaval syndrome.[15-19]

The most common paraneoplastic syndrome associated with mediastinal masses is hypercalcemia. Up to 50% of canine patients with hypercalcemia have cranial mediastinal lymphoma.[20,21] The hypercalcemia may cause clinical signs, such as polyuria/polydipsia, that would prompt a client to seek veterinary care. Hypercalcemia is not only related to lymphoma, but has also been reported with other mediastinal masses including thymoma.[13,22] See Box 21-2 for reported paraneoplastic syndromes associated with thymoma.[12-14,22-31] Paraneoplastic myasthenia gravis occurs sporadically in cats and in up to 40% of canine patients with thymoma.[12-14,23-28]

Diagnosis and Staging

Establishing the definitive diagnosis for a mediastinal mass is imperative for appropriate treatment recommendations to be made. Cytologic or histologic samples are necessary to establish a diagnosis.

Blood Work

Although rarely diagnostic, neoplastic lymphocytes may be present in the circulation, supporting a diagnosis of lymphoma. Paraneoplastic hypercalcemia may be noted and supports a diagnosis of lymphoma or thymoma in pets with known mediastinal masses. Acetylcholine receptor antibody testing should be considered in all cats with thymoma, since they may be asymptomatic for myasthenia gravis. Dogs presenting with clinical signs such as megaesophagus, aspiration pneumonia, or generalized weakness should also be tested.

Imaging Studies

Tracheal elevation on the lateral radiographic images is a consistent sign of a mediastinal mass (Figure 21-2). Positioning can also cause tracheal deviation; a mass that

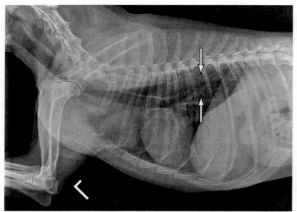

FIGURE 21-2 Lateral radiograph of a dog with a cranial mediastinal mass as evidenced by tracheal elevation. Note the presence of megaesophagus (arrows). (Courtesy Dr. Greg Almond, Auburn University.)

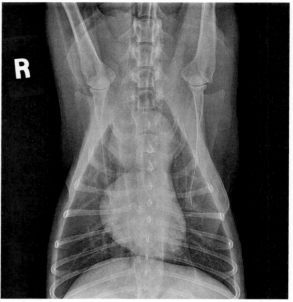

FIGURE 21-3 A widened cranial mediastinum suggests the presence of a mediastinal mass. In this case, the diagnosis was thymoma. (Courtesy Dr. Greg Almond, Auburn University.)

deviates the trachea should be obvious. Differentiating a pulmonary or chest wall mass from a mediastinal mass is best done with the V-D image. The normal mediastinum should be twice the width of the spine in the dog, and the width of the sternum in the cat. A widened mediastinum suggests the presence of a mass (Figure 21-3); however, fat can widen the mediastinum in the absence of a true mass. Pulmonary masses are usually lateral to the mediastinum, and chest wall masses tend to be peripheral, causing rib lysis or spreading. Malignant or chylous pleural effusion resulting from obstruction or invasion of the thoracic duct and other lymphatics may be present.[32,33] Esophagrams and angiograms (Figure 21-4) may be useful in determining invasiveness, and thus resectability of mediastinal masses.[16] An esophagram can also be used to confirm megaesophagus if not apparent on plain films. Ultrasound of the cranial mediastinum can be useful in differentiating a cranial mediastinal mass from pleural fluid and may be helpful in determining the best aspiration or biopsy site.[34] Lymphoma is generally homogenous in echotexture, whereas thymomas and other masses are more frequently mixed with areas of cavitation.[35] CT scan or MRI is useful for determining invasiveness of thymomas or other masses in order to plan surgical resection or radiation treatment of the tumor.[36]

Fine-Needle Aspiration and Cytology
Aspiration cytology may be helpful in determining the diagnosis for a mediastinal mass and can differentiate thymoma from lymphoma in many instances. Thymomas

should contain three cell types: mature lymphocytes, neoplastic epithelial cells, and mast cells. Cytologic diagnosis is difficult when all three components are not present in the aspiration sample. Lymphomas are usually lymphoblastic, with large, immature lymphocytes. Flow cytometry of the mass aspirate to determine a clonal neoplastic population may be useful to confirm a diagnosis of lymphoma.[37] Cytology of pleural effusion can also be diagnostic for lymphoma if exfoliated lymphoblasts are present.[32,33]

Histopathology and Immunohistochemistry
Histopathology is the definitive diagnostic test for mediastinal masses. Thymomas can be cystic, so a blind biopsy may give non-diagnostic results. Open surgical biopsy, ultrasound, or CT guidance will often provide the best sample. Multiple samples should be obtained since cystic areas may be filled with hemorrhage and necrotic debris. In addition, the morphology of the samples may be highly variable depending on the area biopsied. Immunohistochemistry (IHC) may facilitate diagnosis. A variety of IHC markers including CD3 (T-cell lymphoma), CD79 (B-cell lymphoma), cytokeratin (thymoma), synaptophysin and chromogranin (neuroendocrine tumors) and TTF-1 (thyroid tumor),

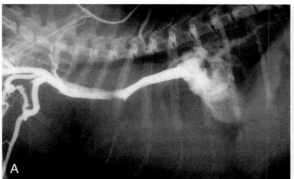 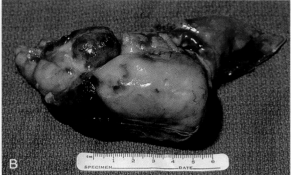

FIGURE 21-4 A, Contrast radiographs (angiogram) showing displacement of the heart by a large mediastinal mass in a cat. **B,** Gross appearance of the mass noted radiographically in *A*. The diagnosis in this case was thymic lymphoma. (Courtesy of the University of Missouri Veterinary Medical Teaching Hospital Oncology Service.)

thyroglobulin (thyroid follicular cell), and calcitonin (thyroid medullary cell) are available to help differentiate among the most likely diagnoses.[5]

Metastasis

Thymomas are generally classified as *invasive* or *non-invasive*,[2,38,39] rather than malignant or benign unless a rare diagnosis of thymic carcinoma or squamous cell carcinoma[1,40,41] is made. Thymomas rarely metastasize, although spread beyond local invasion has been reported.[42-44] Thymic carcinomas can be metastatic to distant sites, including lymph nodes, other mediastinal sites, pleura, and lungs.[1] Cranial mediastinal carcinomas have also been reported to metastasize, namely to the lungs and mediastinal lymph nodes.[5]

Treatment Modalities

With the exception of lymphoma, surgical resection is the treatment of choice for tumors of the mediastinum. Radiographic imaging of the thoracic cavity may not indicate the invasiveness of these tumors, and advanced imaging (CT or MRI) is advised. The presence of effusions should not rule out exploratory surgery.[2,5] Exploratory surgery is often the best way to determine resectability.

Lymphoma

Lymphoma is generally considered a systemic disease; surgery is used primarily in the diagnostic setting. Radiation has utility in palliation of disease; however, chemotherapy is the mainstay of treatment. Several chemotherapy protocols are available and are reviewed in Chapter 25, Section A.

Thymoma

Surgery is the treatment of choice for thymomas. Even tumors with precaval thrombi can be removed by a skilled surgeon.[2,16] Approximately 30% of thymomas are not surgically resectable.[2] Radiation therapy may be useful, either as solitary therapy or an adjunct to incomplete removal.[39,45,46] Prednisone may contribute to remissions[39,45] and is useful in the management of myasthenia gravis, along with anticholinesterase drugs. Chemotherapy protocols for lymphoma may have utility in lymphocyte-rich thymomas. Cisplatin alone or in combination is used most frequently in people.[47] Other drugs to consider are carboplatin, ifosfamide, and doxorubicin.[39,47]

Prognosis and Survival

Lymphoma

Remission rates for cats with mediastinal lymphoma range from 50% to 90% and are similar regardless of FeLV status.[9,48-52] Median survival times with chemotherapy with or without radiation therapy range from 2 to 9 months.[9,48-52] Mediastinal location and hypercalcemia have been negative prognostic indicators in dogs with lymphoma.[53,54] The reader is referred to Chapter 25, Section A, for a thorough discussion of lymphoma prognosis.

Thymoma

Dogs without megaesophagus and completely resected disease have a greater than 80% 1-year survival rate.[12,13,15] Animals with megaesophagus treated with surgery often have very short survival times, reported to be less than 1 week in two thirds of patients.[13] Surgery may be contraindicated because of the morbidity and mortality associated with postoperative recovery.[2] Cats with uncomplicated cases also have a prolonged survival with surgical excision (6-36–month follow-up), although perioperative hemorrhage can be a fatal complication.[24,29] Paraneoplastic syndromes associated with thymoma may or may not resolve with therapy, and may occur later in life despite successful therapy.[13,14,28,30,54] For those not amenable to surgical resection, approximately 75% appear to respond to radiation, although complete remission is achieved in only 20% of patients.[39] Partial remission and temporary relief of clinical signs is common.[39,45] An unresectable thymoma may be consolidated with radiation therapy, thus facilitating surgical excision.[2] Median survival times for 17 dogs and 7 cats with unresectable thymomas treated with variable courses of radiation with or without surgery and/or chemotherapy was 248 days and 720 days, respectively.[39] Reports of prolonged survival in animals with no therapy exist, which may indicate the slow-growing nature of some thymomas.[12]

Mediastinal Carcinomas

A manuscript describing nine dogs with cranial mediastinal carcinomas reported a 243-day median survival time. Degree of local invasion, pleural effusion, and metastasis did not have a significant impact on survival in this case series.[5]

Selected References*

Atwater SW, Powers BE, Park RD, et al: Thymoma in dogs: 23 cases (1980-1991), *J Am Vet Med Assoc* 205:1007, 1994.
This retrospective study discusses the presentation, clinical findings, histologic findings, treatments, and survival of 23 dogs with thymoma. It is the largest study of thymomas in dogs. Paraneoplastic syndromes are discussed, and prognostic implications of these syndromes are evaluated.

Gores BR, Berg J, Carpenter JL, et al: Surgical treatment of thymomas in cats: 12 cases (1987-1992), *J Am Vet Med Assoc* 204:1782, 1994.
This is a small retrospective study of feline thymomas treated with surgical resection alone. Paraneoplastic conditions, surgical complications, and survival are discussed.

Liptak JM, Kamstock DA, Dernell WS, et al: Cranial mediastinal carcinomas in nine dogs, *Vet Comp Oncol* 6:19, 2008.
This manuscript reports on a case series of 9 dogs with cranial mediastinal carcinomas, which does not exist elsewhere in the veterinary literature. Treatments and survival times as well as factors associated with prognosis are discussed.

Smith AN, Wright JC, Brawner WR Jr, et al: Radiation therapy in the treatment of canine and feline thymomas: a retrospective study (1985-1999), *J Am Animal Hosp Assoc* 37:489, 2001.
A retrospective evaluation of radiation therapy for the treatment of thymomas in dogs and cats.

*For a complete list of the references cited in this chapter, please go to www.smallanimaloncology.com.

SECTION C: Metastatic Respiratory Tumors

A. Elizabeth Hershey

KEY POINTS

- Tumors with a high rate of pulmonary metastasis include melanoma, osteosarcoma, mammary carcinoma, histiocytic tumors, hemangiosarcoma, renal cell carcinoma, high-grade sarcomas, lymphoma, and pulmonary carcinoma.
- Once macroscopic metastatic disease has developed, treatment is difficult and durable remissions or cures are uncommon.
- Palliative care of the patient with metastatic lung cancer is aimed at improving appetite, decreasing coughing, and addressing paraneoplastic syndromes.

Incidence, Etiology, and Risk Factors

Metastatic respiratory tumors are more common than primary lung tumors in dogs and cats. Metastasis to the lungs may occur by either the lymphatic or hematogenous routes, with incidence varying according to the primary cancer type. Tumors with high incidence of metastases to lung parenchyma include melanoma, osteosarcoma (OSA), mammary carcinoma, histiocytic tumors, hemangiosarcoma (HSA), renal cell carcinoma, high-grade sarcomas, lymphoma, and pulmonary carcinoma. Occasionally, patients will present with occult lung metastases without history or evidence of a primary tumor.

Clinical Features

Symptoms of metastatic lung disease may include weight loss, poor appetite, lethargy, exercise intolerance, cough, hemoptysis, and/or dyspnea. Occasional patients may be presented peracutely because of hemothorax, pneumothorax, or malignant pleural effusion (MPE).[1] Paraneoplastic syndromes associated with metastatic lung cancer are rare in dogs and cats, with the most common being HO.[2] When this syndrome occurs, patients will be presented for lameness and/or limb swelling (see Chapter 11).

Diagnosis and Staging

Identification of lung metastases is most commonly made by thoracic radiography. Both right and left lateral and ventrodorsal views are recommended for evaluation of lung metastases. Lung metastases often take the form of discrete nodules on the thoracic radiograph (Figure 21-5). For tumors that spread via the lymphatics, such as lymphoma, a more diffuse pattern of metastases is observed (Figure 21-6). CT of the thorax may be useful for detecting lung metastases at an earlier stage than what can be detected by radiography.[3] However, the higher cost and limited availability of CT currently restrict its use as a routine screening tool for lung metastases in the veterinary patient.

Definitive diagnosis of lung metastases may be made by cytologic or histopathologic examination. For large masses located peripherally in the lung, ultrasound may be used to guide needle aspiration or biopsy. However, it is not unusual for lung masses to have a necrotic center that may confound cytologic interpretation.[4] Transtracheal or bronchoalveolar lavage is rarely diagnostic, since most lung masses do not extend or exfoliate into the bronchoalveolar space. More diffuse lung lesions may be sampled via a surgical "key hole" biopsy.[5] For most patients, knowledge of a current or previously treated primary tumor with the presence of multiple pulmonary masses is sufficient for the presumptive diagnosis of lung metastases, and further diagnostic tests are not necessary.

Therapy and Prognosis

The probability of metastatic spread to the lungs is often assessed by prognostic factors of the primary tumor, such as poor differentiation of tumor cells and presence

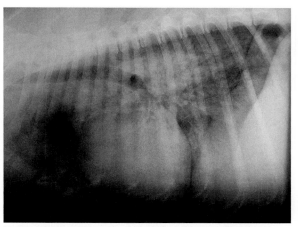

FIGURE 21-6 Diffuse pattern of pulmonary metastasis in a dog with lymphoma. This pattern can be seen with tumors that spread via the lymphatics.

of tumor cells in lymphatic or blood vessels. The presence of these factors can help guide treatment decisions designed to reduce the likelihood of metastases developing. However, once macroscopic lung metastases have developed, treatment is difficult and durable remissions or cures are uncommon.

The role of pulmonary metastasectomy has been well defined in human cancer therapy.[6,7] Major prognostic factors for resection of pulmonary metastases are tumor type, time from treatment of primary tumor to lung metastasis, number of lung metastases, tumor doubling time, existence of extrapulmonary metastases, and general medical condition of the patient.[7] Pulmonary metastasectomy has been evaluated as a method to improve disease-free interval in dogs with OSA[8] and as palliation for HO.[9] Pulmonary metastasectomy is advocated for dogs with OSA when primary local disease has been controlled for greater than 300 days, fewer than three pulmonary lesions are present, and tumor doubling time exceeds 45 days. In patients fitting these criteria, the median disease-free interval following metastasectomy was 128 days.[8] In four patients undergoing pulmonary metastasectomy for palliation of HO, clinical signs of HO resolved within 24 hours, with remissions ranging from 50 to 294 days.[9] The benefit of pulmonary metastasectomy for other tumor types in dogs and cats has not been evaluated.

Few published reports exist describing the use of systemic chemotherapy for the treatment of metastatic lung cancer. One report describes a 12% response rate in dogs with metastatic lung cancer treated with vinorelbine.[10]

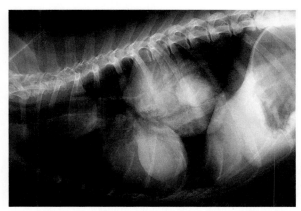

FIGURE 21-5 Lung metastases often take the form of discrete nodules as seen in these thoracic radiographs from a dog with metastatic fibrosarcoma.

Another describes 1 of 45 dogs with metastatic OSA achieving a partial response for 21 days with doxorubicin.[11] Selection of chemotherapy drugs should be based on the primary tumor type. The reasons for treatment failure with systemic chemotherapy in metastatic lung cancer are diverse, but one possibility may be the inability to achieve adequate concentrations of drug at the tumor site with systemic administration. Inhaled delivery of chemotherapeutics offers the theoretical advantage of achieving high local concentration of drug within the lung while minimizing systemic side effects. The safety and efficacy of inhaled therapeutics have been demonstrated for both liposomal interleukin 2 (IL-2) and doxorubicin and taxol chemotherapy.[12,13]

The last two decades have witnessed significant progress in the understanding of the basic mechanisms involved in tumor growth and metastases. Future treatment of metastatic disease will likely target not only metastatic tumor cells but the homeostatic mechanisms that favor metastatic growth and survival. Both immunotherapy and gene therapy offer promising new strategies for the treatment of metastatic cancer in dogs and cats. A recent study has demonstrated systemic immune activation and significantly improved survival time in dogs with OSA lung metastases receiving liposome-DNA complexes encoding the IL-2 gene.[14]

Palliative care of the patient with metastatic lung cancer is aimed at improving appetite, decreasing coughing,

TABLE 21-1   PALLIATIVE TREATMENT OF METASTATIC LUNG CANCER

Drug	Indication	Dose	How Supplied
Prednisone (Should be used in cats)	Anti-inflammatory, appetite stimulant	Cats and dogs: 0.25–1.0 mg/kg SID-BID	1 5, 20, 50 mg tablets; 1 and 5 mg/ml oral suspension
Dexamethasone	Anti-inflammatory, appetite stimulant	0.25–1 mg/kg daily	0.25, 0.5, 0.75, 1, 1.5, 2, 4, and 6 mg tablets; oral elixir solution: 0.5 mg/5 ml
Piroxicam (Feldene)	Anti-inflammatory	Cats and dogs: 0.3 mg/kg PO EOD to SID (EOD recommended in cats)	10 and 20 mg capsules, can be compounded into oral suspension or smaller capsule sizes
Meloxicam (Metacam)	Anti-inflammatory	Cats and dogs: 0.1 mg PO SID	1.5 mg/ml oral suspension; can also be compounded into capsules
Deracoxib (Deramaxx)	Anti-inflammatory	Dogs: 1-2 mg/kg PO SID	25 mg, 100 mg tablets
Hydrocodone	Antitussive	Dogs: 0.25 mg PO BID–QID Cats: 1.25–5 mg per cat PO q 12 hr	Hydrocodone/homatropine 5 mg/1.5 tablets; hydrocodone/homatropine 5 mg/1.5 mg/5 ml syrup
Codeine	Antitussive	1–2 mg/kg PO q 6–12 hr	Codeine sulfate oral tablets: 15, 30, 60 mg; codeine phosphate oral solution: 15 mg/5 ml; codeine with guaifenesin: 10/300;10/100;2.5/75
Dextromethorphan	Antitussive	1–2 mg/kg BID	15 mg gelcaps; dextromethorphan/guaifenesin syrup 10 or 30 mg/5 ml
Butorphanol	Antitussive	0.5–1 mg/kg PO BID–QID	1, 5, 10 mg tablets
Cyproheptadine (Periactin)	Appetite stimulant	Cats: 2–4 mg/cat SID–BID	4 mg tablets, 2 mg/5 ml oral suspension
Megestrol acetate (Megace)	Appetite stimulant	Cats: 5 mg SID for 7 days, then 5 mg EOD Dogs: 5–20 mg SID for 7 days, then 5 mg PO EOD	20 and 40 mg tablets; 40 mg/ml oral suspension
Mirtazapine (Remeron)	Appetite stimulant	Dogs: 0.6 mg/kg PO once daily, with daily max. of 30 mg Cats: 3-4 mg PO every 3 days	15, 30, and 45 mg tablets
Dronabinol (Marinol)	Appetite stimulant	Cats 2.5 mg dailyDogs 5–10 mg daily	2.5, 5, and 10 mg capsules

EOD, every other day.

and addressing paraneoplastic syndromes such as HO. Use of non-steroidal or steroidal anti-inflammatories will help decrease respiratory symptoms of cough, in addition to decreasing pain associated with HO. Effective antitussive agents in dogs and cats include butor-phanol, hydrocodone, codeine, and dextromethorphan. Effective appetite stimulants include prednisone or dexamethasone, cyproheptadine (cats), megestrol acetate, mirtazapine, and dronabinol (Marinol). See Table 21-1 for dosing information.

Selected References*

Dow S, Elmslie R, Kurzman I, et al: Phase I study of liposome-DNA complexes encoding the interleukin-2 gene in dogs with osteosarcoma lung metastases, *Hum Gene Ther* 16:937-946, 2005.

This article demonstrates that repeated infusion of liposome DNA complexes in dogs with spontaneous lung tumor metastases is safe and well tolerated and may be capable of eliciting anti-tumor activity in some patients.

Hershey AE, Kurzman ID, Forrest LJ, et al: Inhalation chemotherapy for macroscopic primary or metastatic lung tumors: proof of principle using dogs with spontaneously occurring tumors as a model, *Clin Cancer Res* 5:2653-2659, 1999.

This article demonstrates that paclitaxel and doxorubicin administered by the inhalation route avoided systemic toxicity while delivering efficacious local drug levels as evidenced by tumor responses in 25% of patients receiving therapy.

Khanna C, Anderson PM, Hasz DE, et al: Interleukin-2 liposome inhalation therapy is safe and effective for dogs with spontaneous pulmonary metastases, *Cancer* 79:1409-1421, 1997.

This article demonstrates that aerosol delivery of interleukin 2 liposomes is nontoxic and biologically effective in dogs with naturally occurring pulmonary metastases and primary lung carcinomas.

Nemanic S, London CA, Wisner ER: Comparison of thoracic radiographs and single breath-hold helical CT for detection of pulmonary nodules in dogs with metastatic neoplasia, *J Vet Intern Med* 20:508-515, 2006.

This article demonstrates that CT is significantly more sensitive than thoracic radiography for detecting soft tissue nodules in dogs.

O'Brien MG, Straw RC, Withrow SJ, et al: Resection of pulmonary metastases in canine osteosarcoma: 36 cases (1983-1992), *Vet Surg* 22:105-109, 1993.

This article demonstrates that prognostic variables exist for dogs with metastatic pulmonary osteosarcoma and help predict survival after metastasectomy—similar to those prognostic variables determined for human patients undergoing pulmonary metastasectomy for osteosarcoma.

Wood EF, O'Brien RT, Young KM: Ultrasound fine-needle aspiration of focal parenchymal lesions of the lung in dogs and cats, *J Vet Intern Med* 12:338-342, 1998.

This article demonstrates that neoplasia was correctly identified by FNA cytology in 10 of 11 animals with no false-positive results.

*For a complete list of the references cited in this chapter, please go to www.smallanimaloncology.com.

SECTION D: Rib and Pleural Tumors

Leslie E. Fox

KEY POINTS

- In dogs and cats, osteosarcoma and chondrosarcoma are the most common primary tumors arising from the rib cage and are locally aggressive and can only be completely resected with wide surgical margins involving one to two ribs on either side of the lesion.
- Biopsy or surgical excision of a suspected primary rib lesion is warranted, since chondrosarcoma and osteosarcoma can look identical on radiographs, yet vary dramatically in prognosis; some rib chondrosarcomas may be completely excised, whereas rib osteosarcomas have probably metastasized (at least microscopically) at the time of diagnosis.
- Advanced imaging with CT and/or MRI greatly improve preoperative tumor visualization.
- Malignant mesothelioma is easily confused with carcinomatosis because finding irregular pleural thickening, intrathoracic masses, and pleural effusion on plain thoracic radiographs is consistent with both diseases.
- Cytology and histopathology are often unable to differentiate between mesothelioma and metastatic carcinoma.

Incidence—Morbidity and Mortality

Thoracic wall tumors are most often locally invasive, aggressive tumors of the rib cage and surrounding soft tissue. In dogs and cats, OSA and chondrosarcoma (CSA) are the most common primary tumors arising from the rib cage. In the dog, fibrosarcoma and HSA are less frequent.[1-5] The same tumors that originate from the skin, subcutaneous, and connective tissue elsewhere in the body can be found in the soft tissues of the thoracic wall. Mast cell tumors and soft tissue sarcomas are most frequently found in dogs and are generally not easily resected. In cats, vaccine-associated sarcomas are more common than rib tumors.

Rib tumors typically affect middle-aged, larger breed dogs as progressively enlarging, sometimes painful, firm masses on the thorax that are often present for more than 10 months before diagnosis.[2] A few dogs have no palpable external swelling but instead have invasion into the thorax.[1,4] Associated clinical signs depend on the location and size of the mass and include forelimb lameness, pain, dyspnea, lethargy, weight loss, exercise intolerance, or coughing.[1-5] Cats have similar signs.

Etiology/Risk Factors

X-ray or radium irradiation of bone may cause spontaneous OSA or CSA following exposure. Molecular factors, such as upregulated expression of COX-2, have been demonstrated in some highly malignant OSAs.[6]

Diagnosis and Staging

Most canine and feline patients are suspected of having a chest wall lesion on the basis of clinical examination and/or plain chest radiographs. Rib tumors are typically extrapleural with a combination of osteolysis and bone proliferation similar to the pattern seen in primary appendicular skeleton malignancies (Figure 21-7).[1-5] A presumptive diagnosis can be made with fine-needle aspirate cytology; however, a definitive diagnosis can only be made with histopathologic examination of a large excisional or wedge biopsy. Tissue obtained via Michele trephine or Jamshidi bone biopsy needle may be insufficient. Like appendicular OSA, tissue obtained from the center of the lesion may be more representative than tissue from the periphery. Care should be taken to select a biopsy site where the biopsy tract can be included in definitive surgical excision at a later date.[7]

Clinical staging includes a minimum of a complete blood count, serum biochemical panel, and urinalysis, as well as thoracic radiographs and regional lymph node

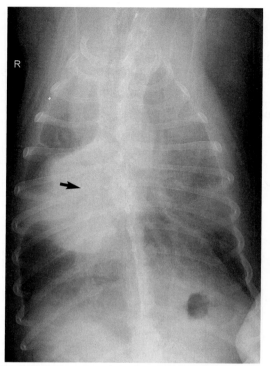

FIGURE 21-7 Dorsoventral thoracic radiograph of a dog with a firm mass over the right thorax showing destruction of bone at the head of the seventh rib *(arrow)* in association with a 5-cm diameter increased soft tissue density separating the right cranial and caudal lung lobes. A moderate amount of pleural effusion obscures the heart. The lung lobes are retracted from the thoracic wall consistent with pleural effusion. Histopathologic examination confirmed an osteosarcoma. (Courtesy of Dr. Elizabeth Riedesel, Iowa State University.)

aspiration and cytology. Cats should also be evaluated for feline leukemia viremia and feline immunodeficiency antibodies, since these diseases may confound the treatment and prognosis of various tumors. Differentiating between tumors of lung origin and rib tumors with secondary lung involvement is critical to treatment planning and may be determined using plain radiography, ultrasonography, or CT/MRI. With thoracic radiographs, air bronchograms seen in an intrathoracic mass are consistent with a pulmonary neoplasm as the cause of the thoracic wall disease.[8] In contrast, an extrapleural soft tissue mass originating from the thoracic wall typically protrudes into the thoracic cavity in association with a well-delineated parietal pleural line that tapers smoothly over the mass to the thoracic wall.[8] The base of an extrathoracic mass is oriented toward the parietal pleura.[8] Ultrasound is useful to delineate the extent of the mass, particularly if pleural effusion is present and can guide a needle biopsy.[9,10]

CT is better than thoracic radiography for documenting the presence and extent of mass lesions involving the thoracic wall and rib (Figure 21-8).[11] CT can be used to guide a biopsy needle (Figure 21-9). In addition to providing more detailed description of the primary tumor, CT or MRI may better evaluate tracheobronchial lymph nodes before surgery than plain radiography. Involvement of additional lymph nodes such as the superficial cervical, axillary, intercostal, retrosternal, and mediastinal lymph nodes should be considered since they drain the thoracic wall, rib cage, and thoracic pleura.[12]

Metastasis

Spread of canine mesenchymal thoracic wall tumors is by local extension into surrounding tissues and to lung and regional lymph nodes.[1,3] The behavior of CSAs is similar to other locations (i.e., locally aggressive, metastasizing

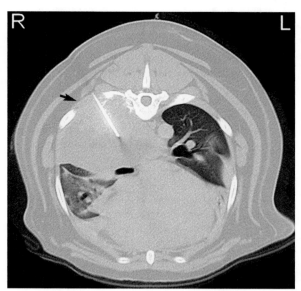

FIGURE 21-9 Computed tomography scan of guided tissue sampling with an 18-g Wescott biopsy needle (white line) in a soft tissue mass attached to the 7th rib *(arrow)*. (Courtesy of Dr. Christine Miles, Iowa State University.)

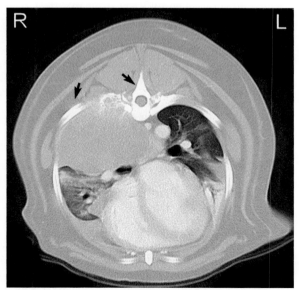

FIGURE 21-8 Computed tomography image of the thoracic cage with contrast enhancement of the same dog at the level of the 7th rib. Note marked bone lysis and increased bone proliferation at the head of the rib (see vector) and associated soft tissue density mass. Visualization of the location and extent of bone involvement are improved when compared with the radiograph in Figure 21-7. (Courtesy of Dr. Christine Miles, Iowa State University.)

late in the course of the disease). OSAs are locally aggressive with rapid pulmonary metastasis, similar to appendicular OSA.

Treatment Modalities

Early, radical surgical excision is the treatment of choice for primary tumors of the thoracic wall in dogs and cats. For tumors involving ribs, the recommended excision is en bloc resection of the thoracic wall including associated muscle, fascia, pleura, and overlying skin with 2- to 3-cm margins and one unaffected rib on each side of the tumor.[1,2,13] Advanced imaging is an essential component of the treatment plan, since local recurrence is frequent and problematic, but may be reduced when more ribs are taken (at least three to four).[1,5,14] For dogs with rib OSA, rapid pulmonary metastasis makes surgical excision alone undesirable without a plan for adjuvant therapy (carboplatin, cisplatin, and/or doxorubicin) aimed at the micrometastatic pulmonary disease that is probably present at the time of diagnosis.[1-5,15]

Recurrence of chest wall and rib tumors is more likely when neoplastic cells extend to the surgical margins but may result even when surgical margins appear free of tumor cells microscopically.[1-3] Survival is increased when conventional radiation therapy is used for dogs with residual microscopic tumor.[2] High-dose, short-term therapy (36 Gy delivered in four fractions) has been used palliatively or in addition to surgical excision.[1]

For cats with axial skeleton OSA (including rib OSA), aggressive excision combined with adjunctive therapy (chemotherapy or radiation therapy) improves survival times compared with excisional biopsy.[16] Because of the risk of fatal pulmonary toxicity associated with cisplatin administration in cats, this drug should not be used as adjuvant therapy in this species.

Prognosis and Survival

Overall, the postoperative median survival times are about 4 months for dogs with OSA, about 6 months for dogs with FSA, and about 14 months for dogs with CSA, compared with a median survival time of about 1 month for dogs receiving no therapy.[1-5,17,18] In one study, dogs with aggressively resected rib CSA had a median survival time of three years.[5] Adjuvant chemotherapy increases post-operative survival times for dogs with OSA (3 vs. 8 months median survival time) and is largely untried for other rib tumors. Completeness of excision and specific histologic diagnosis are identified most consistently as prognostic factors.[1-5,7,14,17]

Mesothelioma

Incidence—Morbidity and Mortality

Mesothelioma generally occurs in older animals, but malignant mesothelioma has been reported in cats and dogs <12 months old.[19,20] There is no apparent gender or breed predilection. Although non-neoplastic diseases more commonly cause pleural effusion, mesothelioma without pleural effusion is rare. Dogs and cats with MPE may exhibit restrictive breathing patterns, increased inspiratory effort and time, delayed expiration, tachypnea, muffled or dull lung sounds, muffled heart sounds, dulled percussion over areas containing fluid, shallow respiration, open mouth breathing, cyanosis, exercise intolerance, lethargy, weight loss, inappetence, and coughing.[12,21,22] Cats with pleural effusion caused by mediastinal lymphoma may have a noncompressible thorax.

Etiology and Risk Factors

Although the molecular mechanism of neoplastic transformation is multifactorial, exposure to asbestos, a group of fibrous silicate minerals, is increased in dogs with malignant pleural mesothelioma (MPM) when compared with non-exposed dogs. Second-hand exposure to asbestos fibers through owners is a demonstrated risk.[23]

Diagnosis and Staging

Finding irregular pleural thickening, possible intrathoracic masses, and pleural effusion on plain thoracic radiographs raises the suspicion for MPM, but this is consistent with metastatic disease (particularly carcinomatosis) as well.[24] The most diagnostic views for detection of pleural effusion are the lateral recumbent and the ventrodorsal views looking for widened fissures; retraction of the lung lobes away from the thoracic wall; rounding of the lungs at the costophrenic angle on the ventrodorsal view; silhouette sign with the heart and diaphragm; and scalloping of the lung edges near the sternum.[25] Thoracic CT is superior to plain radiography or ultrasound imaging for anatomic localization and the extent of disease.

A tissue biopsy is usually required for a diagnosis of mesothelioma, because cytologically, mesothelial neoplasia is not readily distinguished from epithelial neoplasia or marked mesothelial hyperplasia.[13] Ultrasound-guided fine needle aspiration (20- to 22-gauge needle) of solid tissue or pleural effusion may be helpful to rule out non-neoplastic diseases and is associated with a low complication rate in dogs and cats.[26,27] However, thoracotomy is often required to obtain sufficient tissue to differentiate mesothelioma from other neoplasms. If the diagnosis is undetermined, presurgical work-up includes a complete blood count, serum biochemical panel, and urinalysis and abdominal radiographs and ultrasound.

Metastasis

Because the MPM is internal, most patients are presented with advanced disease.[24,28] Mesothelioma spreads by extension and can metastasize to lymph nodes, lung parenchyma, and heart, although most dogs do not have metastasis beyond the thorax.[24]

Treatment Modalities

Pleural mesothelioma is rare in cats and dogs; thus, the most effective therapy is undetermined. Supportive and palliative care is needed. Intermittent thoracocentesis may be helpful in easing respiratory effort in dogs and cats with pleural effusion; however, they are often euthanized because thoracocentesis is required too frequently. Pleurodesis and intracavitary chemotherapy with cisplatin in dogs or carboplatin in cats have helped reduce pleural effusion and stabilize tumor growth.[29,30] Since MPM is largely chemotherapy resistant, new agents are needed that target malignant mesothelial cell proliferation and survival-like selective inhibitors of factors known to control angiogenesis and cell proliferation.[31]

Malignant Pleural Effusions

Pleural effusion of almost any type can be found in association with a tumor. However, MPE is found much less frequently than pneumothorax, diaphragmatic hernia, cardiac disease, trauma, chylothorax, lung lobe torsion, and hypoproteinemia, which are more common causes of the respiratory distress associated with pleural effusion in dogs than malignant causes (thymoma, mediastinal lymphoma, metastatic carcinoma, lymphoma, and mesothelioma).[32] In a group of 82 cats with pleural fluid accumulation, the most frequently encountered diseases were chylothorax, pyothorax, intrathoracic neoplasia, hypertrophic cardiomyopathy, and feline infectious peritonitis.[22]

Pleural fluid should be placed immediately into a sterile red-top tube and a purple-top tube containing EDTA for biochemical and cytological evaluation. Collected fluid is analyzed for color, turbidity, odor, clot formation, total protein, specific gravity by refractometer, total nucleated cell count, and differential cell count followed by cytologic evaluation of direct smears.[12] An aerobic and anaerobic culture with antimicrobial sensitivity is indicated. A packed cell volume may help identify malignant effusions. Malignant effusions typically have a PCV of less than 5% and are nonclotting; however, if the PCV is near the PCV of peripheral blood clots or is acute in onset, then trauma, an HSA, or other neoplasms that infiltrate large blood vessels are possible diagnoses.[12] Effusions associated with lymphoma in cats are typically chylous.[12]

Neoplastic effusions are most often classified as modified transudates (protein of 3–5 gm/dl, 1000–5000 cells/µl) or exudates (protein of >3.5 g/dl, >5000 cells/µl), or consistent with hemothorax or chylothorax.[12,22] Macrophages and mesothelial cells are typical. Lymphoblasts are usually observed with lymphoma in cats and dogs.[12,22] Unfortunately, other neoplastic cells are not often visualized within effusions.

Prognosis

Poor performance status, lack of epithelial histology, weight loss, male gender, older age, high platelet and leukocyte counts, tumor growth through the diaphragm, involvement of mediastinal lymph nodes, and invasion into visceral pleura are related to a poor prognosis.[33]

Selected References*

Baines SJ, Lewis S, White RA: Primary thoracic wall tumours of mesenchymal origin in dogs: a retrospective study of 46 cases, *Vet Rec* 150:335-339, 2002.
An excellent review of the literature and survival outcome for dogs with four primary rib tumor types.
Charney SC, Bergman PJ, McKnight JA: Evaluation of intracavitary mitoxantrone and carboplatin for treatment of carcinomatosis, sarcomatosis and mesothelioma, with or without malignant effusions: a retrospective analysis of 12 cases (1997-2002), *Vet Comp Oncol* 3:171-181, 2005.
A retrospective study of intracavitary chemotherapy for the treatment of malignant pleural and peritoneal neoplasms that present with and without effusion.
Davies C, Forrester SD: Pleural effusion in cats, *J Small Anim Prac* 37:217-224, 1996.
Eighty-two cases of feline pleural effusion were evaluated with respect to clinicopathologic findings, predisposing conditions, and response to treatment.
Popvitch CA, Weinstein MJ, Goldschmidt MH, et al: Chondrosarcoma: a retrospective study of 97 dogs (1987-1990), *J Am Anim Hosp Assoc* 30:81-85, 1994.
Disease description and treatment outcome for dogs with chondrosarcomas of all locations.
Prather AB, Berry CR, Thrall DE: Use of radiography in combination with computed tomography for the assessment of noncardiac thoracic disease in the dog and cat, *Vet Rad Ultrasound* 46:114-121, 2005.
An evaluation of 28 dogs and cats comparing information from plain thoracic radiographs followed by CT in which the diagnosis in 40% of dogs changed as a result of the CT.

▊ *For a complete list of the references cited in this chapter, please go to www.smallanimaloncology.com.

SECTION E: Cardiac and Heart-Based Tumors

Deborah M. Fine and Kathryn J. Atkinson

KEY POINTS

- Primary cardiac tumors are uncommon in dogs and cats.
- Clinical signs result from pericardial effusion and include weakness, lethargy, and syncope.
- Thoracic radiography and echocardiography are integral to the diagnosis of cardiac tumors.

Cardiac tumors are uncommon in dogs and exceedingly rare in cats.[1-3] The most common cardiac tumors are HSA, chemodectoma, mesothelioma, and lymphoma. Other reported cardiac tumors include rhabdomyoma/sarcoma, fibroma/sarcoma, chondroma/sarcoma, and myxoma/sarcoma.

COMMON CLINICAL FEATURES

Patients with cardiac and heart base tumors almost always present for clinical signs resulting from pericardial effusion.[4] Common physical examination findings are shown in Table 21-2. Presenting complaints may include weakness, lethargy, anorexia, coughing, and syncope.

HEMANGIOSARCOMA

Incidence, Etiology, and Risk Factors

HSA is the most common cardiac tumor of dogs, accounting for about 40% of all cardiac neoplasia.[1,3] HSA is less common in cats.[5] In one necropsy survey, only 3 of 18 cats with HSA had cardiac involvement.[6] In another study of 31 HSA cases, no cat had cardiac involvement.[7] German shepherd dogs, golden retrievers, Labrador retrievers, and poodles are among the breeds most commonly affected.[1] No breed predilection has been found in cats.[6,7] The mean age of dogs and cats with HSA is 8 to 10 years.[7,8]

Diagnosis and Staging

Imaging of the thorax and heart is integral to diagnosis of cardiac HSA. Radiographs will often show multiple pulmonary nodules indicative of metastatic disease. The heart may appear enlarged and the caudal vena cava distended if a large volume of pericardial effusion is present. However, thoracic radiographs can appear normal if only a small volume of effusion is present, or metastases are small. On echocardiogram, HSA is most commonly associated with the right atrium or auricle, but it can be

found anywhere in the heart.[9] The size of the tumor varies considerably, and small, multiple hypoechoic cystic regions are frequently observed within the mass. HSAs exfoliate poorly; thus, cytology of the effusion is usually non-diagnostic. However, serum cardiac troponin I concentrations are significantly higher in dogs with pericardial effusions because of HSA compared with idiopathic effusion.[10] Because of the metastatic nature of HSA, complete tumor staging should include abdominal ultrasound to assess for concurrent lesions in the spleen, liver, or other organs. See Chapter 22, Section D, for more staging information related to splenic HSA.

Biological Behavior/Metastasis

Canine HSA is highly metastatic and may be found in many other tissue types, particularly the spleen, and cutaneous tissues.[8,11] One report suggests that approximately 25% of dogs with splenic HSA have concurrent right atrial HSA.[12]

Therapy and Prognosis

Treatment options for cardiac HSA include chemotherapy, surgical resection, and pericardiectomy.[13-16] No single chemotherapeutic regimen for cardiac HSA has been established. Various doxorubicin-based chemotherapy protocols have been published with survival times ranging from 4.6 to 6.7 months.[14] The average survival time for dogs treated with surgery alone ranges from 1 to 4 months.[11,16] Adding chemotherapy increases the survival to approximately 6 months.[16] Pericardiectomy or percutaneous balloon pericardiotomy may be used to palliate clinical signs but is unlikely to improve survival time unless coupled with chemotherapy.[15,17,18]

HEART-BASED TUMORS

Incidence, Etiology, and Risk Factors

The term *heart base tumor* describes any tumor found at the base of the heart, with chemodectoma being the most common.[1] These tumors are also referred to as aortic body tumors and nonchromaffin paragangliomas. Other heart base tumors include thymoma, ectopic thyroid and parathyroid carcinomas, and HSA. Chemodectomas account for 7% to 17% of all reported cardiac tumors and most commonly affect brachycephalic dogs (boxers, bulldogs, and Boston terriers).[1,3,19] The brachycephalic

TABLE 21-2   DIAGNOSTIC APPROACH TO PERICARDIAL EFFUSION

Test	Common Findings
Physical examination	Muffled heart sounds, jugular distension, tachycardia, arrhythmias, weak femoral pulses, pulsus alternans, hepatomegaly, ascites
Thoracic radiographs	Enlarged cardiac silhouette
	Distended caudal vena cava
	Metastases (+/−)
Electrocardiography	Sinus tachycardia
	Small QRS complexes
	Electrical alternans
	Atrial or ventricular premature complexes
Echocardiography	Pericardial effusion appears as hypoechoic space between the pericardium and heart
Hemangiosarcoma	Multi-cystic mass at the right atrium, atrioventricular junction, or right ventricle
Chemodectoma	Large homogenous mass encircling the ascending aorta
Mesothelioma	No visible mass
Lymphoma	No visible mass; myocardium may appear hypertrophied, irregular, and hyperechoic
Fluid cytology	Gross appearance usually identical to venous blood regardless of etiology
Hemangiosarcoma	Non-diagnostic
Chemodectoma	Non-diagnostic
Mesothelioma	Non-diagnostic
Lymphoma	Lymphoblastic cells frequently present

conformation is thought to create a hypoxic state, resulting in chronic stimulation of the chemoreceptors. This hypothesis is supported by the increased incidence of chemoreceptor tumors in humans living at high altitude. Within the brachycephalic breeds, there appears to be a male predisposition, but this is not seen in other breeds. The average age at presentation for dogs is 10 years. Chemodectoma is very rare in cats.[20]

Diagnosis and Staging

Heart base tumors usually appear as large, relatively homogenous masses on echocardiogram.[9] Lesions are closely associated with the ascending aorta and may completely encircle it. The tumor may also invade the atria, although this is not common. Chemodectomas are poorly exfoliative and therefore unlikely to be diagnosed by cytological examination of the effusion.

Biological Behavior/Metastasis

Metastatic disease with heart-based tumors is relatively uncommon. However, approximately 50% of dogs with aortic body tumors will have another tumor present, often of endocrine origin.[19,21]

Therapy and Prognosis

Optimal therapy of chemodectoma is unknown. Their location makes complete resection impossible, although debulking can be done. The most common approach is palliative pericardiectomy. Reported survival times after pericardiectomy average about 2 years.[15,22,23]

MESOTHELIOMA

Incidence, Etiology, and Risk Factors

Mesothelioma accounts for 5% to 21% of all canine neoplastic pericardial effusions.[24,25] Pericardial mesothelioma is exceedingly rare in cats.[2] Mesothelioma is a neoplastic proliferation of the serosal cell layer lining the peritoneal, pericardial, or pleural spaces. No breed or gender predilection has been identified in dogs.[25] Exposure to asbestos is a known risk factor for development of mesothelioma in people and may also place dogs at higher risk.[26]

Diagnosis and Staging

Mesothelioma presents a diagnostic challenge. It forms as numerous small proliferations that are usually too small to visualize on echocardiogram, so it is common to erroneously diagnose mesothelioma as idiopathic pericarditis. Fluid cytology is usually non-diagnostic. Mesothelial cells are typically found in abundance in pericardial effusion, but reactive mesothelial cells will demonstrate many features of malignancy regardless of the etiology. Even with histopathology, mesothelioma may be incorrectly diagnosed as idiopathic because of its reactive appearance.[26,27] The diagnosis of mesothelioma may be revealed after therapeutic pericardiectomy results in metastatic spread to the pleural cavity with subsequent development of pleural effusion.[26,28] This is not a characteristic of idiopathic pericarditis after pericardiectomy.

Therapy and Prognosis

Although optimal therapy is unknown, pericardiectomy, doxorubicin, and intrathoracic cisplatin have resulted in survival times ranging from 4.3 months to greater then

27 months.[29,30] Pericardiectomy alone does not appear to improve survival.[15]

LYMPHOMA

Incidence

It is relatively common for lymphoma to metastasize to the heart but uncommon for it to result in pericardial effusion.[2,31,32] A multi-center review of 7248 canine records revealed 12 cases of cardiac lymphoma with pericardial effusion (0.17%).[31]

Diagnosis and Staging

On echocardiogram, the myocardium may appear hypertrophied with regions of hyperechogenicity corresponding to areas of cellular infiltration. Unlike most other cardiac neoplasia, lymphoma can usually be diagnosed by cytological examination of the effusion.

Therapy and Prognosis

Optimal therapy of cardiac lymphoma is unknown, but use of multi-agent chemotherapy is advised (see Chapter 25, Section A). Median survival time for dogs in the study just described was 41 days.[31] Dogs that were not treated or received only prednisone had a median survival of 22 days. Dogs that received multi-agent chemotherapy had a median survival of 157 days. There are very few case reports of feline cardiac lymphoma, and most have reported very short survival times.[33,34] However, one cat

was reported to have survived >6 months after treatment with thoracocentesis, pericardiocentesis, and the University of Wisconsin Madison chemotherapy protocol.[35]

Selected References*

Ehrhart N, Ehrhart EJ, Willis J, et al: Analysis of factors affecting survival in dogs with aortic body tumors, *Vet Surg* 31:44, 2002.
A retrospective review of 24 dogs with heart base tumors.
Stafford Johnson M, Martin M, Binns S, et al: A retrospective study of clinical findings, treatment and outcome in 143 dogs with pericardial effusion, *J Small Anim Pract* 45:546, 2004.
One of the largest case studies of dogs with pericardial effusions of various causes.
Stepien RL, Whitley NT, Dubielzig RR: Idiopathic or mesothelioma-related pericardial effusion: clinical findings and survival in 17 dogs studied retrospectively, *J Small Anim Pract* 41:342, 2000.
This retrospective study provides information on the clinical presentation and prognosis for dogs with pericardial effusions.
Thomas WP, Sisson D, Bauer TG, et al: Detection of cardiac masses in dogs by two-dimensional echocardiography, *Vet Radiol Ultrasound* 25:65, 1984.
This manuscript reviews echocardiographic findings in dogs with cardiac masses.

█ *For a complete list of the references cited in this chapter, please go to www.smallanimaloncology.com.

22 Tumors of the Abdominal Cavity

SECTION A: Stomach Tumors

Leslie E. Fox

KEY POINTS

- Stomach cancer should be suspected in geriatric dogs or cats with a history of chronic vomiting, inappetence, and weight loss.
- Carcinomas are typically located in the lesser curvature or pyloric antrum, whereas smooth muscle tumors are found in the area of the cardia.
- Aggressive surgical excision cures benign tumors such as leiomyoma but is primarily palliative for dogs with gastric adenocarcinoma.

Incidence/Mortality

Gastric tumors are uncommon and comprise less than 1% of all neoplasms in dogs and cats.[1-4] The most common malignant gastric tumor in dogs is adenocarcinoma (ACA). Other malignancies affecting the stomach include leiomyosarcoma (LMS), gastrointestinal stromal tumor (GIST), lymphoma, mast cell tumor (MCT), extramedullary plasmacytomas, scirrhous carcinoma, histiocytic sarcoma, and others.[1,3,5] Non-retrovirus–associated lymphoma is the most common gastric tumor in cats followed by LMS, ACA, MCT, extramedullary plasmacytomas, carcinoid, GIST, and others.[2,4,6-11] Benign lesions include gastric adenoma, adenomatous polyps, and leiomyoma.[2,3,9,12] Carcinoids are very rare neuroendocrine tumors of the gastrointestinal tract that are reported only as single case reports in dogs and cats.[13,14] Most dogs and cats with gastric tumors are geriatric (average, 10 years old). Dogs with leiomyoma are usually older (average, 16 years old), and dogs with LMS tend to be younger (7 years old).[1-3,5,7,9,12,15] Gastrointestinal lymphoma and MCT are typically diffuse within both the stomach and intestines in cats and dogs. They are discussed in Chapter 25, Section A and Chapter 23, Section D, respectively.

Etiology/Risk Factors

Breed predilections for ACA include Chow Chows, Rough Collies, Staffordshire terriers, Belgian shepherds, and Norwegian Lundehunds.[1,3,16-18] In most reports, male dogs are more frequently affected.[1,3,17] In general, cats do not appear to have breed or gender predilection.[4,6,7,9,10] Recently, the simultaneous occurrence of gastric ACA was diagnosed in two related Persian cats living in the same household.[16] Dietary factors contribute to the development of stomach cancer in humans and may play a similar role in dogs.[19] Gastric ACA may be experimentally induced in dogs by chronic feeding of nitrosamines.[20] It has been hypothesized that the association found between *Helicobacter heilmannii* infection in pet cats and lymphoblastic or lymphocytic lymphoma of mucosa-associated lymphoid tissue is similar to *H. heilmannii*–associated gastric lymphoma in humans, which resolves when the infection is eradicated with antimicrobial therapy.[21,22]

Clinical Features

Clinical signs develop over weeks to many months and include chronic vomiting, anorexia (often the first clinical sign observed), lethargy, and weight loss.[1,3,5-7,9,10] Additional signs may include abdominal discomfort, ptyalism, anemia, hematemesis, and melena; they may reflect the presence of metastatic disease in other organs. Cats and dogs with gastric polyps are often asymptomatic.[13,23] Physical examination may be unremarkable except for weight loss or may include a palpable abdominal mass, pale mucous membranes, and pain on abdominal palpation. Differential diagnosis for chronic vomiting, inappetence, and weight loss are gastritis, fungal or inflammatory granulomas, foreign body, gastric ulceration, motility disorders, malignant and benign tumors, and pyloric outflow obstruction or dysfunction. Clinicopathologic data are generally normal or have non-specific changes. A non-regenerative, microcytic, hypochromic anemia resulting from chronic blood loss may occur, whereas persistent vomiting may alter electrolytes. Paraneoplastic hypoglycemia has been reported in dogs with gastric leiomyoma and LMS.[24,25]

Diagnosis and Staging

Stomach cancer should be suspected in a geriatric dog or cat with weight loss, chronic vomiting, and inappetence. Survey abdominal radiography with or without contrast is often unremarkable and is considered relatively insensitive for detecting gastric wall changes.[23,26,27] When present, abnormalities include alteration in normal stomach axis (should be parallel to the 10th or 11th ribs in dogs), distention with fluid, masses and/or filling defects, calcified masses, and delayed gastric emptying (>10–12 hours in dogs).[26] Thoracic radiographs should be evaluated for complete staging, but they are typically normal.

Ultrasound examination is preferred for evaluation because stomach wall thickness, gastric lumen structure, focal motility abnormalities, lumen contents, and regional lymph nodes are visualized rapidly, in real time, without special patient preparation or positioning.[27-29] Loss of normal five-layer gastrointestinal tract wall structure and/or wall thickness greater than 7 mm, and decreased wall motility (<4-5 contractions/minute) are consistent with gastric wall infiltration, although confirming the cause (necrosis, neoplasia, hemorrhage, edema, inflammation) requires histopathologic examination.[26] Ultrasound-guided, percutaneous fine-needle aspiration (FNA) cytology, or needle tissue biopsy can be performed with minimal invasiveness.[27-29] Cytologic examination of a FNA sample may support a diagnosis of gastric neoplasia, particularly if the slide is appropriately prepared and the tumor exfoliates well, such as with lymphoma, MCT, or some ACAs.[28] Hypoechoic and hyperechoic lesions in the liver and spleen and enlarged locoregional lymph nodes are consistent with metastatic tumor; however, normal-sized gastric lymph nodes should be evaluated microscopically for metastasis.[23,26]

Endoscopy is minimally invasive and allows direct visualization and sampling of the mucosa. The gastric wall can be diffusely affected and look normal; therefore, multiple biopsy samples are needed, regardless of the mucosal appearance. Gastric lesions may appear diffusely infiltrative or localized and discrete.[1,3,26,27] They may be smooth or ulcerative, proliferative, and/or polypoid.[1,3,26,27] Generally, ACAs are highly invasive, often through the serosa, and are proliferative and ulcerative, whereas adenomatous polyps, leiomyomas, and LMSs are typically covered with intact mucosa.[1] Carcinomas are typically located in the lesser curvature or pyloric antrum, whereas smooth muscle tumors are found in the area of the cardia.[1,3] Peritumoral inflammation, food retention, and necrosis associated with ulceration make definitive histologic diagnosis from mucosal pinch biopsies difficult; however, sampling at the edges of the lesion optimizes tumor identification. Abdominal exploratory may be needed to assess the extent of disease and obtain sufficient tissue (full-thickness biopsy) for diagnosis.

Metastasis

Because ACAs are often detected late in the course of the disease, the locoregional metastatic rate is greater than 70% to 80%.[1,3,17] Metastasis may be through the lymphatic route and/or tumor cell exfoliation directly into the abdominal cavity. Carcinomas metastasize to the gastric lymph nodes (most often affected), liver, spleen, peritoneum, lungs, duodenum, pancreas, esophagus, and adrenal glands.[3] Mesenchymal tumors metastasize to similar sites, but more slowly.[5]

Treatment Modalities

Complete surgical excision is the treatment of choice for focal gastric tumors and may be necessary in order to obtain tissue for histologic diagnosis.[1,3,12,23,30,31] Cytologic examination of tumor tissue impression smears relates well to histologic diagnosis and may provide useful information for intraoperative planning for the aggressiveness of tumor excision.[27] Segmental resection and anastomosis of the stomach with 1 to 3 cm surgical margins can be curative for dogs with benign antral polyps, adenomas, and leiomyomas.[1,12] Adequate control of large, invasive antral carcinomas requires resection of the pyloric antrum and anastomosis of the pylorus to the stomach while sparing the visible biliary tree (Bilroth I surgery). For some patients, more aggressive resection is required (Bilroth II).[1,3,17] Postoperative supportive care consists of antiemetics, fluid therapy, possible blood transfusions, and pain control. For dogs and cats with significant resection, a jejunostomy tube placed during laparotomy or total parenteral nutrition (TPN) can provide nutrition for 3 or 4 days after surgery, followed by a low-residue diet.

Surgical excision can also be palliative.[3] Partial gastrectomy decreases bleeding, ulceration, and outflow obstruction. Immediate relief from vomiting for up to 8 months has been reported with partial tumor excision.[3] Neuroglycopenic signs exhibited by dogs with paraneoplastic hypoglycemia resolve within hours of tumor excision.[24,25]

Adjuvant therapy is needed for dogs with malignant disease; however, little information is available regarding treatment selection or outcome with chemotherapy. The FAC protocol (5-fluorouracil [5-FU], doxorubicin, cyclophosphamide), gemcitabine, mitoxantrone, and cisplatinum/carboplatinum have been tried with little success.[1,3] There is some risk of gastrointestinal perforation with chemotherapy. Intestinal carcinomas express COX-2, but normal small intestine mucosa does not, suggesting an anti-cancer role for COX-2 inhibitors in the palliative treatment of dogs with gastrointestinal carcinoma.[32] Piroxicam (0.3 mg/kg, PO, SID) may be useful.[33]

Recently, many canine gastrointestinal tumors previously identified as LMS were reclassified as GIST, thus originating from gastrointestinal pacemaker cells.[34,35] Application of immunohistochemical stains for smooth muscle actin, desmin, S-100, vimentin and c-kit (CD-117) helps identify these heterogenous mesenchymal cell tumors.[34] Most human and canine GIST, but not LMS, express the c-kit protein, a transmembrane receptor with a tyrosine kinase component believed to be responsible for oncogenesis.[35] In humans, the c-kit–positive GIST is quite resistant to chemotherapy but responds to receptor tyrosine kinase inhibitors (TKIs).[19,36] Orally administered receptor TKIs have become available for veterinary use and may prove to have a role in the treatment of nonresectable or metastatic c-kit–positive GIST.[19]

Prognosis and Survival

Prognosis is highly dependent on tumor type and extent. Postsurgical prognosis for dogs with gastric leiomyoma, adenoma, and hypertrophic polyps is excellent with aggressive excision.[1,2,7,17,31] The few dogs and cats reported with gastric plasmacytomas responded favorably to surgical excision and various combinations of chemotherapy, including doxorubicin, melphalan, prednisone, and cyclophosphamide in dogs, and vincristine, chlorambucil, cyclophosphamide, and prednisone in cats.[8,11] In contrast, most dogs with ACA die or are euthanized for progressive disease and intractable vomiting within 2 to 4 months if untreated.[1,3,17,31] With

surgical excision, survival may be extended by months, although there are rare cases of long-term survival.[3,30] Dogs with gastrointestinal LMS that survive the immediate postoperative period have a reported median survival time of about 21 months, even with metastasis.[5] When located in the stomach, GIST may have a better prognosis than LMS.[36]

Selected References*

Bonfanti U, Bertazzolo W, Bottero E, et al: Diagnostic value of cytologic examination of gastrointestinal tract tumors in dogs and cats: 83 cases (2001-2004), *J Am Vet Med Assoc* 229:1130, 2006.
This paper increases awareness of the utility of impression smears for gastric tumor identification.
Dennis MM, Bennett N, Ehrhart EG: Gastric adenocarcinoma and chronic gastritis in two related Persian cats, *Vet Pathol* 43:358, 2006.
This paper discusses gastric carcinoma and the potential influences of Helicobacter *spp. and* Ollulanus tricuspis.
London C: The role of small molecule inhibitors for veterinary patients, *Vet Clin North Am* 37:1121, 2007.
Discusses the application of kinase inhibitors to veterinary patients that have cancer.
Russell KN, Mehler SJ, Skorupski KA, et al: Clinical and immunohistochemical differentiation of gastrointestinal stromal tumors from leiomyosarcomas in dogs: 42 cases (1990-2003), *J Am Vet Med Assoc* 230:1329, 2007.
This paper distinguishes GIST from tumors previously diagnosed as leiomyosarcoma, which may be clinically relevant.
Swann HM, Holt DE: Canine gastric adenocarcinoma and leiomyosarcoma: a retrospective study of 21 cases (1986-1999) and literature review, *J Am Anim Hosp Assoc* 38:157, 2002.
An excellent review of canine gastric adenocarcinomas and leiomyosarcomas with clinical outcome.

*For a complete list of the references cited in this chapter, please go to www.smallanimaloncology.com.

SECTION B: Intestinal Tumors

Kerry Rissetto and Kim A. Selting

KEY POINTS

- Intestinal tumors are uncommon in dogs and cats, with lymphoma and adenocarcinoma reported most often.
- Feline intestinal tumors are more commonly found in the small intestine, whereas colorectal tumors predominate in dogs.

- Differentiating lymphoma from lymphocytic-plasmacytic enteritis, although challenging, can be accomplished via full-thickness biopsies, immunohistochemical staining, and polymerase chain reaction (PCR) to detect neoplastic cell antigen receptor rearrangements. With the development of tyrosine kinase inhibitors, gastrointestinal stromal tumors (GIST) expressing c-KIT should be differentiated from smooth muscle tumors to determine if this targeted therapy is an option.

Incidence

Intestinal tumors account for less than 10% of all neoplasms and 20% to 30% of alimentary tumors of dogs and cats in the United States.[1-3] In most reports, lymphoma (LSA) is most common[3-12] and adenocarcinoma (ACA) the second most common intestinal tumor in both species.[13-15] As with many cancers, incidence of intestinal neoplasia increases with age. The mean age at diagnosis for all intestinal tumors ranges between 10 and 12 years in cats and 6 and 9 years in dogs; for dogs with leiomyosarcoma (LMS), the mean age is 12.[3,8,12,14-25] Young, FeLV-positive cats may develop LSA of any site, including the intestines, although extra-intestinal sites are more common.[8,11,26-31] With the exception of feline large granular LSA,[21] a male predilection is reported for development of intestinal tumors (50%–90%) in both dogs and cats.[15,17,18,20,28,29,32-42] Siamese cats appear to be predisposed to develop intestinal ACA and, perhaps, LSA.[3,8,14,32,43] Male cats and those of Asian ancestry are overrepresented in reports of benign intestinal polyps.[22,44-48] Large breed dogs are more commonly affected with smooth muscle intestinal tumors than are smaller breeds,[39] and collies and German Shepherd dogs may be predisposed to intestinal masses, especially ACA, rectal carcinoma, and polyps.[15,49,50] Mast cell tumors (MCT) are the third most common feline intestinal tumor (Figure 22-1) and, in dogs, have been reported primarily in Maltese, among other miniature breeds. Over 50% of cases in two Japanese reports were Maltese dogs, with males predominating.[51,52]

Epithelial, mesenchymal, neuroendocrine, and round cell neoplasia can all occur in the intestinal tract (Table 22-1). The majority of canine intestinal tumors occur in the distal colon, whereas feline intestinal neoplasia is more often reported to occur in the small intestine (SI), primarily in the ileum or jejunum.[2,3,5,6,8,10,15,16,32,34,35,43,53,54] Most SI neoplasia is malignant in dogs, whereas rectal or colonic canine tumors are more likely to be benign polyps, adenomas, or carcinoma *in situ*.[41,55] Recently, evaluation of intestinal smooth muscle tumors has resulted in the reclassification of many of these tumors to gastrointestinal stromal tumors (GIST) (Table 22-2). The GISTs are anatomically more likely to occur in the large intestine (LI), especially cecum (Figure 22-2), compared

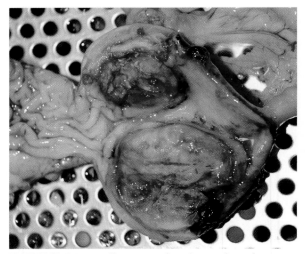

FIGURE 22-1 Mast cell tumors such as the one shown here are the third most common intestinal neoplasm in cats. They also affect small breed dogs, especially Maltese.

with the stomach for leiomyomas.[36,56-58] The advent of tyrosine kinase inhibitors (TKIs) as therapeutic agents suggests that differentiation of GIST and LMS is clinically important. Tumors of globule leukocytes originate from leukocytes found between intestinal epithelial cells. They are extremely rare granulated round cell tumors that only occur in cats, commonly in the ileum.[59-62] Few attempts at therapy have been reported, although one cat did well for over a year following surgical resection until the tumor recurred.[62] Isolated case reports mention other rare intestinal tumors including a rectal ganglioneuroma, mesojejunal liposarcoma, and intestinal melanoma.[63-65]

Etiology

Molecules involved in anti-adhesion and motility such as tenascin, versican, and hyaluronan have been investigated in canine intestinal tumors and may have differential expression in benign and malignant lesions.[55,66,67] All colorectal adenomas and almost half the carcinomas in one study stained positively for β-catenin, suggesting a role in carcinogenesis similar to that shown in human colorectal adenomatous polyposis coli.[68]

Alterations in other molecular processes offer clues as to the pathogenesis of intestinal neoplasia. The tumor suppressor gene p53 has been identified in 15%-50% of canine GI tumors, but does not aid in differentiation of benign from malignant tumors.[68,69] Measures of cellular proliferation such as argyrophilic

TABLE 22-1   DESCRIPTION OF COMMON INTESTINAL TUMORS OF DOGS AND CATS

Tumor Type	Species	Location	Characteristics	References
Lymphoma (most common overall)	Dog	Stomach = small intestine > large intestine	• Diffuse; infiltration into submucosa and lamina propria • LGL subtype is rare.	117
	Cat		• Subtypes: lymphocytic, lymphoblastic, epitheliotropic (T cell only) and LGL (rapidly fatal) types • T ≥ B cell origin, no association with FeLV status • Unique subtypes usually FeLV negative	25,33,61,118,119
Adenocarcinoma	Dog	Colon and rectum	• Often pedunculated (especially in the distal rectum), cobblestone (middle rectum), or annular (middle rectum) appearance, which may relate to behavior and prognosis.	13,54,89,95
	Cat	Small > large, but in large it is the most common tumor	• Colonic = only intestinal tumor for which sx + doxorubicin chemotherapy yields a survival advantage.	2,3,5,6,10,12, 34,43,54, 120-123
Mast cell tumor	Dog	Stomach and small intestine	• Typically poorly granulated • Often positive on IHC for toluidine blue, c-kit, and tryptase • Intestinal mast cells may be structurally distinct from cutaneous	51
	Cat	Distal small intestine and colon	• Third most common intestinal tumor in cats • Similar to, but distinct from, carcinoids • May present as eosinophilic enteritis	4,124-126
Leiomyosarcoma (LMS)	Dog (rare in cats)	Cecum		2,4,5,12,17,43,95
Gastrointestinal stromal tumor (GIST)	Dog	Cecum	• Ultrastructural appearance and c-kit (CD117) staining can distinguish from LMS. • Arises from interstitial cells of Cajal, which regulate intestinal motility via an autonomic pacemaker effect.	17,36,56-58,95
Carcinoids	Dog	Large and small intestines	• From the diffuse endocrine system • Histologic similarity to carcinomas • Contain secretory granules that may contain substances such as 5-hydroxytryptamine (serotonin), secretin, somatostatin, and gastrin Immunohistochemistry for cytokeratin and for secretory substances such as serotonin may be positive. • Follow an aggressive and debilitating course and often metastasize to the liver	3,57,95,127
Extramedullary plasmacytoma	Dog and cat	Most in the oral cavity	• Rare • No systemic signs of multiple myeloma • Slowly progressive and complete excision often gives long-term control.	128

(Continued)

TABLE 22-1   DESCRIPTION OF COMMON INTESTINAL TUMORS OF DOGS AND CATS—CONT'D

Tumor Type	Species	Location	Characteristics	References
Extraskeletal osteosarcoma	Cat	Duodenum	Uncommon (3/145 feline OSA)	129,130
Hemangiosarcoma	Cat	No site predilection	Aggressive, all cats dead within 1 week of surgery (n = 4)	131,132
Polyps	Dogs	Rectum	Most are solitary, but multiple, diffuse lesions are more likely to recur.	41
	Cats	Duodenum	Solitary, but multiple large masses may be caused by *Strongyloides tumefaciens* infection	45-48

TABLE 22-2   SUGGESTED RECLASSIFICATION OF INTESTINAL STROMAL AND SMOOTH MUSCLE TUMORS[58]

	Histologic Malignancy	Stain Positive	Stain Negative	+/−
LM	Benign	• SMA and/or desmin	• S-100 • KIT	• Vimentin
LMS	Malignant	• SMA and/or desmin	• S-100 • KIT	• Vimentin
GIST	Benign or malignant	• Kit • Vimentin	•	• SMA • Desmin • S-100
GIST-like	Benign or malignant	• Vimentin	• KIT	• SMA • Desmin • S-100

GIST, Gastrointestinal stromal tumor; *LM*, leiomyoma; *LMS*, leiomyosarcoma.

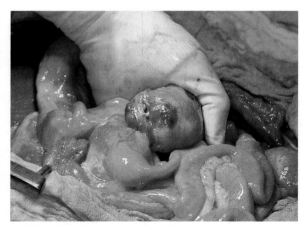

FIGURE 22-2 The cecum is the most common site for gastrointestinal stromal tumors (GISTs), which may become quite large and lead to perforation and peritonitis at the time of presentation.

nucleolar organizer regions (AgNOR) did not correlate with remission rate, duration, or survival time in feline intestinal lymphoma.[24] COX-2 is inconsistently expressed in both benign and malignant small intestinal and colorectal epithelial tumors in dogs, but not in intestinal tumors in cats,[70-72] suggesting a greater value of COX-2 inhibitors in our canine patients.

With the exception of retroviral influence (FeLV and FIV) on the development of feline lymphoma, there are no known etiologic organisms or chemical agents that have been convincingly linked to development of spontaneously occurring intestinal neoplasia in dogs or cats.[14,32] Although previous reports show that older cats with intestinal lymphoma are usually negative for FeLV on serology, one in four of those patients will be PCR tumor positive for FeLV, suggesting a role of FeLV in the pathogenesis of intestinal lymphoma in older seronegative patients.[73] Induction of feline lymphoma in a cat that is serologically negative for FeLV may result from latent, replication-deficient, or partial genome virus infection, or from a "hit and run" incident in which the virus is not incorporated into the host genome.[73] Whereas *Helicobacter pylori* infection is associated with increased risk of gastric cancer in people, no such association has been confirmed in domestic animals. Concurrent LSA and *Helicobacter* infection has been reported in a cat, but cause and effect has not been confirmed.[74] Multiple gastroduodenal ACAs and a rectal adenoma were found in a cougar with concurrent *Helicobacter*-like organisms and spirochetes; whether it was causative or coincidental is unknown.[75] Because some cats shed *Helicobacter* species in the feces,[76] this may represent normal flora rather than pathogens.

An association exists between cyclosporine use in human transplant patients and the development of LSA. Multicentric lymphoma has been reported in one dog 4 weeks after initiation of cyclosporine and ketoconazole therapy for anal furunculosis, but a causative relationship could not be proven.[77]

Clinical and Laboratory Abnormalities

The duration of clinical signs prior to presentation for animals with intestinal tumors averages 6 to 8 weeks, but can range from less than 1 day to several months.[17-19] Clinical signs include weight loss, diarrhea, vomiting, and anorexia, and, less frequently, melena, anemia, and hypoglycemia (with smooth muscle tumors).[3,14,19,28,33,35,37,43] Clinical signs often relate to location of the tumor within the GI tract. Proximal intestinal tract tumors commonly result in vomiting and weight loss, cecal tumors in perforation and peritonitis, and large bowel tumors in hematochezia and tenesmus.[32,40,58] The higher incidence of weight loss associated with SI tumors may result in earlier presentation, smaller size of tumors at the time of diagnosis, and a lower risk of perforation compared with those of the cecum and LI.[58] Russell et al.[57] proposed that the cecal wall is thinner compared with other areas of the intestinal tract and that the tumors commonly found there (GISTs) are more locally invasive compared with other cecal tumors. Because smooth muscle tumors are located within the muscular layer of the intestines, and not within the lumen, evidence of GI bleeding is often absent, but anemia and melena have been reported.[17,20] Anemia is common in dogs and cats with intestinal tumors other than leiomyosarcomas and may occur in conjunction with melena and elevated BUN.[17,19,20,23,32,33,40] Leukogram changes are also common, including leukocytosis in 25% to 70% of dogs and 40% of cats, as well as a left shift and monocytosis.[14,19,20,32,33]

Biochemical abnormalities are similar between dogs and cats with intestinal tumors, with malabsorption-related hypoproteinemia affecting 25% to 33% of patients.[14,19,20,23,37,40] Other common abnormalities include elevated liver enzymes, specifically alkaline phosphatase in 15% to 33% of dogs and up to 85% of cats with non-lymphomatous neoplasia.[19,20,32,33,40] Dogs may also have increased amylase and electrolyte disturbances,[40] and patients with lymphoma may be hypercalcemic.[23]

Paraneoplastic syndromes are uncommon but can occur with intestinal neoplasia. Neutrophilic leukocytosis has been reported in two dogs with rectal tumors as well as one dog with an intestinal sarcoma, which resolved after treatment.[77-80] Although some cats may present with hyperglycemia,[32] smooth muscle tumors in cats and dogs can cause up to 55% of patients to be hypoglycemic as a result of insulin-like growth factor secretion.[17,81] Hypereosinophilic syndrome has been reported in dogs and one cat with intestinal T cell lymphoma; the suggested cause was interleukin-5 secretion by the neoplastic lymphocytes.[82-84] Extramedullary plasmacytoma may lead to hyperviscosity syndrome resulting from overproduction of immunoglobulin.[85] Additional signs deemed paraneoplastic by their resolution with treatment or identification of an underlying mechanism include erythrocytosis (cecal leiomyosarcoma), nephrogenic diabetes insipidus (leiomyosarcoma), and collapse caused by paroxysmal ventricular tachycardia (neuroendocrine tumor).[86-88]

Diagnosis and Staging

Abdominal palpation is a reliable method of identifying an abdominal mass in approximately 20% to 50% of dogs with intestinal tumors[18,19,32,37,40] and 50% to 86% of cats.[14,23,32,33] Other physical findings include pain and fever.[18] Digital rectal examination may identify masses or annular strictures due to rectal tumors or polyps in up to 63% of dogs.[13,40] Dehydration is common in cats with non-lymphomatous tumors.[14,32] In dogs and cats with intestinal lymphoma, concurrent enlargement of liver, spleen, and/or mesenteric lymph nodes may be seen.[18]

When intestinal tumors metastasize, sites of predilection in decreasing frequency include mesenteric lymph nodes (especially ACA), liver (especially LMS), mesentery, omentum, spleen, kidney, bone, peritoneum, and lung.[19,32,34,89] Other rare sites of metastasis include testicles, skin, and other visceral organs.[90-92] Lymphoma is often a systemic disease, and 25% of dogs and 80% of cats with gastrointestinal lymphoma have concurrent involvement of other organs.[8,18] Abdominal radiographs reveal a mass in approximately 40% of dogs and cats with intestinal tumors, although some reports are higher for solid tumors and lower for lymphoma because of the diffuse nature of the disease.[14,18-20,23,32] Effusions or visceral organ involvement causing decreased serosal detail may result in decreased radiographic sensitivity. An obstructive pattern may be seen on plain radiographs with incidence ranging from 10% to 75%.[19,20,32,40]

Contrast radiography can help visualize an obstruction, localize a tumor, and view areas of the GI tract that are difficult to image with ultrasonography because of gas accumulation. Filling defects may be seen in approximately half of the cats and dogs with GI neoplasia, and most cases will have abnormal contrast series.[14,18,32]

Thoracic radiographs are critical to the complete evaluation of the cancer patient; however, for dogs with non-lymphomatous intestinal tumors, pulmonary metastasis is uncommon.[14,17,19,20,32,40,58] For cats and dogs with LSA, enlarged sternal or perihilar lymph nodes, pleural effusion, or diffuse interstitial changes may be seen.[18,23]

Ultrasound allows for more sensitive localization of a tumor and evaluation of other abdominal organs for metastasis or involvement. In addition, it can assist with guidance for needle aspiration and needle biopsy.[17,19,39,93] Ultrasound findings that are most consistent with intestinal neoplasia include bowel wall thickening and loss of normal intestinal wall layers.[40,93,94] Intestinal LSA in dogs often results in long segments of thickened bowel, and in cats either a solitary mass or diffusely thickened intestines. In cats with intestinal ACA, asymmetric mixed echogenic masses have been reported, whereas in dogs, hypoechoic masses with an irregular lumen, proximal fluid accumulation, decreased motility, and regional lymphadenopathy have been reported.[35,40,93-95] Smooth muscle tumors are characteristically large (median diameter 4.8 cm) and anechoic to hypoechoic; a muscular layer origin may be evident. Leiomyomas often have a smooth contour.[39]

Although not diagnostic alone, ultrasound has proven helpful in differentiating neoplastic from non-neoplastic intestinal disease. Dogs with tumors have significantly thicker intestinal walls, and 99% have a loss of wall layering compared with a maintenance of wall layering in 88% of dogs with non-neoplastic disease. In addition, dogs with walls thicker than 1 cm are nearly 4 times as likely to have a tumor, and those with focal lesions are nearly 20 times as likely.[94] Cats with carcinomatosis typically have masses in the double sheet portion of peritoneum and free peritoneal fluid.[38]

Endoscopic findings in dogs with intestinal lymphoma include an irregular cobblestone or patchy erythematous appearance to the duodenal mucosa and poor distensibility and elasticity of the duodenal wall.[37] Endoscopically obtained tissues often facilitate diagnosis; however, partial thickness biopsy samples may limit a diagnosis yield, since transmural neoplastic lymphoid cell infiltration must be identified in order to differentiate GI lymphoma from lymphocytic-plasmacytic enteritis (LPE).[40,53,96,97]

When non-invasive or minimally invasive techniques fail to confirm a diagnosis, an exploratory laparotomy may be indicated for a dog or cat with persistent signs of GI disease. Benefits include direct visualization of all abdominal viscera and the ability to collect full-thickness biopsy samples. Surgery may provide both a diagnosis and treatment in those with resectable tumors and can facilitate the diagnosis and evaluation of carcinomatosis. It should be noted that carcinomatosis should not always be seen as a death sentence, since long-term survival has been reported in cases treated with chemotherapy.[14]

Immunocytochemistry and IHC for markers such as CK7 may differentiate benign from malignant GI tumors.[98] Likewise, lymphocyte markers and polymerase chain reaction (PCR) can determine clonality of intestinal lymphoma as well as distinguish lymphoma from inflammatory bowel disease.[99,100]

Treatment

With the exception of LSA and potentially MCT cases,[51,52] surgical resection is the primary treatment for intestinal tumors and complete excision is often possible (Figure 22-3).[101,102] In the absence of metastasis, long-term survival is possible following surgical resection. The overall 1-year survival rate is approximately 40% for dogs with surgically treated solid (non-lymphoma) SI tumors.[19] Approximately 50% of intestinal ACAs in cats will metastasize to the local lymph nodes, 30% to the peritoneal cavity (carcinomatosis), and up to 20% to the lungs.[3,32,34] Similar lymph node metastasis rates are noted with canine ACA and LMS, although the liver is the second most frequent metastatic site.[19,32,95] Perioperative mortality approaches 30% to 50% as a result of sepsis, peritonitis, or euthanasia for non-resectable intestinal tumors.[17,19]

Dogs with colorectal tumors can fare well following surgical removal, with a reported median survival time (MST) of 15 months for extramedullary

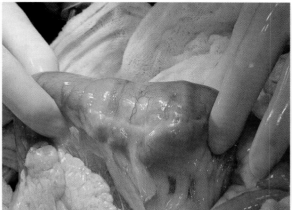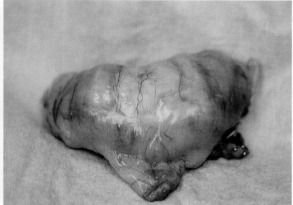

FIGURE 22-3 Surgical resection is the treatment of choice for most intestinal malignancies, such as this duodenal ACA.

plasmacytomas, 22 months for colorectal ACA, and 2 years for polyps.[13,49] In contrast, reported survival for dogs with small intestinal ACA is only 12 days without treatment and 4 to 10 months with surgical resection.[19,32,40,103]

Dogs with LMS who survive the perioperative period have reported MST ranging from 7.8 to 21.3 months.[17, 20] Those with GISTs also do well, with MST greater than 3 years reported.[57] No significant difference in recurrence free period or overall survival time was found when comparing tumor location (SI or cecum) or tumor type (LMS or GIST).[57,58]

Excision of discrete, solitary intestinal lymphoma masses is controversial. Although some clinicians favor excision to prevent a possible post-chemotherapy perforation, others prefer chemotherapy alone with close monitoring of the intestines. When considering intestinal mast cell disease in dogs, the benefit of surgery is questionable. In two case series, the majority of dogs died within 1 month of surgery with only 2 of 49 dogs living longer than 180 days.[51,52]

Distal colorectal carcinomas may be excised via pull-through technique. Although short-term complications such as rectal bleeding, tenesmus, stricture, and, uncommonly, chronic fecal incontinence may occur, long-term survival has been reported.[104,105] In one report, bilateral pubic and ischial osteotomy in the surgical management of caudal colorectal masses resulted in no associated complications, and all patients were ambulatory within 3 days of surgery.[106] Because of slower cecal wall healing, staples are indicated in typhlectomies to provide greater resistance against tension, thus minimizing the risk of dehiscence.[107] Colostomy

is reported to aid in the management of dogs with non-resectable rectal tumors. In one report, skin excoriation was the most common complication, but colostomy bags were maintained for up to 7 months.[108]

Benign canine rectal tumors can be removed endoscopically or surgically, resulting in improvement in quality of life. However, clinical signs recur in 41% of dogs, and transition to malignancy has been reported in 18% of patients.[41,109] Surgical removal of duodenal polyps in cats typically affords a cure.[22]

Cats with small intestinal ACA who survive the perioperative period may experience long-term control with surgery alone, with mean survival times ranging from 5 to 15 months.[14,43] Without surgery, all patients in two studies were dead within 2 weeks of diagnosis.[14,32] In cats with LI neoplasia, survival following surgery alone was approximately 3.5 months for lymphoma, 4.5 months for ACA, and 6.5 months for mast cell tumor. Adjuvant chemotherapy improved survival for cats with ACA, but not for cats with lymphoma.[12] Colonic stenting may also be an option for maintaining quality of life in patients with ACA.[110] Following removal of a primary intestinal ACA, two cats with carcinomatosis lived 4.5 and 28 months after surgery.[14] Feline LSA is primarily treated with chemotherapy, with the exception of intestinal obstruction, intestinal perforation, or when the need for a full-thickness biopsy necessitates surgery.

No randomized studies exist to confirm or deny any benefit of adjuvant chemotherapy following resection of intestinal tumors. When attempted, adjuvant chemotherapy for solid intestinal tumors (non-lymphoma) typically includes doxorubicin. Prolonged survivals have been noted in dogs with intestinal LMS and ACA that were treated with chemotherapy after surgery; however, dogs that do not receive chemotherapy may fare equally well.[17,40]

Multidrug protocols are used for treatment of lymphoma, but outcome is poor in dogs, with reported survival times of less than 14 weeks.[18,111] Cats do better, with MST typically around 6 to 9 months.[23,28] Surgery and chemotherapy did not improve survival compared with chemotherapy alone for cats with alimentary lymphoma.[25] Cats with small cell, lymphocytic intestinal lymphoma did very well with chlorambucil and prednisone treatment.[35] Large granular lymphoma in cats, however, is an aggressive form of lymphoma with MST of only 57 days with treatment.[112]

For carcinomatosis, intracavitary treatment with carboplatin in cats, and cisplatin, carboplatin, mitoxantrone, or 5-flourouracil in dogs may be beneficial.[113,114] Dogs with carcinomatosis, sarcomatosis, or mesothelioma treated with intracavitary carboplatin or mitoxantrone had a significantly improved survival (332 days) compared with those in the untreated group (25 days); pleural and peritoneal effusion had no effect on prognosis.[113]

A significant reduction in the size and clinical signs of rectal polyps was noted in eight dogs after receiving piroxicam therapy, either orally or in suppository form, regardless of the presence of tumor-associated inflammation.[71]

Radiation Therapy

Radiation therapy is seldom used in the treatment of intestinal tumors for a variety of reasons. In addition to the concern for normal tissue toxicity, radiation is often unnecessary, since local disease control is surgically possible. In a recent retrospective evaluation of complications in dogs undergoing definitive pelvic irradiation for a variety of neoplasms, the authors found an increase in complications in dogs with large radiation fields and those with perineal tumors.[115]

Prognosis

Intestinal perforation does not appear to be a negative prognostic factor for LMS, since dogs surviving the perioperative period enjoyed prolonged survival in one series.[17] For colorectal tumors, treatment is prognostic, with local excision significantly better than palliative care. Dogs with annular, obstructing masses survived a mean of 1.6 months, those with nodular or cobblestone masses 12 months, and those with single, pedunculated masses 32 months.[13]

For nonlymphomatous SI tumors in dogs, metastasis at the time of surgery results in significantly shorter survival times (3 vs. 15 months) with 1-year survival for dogs with lymph node metastasis only 20% versus 67% without.[19] Patients with visceral metastasis from LMS enjoyed prolonged survival following resection of the primary tumor (over 21 months).[17] In one study, males fared significantly better than female dogs with small intestinal ACA, although the number of females was small.[40]

Within a diagnosis of feline intestinal lymphoma, tumor subtype impacts behavior. Cats with lymphocytic small cell lymphoma experienced a 69% complete remission rate with prednisone and chlorambucil for an MST of nearly 2 years, whereas cats with lymphoblastic lymphoma had only an 18% complete remission rate and MST less than 3 months with combination chemotherapy.[35] As with other forms of LSA, the strongest prognostic factor for the intestinal form of the disease in cats is response to treatment. Cats achieving a complete remission indicated by resolution of clinical signs typically fare significantly better than those that do not.[25,33,116] Of 103 cats with lymphoma, 28 of which were intestinal, negative prognostic factors included advanced stage of disease and FeLV status in early stage disease (MST = 3 months if FeLV+ and 17 months if FeLV-)[29] Unlike the case in dogs, immunophenotype does not appear to be a prognostic factor for cats with intestinal lymphoma.[25] If surgery is attempted for feline colonic lymphoma, adjuvant chemotherapy appears to offer no advantage (MST of just over 3 months in both groups). Cats with ACA, however, survive significantly longer if they receive subtotal colectomy (138 days vs. 68 days with mass excision), postoperative doxorubicin (280 days with vs. 56 days without), and have negative lymph nodes at surgery (259 days negative vs. 49 days positive).[12]

Selected References*

Bonfanti U, Bertazzolo W, Bottero E, et al: Diagnostic value of cytologic examination of gastrointestinal tract tumors in dogs and cats: 83 cases (2001-2004), *J Am Vet Med Assoc* 229:1130–1133, 2006.
This report supports the necessity for histopathology to diagnose gastrointestinal tract tumors in our small animal patients.
Evans SE, Bonczynski JJ, Broussard JD, et al: Comparison of endoscopic and full-thickness biopsy specimens for diagnosis of inflammatory bowel disease and alimentary tract lymphoma in cats, *J Am Vet Med Assoc* 229:1447–1450, 2006.
This is a good study determining the efficacy of endoscopic biopsies versus full-thickness biopsies in determining a histologic diagnosis of lymphoma.

Maas CP, ter Haar G, van der Gaag I, et al: Reclassification of small intestinal and cecal smooth muscle tumors in 72 dogs: clinical, histologic, and immunohistochemical evaluation, *Vet Surg* 36:302–313, 2007.
This recent review discusses the histologic and immunohistochemical criteria for classifying smooth muscle tumors of the intestinal tract. It also provides a brief review of the two prior studies (Frost and LaRock) discussing similar reclassification criteria.

Paoloni MC, Penninck DG, Moore AS: Ultrasonographic and clinicopathologic findings in 21 dogs with intestinal adenocarcinoma, *Vet Radiol Ultrasound* 43:562–567, 2002.
This provides a good description not only of ultrasonographic findings of intestinal adenocarcinoma, but signalment, clinical presentation, laboratory findings, treatment, as well as outcome.

Waly NE, Gruffydd-Jones TJ, Stokes CR, et al: Immunohistochemical diagnosis of alimentary lymphomas and severe intestinal inflammation in cats, *J Comp Pathol* 133: 253–260, 2005.
This paper reviews immunohistochemical stains as an adjunctive diagnostic tool to differentiate lymphoma from lymphocytic-plasmacytic enteritis in cats, as well as determine immunophenotype.

■ *For a complete list of the references cited in this chapter, please go to www.smallanimaloncology.com.

SECTION C: Liver, Gall Bladder, and Non-Endocrine Pancreatic Tumors

Bonnie Brugmann and Mary Lynn Higginbotham

KEY POINTS

- Primary hepatic tumors are uncommon in dogs and cats; metastatic hepatic neoplasia and liver involvement of lymphoma and mast cell disease are more common.
- If resectable, long-term survival with massive hepatocellular carcinoma is common, but nodular and diffuse tumors carry a poor prognosis.
- Exocrine pancreatic tumors are typically aggressive in both dogs and cats, with metastatic disease common at the time of diagnosis.

Incidence—Morbidity and Mortality

Primary hepatobiliary tumors are uncommon in companion animals. They have been reported to comprise between 0.6% and1.3% of all canine neoplasms and between 1.5% and 6.9% of all feline neoplasms.[1-6] Metastatic disease to the liver occurs three times more often than primary neoplasia in the liver of dogs.[3] Other common neoplastic diseases that may involve the liver include lymphoma, mast cell tumors, and histiocytic diseases. The reader is referred to chapters specific to these tumors for detailed information.

Etiology and Risk Factors

The cause of hepatobiliary tumors in companion animals is largely unknown. Chronic diseases of the liver, such as hepatitis B or C infection and cirrhosis, are often associated with hepatocellular tumors in humans[7]; however, they have not been associated with these tumors in companion animals.[8] A possible association between cholangiocarcinoma and hookworm or whipworm infestation[9] was reported, but this association has not been substantiated. Hepatobiliary tumors tend to occur in geriatric animals, with the majority of animals being 10 years of age or older.[1,10,11]

Clinical Features of Canine Hepatobiliary Tumors

Four general categories of primary hepatic tumors exist: hepatocellular tumors, bile duct tumors, neuroendocrine tumors, and sarcomas. Hepatobiliary tumors are also categorized based upon their gross appearance: *massive,* involving only one liver lobe; *nodular,* multiple and involving more than one liver lobe; or *diffuse,* effacement of the hepatic tissue. A summary of the incidence of canine hepatobiliary tumors can be found in Table 22-3.

Hepatocellular Tumors

Hepatocellular adenoma, or hepatoma, is a benign tumor that has infrequently been reported and must be histologically differentiated from nodular hyperplasia and low-grade hepatocellular carcinoma (HCC).[12] Hepatocellular carcinoma is the most common canine liver tumor,[1] and there appears to be a predilection for the left liver lobe with massive HCC.[1,13,14] Multiple histologic types of HCC have been identified but do not aid in determining prognosis.[8] There is an overall reported metastatic rate of 61% for HCC in dogs, most frequently to the lymph nodes, lungs, and peritoneum.[8]

TABLE 22-3   INCIDENCE, METASTATIC RATE, AND SURVIVAL DATA OF DOGS WITH HEPATOBILIARY TUMORS

Tumor Type	Incidence	Metastatic Rate	Treatment	Survival	Reference
Hepatocellular carcinoma	55/110 = 50%				1
Massive	61%	4.8%–6.6%	surgery vs. no treatment	>1460 days vs. 270 days	8, 25
Nodular	29%	93%	NR	NR	8
Diffuse	10%	100%	NR	NR	8
Biliary carcinoma	24/110 = 22%	27%–88%	NR	NR	1, 9, 14
Massive	50%	NR	NR	NR	14
Nodular	28%	NR	NR	NR	14
Diffuse	22%	NR	NR	NR	14
Neuroendocrine tumors	15/110 = 14%	93%	NR	NR	1, 15
Massive	0%	NR	NR	NR	15
Nodular	33%	NR	NR	NR	15
Diffuse	66%	NR	NR	NR	15
Mesenchymal tumors	14/110 = 13%	86%	NR	NR	1
Leiomyosarcoma	10/14 = 9%	100%	surgery	euthanized at surgery	1, 21
Fibrosarcoma	3/14 = 3%	NR	NR	NR	1
Osteosarcoma	1/14 = 1%	NR	NR	NR	1
Hemangiosarcoma	6/104 = 6%	NR	NR	NR	19

NR, Not reported.

Bile Duct Tumors

The majority of feline and canine biliary carcinomas are intrahepatic in origin rather than extrahepatic or of the gall bladder in origin, as they are in people.[9,12,15] Benign intrahepatic biliary tumors, or cholangioma, have been reported in the dog but occur less frequently than the malignant cholangiocarcinoma. Cholangiocarcinomas accounted for 22% of primary hepatic tumors in one study.[16] Biliary tumors in general may be solid or cystic in nature.[12] In dogs, cholangiocarcinomas have a reported metastatic rate of 88%, and the most frequent metastatic sites are the lymph nodes, lungs, and peritoneum.[16]

Neuroendocrine Tumors

Neuroendocrine tumors, also termed *carcinoids,* are of neuroectodermal origin and are rare in domestic species.[1,2,17] They occur throughout the gastrointestinal tract and have been reported in the liver[1,12,17,18] and gall bladder[1,12,17,19] in dogs. In a study of 15 dogs with hepatic carcinoid tumors, a 93% extrahepatic metastatic rate was reported, with the lymph nodes and peritoneum most frequently affected.[17]

Sarcomas

Primary liver sarcomas are rare, but predominantly include leiomyosarcoma, hemangiosarcoma (HSA), and fibrosarcoma (FSA).[1,12,20] Primary hepatic chondrosarcoma has been reported in one dog.[21] Although the liver is more commonly a site of metastatic HSA than primary HSA, approximately 5% originate in the liver.[22] No breed predilection has been reported for primary hepatic sarcomas, but males may be at an increased risk.[1] The behavior of these tumors is aggressive with metastatic rates of 57% to 100% reported.[1,22,23] Primary hepatic leiomyosarcomas are uncommon, yet aggressive, tumors. In a report of leiomyosarcomas, 5 of 44 cases occurred in the liver, and all five of those dogs had evidence of metastasis at the time of surgery.[24]

Clinical Features of Feline Hepatobiliary Tumors

Hepatocellular, bile duct, neuroendocrine, and mesenchymal tumors have also been reported in cats. Malignant hepatobiliary tumors are more likely to be multifocal (nodular or diffuse) in the cat.[25] A summary of the incidence of feline hepatobiliary tumors can be found in Table 22-4.

Bile Duct Tumors

Tumors involving the bile duct are more common than hepatocellular tumors in cats and extrahepatic biliary tumors occur more frequently than in the dog.[25] Biliary adenomas are the most common primary hepatic neoplasm in the cat.[10-12,25] A 67% distant metastatic rate has been reported for feline biliary adenocarcinomas.[25]

TABLE 22-4   INCIDENCE, METASTATIC RATE, AND SURVIVAL DATA OF CATS WITH HEPATOBILIARY TUMORS

Tumor Type	Incidence	Metastasis	Treatment	Survival	Reference
Hepatocellular adenoma	9/41 = 22%				11
		25%			
	8/47 = 17%				
	2/25 = 8%				
Hepatocellular carcinoma	1/41 = 2%		NR	NR	10, 22
Hepatobiliary cystadenoma	NR	0%	Surgery (n = 5)	12–44 months	11, 30
	5/41 = 12%				
Bile duct					
Biliary adenoma	16/47 = 34%	0%	NR	NR	10, 11, 22
	13/25 = 52%				
	13/41 = 32%				
Biliary adenocarcinoma	13/47 = 28%	77%	NR	NR	10, 11, 22
	6/25 = 24%				
	10/41 = 24%				
Gall bladder adenocarcinoma	2/47 = 4%	100%	NR	NR	22
Neuroendocrine	2/47 = 4%	100%	NR	NR	10, 22
	1/25 = 4%				
Mesenchymal	6/47 = 13%		NR	NR	10, 22
	3/25 = 12%				
Hemangiosarcoma	5/47 = 11%	60%	NR	NR	11, 22
	2/41 = 5%				
Leiomyosarcoma	1/47 = 2%	100%	NR	NR	22
Fibrosarcoma	1/41 = 2%	NR	NR	NR	11

NR, Not reported.

Hepatocellular Tumors

Although hepatocellular adenomas have been reported in cats, hepatocellular carcinomas are more frequent and are the second most common primary hepatic tumor in cats.[10,11,20,25] A distant metastatic rate of 25% has been reported.[25]

Myelolipoma

Myelolipoma is a benign primary hepatic tumor that occurs in cats. The etiology is unknown, but they are composed of well-differentiated adipose and myeloid tissues. They may be single or multiple in nature and may involve multiple lobes of the liver. Most cats are asymptomatic for these tumors, since they are typically incidental findings.[12]

Diagnosis and Staging

Clinical Findings

Most animals with primary liver tumors present for non-specific signs such as lethargy, weakness, anorexia, vomiting, and polyuria-polydipsia,* yet other animals are

*References 1,3,6,8,10-12,13,16,20,25,26.

asymptomatic.[13] Physical examination reveals hepatomegaly or a cranial abdominal mass in greater than 50% of animals with primary hepatobiliary tumors.[1,3,8,13,26] Less common is the presence of icterus or ascites.[1,10,11] Hepatic encephalopathy and paraneoplastic hypoglycemia have been associated with hepatic tumors and may be a cause for weakness, seizures, or other neurologic signs.[1,3]

Blood Work Findings

Common CBC abnormalities for patients with hepatic tumors include a normocytic-normochromic non-regenerative anemia, consistent with chronic disease, and a mature neutrophilia. Thrombocytosis was recently reported to occur in approximately 50% of dogs diagnosed with massive HCC; however, the significance of this is unknown.[14] The biochemical profile typically reflects changes consistent with liver disease. Non-specific liver enzyme elevation is often present with primary hepatobiliary tumors, and in a recent study of canine massive hepatocellular carcinomas, 95% had ALP elevation, 88% had ALT elevation, 66% had AST elevation, and gamma-glutamyl transferase (GGT) was elevated in 54% of dogs.[14] Abnormal clotting profiles have been identified in dogs with hepatic masses; however, the clotting abnormalities are rarely clinically significant.[14,27]

Imaging Studies

Radiography and ultrasonography are beneficial in evaluating for the presence of a mass, the extent of involvement, and potential metastatic lesions. A hepatic mass or enlargement typically results in caudolateral displacement of the gastric axis on radiographs.[13,14,26] Peritoneal effusion may result in loss of abdominal detail. Three-view thoracic radiographs should be evaluated for pulmonary metastatic disease or other abnormalities. Abdominal ultrasonography is helpful in identifying hepatic masses; however, a strong correlation between histologic type and ultrasonographic appearance has not been found.[28,29] A recent study using MRI to differentiate benign and malignant focal hepatic lesions found a 94% accuracy rate.[30]

Fine-Needle Aspiration and Cytology

Abdominal effusion associated with a hepatic mass may be ascites, or it may be a malignant effusion if peritoneal carcinomatosis is present. A modified transudate is often described, and malignant cells may be present with carcinomatosis. Ultrasound-guided FNA or needle-core biopsy may be helpful in determining the etiology of hepatic masses. Prior to surgical intervention, FNA cytology is recommended if lymphoma or mast cell disease is a strong consideration.

Treatment Modalities

The mainstay of treatment for any primary hepatic mass is surgery. Unfortunately, even with advanced imaging, the resectability of a massive hepatobiliary tumor is difficult to determine preoperatively; thus, exploratory laparotomy is often necessary.[14] The likelihood of complete resection of a nodular or diffuse hepatobiliary tumor is poor, due to the extensive liver involvement. However, because benign hepatic lesions may appear similar to severe, diffuse malignant lesions on gross evaluation, biopsy and histopathological evaluation are warranted prior to final treatment and prognosis discussions with the pet owner. Adjunctive chemotherapy for malignant primary hepatobiliary tumors has not been adequately evaluated.

Prognosis and Survival

Because of their extensive nature and likelihood for metastasis, the prognosis for mesenchymal, neuroendocrine, nodular, or diffuse primary, malignant hepatobiliary tumors in the dog and cat is poor. No reports exist in the veterinary literature evaluating survival of dogs with biliary carcinomas. The outcome for massive hepatocellular carcinomas in dogs, however, appears to be relatively good with surgery, and a recent study of massive HCC in dogs showed a MST of greater than 1460 days in dogs treated with surgery versus 270 days for those not treated.[14] A previous study showed similar results for those that survived the immediate post-operative period.[13] Reported MST for cats with malignant hepatobiliary tumors is 0.1 month.[11] Survival of 12 to 44 months with no recurrence was reported in five cats treated with surgery for benign hepatobiliary tumors.[11,31]

EXOCRINE PANCREATIC TUMORS

Incidence—Morbidity and Mortality

Exocrine pancreatic tumors are rare, with a reported incidence of 17.8 and 12.6 per 100,000 patient years at risk in the dog and cat, respectively.[32] They are typically of epithelial origin, and malignant tumors (carcinoma, adenocarcinoma) are more common than benign adenomas.[33] Benign nodular hyperplasia is a common incidental finding in older animals, which can appear as solitary or multi-focal mass-like lesions.[33] Pseudocysts and necrosis have also been described as masses in the pancreas associated with pancreatitis in dogs and cats.[34,35]

Etiology and Risk Factors

There is no apparent sex predilection for exocrine pancreatic tumors.[32] Advanced age is a risk factor for exocrine pancreatic carcinomas.[32] Airedale terriers are reportedly at an increased risk.[32] Although there is no known natural cause, experimental intraductal N-ethyl-N'-nitro-N-nitrosoguanidine administration has reportedly induced pancreatic adenocarcinoma in dogs.[36] Exocrine pancreatic carcinoma was reported in 8 of 37 cats with diabetes mellitus,[37] which is a risk factor for the development of pancreatic cancer in people.[38] Although suspicious, the relationship has not been proved in cats.

Clinical Features

Clinical signs of exocrine pancreatic tumors in both the dog and cat are non-specific in nature and are often similar to those accompanying pancreatitis. A list of clinical signs and common examination findings can be found in Boxes 22-1 and 22-2. Paraneoplastic conditions have been reported for dogs and cats with exocrine pancreatic tumors[39-45] and are listed in Box 22-3. The cause of these conditions is poorly understood; however, panniculitis and steatitis are thought to occur because of

Box 22-1   **CLINICAL SIGNS REPORTED WITH PANCREATIC TUMORS IN DOGS AND CATS**

- Weight loss
- Vomiting
- Anorexia
- Lethargy
- Palpable abdominal mass
- Abdominal effusion
- Painful abdomen
- Icterus

Box 22-2   **COMMON BLOOD WORK FINDINGS ASSOCIATED WITH PANCREATIC TUMORS IN DOGS AND CATS**

- Neutrophilia
- Non-specific liver enzyme elevation
- Hyperlipasemia
- Hyperamylasemia

Box 22-3   **PARANEOPLASTIC CONDITIONS ASSOCIATED WITH PANCREATIC TUMORS IN DOGS AND CATS**

Cats
- Alopecia—symmetrical, ventrum and may extend to the head and medial aspect of extremities[38,39,41]
- Panniculitis[44]
- Steatitis[44]

Dogs
- Panniculitis[42,43]
- Steatitis[42,43]
- Osteomyelitis[45]
- Polyarthritis[45]

hydrolysis of fat by circulating digestive enzymes such as lipase.[43-46] Resolution of paraneoplastic conditions associated with exocrine pancreatic tumors has only been reported in one cat after surgical resection of pancreatic carcinoma[42] and should not be expected, because of the advanced stage of most exocrine pancreatic tumors at the time of diagnosis.

Diagnosis and Staging

Neutrophilia, liver enzyme elevation, and hyperlipasemia[47] are frequently noted with exocrine pancreatic tumors; however, no specific blood work abnormalities are diagnostic. Radiographic imaging may reveal an abdominal mass or loss of abdominal detail if effusion is present. Ultrasonography is typically of more benefit since it allows for evaluation of the pancreas, liver, and other potential metastatic sites and has been shown to be more sensitive in the detection of pancreatic tumors.[48] Ultrasound imaging may also aid in percutaneous aspiration or biopsy of identified masses for cytologic or histopathologic evaluation.[49] Exploratory celiotomy may be necessary for biopsy procurement for definitive diagnosis. Prior to celiotomy, thoracic radiographs should be performed to evaluate for possible pulmonary metastatic disease.

Metastasis

The biological behavior of pancreatic carcinomas and adenocarcinomas is highly aggressive in both dogs and cats. The presence of metastatic disease is common at the time of diagnosis to the liver and lymph nodes, and widespread metastasis has been reported,[33,45,46,48-51] including intracranial locations.[51]

Treatment Modalities

Because of the extensive nature of these tumors and the likelihood that most animals have metastatic disease at the time of diagnosis, treatment is often unrewarding. Complete pancreatectomy or pancreaticoduodenectomy, referred to as Whipple's procedure, can be considered, but carries significant risks with minimal benefit in light of the aggressive nature of this disease. Before consideration, all efforts should be made to confirm the disease is early stage and localized within the pancreas. Adjuvant therapy is used for human pancreatic carcinoma, but the efficacy of radiation therapy or chemotherapy has not been evaluated for exocrine pancreatic carcinomas in companion animals. 5-FU and gemcitabine are chemotherapeutic agents discussed in people.[52] However, due to fatal neurotoxicity, 5-FU should not be considered for use in cats.

Prognosis and Survival

The prognosis for patients diagnosed with malignant exocrine pancreatic tumors is poor. No long-term reports of survival exist to the authors' knowledge. A single report exists of a cat with pancreatic carcinoma that survived 18 weeks after resection. Although no evidence of metastasis was found at the time of surgery, metastatic disease was noted on post-mortem examination.[42]

Selected References*

Lawrence HJ, Erb HN, Harvey HJ: Nonlymphomatous hepatobiliary masses in cats: 41 cases (1972-1991), *Vet Surg* 23:365, 1994.

Largest clinical study of hepatobiliary masses in cats that discusses diagnosis as well as clinical findings and general survivals.

Liptak JM, Dernell WS, Monnet E, et al: Massive hepatocellular carcinoma in dogs: 48 cases (1992-2002), *J Am Vet Med Assoc* 225:1225, 2004.

Large clinical evaluation of massive hepatocellular carcinomas in the dog. Discusses clinical findings and survival.

Patnaik AK, Hurvitz AI, Lieberman PH: Canine hepatic neoplasms: a clinicopathologic study, *Vet Pathol* 17:553, 1980.

Comprehensive case study of hepatic tumors in dogs.

Seaman RL: Exocrine pancreatic neoplasia in the cat: a case series, *J Am Anim Hosp Assoc* 40:238, 2004.

Clinical evaluation of exocrine pancreatic tumors in the cat. Discusses clinical findings and paraneoplastic conditions associated with this disease in cats.

▮ *For a complete list of the references cited in this chapter, please go to www.smallanimaloncology.com.

SECTION D: Splenic Tumors

Kim D. Johnson

KEY POINTS

- Dogs with splenomegaly generally follow a law of two thirds: two thirds have splenic neoplasia, and two thirds of those have hemangiosarcoma.
- Dogs presenting with splenomegaly, along with anemia, nucleated red blood cells, abnormal red cell morphology, or splenic rupture have a significantly greater chance of having splenic neoplasia than a non-neoplastic disease.
- Mast cell tumor and lymphoma are the predominate tumors of the feline spleen.
- Splenectomy may provide long-term remission for cats with splenic mast cell tumor.

Introduction and Clinical Behavior

Splenic neoplasia may arise from any of the various tissues comprising the spleen, including blood vessels, lymphoid tissues, smooth muscle, or the connective tissue that makes up the fibrous stroma. Common splenic tumors include hemangiosarcoma (HSA), mast cell tumors (MCTs), lymphoma (LSA), and various sarcomas.[1-3] Hematomas are the most common benign splenic masses in dogs. Of the non-lymphoid primary splenic tumors, HSA predominates in dogs and MCT predominates in cats.[1-3] Splenic LSA primarily occurs as part of multisystemic LSA but may be limited to the spleen in some cases. Feline splenic disease is more likely to be neoplastic, compared with canine splenic disease.[4] In general, dogs with splenomegaly follow a law of two thirds: two thirds have splenic neoplasia, and two thirds of those have HSA.[5]

Etiology/Risk Factors

Splenic tumors usually occur in medium to large breed dogs, with the German shepherd dog ranking first in breed prevalence for splenic diseases such as hyperplastic nodule/hematoma, HSA and LSA. Golden retrievers and Labrador retrievers rank second and third, respectively.[4]

Clinical Features of Canine Splenic Tumors

Splenomegaly in dogs is readily detectable through abdominal palpation, radiography, and ultrasonography. Differential diagnoses are shown in Box 22-4. Clinical signs are often vague and vary with the extent of disease. Dogs may be presented for treatment of abdominal enlargement, anorexia, lethargy, depression, diarrhea, or vomiting; alternatively, they may have acute signs of weakness and hypovolemic shock as a result of splenic rupture and hemorrhage.[1,3,6] In a report of 39 dogs with acute non-traumatic hemoabdomen, 24/30 (80%) dogs with definitive diagnosis had malignant neoplasia and 21 of the 24 (88%) malignant masses were diagnosed as HSA.[7]

Hemangiosarcoma

Hemangiosarcoma is a common, aggressive malignant neoplasm of dogs that arises from transformed vascular endothelial cells.[1] It occurs more frequently in dogs than any other species and is characterized by local infiltration and systemic metastases to organs such as the liver and lung and, less commonly, to the omentum, mesentery, brain, muscle, and bone (Figure 22-4).[1,6,8-10] This tumor typically affects older dogs, with a mean age range from 8 to 13 years.[11] German shepherds and golden retrievers are at greater risk.[11,12] More than half

Box 22-4 PATHOLOGIC CAUSES OF SPLENOMEGALY IN THE DOG

Non-neoplastic
  Hyperplastic nodule
  Hematoma
  Splenitis
    Abscess
    Granulomatous
  Congestion
    Torsion
    Right-sided heart failure
    Gastric dilatation and volvulus
    Drugs
  Infection
    Fungal
    Bacterial
    Viral
  Immune-mediated disease

Neoplastic
  Benign
    Hemangioma
    Lipoma
    Leiomyoma
    Myelolipoma
  Malignant
    Hemangiosarcoma
    Lymphoma
    Undifferentiated sarcoma
    Fibrosarcoma
    Leiomyosarcoma
    Malignant histiocytosis
    Plasma cell tumor
    Mast cell tumor
    Liposarcoma
    Mesenchymoma
    Myxosarcoma
    Histiocytic sarcoma
    Osteosarcoma
    Metastatic carcinoma

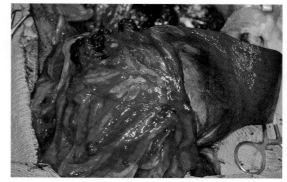

FIGURE 22-4 Appearance of splenic hemangiosarcoma in a 5-year-old castrated Doberman with a history of weight loss and lethargy. Metastases were grossly evident on the liver and omentum.

solution, cyclophosphamide, and piroxicam was shown to be comparable to conventional doxorubicin chemotherapy for dogs with Stage II disease.[18] See Table 22-5 for further information on chemotherapy options.

Lymphoma
Lymphoma most commonly occurs in the spleen as part of multisystemic LSA. However, some canine LSA, especially the marginal zone and mantle cell subtypes of indolent nodular LSA, may occur as solitary splenic nodules.[21] See Chapter 25, Section A, for more information on LSA.

Malignant Histiocytosis
Malignant histiocytosis is an uncommon neoplastic process characterized by progressive, systemic invasion of multiple organs by morphologically atypical histiocytes.[22] The spleen, liver, bone marrow, and lymph nodes are commonly affected, and there is a reported familial predilection in Bernese mountain dogs.[23] See Chapter 23, Section F, for more information.

Mast Cell Tumors
The visceral form of MCT is often referred to as disseminated mastocytosis and is almost always preceded by an undifferentiated primary cutaneous lesion in dogs. Tumors of primary visceral origin are rare. Splenectomy, along with adjunctive chemotherapy (vinblastine/prednisone or lomustine), may improve survival times.[24] See Chapter 23, Section D, for more information on MCTs.

Fibrohistiocytic Nodules
Fibrohistiocytic nodules include a distinct population of spindle and/or histiocytoid cells (fibrohistiocytic cells)

of affected dogs have gross evidence of metastatic disease on initial presentation. Reported MST in dogs treated with surgery alone ranges from 3 weeks to 2 months and improves to 3 to 6 months with the addition of chemotherapy.[4,6,9,11-20] Doxorubicin-based protocols have been the mainstay of chemotherapy for canine HSA for many years. Recently, an oral continuous low-dose chemotherapy protocol using etoposide prepared as a

TABLE 22-5   REPORTED OUTCOME WITH VARIOUS TREATMENT PROTOCOLS FOR CANINE SPLENIC HEMANGIOSARCOMA

Treatment	No. of Dogs	Median Survival (days)	Reference
Splenectomy	59	19	13
Splenectomy	21	65	9
Splenectomy	19	56	5
Stage I	4	91	5
Stage II	1	168	5
Stage III	14	56	5
Splenectomy	32	86	11
Splenectomy + MBV	10	91	9
Splenectomy + MBV + VMC	10	117	9
Splenectomy + VAC ± ChM	6	145	15
Splenectomy + VAC	3	140	5
Splenectomy + AC	6	180	16
Splenectomy + AC	16	141	17
Stage I	7	166	17
Stage II	9	96	17
Splenectomy + AC + L-MTP-LE	16	273	17
Splenectomy + CLDC	9	178	18
splenectomy + doxorubicin q21d × 5	46		19
Complete resection	27	172	19
Incomplete resection	19	60	19
*Splenectomy + doxorubicin q14d × 5	20		20
Stage I	5	257	20
Stage II	9	210	20
Stage III	6	107	20

AC, Doxorubicin; *ChM*, chlorambucil, methotrexate; cyclophosphamide; *CLDC*, continuous low-dose chemotherapy (etoposide, cyclophosphamide, piroxicam); *L-MTP-PE*, liposome-encapsulated muramyl tripeptide-phosphatidylethanolamine; *MBV*, mixed bacterial vaccine; *VAC*, vincristine, doxorubicin, cyclophosphamide; *VMC*, vincristine, methotrexate, cyclophosphamide.

*20 dogs (14 splenic, 4 subcutaneous, 1 right atrium, 1 renal).

that represent a transitional form of splenic nodular lesions. There is a possible female sex predilection among German shepherd dogs, cocker spaniels, Labrador retrievers, golden retrievers, and poodles. Splenectomy is the treatment of choice and improves survival to approximately 12 months; however, grade affects survival with ranges from 3.5 to 12 months for dogs with grades I and II fibrohistiocytic nodules.[25]

Splenic Sarcoma

Several types of canine splenic sarcoma have been reported, including fibrosarcoma, leiomyosarcoma, osteosarcoma, mesenchymoma, myxosarcoma, liposarcoma, histiocytic sarcoma, and undifferentiated sarcoma. It has been suggested that the biological behavior of splenic non-angiomatous, non-lymphomatous sarcomas is best predicted by mitotic index (MI), with a MI greater than 9 associated with significantly shorter survival times. Splenic sarcomas tend to be fatal within 1

year of diagnosis, with the exception of mesenchymoma, for which the 1-year survival rate is 50%.[26] Splenic leiomyosarcoma, despite a relatively high metastatic rate, is associated with MSTs of 8 months after splenectomy for dogs surviving the initial post-surgical period.[27]

Clinical Features of Feline Splenic Tumors

Palpable splenomegaly is often easily appreciable in cats but is a non-specific finding that warrants further investigation. The feline spleen is non-sinusoidal and has slightly less blood storage capacity compared with dogs.[28] This anatomic difference suggests that severe splenomegaly would less likely be physiologic in the cat (Box 22-5).

Mast Cell Tumors

Up to 50% of feline MCT occur in visceral sites.[2] In a series of 455 pathologic specimens, the splenic form (or lymphoreticular MCT) was the most common differential diagnosis for splenic disease in cats,

Box 22-5   PATHOLOGIC CAUSES OF SPLENOMEGALY IN THE CAT

Non-neoplastic
  Congestion
  Splenitis
  Hypereosinophilic syndrome
  Hematoma
  Extramedullary hematopoiesis
Neoplastic
  Mast cell tumor
  Lymphoma
  Myeloproliferative disease
  Hemangiosarcoma

accounting for 15% of submissions.[29] The mean age of affected cats is approximately 10 years, with no known breed or gender predilection.[2] Widespread dissemination and metastasis are common. Clinical signs may include anorexia, weight loss, and a history of chronic vomiting related to histamine release by the MCT and subsequent hypergastrinemia and GI ulceration.[30] Palliative medical treatment rarely results in significant clinical improvement; therefore, splenectomy is the treatment of choice, producing an MST of 12 months. The role of chemotherapy has not been adequately assessed.[3,30,31]

Hemangiosarcoma

While the spleen has been reported as a primary site for HSA, this is not a common splenic malignancy in cats.[32] Tumors may be solitary or multiple and are of variable size.[1] The liver is the most common site of metastasis, although metastasis to the lymph nodes, heart, lung kidney, and brain has been reported.[33] Splenectomy is the initial treatment of choice, and adjuvant chemotherapy has not been reported to improve survival.[3]

Diagnosis and Staging

Clinical staging is necessary in order to establish the extent of disease, most appropriate treatment plan, and parameters by which to evaluate response to treatment. Complete clinical staging procedures include a complete blood count (CBC), chemistry panel, urinalysis, three-view thoracic radiographs, abdominal radiographs and/or ultrasound, and echocardiography if HSA is suspected. Cytologic or histologic samples are necessary to confirm a diagnosis.

Complete Blood Count

Hematologic abnormalities may support the tentative diagnosis of splenic neoplasia. Dogs appearing with splenomegaly that also have anemia, nucleated red blood cells, abnormal red blood cell morphology, or splenic rupture are more likely to have splenic neoplasia than a non-neoplastic process.[5] Anemia may occur as a result of splenic neoplasia by several mechanisms, including hemorrhage into the peritoneal cavity from tumor rupture. Neutrophilic leukocytosis may be present in some dogs. Other hematologic abnormalities include Howell-Jolly bodies, poikilocytosis, acanthocytosis, schistocytosis, and/or thrombocytopenia. Presurgical evaluation of a coagulation profile is warranted whenever HSA is suspected, because of the association of disseminated intravascular coagulation with this disease.

Imaging Studies

Three-view thoracic radiographs are indicated to assess for pulmonary metastasis and pleural fluid. Abdominal ultrasound is the imaging modality of choice for splenic lesions, since it allows detailed visualization of the abdominal organs and is less affected than radiography by the presence of peritoneal effusion. MRI provides soft-tissue contrast that is superior to either ultrasound or CT.[34] See Chapters 9 and 10 for additional information on imaging.

Fine-Needle Aspiration and Cytology

Ultrasound-guided cytologic specimens may yield information that precludes the need for surgery, especially for patients with lymphoma or non-neoplastic disorders for which surgery is not indicated. However, even with ultrasound guidance, non-representative tissues may be inadvertently sampled, making the distinction between reactive, benign, and neoplastic conditions impossible. In a retrospective study of 32 cases (29 dogs and 3 cats) where FNA was performed to assess splenic lesions identified on ultrasound, cytologic diagnoses corresponded with histologic diagnoses in 61% of the cases.[35] No complications resulting from the aspiration procedure were reported. Prior to splenic aspiration in cats suspected of having MCT, the authors advise pretreatment with diphenhydramine to reduce the potential for life-threatening consequences of systemic histamine release from the manipulated tumor.

Cardiac Evaluation

As many as 45% of dogs with splenic HSA may have concurrent right atrial HSA; therefore, an echocardiogram is indicated as part of the diagnostic process.[1] In addition, cardiac arrhythmias often occur as a result of both benign and malignant splenic lesions in dogs. Thus, a complete evaluation for rhythm disturbances prior to surgery will assist with selecting appropriate anesthetic drugs and developing a plan for patient monitoring.[36]

Treatment Modalities

Therapeutic options are aimed at slowing the progression of disease, controlling clinical signs, and maintaining quality of life for as long as possible. Splenectomy is the treatment of choice for animals lacking evidence of extensive metastasis or other organ failure that would preclude the short-term benefits of removing the enlarged or ruptured spleen. However, even at surgery, it is often impossible to distinguish various diseases on the basis of gross appearance of the spleen. Unless a firm diagnosis can be made by aspiration cytology or frozen section biopsy, splenectomy is usually performed before establishing a definitive diagnosis, and it is the mainstay of therapy for all splenic tumors except lymphoma. Adjuvant chemotherapy is recommended for treatment of canine splenic HSA. Reported treatment outcomes are summarized in Table 22-5.

Prognosis and Survival

Dogs with primary and metastatic splenic malignancy generally have a grave prognosis, with 1-year survival rates less than 10%.[11,14] Notable exceptions are splenic leiomyosarcoma, mesenchymoma, and indolent lymphoma, for which longer survival times may be expected. Likewise, despite a lack of demonstrated successful medical options for cats with splenic MCT, splenectomy alone may provide for prolonged survival.

Selected References*

Clifford CA, Mackin AJ, Henry CJ: Treatment of canine hemangiosarcoma: 2000 and beyond, *J Vet Intern Med* 14:479, 2000.
This review of canine hemangiosarcoma provides a brief historical overview of treatment options, examines recent treatment options, and identifies future potential therapies.
Johnson KA, Powers BE, Withrow SJ, et al: Splenomegaly in dogs. Predictors of neoplasia and survival after splenectomy, *J Vet Intern Med* 3:160, 1989.
This retrospective study includes a relatively large group of dogs with splenomegaly and evaluates survival times and the usefulness in differentiating neoplastic from non-neoplastic splenic disease.
Lana S, U'ren L, Plaza S, et al: Continuous low-dose oral chemotherapy for adjuvant therapy of splenic hemangiosarcoma in dogs, *J Vet Intern Med* 21:764, 2007.
This manuscript reports on the use of an oral low-dose continuous chemotherapy protocol found to be comparable with conventional doxorubicin chemotherapy for treatment of canine splenic hemangiosarcoma.
Spangler WL, Culbertson MR: Prevalence, type, and importance of splenic diseases in dogs: 1,480 cases (1985-1989), *J Am Vet Med Assoc* 200:829, 1992.
This retrospective study includes a large group of dogs with splenic diseases and evaluates the importance of neoplasia in the canine spleen relative to the prevalence and importance of non-neoplastic splenic diseases.
Spangler WL, Kass PH: Pathologic factors affecting postsplenectomy survival in dogs, *J Vet Intern Med* 11:166, 1997.
This study examines splenic lesions in dogs and correlates the pathologic diagnosis with postoperative patient survival.

▮ *For a complete list of the references cited in this chapter, please go to www.smallanimaloncology.com.

SECTION E: Female Reproductive Tumors

Kathryn H. Taylor

KEY POINTS

- The majority of canine ovarian tumors are derived from epithelial or sex-cord stromal tissues and may be benign or malignant in nature; most sex-cord stromal tumors are granulosa-cell tumors and more than 70% are functional, resulting in clinical signs of excessive sex hormone production.
- The majority of feline ovarian tumors are sex-cord stromal tumors and malignant in nature; epithelial ovarian tumors are uncommon in the cat.

- Leiomyoma is the most common canine uterine tumor; epithelial uterine tumors are rare in dogs but are generally malignant when they occur. Malignant epithelial tumors are the most common feline uterine tumor.
- An inherited syndrome of concurrent bilateral renal cystadenocarcinoma, nodular dermatofibrosis, and multiple uterine leiomyomas has been reported in German shepherd dogs.

OVARIAN TUMORS

Incidence

Canine ovarian tumors have a reported incidence of 6.3% in the entire female.[1] However, because of the large number of spayed animals in the United States, the incidence in all female dogs has been reported as 0.5 to 1.2%[2-4] and 0.7% to 3.6% in cats.[3,4] Ovarian tumors usually occur in older animals with a median age at diagnosis of 10 to 12 years in dogs.[5-8] Teratomas are an exception and usually occur in dogs less than 6 years of age.[6,9-12] Ovarian tumors have been reported in cats as young as 2 years of age.[13]

Etiology/Risk Factors

The etiology of ovarian neoplasia in veterinary medicine is unknown. The risk of human ovarian tumor development increases with mutations in tumor suppressor genes and in the mismatch repair genes responsible for DNA damage repair. The hormonal influence of estrogen during continuous cycling in nulliparous women increases the risk of ovarian tumors. Pregnancy, lactation, and oral contraceptives appear to be protective against ovarian tumors in women.[14] These factors have not been fully investigated in veterinary medicine. Pointer breeds are at an increased risk for the development of epithelial ovarian tumors, and English Bulldogs may have an increased risk for development of granulosa-theca cell neoplasia.[15]

Most ovarian tumors develop from one of three tissue types within the ovary: epithelial tissues, sex-cord stromal tissues, or germ cell tissues (Table 22-6). Mesenchymal and metastatic tumors of the ovary are rare. Epithelial and sex-cord stromal tumors account for the majority of ovarian neoplasia in dogs. Papillary adenomas and adenocarcinomas may be bilateral[5,6,7,16-22] whereas cystadenomas are generally unilateral.[7,16] Sex-cord stromal tumors may be functional, producing excessive sex hormones including estrogen, progesterone, and rarely testosterone. Granulosa cell tumors are the most common sex-cord stromal tumor, and more than 70% are functional.[18] Germ cell tumors are uncommon tumors of the canine ovary. Dysgerminomas can be bilateral. Teratomas may have both mesenchymal and epithelial components. Mesenchymal or metastatic tumors are sporadically reported to occur within the ovary. Hemangiomas, lipomas, leiomyomas, and hemangiosarcomas have been reported as primary tumors of the ovary, and reported metastatic tumors include mammary carcinoma, intestinal carcinoma, pancreatic carcinoma, lymphoma, and melanoma.[1,3,16,18]

Sex-cord stromal tumors account for more than 50% of feline ovarian tumors.[13,17,18] Granulosa cell tumors are the most common, and more than 50% are malignant.[13,16,23-26] Other reported sex-cord stromal tumors in cats include interstitial gland tumors, thecomas, Sertoli cell tumor of the ovary, and Leydig

TABLE 22-6   SUMMARY OF CANINE OVARIAN NEOPLASIA[1,3,5-7,10,15,16,18-20,21]

Tumor	Epithelial	Germ Cell	Sex Cord-Stromal	Other
Benign	Papillary adenoma Cystadenoma	Teratoma Dysgerminoma	Granulosa cell Sertoli-Leydig cell Thecoma Interstitial gland	Hemangioma Leiomyoma Lipoma
Malignant	Papillary adenocarcinoma Undifferentiated carcinoma	Teratocarcinoma	Malignant granulosa cell tumor	Hemangiosarcoma Any metastatic tumor
Percentage of ovarian tumors	40%–50 %	10%–15%	30%–50%	<5%
Clinical signs	Space-occupying mass Effusion if malignant	Space-occupying mass	Space-occupying mass Excessive hormone production	Space-occupying mass if benign Systemic illness if metastatic
Treatment	OHE Consider chemotherapy if malignant effusion or metastasis	OHE Consider chemotherapy if malignant effusion or metastasis	OHE Supportive care if illness associated with excessive hormone production	OHE Consider chemotherapy if malignant effusion or metastasis

cell tumors, which are all generally benign.[13,23,27,28] Germ cell tumors account for approximately 15% of feline ovarian tumors of which dysgerminomas are the most common. Teratomas are rare in cats.[29,30] Unlike human and canine ovarian tumors, epithelial ovarian tumors are rare in the cat. Carcinomas have been reported more often than benign adenomas or cystadenomas.[13,23,31,32]

Clinical Features

Clinical signs associated with ovarian tumors are usually related to a space-occupying mass within the abdomen (Figure 22-5) or excessive hormone production by the tumor. Clinical signs may be associated with abdominal hemorrhage if the mass is eroding through vessels within the ovarian pedicle.[18] Malignant epithelial tumors may present with malignant abdominal effusion.[7,33] Sex cord–stromal tumors may cause signs of excessive estrogen, progesterone, or testosterone production.[5-8] See Table 22-7 for clinical signs associated with excessive hormone production.

Diagnosis/Staging

See Table 22-8 for minimum database, diagnostics, and staging of ovarian tumors.

Metastasis

Adenocarcinomas and undifferentiated carcinomas frequently metastasize through peritoneal implantation, resulting in carcinomatosis and malignant

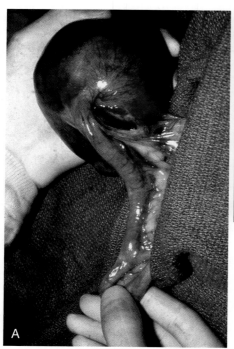
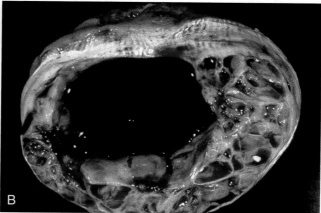

FIGURE 22-5 A, A large space-occupying mass in an adult female dog that was resected with ovariohysterectomy. Histopathology revealed an ovarian carcinoma. **B**, Cross-section evaluation of the ovarian carcinoma in **A**. No evidence of carcinomatosis was present during exploratory laparotomy; however, note the cystic nature of the mass.

TABLE 22-7   CLINICAL SIGNS ASSOCIATED WITH EXCESSIVE SEX HORMONE PRODUCTION

| | HORMONE | | |
	Estrogen	Progesterone	Testosterone
Clinical signs	Bone marrow suppression Alopecia Persistent estrus Pyometra	Mammary gland hyperplasia Cystic endometrial hyperplasia	Masculinization Aggression

TABLE 22-8   DIAGNOSIS AND STAGING OF OVARIAN AND UTERINE TUMORS

Diagnostic Test	Purpose/Findings
Physical examination	Many ovarian and uterine masses are palpable
CBC, chemistry panel, urinalysis (FeLV/FIV test—cats)	Determine general health reserves of patient and rule out estrogen toxicity
Three-view chest radiographs	Rule out metastasis, preanesthetic screening
Abdominal radiographs	Localize the mass
Abdominal ultrasound	Confirm location; check for evidence of metastasis
Cytology of mass or effusion	Evaluate for malignant cells
Biopsy and histopathology	Definitive diagnosis

peritoneal effusion. Pulmonary metastasis of carcinomas can also result in malignant pleural effusion.[18,19] Up to 30% of teratomas have a malignant epithelial component.[6,10,18] Between 10% and 30% of dysgerminomas[5,10,16,18,21,34] and 10% and 20% of granulosa cell tumors are malignant.[2,5-8,16-18] Thecomas and interstitial gland tumors are benign, but cases of malignant Sertoli-Leydig cell tumors have occasionally been reported.[16,17,35]

Treatment Modalities

- Complete ovariohysterectomy (OHE)
- Abdominal exploratory and biopsy of abnormal findings
- Supportive care if evidence of marrow suppression or pyometra
- Consider adjunctive chemotherapy if malignant

Many dogs with ovarian tumors have secondary pathologic changes within their uterus, including cystic endometrial hyperplasia and pyometra, suggesting that an OHE should be performed.[6,10] Histopathology should be performed on the entire uterus and ovaries in all patients that undergo OHE for pyometra, even if gross evidence of an ovarian tumor is not present.[36] The survival benefit for patients receiving chemotherapy to prevent or delay the development of metastasis of malignant ovarian tumors is unclear. Human carcinomas are often chemo-responsive to platinum compounds, gemcitabine, doxorubicin, and taxanes. For dogs with evidence of metastasis, reports of short-term responses (3-6 months) to intracavitary cisplatin, systemic platinum-based chemotherapy, and alkylating agents, such as cyclophosphamide, have been reported.[2,33,37-39] Adjunctive treatment with chemotherapy for malignant feline ovarian tumors has not been reported, although the use of carboplatin has been suggested.[40] Because of the potential for fatal toxicity, cisplatin should not be used in cats.

Survival

Prognosis is excellent for complete excision of benign ovarian tumors[10] but is guarded for malignant ovarian tumors because of the potential for metastasis. Prognosis for patients with evidence of metastatic disease and/or malignant effusions is poor. Prognosis for patients with bone marrow suppression caused by estrogen toxicity is guarded for full recovery of normal marrow function.

The most common ovarian tumor in cats—granulosa cell tumor—is frequently malignant and carries a guarded prognosis. Approximately 50% of cats develop metastatic disease within 5 to 10 months of diagnosis.[24-26] Dysgerminomas may carry a favorable prognosis in cats with early surgical excision, since metastasis occurs late in the course of disease. Epithelial tumors in cats are frequently carcinomas, which carry a poor prognosis.

UTERINE TUMORS
Incidence/Etiology/Risk Factors

The incidence of canine and feline uterine tumors is low (0.3%–0.4% and 0.2%–1.5%, respectively), because of the high number of spayed animals in the United States.[4,7,41-43] The incidence of uterine tumors in the population of intact females is likely higher but has not been reported.

The etiology of uterine tumors in companion animals has not been fully investigated. Similar to human uterine leiomyomas, canine uterine leiomyomas may be hormone dependent.[44] Risk factors for human leiomyoma growth include nulliparity and obesity.[45] Oral contraceptives appear to reduce the risk of tumor development but can increase the risk of cervical carcinoma development in women.[45,46] Human cervical carcinomas are most commonly caused by the human papilloma virus.[46] On the contrary, carcinomas are rare in dogs and have not been correlated to progestin use or to papilloma viral infection. A single report of a 2-year-old mixed-breed dog developing a uterine carcinoma after treatment with an estradiol/testosterone preparation and megestrol acetate has been published; however, a direct cause-and-effect relationship could not be confirmed.[47] The role of sex hormones in the development of feline uterine neoplasia has not been fully investigated. Adenocarcinomas, mixed Müllerian tumors, and leiomyomas express estrogen receptor alpha in cats. At least one case of a uterine stump adenocarcinoma has been reported in a cat after OHE, suggesting that this individual tumor developed in the absence of ovarian sex hormone influence.[48]

German shepherd dogs are the only breed reported to have a genetic predisposition for the development of uterine tumors. They may inherit the syndrome of concurrent bilateral renal cystadenocarcinoma, nodular dermatofibrosis, and multiple uterine leiomyomas.[49] The median age at diagnosis for these dogs is 6 years. Most dogs develop metastatic disease of the renal adenocarcinoma, resulting in illness and death an average of 3 years after diagnosis.[49] Uterine tumors are mesenchymal or epithelial in origin. Leiomyomas account for 85% to 90% of canine uterine tumors, are benign, and are often an incidental finding. Leiomyosarcomas represent approximately 10% of uterine tumors[50,51] and can be both locally aggressive and metastatic. Other mesenchymal uterine tumors are rare, including hemangiosarcoma and angiolipoleiomyoma.[52,53] Epithelial uterine tumors are extremely uncommon in the dog but generally malignant when they occur. A single report of a canine uterine plasmacytoma has been published.[54]

Epithelial tumors are most commonly reported in cats and are generally adenocarcinomas.[55,56] Uterine squamous cell carcinoma (SCC) has been reported in a single cat.[57] Mixed Müllerian tumors (carcinosarcomas, metaplastic carcinomas, adenosarcoma) have been reported in the cat and have a malignant behavior.[58-60] Mesenchymal tumors are less frequently reported in the cat and include leiomyoma, fibroma, hemangioma, lipoma, leiomyosarcoma, and fibrosarcoma.[56] Lymphoma has also been reported to occur in the feline uterus.[61]

Clinical Features

Benign tumors are often an incidental finding. The presence of a mass within the uterus may result in chronic inflammation causing a mucoid, purulent or blood-tinged vaginal discharge, or pyometra. Large tumors, whether benign or malignant, may cause abdominal distension. Malignant tumors are more likely to cause abdominal effusion, anorexia, weight loss, and general malaise.

Diagnosis/Staging

See Table 22-8 for minimum database, diagnostics, and staging of uterine tumors.

Treatment Modalities

- Complete OHE
- Abdominal exploratory and biopsy of abnormal findings
- Supportive care if evidence of pyometra
- Consider adjunctive chemotherapy if malignant

Histopathology should be performed on the entire uterus and ovaries in all patients that undergo OHE for pyometra, even if gross evidence of a tumor is not present.[36] The survival benefit for patients receiving chemotherapy to prevent or delay the development of metastasis of malignant uterine tumors is unclear. Adjunctive chemotherapy with epirubicin has been performed in a 10-month-old golden retriever with uterine carcinoma, resulting in a greater than 2-year survival.[62] The use of doxorubicin or carboplatin has been suggested for cats with malignant uterine tumors.[40]

Metastasis/Survival

Leiomyomas carry an excellent prognosis with OHE. Leiomyosarcomas and carcinomas carry a guarded prognosis with the potential for the development of metastatic disease. However, long-term survivals have been reported.[47,62] Dogs with evidence of metastatic disease at the time of diagnosis have a poor prognosis.

Uterine carcinomas and mixed Müllerian tumors in the cat are highly malignant with a poor prognosis. Carcinomatosis is common, and distant metastasis to the lungs, eye, and brain has been reported. Most cats develop metastatic disease within 6 months of diagnosis.[24,48,55] Leiomyosarcomas have a guarded prognosis. The presence of metastatic disease at the time of diagnosis is less common for leiomyosarcoma than carcinomas, but future metastases may develop.[48]

CANINE VAGINAL/VULVAR TUMORS
Incidence/Etiology/Risk Factors

Vaginal and vulvar tumors are the most common reproductive tract tumors in the dog with an incidence of 2.4% to 3.0%,[4,41] but only rare reports exist in the cat. More than 86% of vaginal and vulvar tumors in the dog are benign.[41,63] They are most common in older nulliparous dogs.[41,50,63] The influence of ovarian hormones is thought to contribute to the development of leiomyomas. Tumor recurrence was not reported in a study of dogs undergoing an OHE with leiomyoma removal; however, dogs that did not have an OHE had a 15% leiomyoma recurrence rate.[63,64]

Leiomyomas are the most common vaginal/vulvar tumor in the dog, accounting for up to 70% of benign tumors.[41] Most leiomyomas arise within the vestibule, and they may be intraluminal or extraluminal[51] (Figure 22-6). Other benign vaginal/vulvar tumors reported in the dog include polyps, fibromas, lipomas, sebaceous adenomas, fibrous histiocytoma, melanoma, and myxoma.[7,41,50,63] Leiomyoma, fibroma, leiomyofibroma, and myxoma have been reported in cats.[24,27,61,65,66] Transmissible venereal tumor (TVT) is a common canine vulvar tumor in endemic areas.[67] Young, sexually intact dogs (median of 5 years of age) are more likely to be exposed to and develop TVT.[67]

Malignant vaginal/vulvar tumors are uncommon. The most commonly reported malignant tumor in the dog is leiomyosarcoma.[7,41,63] Other reported malignant tumors in dogs include adenocarcinoma, squamous cell carcinoma, hemangiosarcoma, osteosarcoma, rhabdomyosarcoma, and mast cell tumor.[7,41,50,51,63] Leiomyosarcoma and granular cell tumors have been reported in cats.[24,68]

Clinical Features

- Space-occupying mass
- Perineal swelling (extraluminal)
- Mass protruding from vulva (intraluminal)

- Excessive licking of the genital region
- Dysuria or tenesmus
- Vulvar bleeding or discharge (more common with malignant tumors or TVT)

Vaginal prolapse caused by vaginal hyperplasia during proestrus is a common differential diagnosis for a vaginal mass in the entire female dog.[69] Transmissible venereal tumors may have a characteristic cauliflower-like appearance. Multiple TVTs may be present, and they are generally friable and bleed easily.[67]

Diagnosis/Staging (Table 22-9)

Treatment Modalities

- Complete surgical excision (exception, TVT)
- Episiotomy may be necessary for visualization
- Vulvovaginectomy and perineal urethrostomy (indicated for large, malignant tumors[70])
- OHE may prevent recurrence of leiomyoma[63,64]
- Radiation therapy—TVT or incompletely excised malignant tumors
- Chemotherapy—TVT or malignant tumors

Transmissible venereal tumors are unlike other vaginal/vulvar tumors. Complete surgical excision is not possible; however, a surgical biopsy may be necessary for diagnosis. Chemotherapy and radiation therapy are treatment options for TVT. Vincristine is the chemotherapy of choice with a complete response rate of greater than 90%. Vincristine should be administered weekly for two doses beyond clinical remission. Transmissible venereal tumors have a low metastatic rate, with reports up to 17%.[67,71-73] Metastases to local lymph nodes often also respond well to vincristine. However, distant metastases may be less responsive

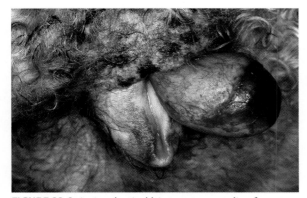

FIGURE 22-6 An intraluminal leiomyoma protruding from the vulva of an intact female poodle. The mass was completely resected and an OHE was performed. Recurrence was not noted in this patient.

TABLE 22-9   DIAGNOSIS AND STAGING OF VAGINAL/VULVAR TUMORS

Diagnostic Test	Purpose/Findings
Physical examination	Evaluate for visible/palpable masses
CBC, biochemical profile, urinalysis	Preanesthetic screening
Two-view thoracic radiographs	Preanesthetic screening
Vaginoscopy	Visualize smaller intraluminal masses
Computed tomography	Surgical planning
Cytology of mass	Evaluate for malignant cells
Biopsy and histopathology	Definitive diagnosis

to chemotherapy. Doxorubicin has been used to treat vincristine-resistant TVT.[67,73] Radiation therapy has also been used to treat TVT with complete response rates near 100%, and responses have been seen in TVTs that are resistant to vincristine therapy.[67,72] Radiation therapy also appears to be effective for metastases. However, there are increased costs and treatment-related side effects associated with radiation therapy that should be considered when making recommendations for treatment of TVT.

Metastasis/Survival

More than 86% of vaginal/vulvar tumors are benign with an excellent prognosis with complete surgical excision. Recurrence of leiomyomas can be prevented with concurrent OHE.[63,64] Malignant tumors have a guarded prognosis with an increased risk for local recurrence and distant metastasis. Leiomyosarcomas and squamous cell carcinomas frequently recur with marginal tumor resection. However, metastasis occurs late in the course of disease. On the contrary, osteosarcomas, hemangiosarcomas, and adenocarcinomas have both a high local recurrence rate and can metastasize early in the disease process. The prognosis for TVT treated with chemotherapy or radiation therapy is generally excellent. Distant metastases to liver, spleen, brain, eye, skin, and muscle, although rare, have been reported. Most patients receiving treatment achieve a complete remission and long-term survival.[67]

FELINE VAGINAL/VULVAR TUMORS

Feline vaginal/vulvar tumors are extremely rare with only scattered reports of individual tumors. Too few reports exist to formulate risk factors or to determine an etiology.

Most reported tumors are benign and include leiomyoma, fibroma, leiomyofibroma, and myxoma.[24,32,61,65,66] Reported malignant tumors include leiomyosarcoma and granular cell tumor.[24,68] Clinical signs are similar to those seen in the dog associated with a space-occupying mass. Dysuria, excessive licking, tenesmus, and constipation may be observed.[68] Owners may notice a swelling or visible mass in the perineum. A minimum database of CBC, chemistry panel with urinalysis, FELV/FIV test, and three-view thoracic radiographs is recommended to determine the overall health of the patient. Complete surgical excision is the treatment of choice. Vulvovaginectomy and perineal urethrostomy may be required for excision of large masses. The prognosis for complete excision of benign tumors is excellent. The prognosis

for malignant tumors should be guarded based on the behavior of malignant tumors in other species. Too few reports of feline malignant vaginal/vulvar tumors exist to determine metastatic rate or accurate estimates of MST.

Selected References*

Miller MA, Ramos-Vara JA, Dickerson MF, et al: Uterine neoplasia in 13 cats, *J Vet Diagn Invest* 15:515, 2003.

This report is a retrospective study evaluating the histologic, immunohistochemical, and clinical outcome of 13 cats with uterine tumors.

Moore AS, Kirk C, Cardona A: Intracavitary cisplatin chemotherapy experience in six dogs, *J Vet Intern Med* 5:227, 1991.

This report describes the technique of intracavitary chemotherapy and the outcome of six dogs undergoing this form of treatment.

Rogers KS, Walker MA, Dillon HB: Transmissible venereal tumor: a retrospective study of 29 cases, *J Am Anim Hosp Assoc* 34:463, 1998.

This retrospective study evaluates the clinical presentation, treatment, and outcome of 29 dogs presented with naturally occurring transmissible venereal tumor. Treatments used include chemotherapy and radiation therapy.

Sforna M, Brachelente C, Lepr E, et al: Canine ovarian tumours: a retrospective study of 49 cases, *Vet Res Comm* 1(27 Suppl):359, 2003.

This retrospective evaluation of canine ovarian tumors reports the methods of histopathologic differentiation and the incidence of various canine ovarian tumors among 49 cases.

Thacher C, Bradley R: Vulvar and vaginal tumors in the dog: a retrospective study, *J Am Vet Med Assoc* 183:690, 1983.

This retrospective study evaluates the clinical presentation, histologic type, and clinical outcome of 99 dogs with vulvar and vaginal tumors. Ovariohysterectomy was found to be effective in preventing recurrence of benign tumors in this study.

■ *For a complete list of the references cited in this chapter, please go to www.smallanimaloncology.com.

SECTION F: Mammary Tumors

Carolyn J. Henry

KEY POINTS

- Mammary tumors in cats are generally malignant, with adenocarcinomas predominating.
- A simple rule of thumb for canine mammary tumors is that approximately 50% are malignant and approximately 50% of the malignant tumors will metastasize.
- Because patients can present with concurrent benign and malignant mammary masses, all excised lesions must be submitted for histopathological examination.
- Inflammatory mammary carcinoma is an extremely aggressive form of mammary cancer for which surgery is unlikely to be of benefit.
- Complete surgical excision via lumpectomy or simple mastectomy in dogs and unilateral or bilateral mastectomy in cats is recommended for patients without evident metastasis at the time of presentation. Unilateral mastectomy reduces the likelihood of subsequent ipsilateral tumor development in intact dogs.

Mammary tumors are some of the most common tumors in dogs and cats. However, the disease varies considerably between the two species, as shown by the comparison in Table 22-10. Tumor types reported in the dog and their relative frequency are listed in Box 22-6. Whereas approximately 50% of canine mammary tumors (CMT) are benign, feline mammary masses are most often malignant, with adenocarcinomas (ACA) predominating.[1,2] Other malignant feline mammary tumors include squamous cell carcinomas (SCC), sarcomas, mucinous carcinomas, and inflammatory mammary carcinoma (IMC). Because there are key differences between the two species in terms of tumor types, prognosis, and therapy recommendations, canine and feline mammary tumors will be considered separately within this section.

CANINE MAMMARY TUMORS

Etiology/Risk Factors

Dog breeds reportedly at increased risk for mammary tumor development include English Springer, Brittany, and Cocker spaniels, toy and miniature poodles, English setters, pointers, German shepherds, Maltese, Yorkshire terriers, and dachshunds.[3-5] Mammary tumors in small breed dogs are more likely to be benign than those that develop in large breed dogs (25% vs. 58%).[6] Middle-aged (9–11 years) female intact dogs are most often affected, with an increased incidence beginning at approximately 6 years of age. It is well accepted that spaying dogs before the age of 2.5 years is protective against the development of mammary cancer. This is based on the work of Schneider et al.[7] that showed that the risk of developing mammary tumors rose to 26% for dogs spayed after their second estrus, compared with 0.5% and 8% for dogs spayed before their first or second estrus, respectively. The protective effect of spaying is not seen after two estrous cycles, likely because sex steroid hormones have already had their primary effect on target cells by this time. Products that contain medroxyprogesterone acetate (progestin and estrogen combination), such as those used for the prevention of estrus or to treat pseudopregnancy, have also been linked to an increased incidence of CMT.[8] Male dogs are not completely protected against CMT development. Approximately 1% of CMT occur in males and may be associated with hormonal abnormalities such as estrogen secretion by a Sertoli cell tumor.[9,10] Other potential risk factors for CMT development include obesity at a young age and feeding homemade diets, as opposed to commercial foods.[11,12] In one study, dogs with CMT had lower serum retinol concentrations compared with control dogs.[12] However, additional research is needed to determine the impact of retinol concentration and other dietary components on CMT development.

Clinical Features

Mammary tumors are often incidental findings during routine wellness examinations in older intact female dogs, or they may be discovered by conscientious owners. In over half of all cases of CMT, dogs appear with multiple mammary masses that may be either simultaneous primary masses or may reflect one primary lesion with regional extension or metastasis.[13] Whereas some studies have suggested that the caudal mammary glands are the most commonly affected in the dog, reports vary. Given the complex pattern of lymphatic drainage for canine mammary tissue, nodal metastasis may occur to either the axillary or inguinal lymph nodes. Of the five pairs of mammary glands (two cranial/thoracic, two abdominal, and one caudal/inguinal), the thoracic glands generally drain to the axillary or sternal nodes, the inguinal

TABLE 22-10 COMPARATIVE ASPECTS OF CANINE AND FELINE MAMMARY TUMORS

		Dog	Cat
Estimated annual incidence in the United States		199/100,000	25/100,000
Percent of benign tumors		50%–70%	10%–20%
Most common malignancy		Complex carcinoma	Adenocarcinoma (tubular, papillary, and solid carcinomas predominate)
Hormone receptor expression in invasive carcinomas		Majority (62.5%) are ERα+	Majority (57%) are ERα- and PR+
Genetic mutations	BRCA1 and BRCA2	Unknown	Unknown
	HER-2/neu	Protein overexpressed in 17.6%-29.7%	Protein overexpressed in 59.6%
	p53	15%–75%	19%–33%
Metastatic behavior		32%–77%, depending on histologic type	>50% metastatic
Poor prognostic factors		Diagnosis of ductal carcinoma, IMC, or sarcoma	High AgNOR count
		Ulceration of skin	Tumor size >3 cm
		Invasive growth; fixed to adjacent tissue	Ki-67 index >25.2
		Increased age at diagnosis	Lymphatic invasion
		German shepherd breed	Increased WHO stage
		Heat shock protein expression	
		Advanced stage	
		Tumor size >3 cm	
		High histologic grade	
		High Ki-67 score	
		High COX-2 levels	
		Nodal metastasis	
		Non-ovariectomized	
		Male gender	
Overall prognosis		Reported mean survival time = 439 days	1-year survival noted for ~⅓ to ½ of cats treated with surgery alone; up to 59% 1-yr survival with adjuvant chemotherapy
		MST = 70 weeks after surgery for malignant vs. 114 weeks for benign tumors	2 year survival is ~15-20% with surgery alone; improves to ~37% with addition of chemotherapy
			Cats with complex carcinomas have a more favorable prognosis (32.6 mos MST vs. 15.5 mos for other carcinomas)

IMC, Inflammatory mammary carcinoma; *MST,* median survival time.

glands are drained by the inguinal nodes, and the two abdominal glands may drain to either site. The presence of lymph node enlargement, lymphedema, skin ulceration, and fixation to underlying tissue are all characteristics that suggest malignancy. A unique clinical entity that warrants an altered approach to diagnosis and case management is IMC (Figure 22-7). This malignancy may be mistaken for mastitis, because affected dogs classically present with warm, erythematous mammary tissue and associated lymphedema, ulceration and vesicles,

and significant pain upon any manipulation of the tissue. Alternatively, the diagnosis of IMC may become apparent only after wound dehiscence occurs as a result of what was anticipated to be a routine mammary mass excision (referred to as secondary IMC).

Diagnosis

Diagnosis of CMT requires histologic examination of incisional or excisional biopsy samples. It is important to remember that benign and malignant mammary masses

Box 22-6 HISTOLOGIC CLASSIFICATION OF CANINE MAMMARY TUMORS

Malignant Tumors
   Non-infiltrating *(in situ)* carcinoma
   Complex carcinoma
   Simple carcinoma
      Tubulopapillary carcinoma
      Solid carcinoma
      Anaplastic carcinoma
   Special types of carcinomas
      Spindle cell carcinoma
      Squamous cell carcinoma
      Mucinous carcinoma
      Lipid-rich carcinoma
   Sarcoma
      Fibrosarcoma
      Osteosarcoma
      Other sarcomas
   Carcinosarcoma
   Carcinoma or sarcoma in benign tumor

Benign Tumors
   Adenoma
      Simple adenoma
      Complex adenoma
      Basaloid adenoma
   Fibroadenoma
      Low-cellularity fibroadenoma
      High-cellularity fibroadenoma
   Benign mixed tumor
   Duct papilloma

(From Misdorp W, Else R, Hellman E, et al: Histologic classification of mammary tumors of the dog and cat. In World Health Organization international histological classification of tumors of domestic animals, series 2, vol 7, no 2, Washington, DC, 1999, Armed Forces Institute of Pathology.)

may occur concurrently. As such, it is necessary to submit all excised masses for histopathological examination, rather than assume that one nodule is representative of all tumors of the mammary tumors that are present.

Staging and Metastasis

Approximately 50% of the malignant canine mammary tumors will metastasize. Therefore, complete tumor staging requires not only a thorough evaluation of the primary tumor with regard to size and gross features (ulceration, fixation, etc), but also a complete assessment for regional and distant metastases. The original clinical staging for CMT was based on a four-stage system

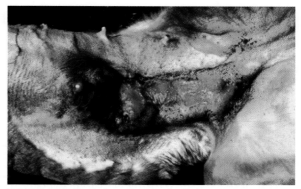

FIGURE 22-7 Typical appearance of inflammatory mammary carcinoma. Erythema, ulceration, and edema are characteristic of this tumor for which surgery is contraindicated.

developed by the World Health Organization (WHO) and reported in 1980.[14] Since that time, a modified staging system has been reported (Table 22-11), with the primary difference being the addition of a Stage V for dogs with distant metastatic disease and the designation of a Stage IV (rather than Stage II or III) for those with nodal metastasis.[9] Either staging system necessitates evaluation of regional lymph nodes as well as assessment of potential distant sites of metastasis, especially distant lymph nodes and lungs. Preoperative cytology of any palpable lymph nodes may aid in determining disease extent prior to surgery. Regardless of preoperative assessment, lymph node tissue removed at the time of surgery should be submitted for histologic examination. Although standard hematoxylin and eosin (H & E) staining of slides from nodal tissue will permit accurate identification of micrometastasis in most cases, cytokeratin immunostaining using an anti-pancytokeratin antibody AE1/AE3 was reported to detect occult micrometastasis in 12 of 131 (9.2%) lymph nodes from dogs judged to have node-negative disease based on H & E results.[15] The impact of micrometastatic disease on prognosis for CMT is unknown at this time. Three-view thoracic radiographs are essential before surgery, since pulmonary metastases warrant a poor prognosis and may dictate therapy decisions. In addition to clinical staging to determine disease extent, there is a histologic staging system outlined in Table 22-12. In this system, Stages 0, I, and II are based on histologic assessment, whereas Stage III is based on clinical assessment of distant metastasis. This system should not be confused with the clinical staging systems proposed in Table 22-11. Although the histologic staging system is not universally applied

TABLE 22-11   COMPARISON OF THE ORIGINAL AND MODIFIED STAGING SYSTEMS FOR THE CLASSIFICATION OF CANINE MAMMARY TUMORS

Stage	Original WHO Staging	Modified WHO Staging
I	T1 (<3 cm) N_0 M_0	T1 (<3 cm) N_0 M_0
II	T2 (<5 cm) N_{1+} M_0 (histologically positive node, but not fixed to underlying tissues)	T2 (3–5 cm) N_0 M_0
III	Any T3 or any tumor with fixed nodal involvement	T3 (>5 cm) N_0 M_0
IV	Distant metastasis (any T, any N, M_1)	Regional node metastasis (any T, N_1 M_0)
V	No Stage V	Distant metastasis (any T, any N, M_1)

TABLE 22-12   HISTOLOGIC STAGING SYSTEM FOR CANINE MAMMARY TUMORS (CMTS)

Stage	Features	Frequency of *De Novo* or Recurrent CMT 2 Years after Surgery
0	Tumor cells are limited to ductal tissue	25%
I	Tumor cells invade stromal tissue	72%
II	Vascular/lymphatic invasion and/or regional lymph node metastasis	95%
III	Systemic metastasis	Not reported; dogs with Stage III disease by definition have no disease-free interval

(Adapted from Gilbertson SR, Kurzman ID, Zachrau RE, et al: Canine mammary epithelial neoplasms: biologic implications of morphologic characteristics assessed in 232 dogs, *Vet Pathol* 20:127, 1983.)

in veterinary medicine, it is highlighted here because it correlated well with clinical outcome in one large study (n = 232) of dogs undergoing mastectomy for CMT.[16]

Treatment Modalities

Surgery

Surgery is the mainstay of therapy for most CMT, with the exception of IMC (see later discussion). In their pivotal study published in 1985, MacEwen et al.[17] demonstrated that type of surgery is not a major prognostic factor for survival of dogs with mammary cancer, provided resection is complete as assessed by histologic examination. Thus, they established the surgical standard of care for CMT to include minimal but adequate tumor excision, usually via lumpectomy or partial mastectomy. Lumpectomy is generally reserved for dogs with lesions less than 0.5 cm.[9,18] The recommendation made by MacEwen et al. have been supported by subsequent studies evaluating survival time as the endpoint.[19] However, a 2008 report by Stratmann et al.[20] demonstrated that 58% of intact dogs undergoing regional mastectomy for a solitary mammary tumor went on to develop a second mammary mass, 75% of which were malignant, in the remaining ipsilateral mammary chain. Although effect on overall survival was not assessed, the authors of the study proposed that unilateral radical mastectomy be recommended because

of the high rate of second tumor development in the remaining ipsilateral tissue. Given the publication of this new information, it is advisable to discuss with owners the possibility of subsequent development of new masses in the remaining mammary tissue and the role that unilateral mastectomy may have in preventing this. However, one must also realize that, were this recommendation applied to the study population in the Stratmann et al. study, 42 of their 99 dogs would have undergone a more extensive surgery than was necessary, based on the known outcome of no ipsilateral tumor recurrence in these dogs. The effect of ovariohysterectomy (OHE) on the rate of second tumor development could not be assessed in the study because enrollment was limited to dogs that remained intact. Controversy has long existed regarding whether or not to perform OHE at the time of mammary tumor excision.[5,21] Given the high rate of ER-positive tumors in dogs, it would seem reasonable to consider hormone ablation via OHE in dogs with mammary malignancy. However, early reports suggested no benefit to OHE at the time of tumor excision. Two more recent studies have shown a survival advantage for dogs that undergo OHE. In the first report, dogs undergoing OHE within 2 years prior to or at the time of CMT removal survived 45% longer than intact dogs or dogs spayed greater than 2 years before CMT excision.[22] A subsequent study demonstrated that dogs undergoing OHE were more likely to survive at least 2 years after surgery than dogs that remained intact. This was especially true for dogs with complex carcinomas.[19] Although practitioners may not know if they are dealing with a malignant versus a benign mass at the time of surgery, these two latter studies support the practice of performing OHE as an adjunct to complete tumor excision when malignant CMT is suspected.

Chemotherapy

Chemotherapy has not been definitively shown to improve survival times for dogs with mammary cancer. Protocols that have been adapted from human oncology are generally recommended for dogs with high-grade tumors or those with evidence of tumor emboli noted on histopathology. Various chemotherapy agents including paclitaxel, 5-FU, doxorubicin, cyclophosphamide, mitoxantrone, and carboplatin have been used, with no clear advantage of one protocol over others for treatment of CMT. A prospective study comparing outcome of dogs (n = 8) treated with 5-FU (150 mg/m² IV) and cyclophosphamide (100 mg/m² IV) once weekly for 4 weeks to that of dogs (n = 8) treated with surgery alone demonstrated a significant improvement in survival for dogs receiving chemotherapy. The MST for the chemotherapy group was 24 months, compared with 6 months for the surgery-only group.[23] In a subsequent prospective study, outcome for dogs treated with postoperative doxorubicin or docetaxel (n = 12) was compared with that of dogs treated with surgery alone (n = 19). There was no significant impact of chemotherapy on recurrence-free interval, time to metastasis, or overall survival.[24] Additional randomized prospective studies are necessary to better define the role of chemotherapy in the clinical management of dogs with mammary cancer.

Radiation Therapy

Although it is an important component of breast cancer treatment in women, radiation therapy remains largely unexplored for the treatment of CMT. Anecdotal reports of palliation for unresectable lesions or for IMC currently serve as the only evidence to support radiation therapy for CMT. Given the efficacy of radiation therapy in women with breast cancer, further evaluation of this treatment modality for CMT is warranted.

Hormonal Therapy

Hormonal therapy has not been widely used in the treatment of CMT, perhaps in part because of the relative difficulty of performing routine estrogen and progesterone receptor assays on canine tissue. Hormone ablation may be accomplished via ovariectomy (as described previously). In addition, tamoxifen is a drug that has been evaluated as hormonal therapy for CMT. Tamoxifen has both estrogenic and antiestrogenic effects and is advocated for treatment of estrogen receptor-positive human breast cancer patients. In a pilot study evaluating outcome of dogs with mammary carcinoma treated with 2.5 to 10 mg (mean dose 0.42 mg/kg q12h, PO) tamoxifen, five of seven dogs that had either metastatic or unresectable mammary carcinoma experienced a decrease in tumor burden.* In another report of 10 dogs with advanced mammary cancer treated with tamoxifen (0.7 mg/kg q24h), no measurable responses were noted.[25] Adverse effects of tamoxifen in dogs may include vaginal discharge, vulvar swelling, urinary incontinence, urinary tract infection, mental dullness, signs of estrus, and partial alopecia. Pyometra occurs in approximately 25% of dogs treated with tamoxifen; thus, clients must be counseled regarding this potential complication of tamoxifen therapy.

Immunotheraphy

Various methods of nonspecific immunomodulation have been investigated for the treatment of CMT, including *Corynebacterium parvum*, Bacillus Calmette-Guerin (BCG), levamisole and liposome-encapsulated muramyl tripeptides (L-MTP-PE).[26-28] However, none have been clearly demonstrated to be of clinical benefit for dogs with CMT.

Therapy for Inflammatory Mammary Carcinoma

Although recommendations for therapy of dogs with IMC vary among veterinary oncologists, there is general agreement that surgery is contraindicated. Wound dehiscence, disseminated intravascular coagulation, and ventral and limb edema are clinical features of IMC that may complicate surgical recovery. The disease is generally not amenable to complete surgical excision. The demonstration of high levels of COX-2 expression in canine IMC suggests that COX-2 inhibition with non-steroidal anti-inflammatory drugs (NSAIDs) may be beneficial.[29] Although there are anecdotal reports of disease palliation with radiation therapy, NSAIDs, and doxorubicin-based chemotherapy protocols, the prognosis for IMC remains poor.

Prognosis and Survival

Of the mammary tumor types encountered in dogs, sarcomas and IMC are associated with the worst prognosis.[3,30,31] Mixed malignant tumors and squamous cell

---

*Kitchell BE, Fidel J: Tamoxifen as a potential therapy for canine mammary carcinoma, *Proc Vet Cancer Soc* p 91, 1992 (unpublished data).

carcinomas are also associated with poor survival times. Of the carcinomas, solid carcinomas have been associated with poorer survival times than either tubular or papillary carcinomas.[31,32] Those carcinomas warranting a better prognosis include carcinoma *in situ* and adenocarcinomas.

Prognostic factors for CMT have been assessed in multiple prospective and retrospective studies. Factors that are shown to correlate with prognosis in multivariate analysis are more compelling than those identified in univariate analysis because the interdependent effects of multiple factors are considered in such analyses. Factors that are generally accepted to have a negative impact on CMT prognosis are listed in Table 22-10.[3,6,23,33-38]

FELINE MAMMARY CANCER

Incidence, Etiology, and Pathogenesis

Mammary cancer is the third most common feline tumor, with only skin tumors and lymphoma being more common.[39,40] As with CMT, mammary tumors in cats may affect both genders. Estrogen and progesterone are both believed to play important roles in feline mammary cancer (FMC) development, although the underlying mechanisms are less clear than for CMT. Intact females and cats regularly exposed to progestins are at increased risk for mammary cancer development.[41] The literature also suggests that, as in dogs, ovariectomy at an early age may lower the risk of FMC development. In one report, cats ovariectomized at 6 months of age had an approximate seven-fold reduction in risk of FMC compared with intact cats.[39] A subsequent report comparing 308 cats with biopsy-proven FMC to a control population of 400 female cats without mammary tumors showed a statistically significant reduction in risk of FMC development in cats spayed prior to 1 year of age compared with intact cats. Specifically, a 91% reduction in risk was reported for those spayed before 6 months of age, and an 86% reduction was demonstrated for those spayed before 1 year of age. Parity was not significantly related to risk of FMC.[42] As such, there is some justification for recommending ovariectomy/OHE prior to 1 year of age in cats.

Clinical Features

Cats with mammary cancer are usually presented for evaluation of a palpable nodule, or the finding may be incidental to routine physical examination. In contrast to canine mammary tumors, the majority (80%-96%) of feline mammary masses are malignant. Lesion ulceration is common and is suggestive of malignancy. As in

the dog, multiple lesions are often present at the time of diagnosis, although cats are less likely to have synchronous benign and malignant lesions.

Diagnosis, Staging, and Metastasis

Cats with suspected mammary carcinoma should be evaluated with a urinalysis, CBC, and serum biochemical evaluation, in anticipation of anesthesia and surgery. Thoracic radiographs (right lateral, left lateral, and ventrodorsal views) and regional lymph node palpation/aspiration are imperative, since the reported metastatic rate for FMC ranges from 25% to as high as 100%, with the most common sites being the lymph nodes and lungs (Figure 22-8).[43-45] In a review of the literature between 1952 and 1996, Waters et al.[46] found 338 cases of extraskeletal metastases in 799 cats with malignant mammary tumors. However, the rate of skeletal metastasis from mammary carcinoma is very low in cats compared with people and dogs.

Histopathologic examination is required to confirm a diagnosis of FMC. Biopsy specimens are often obtained at the time of definitive surgery rather than as part of a presurgical evaluation. The majority of mammary tumors in cats are diagnosed as adenocarcinomas, specifically of tubular, papillary, solid, or cribriform type. Less common malignancies include squamous cell carcinoma, sarcoma, mucinous carcinoma, and complex carcinomas. The latter are characterized by the presence of both luminal epithelial and myoepithelial cells

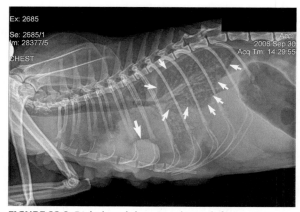

FIGURE 22-8 Right lateral thoracic radiograph from a 12-year-old domestic short hair (DSH) with metastatic mammary carcinoma. Pleural effusion has caused lung lobe retraction (*small arrows*), and a diffuse metastatic pattern is evident within the lung parenchyma. Larger masses (*large arrow*) are extrathoracic, originating within the mammary tissue.

and are associated with a better prognosis than other FMC.[47] Inflammatory mammary carcinoma was first described in cats in 2004, with three cats described as having lesions typical in gross appearance to that of human and canine IMC and with a similar poor prognosis.[48] Lesions in these cats differed from those typical of human or canine IMC in that they stained positive for ER-α, occurred only after prior mastectomy, and were associated with severe inflammation of the dermis and subcutaneous tissue.

Fine needle aspiration and cytology of mammary lesions in cats are seldom useful, but may be considered if cutaneous or subcutaneous lesions of non-mammary tissue origin, such as mast cell tumors, are suspected. Cytologic evaluation of pleural effusion fluid or of aspirates from enlarged lymph nodes is warranted when these conditions are present. The staging system for FMC has been modified from the original system proposed by Owen in 1980. The modified system limits nodal metastasis to Stage III or IV, whereas the original system placed cats with histologically confirmed nodal metastasis but without fixation of nodes to surrounding tissue into Stage II. A comparison of the staging systems is outlined in Table 22-13.

Treatment Modalities

Surgery

Surgery is the primary treatment for FMC, often with adjuvant chemotherapy. Unilateral or bilateral mastectomy is generally considered the preferred surgical method in cats. Although it is unclear if radical mastectomy provides a survival advantage in cats, the procedure has been shown to significantly decrease the recurrence rate of FMC. When bilateral radical mastectomy is performed, it may be done as one surgical procedure or as a staged procedure, with the second unilateral mastectomy scheduled 2 to 6 weeks after the first. The inguinal lymph node is removed with the caudal mammary glands; however, axillary node excision is not a routine part of the radical mastectomy. Removal of the axillary node is only recommended if it is suspected to have metastatic disease, because prophylactic axillary node excision is unlikely to benefit the patient.

Chemotherapy

Few studies have assessed the role of chemotherapy for the primary or adjuvant treatment of FMC. Doxorubicin-based protocols have been evaluated most frequently. Approximately one third to one half of cats with stage III or IV disease (see Table 22-13 for staging criteria) have measurable responses to the combination of doxorubicin and cyclophosphamide. In a retrospective study of 67 cats with mammary adenocarcinoma receiving adjuvant doxorubicin chemotherapy (1 mg/kg q21d, IV for an intended five treatments) beginning at the time of suture removal, the MST was 448 days and the 1- and 2-year survival rates were 58.9% and 37.2%, respectively.[49] The author and others carried out a randomized, prospective clinical trial comparing mitoxantrone (5 mg/m² q21d, IV for four total doses) to doxorubicin (four doses at 20 mg/m² q21d, IV) for adjuvant therapy of FMC after radical (unilateral or bilateral) mastectomy. Data analysis indicated no significant difference in outcome between the two groups (MST and metastasis-free interval [MFI] both = 747 days for mitoxantrone; MST = 484 days and MFI = 940 days with doxorubicin).[50] The literature supports use of adjuvant chemotherapy for advanced stage FMC, although its role for treatment of Stage I tumors is not clear.

Prognosis

Tumor size (and, therefore, T stage according to the WHO staging system) is the single most reliable prognostic indicator for cats with mammary cancer. In one report, the MST for cats with tumors greater than 3 cm was 12 months, compared with 21 months for cats with lesions less than 3 cm.[51] Other prognostic factors and a summary of the literature regarding survival times are shown in Table 22-10.[47,52-58]

TABLE 22-13 COMPARISON OF THE ORIGINAL AND MODIFIED STAGING SYSTEMS FOR THE CLASSIFICATION OF FELINE MAMMARY CANCER (FMC)

Stage	Original WHO Staging for FMC	Modified WHO Tumor Staging System for FMC
I	T1 (<1 cm) N_0 M_0	T_1 (<2 cm) N_0 M_0
II	T2 (<3 cm) N_{1+} M_0 (histologically positive node, but not fixed to underlying tissues)	T_2 (2–3 cm) N_0 M_0
III	Any T3 or any tumor with fixed nodal involvement	Regional node metastasis or T3 (>3 cm) lesion, or both, but no distant metastasis
IV	Distant metastasis (any T, any N, M_1)	Distant metastasis (any T, any N, M_1)

Selected References*

Chang S, Chang C, Chang T, et al: Prognostic factors associated with survival two years after surgery in dogs with malignant mammary tumors: 79 cases (1998-2002), *J Am Vet Med Assoc* 227:1625, 2005.
A retrospective evaluation of prognostic factors in 79 dogs with mammary cancer, this paper provides support for the practice of spaying dogs at the time of mammary tumor resection.

Gilbertson SR, Kurzman ID, Zachrau RE, et al: Canine mammary epithelial neoplasms: biologic implications of morphologic characteristics assessed in 232 dogs, *Vet Pathol* 20:127, 1983.
A retrospective review of pathologic features of canine mammary tumors, including a description of the histologic grading scheme proposed for use in dogs.

MacEwen EG, Harvey HJ, Patnaik AK, et al: Evaluation of the effect of levamisole and surgery on canine mammary cancer, *J Biol Resp Mod* 25:540, 1985.
A prospective study comparing simple mastectomy to radical mastectomy, this report was the first to show the equivalency of surgery type (radical vs. minimal complete resection) with regard to outcome in dogs with mammary cancer.

Novosad CA, Bergman PJ, O'Brien MG, et al: Retrospective evaluation of adjunctive doxorubicin for the treatment of feline mammary gland adenocarcinoma: 67 cases, *J Am Anim Hosp Assoc* 42:110, 2006.
This is one of the few published reports evaluating outcome for cats treated with adjuvant chemotherapy for mammary cancer.

Overley B, Shofer FS, Goldschmidt MH: Association between ovariohysterectomy and feline mammary carcinoma, *J Vet Intern Med* 19:560, 2005.
A report including 308 cats with mammary cancer and 400 control cats that demonstrated that cats spayed before 1 year of age were at decreased risk of developing mammary cancer.

Schneider R, Dorn CR, Taylor DON: Factors influencing canine mammary cancer development and postsurgical survival, *J Natl Cancer Inst* 43(6):1249, 1969.
The seminal paper demonstrating the protective effect of early OHE against canine mammary cancer development.

Sorenmo KU, Shofer FS, Goldschmidt MH: Effect of spaying and timing of spaying on survival of dogs with mammary carcinoma, *J Vet Intern Med* 14:266, 2000.
The first report to demonstrate a survival advantage for dogs undergoing OHE at the time of mammary tumor excision, compared with those that were not spayed at the time of resection.

Waters DJ, Honeckman A, Cooley DM, et al: Skeletal metastasis in feline mammary carcinoma: case report and literature review, *J Am Anim Hosp Assoc* 34:103, 1998.
A comprehensive review of reported cases of metastatic disease associated with mammary carcinoma in 799 cats.

■ *For a complete list of the references cited in this chapter, please go to www.smallanimaloncology.com.

SECTION G: Male Reproductive Tumors

Kathryn H. Taylor

KEY POINTS

- The majority of canine testicular tumors are benign in nature.
- Cryptorchidism significantly increases the risk of testicular tumor development; cryptorchid testicular tumors are more likely to be malignant and estrogen secreting when compared with tumors occurring in descended testicles.
- Surgical resection is the treatment of choice for most testicular, penile, preputial, and scrotal tumors in dogs and cats. Adjunctive treatment with chemotherapy or radiation therapy may be indicated for malignant tumors.
- Transmissible venereal tumors are transplantable canine tumors that most often occur in the perineal region and are often curable with vincristine chemotherapy.

CANINE TESTICULAR TUMORS

Incidence

Testicular tumors are the second most common site of tumor development in the male dog with an incidence between 7% and 16%.[1-3] More than 40% of dogs have multiple testicular tumors at the time of diagnosis.[3] The incidence of testicular tumors increases with age with a mean age at diagnosis of 10 years.[4-6]

Etiology/Risk Factors

The etiology of testicular tumors remains unknown. Risk factors for their development have been investigated, including increasing age, breed, cryptorchidism, and environmental factors. Dogs less than 6 years of age have a low risk of tumor development. Breed-specific risks for the development of testicular tumors

TABLE 22-14   BREEDS AT INCREASED RISK FOR TESTICULAR TUMOR DEVELOPMENT[8]

All Testicular Tumors	Seminoma	Sertoli Cell Tumor	Interstitial Cell Tumor
Siberian Husky	Siberian Husky	West Highland white terrier	Siberian Husky
Norwegian elkhound	Norwegian elkhound	Norwegian elkhound	Bull terrier
Afghan hound	Keeshond	Afghan hound	Afghan hound
Shetland sheepdog	Great Dane	Shetland sheepdog	Shetland sheepdog
Fox terrier	Fox terrier	Fox terrier	Fox terrier
	Weimaraner	Weimaraner	Dalmatian
	Old English sheepdog	Airedale terrier	Old English sheepdog
	Samoyed	Pekingese	
	Scottish terrier		
	Bulldog		

have been evaluated in several studies[1,7] (Table 22-14). Cryptorchidism is a significant risk factor for the development of Sertoli cell tumors and seminomas, increasing the risk of these tumors 8.8 and 16 times, respectively, when compared with a scrotal testicle.[9] Unknown environmental factors are thought to influence testicular tumor development, based on the increased incidence of testicular tumors in German shepherd working dogs serving in Vietnam compared with those in the United States.[10]

Clinical Features

The most common testicular tumors arise from three cell types: Sertoli cell tumors from the sustentacular cell of the seminiferous tubules, seminomas from the germinal epithelial cells of the seminiferous tubules, and interstitial cell tumors from the Leydig cells between the seminiferous tubules. Other rare testicular tumors include gonadoblastomas, adenocarcinomas, and sarcomas.[11,12] Most testicular tumors are an incidental finding. However, up to 45% of Sertoli cell tumors and occasional seminomas may produce estrogen-causing clinical signs and illness (Table 22-15). Cryptorchidism increases the risk of hormone production by tumors of retained testicles.[9,13] Estrogen toxicity is a serious complication with as few as 20% of patients experiencing a full recovery. Improvements in myelosuppression are usually seen within 2 to 4 weeks, and full recovery may take up to 5 months.[14,15] Recurrence of myelosuppression after marrow recovery may indicate the development of metastatic disease. Interstitial cell tumors may produce excessive testosterone contributing to the incidence of perineal hernia, prostatic hyperplasia, and perianal gland hyperplasia in male dogs.[1,16,17] The general characteristics of testicular tumors are summarized in Table 22-16.

TABLE 22-15   CLINICAL SIGNS AND TREATMENT RECOMMENDATIONS FOR TESTICULAR TUMORS WITH EXCESSIVE ESTROGEN PRODUCTION

CLINICAL SIGNS	TREATMENT
Gynecomastia	1. Castration to remove the affected testicle
Pendulous prepuce	
Galactorrhea	2. Supportive care
Symmetrical alopecia and hyperpigmentation	with blood products or broad spectrum antibiotics, if significant myelosuppression
Atrophy of scrotum and opposite testicle	
Myelosuppression	3. Adjunctive chemotherapy or radiation therapy if evidence of metastasis

Diagnosis and Staging

The majority of canine testicular tumors are benign. Rare malignant tumors may require further staging to evaluate the thorax, liver, and lumbar lymph nodes for metastasis. A complete physical examination, including rectal examination, should be performed. A CBC to evaluate for myelosuppression resulting from hyperestrogenemia as well as chemistry panel and urinalysis are recommended. Three-view thoracic radiographs and abdominal ultrasound should be performed on cryptorchid patients or those with a known malignant tumor. Fine needle aspiration and cytology may be helpful to differentiate inflammatory causes of testicular enlargement.

Metastasis

Metastasis, although rare, may affect the regional lymph nodes, liver, kidney, spleen, adrenal gland, pancreas, and brain (see Table 22-16).[3,16,18,19] Peritoneal dissemination may occur with malignant tumors of intra-abdominal testicles. Cryptorchid tumors appear to metastasize more

TABLE 22-16   GENERAL CHARACTERISTICS OF CANINE TESTICULAR TUMORS

	Sertoli Cell Tumor	Seminoma	Interstitial Cell Tumor
Clinical findings	Large and palpable signs of feminization are common	Most tumors are <2 cm in diameter	Small to microscopic, generally an incidental finding May have concurrent perineal hernia, perianal gland hyperplasia, or prostatic hyperplasia
Behavior	9%–14% metastasize	<10% metastasize	Considered benign
Hormone production	Up to 45% produce estrogen	Occasionally reported to produce estrogen	May produce excessive testosterone Very rarely reported to produce excessive estrogen

often, possibly because these tumors are diagnosed later in the course of disease.[20]

Treatment Modalities

Castration for tumor removal is usually curative. More than 40% of affected dogs have multiple testicular tumors, such that bilateral orchiectomy is recommended, especially in dogs with clinical signs related to excessive hormone production. In addition to castration, dogs with estrogen toxicity may require supportive care with blood products or broad-spectrum antibiotics, if myelosuppression is severe.

Malignant testicular tumors may warrant adjunctive chemotherapy or radiation therapy. The development of metastatic disease as long as 8 years after castration has been reported.[20] Platinum-based chemotherapy drugs are used in aggressive human testicular neoplasia and have shown efficacy in individual case reports of dogs with metastatic testicular tumors with survival times ranging from 6 to 31 months.[20] In addition, cyclophosphamide, methotrexate, and vinblastine have been used in dogs.[21] External beam radiation therapy for the treatment of metastatic seminoma has resulted in complete remission in four dogs for more than 36 months.[22]

Prognosis and Survival

The prognosis for canine testicular tumors is usually excellent, since most tumors are cured with surgical excision. If there is evidence of malignant or metastatic disease, or estrogen toxicity, the prognosis is guarded.

CANINE PENILE AND PREPUTIAL TUMORS
Incidence/Etiology/Risk Factors

Penile and preputial tumors in the dog are uncommon. Although circumcision appears to be a protective factor against preputial carcinomas in men, risk factors for the development of preputial or penile tumors in dogs have not been fully investigated.[23] Ultraviolet light exposure is thought to contribute to squamous cell carcinoma (SCC) and hemangiosarcoma (HSA) development within the skin of the ventral abdomen, including the prepuce.[24,25]

Clinical Features

The most common preputial tumors in dogs include SCC, transmissible venereal tumor (TVT), and mast cell tumor (MCT). Any skin tumor common to haired skin may occur within the prepuce. Papilloma, hemangioma, fibroma, sebaceous adenoma, fibrosarcoma, and HSA have been reported within the prepuce.[26] The most common penile tumors in dogs are TVT and SCC. Other tumors reported to affect the penis include papilloma of the glans penis, chondrosarcoma of the os penis, and lymphoma.[27-29]

Preputial tumors are commonly visible to owners, and dogs may present due to a visible mass, hematuria, dysuria, or excessive licking. Penile tumors may not be visible and dogs usually present for dysuria, stranguria, or hematuria.

Transmissible venereal tumors are the most common penile and preputial tumors of the dog. Dogs less than 6 years of age are more commonly affected. They are endemic in many tropical climates and in areas with large numbers of free-roaming dogs.[30] The glans penis and prepuce are often concurrently affected. Transmission occurs via exfoliation and implantation of cells within the genital epithelium.[31] Masses may have a cauliflower-like appearance or be friable and bleed easily.[30] Squamous cell carcinoma of the penis and prepuce resembles SCC of the skin and may be raised, plaque-like, ulcerated, or necrotic. Mast cell tumors may have a variable appearance from raised and ulcerated to soft and freely moveable. Papillomas of the glans penis may be mistaken for TVT because of a similar cauliflower-like appearance. Hemangioma and HSA are usually dark, blood-filled lesions that may be dermal or subcutaneous.

Diagnosis and Staging

The diagnosis of a penile or preputial tumor usually requires histopathology. FNA and cytology may be adequate for the diagnosis of TVT or well-granulated MCTs. Before definitive therapy for a penile or preputial tumor, the general health of the dog should be evaluated. Diagnostics include physical examination, CBC, chemistry panel with urinalysis, and two-view thoracic radiographs. Further staging may be required for malignant tumors, including lymph node aspirates, three-view thoracic radiographs, or ultrasound. Complete staging recommendations for malignant tumors may be found in the chapters related to each tumor type.

Metastasis

Transmissible venereal tumors are the most common penile and preputial tumors and have a low metastatic rate. Less than 10% of TVTs will metastasize.[30] However, distant metastasis of TVT to liver, spleen, lung, skin, muscle, brain, and eye has been reported.[32,33] Tumors with moderate metastatic potential include SCC and poorly differentiated MCTs. Subcutaneous HSAs have high metastatic potential.[34] A thorough discussion of metastatic potential may be found for each tumor type in their respective chapters.

Treatment Modalities

The treatment of choice for most penile and preputial tumors is complete surgical resection; TVTs are an exception where vincristine chemotherapy is recommend as the primary treatment (Figure 22-9). Treatment should continue for two doses beyond complete remission of the tumor. Vincristine is also effective for the treatment of lymph node metastasis of TVT. Radiation therapy has resulted in a 100% complete remission rate for the treatment of TVT and has also been effective for treating vincristine-resistant TVTs.[30,35]

Surgical excision of small preputial tumors may be performed with little reconstruction. Excision of large preputial tumors may require rotation flaps to reconstruct the prepuce. If reconstruction is not possible, partial or complete penile amputation may be required. Benign penile tumors may be removed with narrow margins and conservation of normal penile anatomy. Excision of large or malignant penile tumors may require partial penile amputation or complete amputation with scrotal or perineal urethrostomy.

Prognosis and Survival

The prognosis for TVT treated with chemotherapy or radiation therapy is generally good with long-term control in over 90% of patients. Patients with local lymph node metastasis may also experience long-term control. However, in rare patients with distant metastasis of TVT, prognosis is guarded.[30,32,35]

Complete surgical excision of benign penile and preputial tumors is thought to be curative. Malignant tumors carry a guarded prognosis. Early stage SCC and low-grade MCTs may have a favorable prognosis with complete excision. However, advanced stages of these tumors carry a guarded to poor prognosis. Treatment

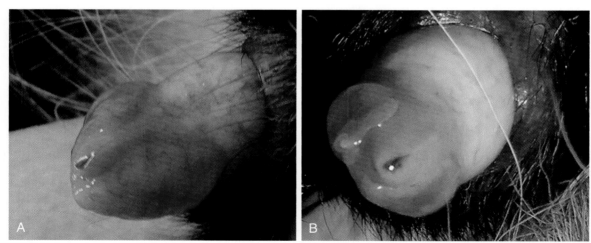

FIGURE 22-9 Penile transmissible venereal tumor (TVT) before **(A)** and 1 week after **(B)** administration of vincristine. Complete resolution of the mass occurred with five doses of vincristine.

and survival of malignant tumors varies with tumor type and stage of disease.

CANINE SCROTAL TUMORS

Any tumor that affects the skin may also affect the scrotum. Mast cell tumors are the most common scrotal tumor comprising 88% of all scrotal tumors in one study.[36] Other reported scrotal tumors include melanoma, histiocytoma, hemangioma, neurofibroma, papilloma, sebaceous adenoma, fibroma, fibrosarcoma, SCC, and apocrine gland tumors.[26]

The etiology and risk factors associated with scrotal tumor development are unknown. Most scrotal tumors are large enough to see or palpate. Dogs generally present for a visible mass, excessive licking, or scrotal bleeding caused by ulceration or trauma of the tumor. Because most scrotal tumors are MCTs, thorough evaluation of the patient for other cutaneous masses is recommended. FNA of the mass may be diagnostic for MCT; however, histopathology should be performed to confirm the diagnosis and obtain a tumor grade.

Staging and treatment of scrotal tumors should be based on tumor type. Prior to definitive therapy, the general health of the patient should be assessed. A CBC, chemistry panel, urinalysis, and chest radiographs may be warranted. Benign tumors may be removed with narrow margins and complete scrotal ablation may not be required. MCTs and malignant tumors may require further diagnostics for complete staging. The treatment of choice for MCTs and malignant tumors is complete scrotal ablation and castration.

The prognosis for dogs with benign scrotal tumors is excellent with complete surgical excision. Some controversy exists regarding the behavior of scrotal MCTs. Several reports suggest a more aggressive behavior of perineal and inguinal MCTs with shorter survival times.[37,38] However, these reports have been refuted, suggesting that dogs with scrotal MCTs have survival times similar to dogs with MCTs in other cutaneous locations.[39,40]

FELINE MALE REPRODUCTIVE TRACT TUMORS

Reproductive system tumors in male cats are rare. Reported testicular tumors include seminoma, Sertoli cell tumor, interstitial cell tumor, teratoma, and carcinoma.[41-45] Only case reports exist, such that etiology, risk factors, metastatic behavior, and survival cannot be accurately assessed. However, metastasis of a seminoma, a teratoma, and two Sertoli cell tumors have been reported in cats.[41-43] Tumors of the penis and prepuce have not been reported in the domestic cat. A single case of a scrotal fibroma has been reported.[46] Staging and diagnosis of these tumors should adhere to basic oncologic principles. Malignant testicular tumors have been reported in the cat, suggesting that cats with testicular tumors should be evaluated for evidence of metastatic disease at the time of diagnosis.

Selected References*

Cahalane AK, Payne S, Barber LG, et al: Prognostic factors for survival of dogs with inguinal and perineal mast cell tumors treated surgically with or without adjunctive treatment: 68 cases (1994-2002), *J Am Vet Med Assoc* 225:401, 2004.
This study reports on perineal and inguinal MCTs and refutes the long-time belief that MCTs in this location have a poorer prognosis than those in other locations.
Rogers KS, Walker MA, Dillon HB: Transmissible venereal tumor: A retrospective study of 29 cases, *J Am Anim Hosp Assoc* 34:463, 1998.
This retrospective study reports tumor location, metastasis, treatment, and outcome of dogs with TVT.
Sherding RG, Wilson GP, Kociba GJ: Bone marrow hypoplasia in eight dogs with Sertoli cell tumor, *J Am Vet Med Assoc* 178:497, 1981.
This report discusses myelotoxicosis and other toxicities associated with estrogen-secreting Sertoli cell tumors in dogs. Symptomatic therapy and outcome of 8 dogs is reported.

▎*For a complete list of the references cited in this chapter, please go to www.smallanimaloncology.com.

SECTION H: Renal Tumors

Jeffrey N. Bryan

KEY POINTS

- Hematuria in the absence of clinical signs may suggest renal neoplasia.
- Second opinions on renal histopathology are recommended, since it is not uncommon for renal

adenoma, carcinoma, and lymphoma diagnoses to be reclassified when slides are reviewed.
- To date, surgery is the only therapy that is associated with prolonged survival in non-lymphoma primary renal tumors. Nephrectomy may be for curative or

palliative intent and facilitates definitive diagnosis, which is necessary for prognosis and therapeutic decisions.
- Renal hemangiosarcoma may have an insidious course and a better overall prognosis than that reported for hemangiosarcoma of other visceral sites.

Primary renal tumors arise from kidney parenchyma of epithelial (carcinoma), mesothelial (sarcoma), or mixed embryonal (nephroblastoma) origin (Box 22-7). As a group, these occur most commonly in older adults.[1,2] Nephroblastomas have been reported in young dogs, similar to the juvenile onset Wilms' tumor in humans.[3] Carcinomas represent approximately 60%, sarcomas 34%, and nephroblastomas 6% of primary renal tumors in dogs.[2] Affected dogs tend to be geriatric.[2] Affected cats tend to be older adults, but young cats may develop

FeLV-related renal lymphoma[4] (Figure 22-10). In a series of 19 cats with non-lymphoma primary renal tumors, carcinomas were overwhelmingly represented with only one sarcoma, one nephroblastoma, and one adenoma.[5] Lymphoma affecting the kidneys should be assumed to be bilateral.[4] Of the tumors of primary renal origin (excluding lymphoma), a review of 82 dogs found that only carcinomas occurred bilaterally.[2] Oncocytoma was reported to be bilateral in a greyhound.[6] As a group, these tumors occur infrequently and have an occult clinical course, resulting in diagnosis at advanced stage. A male predominance has been reported for renal carcinomas in dogs, but is inconsistent across the literature.[1,3,7] The dermatologic condition, nodular dermatofibrosis, has been associated with bilateral renal cystadenocarcinomas in German Shepherd dogs.[8] A gene mutation in the Birt-Hogg-Dube gene is responsible for this syndrome.[9] No other breed predispositions have been identified.[2]

Clinical Features

Primary renal tumors are typically associated with few clinical signs in early stages. Although dogs or cats with renal lymphoma may appear with clinical signs of illness or renal failure, most primary renal tumors cause vague and non-specific clinical signs (Table 22-17). Acute

Box 22-7   REPORTED TYPES OF PRIMARY RENAL TUMORS

Renal carcinoma
Transitional cell carcinoma
Transitional cell papilloma
Tubular adenocarcinoma
Tubular and papillary adenocarcinoma
Renal adenocarcinoma
Sarcomatoid renal adenocarcinoma[20]
Renal tubular carcinoma
Renal papillary carcinoma
Clear cell renal carcinoma
Papillary cystadenocarcinoma
Renal adenoma
Spindle cell sarcoma
Osteosarcoma[21]
Hemangiosarcoma[16,22]
Hemangioma[11]
Renal sarcoma
Leiomyosarcoma[20]
Malignant fibrous histiocytoma
Fibroleiomyosarcoma
Fibroma
Lymphoma
Nephroblastoma
Giant cell tumor[24]
Oncocytoma[6,25]
Mixed mesenchymal tumor
Angiomyolipoma[26]

(Reported in Bryan 2006, Klein 1987, or Henry 1999 unless otherwise noted.)

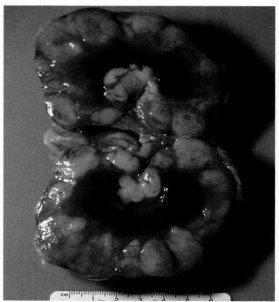

FIGURE 22-10 Renal lymphoma from a feline patient. Lymphoma of the kidneys should be assumed to be bilateral and is not a surgical disease.

collapse, hemoabdomen, or severe renal failure may cause animals with primary renal tumors to appear on an emergent basis. More typically, however, complaints of lethargy, hematuria, an abdominal mass, inappetence, or weight loss prompt initial evaluation.[1,2] Physical examination findings of nephromegaly, abdominal mass,

pale mucous membranes, abdominal distension with fluid wave, or flank pain could be present. Such pain may be more commonly associated with the presence of a sarcoma, but is not likely highly specific.[2] Changes on CBC are non-specific, although polycythemia in an older animal is highly suggestive of a renal tumor. This is an uncommon finding, however, and anemia is much more common.[1,2] Central nervous system signs including seizures have been reported in dogs and cats with paraneoplastic polycythemia and may resolve when polycythemia is reversed.[5,10] Serum chemistry changes are similarly non-specific with abnormalities shared by fewer than 25% of affected individuals.[2] Hypoalbuminemia was reported to be less common in sarcomas than in carcinomas or nephroblastomas.[2] Urinalysis frequently reveals proteinuria, hematuria, or pyuria, often suggestive of a bacterial cystitis.[2] Patients should be screened carefully for the presence of potential septicemia sources such as a urinary tract infection.

Diagnosis and Staging

Imaging studies are the primary modality used to detect these neoplasms. Ultrasound has appeared to be more sensitive than plain radiographs for detection of these tumors with intravenous pyelography also improving detection over plain films (Figure 22-11).[1,2] CT or MRI would be expected to reveal such tumors as well, and provide improved three-dimensional reconstruction for surgical planning. See Table 22-18 for suggested diagnostic examinations. The veterinary bladder tumor antigen (V-BTA, Alidex Inc., Redmond, WA) test may have application in

TABLE 22-17   CHARACTERISTICS OF DOGS WITH PRIMARY RENAL TUMORS

	BRYAN ET AL., 2006	KLEIN ET AL., 1987
Carcinomas	60%	85%
Sarcomas	34%	11%
Nephroblastomas	6%	4%
Median survival carcinoma	16 mos	8 mos
Median survival sarcoma	9 mos	NR
Median survival nephroblastoma	6 mos	NR
Thoracic mets at dx	16%	48%
Mets at death	77%	85%
Mean age at diagnosis	8.1 yrs	9.1 yrs
Bilateral disease	4%	32.4% Necropsied
CLINICAL SIGNS		
Hematuria	32%	26%
Palpable abdominal mass	20%	41%
Inappetence	27%	50%
Pain	7%	15%
Weight loss	20%	39%
CBC RESULTS		
Anemia	33%	26%
Leukocytosis	20%	11%
Polycythemia	4.50%	2%
CHEMISTRY RESULTS		
Elevated alkaline phosphatase	22%	15%
Elevated BUN	22%	26%
Elevated creatinine	20%	9%
Decreased albumin	19%	NR
URINALYSIS RESULTS		
Hematuria	57%	33% G, 50% M[*]
Pyuria	53%	NR
Proteinuria	48%	61%
Isosthenuria	36%	NR

[*]*G*, Gross; *M*, microscopic.

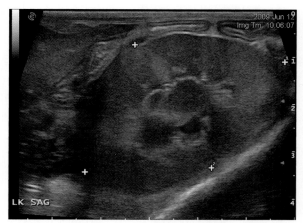

FIGURE 22-11 Ultrasound image of a feline kidney affected by lymphoma with loss of corticomedullary distinction and normal architecture. *(Courtesy of WSU Oncology Service.)*

TABLE 22-18   DIAGNOSTIC EVALUATION OF PRIMARY RENAL TUMORS

Test	Suggestive Results
CBC	Anemia, polycythemia
Chemistry profile	Azotemia, hypoproteinemia, hypoalbuminemia, elevated alkaline phosphatase
Urinalysis	Proteinuria, hematuria, pyuria, isosthenuria
Thoracic radiographs	Metastatic disease
Abdominal radiographs	Mid to dorsal abdominal mass, renomegaly, peritoneal effusion, retroperitoneal effusion
Abdominal ultrasound	Renal mass, metastatic disease (all organs possible)
Fine-needle aspirate	May differentiate carcinoma, sarcoma, lymphoma
Needle biopsy	May yield definitive diagnosis
Echocardiogram*	Rule out heart-based mass if hemangiosarcoma
V-BTA*	May be positive in renal TCC
Renal scintigraphy*	Confirm adequate renal function

*Additional/auxiliary tests.

detecting intraluminal carcinomas of the kidney.[11] Several reviews have documented the difficulty in differentiating between benign (adenoma) and malignant (carcinoma) epithelial renal neoplasms on histopathology.[5,12] On occasion, feline renal lymphoma has also been misdiagnosed as carcinoma.[5,12] Accordingly, one is advised to request a second opinion when these diagnoses are reported.

Biological Behavior/Metastasis

Lymphoma, although not of renal tissue origin, can arise primarily within the kidney. This may occur spontaneously in both dogs and cats or be associated with FeLV infection in felines.[4] Metastasis to the central nervous system has been reported with renal lymphoma in dogs and cats.[4,13] Carcinomas can arise from the transitional urothelial lining or from the renal epithelium in simple carcinoma or adenocarcinoma with tubular or papillary differentiation. Clear cell renal carcinomas are characterized by clear cytoplasm caused by glycogen and lipid content.[14] They tend to be a variant of simple or solid carcinoma.[14] The associated polycythemia that has been reported may be a result of tumor production of erythropoietin or renal hypoxia, causing the remaining normal tissue to over-produce erythropoietin.[15] The metastatic

rate has been reported to be as high as 48% at diagnosis with metastasis at death reported in 69% of cases.[1,2] Sarcomas can arise from any of the mesenchymal cell populations within the tumor. It is important to stage patients carefully, since sarcomas may be metastatic from other sites. The overall metastatic rate for primary renal sarcomas has been reported to be 88%.[2] Primary renal hemangiosarcoma (HSA) has a lower metastatic rate than HSA of the spleen or right atrium. In one report of 14 dogs with renal HSA, only one had metastasis detected at the time of diagnosis. The MST for these dogs was 278 days, suggesting that the prognosis is better for dogs with renal HSA than for those with HSA of other visceral sites.[16] Nephroblastomas can occur in any age dog. The biological behavior of these neoplasms appears to be similarly aggressive to carcinomas and sarcomas with a reported metastatic rate of 75%.[2] Benign tumors of the kidney, including hemangioma, adenoma, fibroma, and leiomyoma have been reported.[1,5,13,17]

Treatment Modalities and Anticipated Outcome

The goals of therapy may be manifold: removing the bleeding mass, resecting the primary tumor entirely, or alleviating clinical signs. Acute therapy must focus on stabilizing the patient by restoring blood volume, raising or lowering the hematocrit to a safe level, or minimizing azotemia, if possible, for surgery. Surgical resection is the only therapy, to date, that has a demonstrated survival benefit for primary non-lymphoma renal tumors in dogs.[2] Dogs undergoing surgery had a median survival of 16 months compared with less than 1 month for those not receiving surgery.[2] Survival for over 4 years has been reported.[2,18] Chemotherapy has only been demonstrated to be beneficial in renal LSA (see Chapter 25, Section A, for protocol).[4,13] The addition of cytosine arabinoside has been associated with a lower rate of CNS metastasis in cats.[4] No chemotherapy has a demonstrated survival benefit in tumors of primary renal origin.[2] Evaluation of antimetabolite-containing protocols such as gemcitabine and 5-FU used in humans has not occurred.[19] Immunotherapy is also standard of care in human renal carcinomas and has been minimally evaluated in dogs or cats.[19]

Selected References*

Bryan JN, Henry CJ, Turnquist SE, et al: Primary renal neoplasia of dogs, *J Vet Intern Med* 20:1155, 2006.
This multi-institutional retrospective study describes clinicopathological findings, tumor behaviour, and case outcome data for 82 dogs with primary renal neoplasia.

Henry CJ, Turnquist SE, Smith A, et al: Primary renal tumours in cats: 19 cases (1992-1998), *J Feline Med Surg* 1:165–170, 1999.

This is a retrospective of 19 cases of primary renal tumors in cats describing the clinical presentations, diagnostics, and outcomes of a variety of tumor types, including hemangiosarcoma.

Klein MK, Cockerell CL, Harris CK, et al: Canine primary renal neoplasms: a retrospective review of 54 cases, *J Am Anim Hosp Assoc* 24:443, 1987.

This is a retrospective of 54 cases of renal tumors in dogs describing clinical features and diagnostic outcomes, but offers minimal survival data.

Lucke VM, Kelly DF: Renal carcinoma in the dog, *Vet Pathol* 13:264, 1976.

This is a review of 33 cases of renal carcinoma in the literature and nine novel cases that describes the clinical features and behavior of renal carcinoma in dogs.

■ *For a complete list of the references cited in this chapter, please go to www.smallanimaloncology.com.

SECTION I: Bladder and Urethral Tumors

Carolyn J. Henry

KEY POINTS

- Urine should not be obtained via cystocentesis when bladder cancer is suspected, since the procedure can transplant tumor cells to unaffected sites within the abdomen.
- Benign lesions may occur in the canine and feline bladder and urethra, but the majority of lower urinary tract tumors in both species are malignant, with transitional cell carcinoma (TCC) predominating.
- The trigone is the most common site for canine TCC of the bladder; thus, complete surgical excision is unlikely.
- Feline bladder TCC is a disease of old cats and is less likely to occur at the trigone compared with canine TCC.
- Mitoxantrone and piroxicam combination therapy is well tolerated and may cause reduction in tumor size, palliation of clinical signs, and prolongation of life in dogs affected with TCC.

Incidence

Lower urinary tract tumors are relatively rare in dogs and cats, comprising fewer than 2% of reported tumors in both species.[1-5] The most common bladder malignancy is transitional cell carcinoma (TCC), with the trigone being the most common site in dogs. In cats, non-trigonal bladder wall sites are often affected. The urethra may be secondarily infiltrated by extension of a primary bladder mass, which occurs in over half of all dogs with urinary bladder TCC.[4,6,7] Alternatively, the urethra may be the initial tumor location. Malignant primary urethral tumors are usually carcinomas, with squamous cell carcinoma and TCC predominating in

dogs.[8,9] Other reported histologies include leiomyoma, adenocarcinoma, hemangiosarcoma, embryonic rhabdomyosarcoma, lymphoma, and chondrosarcoma.[8,10-14] In the scant literature regarding feline primary urethral tumors, transitional cell carcinoma and leiomyoma are reported.[15-17]

Etiology/Risk Factors

The etiology of lower urinary tract cancer, as with other malignancies, is likely multifactorial. Identified risk factors for canine bladder cancer include obesity, exposure to topical flea and tick insecticides, exposure to marshes that have been sprayed with mosquito control products, and possibly treatment with cyclophosphamide.[5,18,19] Although early surveys indicated no gender predisposition in dogs[20,21] multiple subsequent reports document that females are predisposed.[2,4,5,22-24] One proposed explanation for the increased risk in females is that male dogs urinate more frequently as a marking behavior, thus limiting the contact time of the bladder mucosa to carcinogens in the urine.[22,25] Conversely, in cats, male gender is a predisposing factor. Most affected cats are quite old, with a reported median age of 15.2 years (range 6.5–18.5 years).[7] Certain dog breeds, including Shetland sheepdogs, beagles, collies, and various terriers including Scottish, Airedale, West Highland white and Wirehaired fox terriers, appear to be predisposed to development of TCC.[2,4,5,22] Of these, Scottish terriers and Shetland sheepdogs are the most frequently affected breeds.[4,5,22]

Clinical Features

Common presenting complaints include pollakiuria, stranguria, hematuria, and tenesmus. In many cases, if antibiotics are administered based on the assumption that the presenting signs are due to a bacterial cystitis, improvement in clinical signs will occur and obscure or delay the diagnosis of neoplasia. As such, it is important to have a raised index of suspicion for bladder cancer in older dogs and cats with urinary tract signs, rather than presume that improvement after antibiotic therapy confers a diagnosis of bacterial cystitis as the underlying pathology.

Diagnosis and Staging

Urinalysis

Urinalysis is often the first test used to diagnose bladder and urethral cancer. One must be cautious when obtaining urine for analysis, since TCC transplantation has been reported in dogs and cats following tumor manipulation via cystocentesis or at the time of surgery.[7,26-30] Accordingly, the author cautions against cystocentesis when bladder cancer is suspected. Urinalysis findings may be indistinct from those noted with cystitis, including white blood cells, red blood cells, and bacteria. Although urine sediment examination may reveal tumor cells in 30% or more of cases,[2,31] reactive, non-neoplastic transitional cells can look quite similar to TCC cells.[32,33] Thus, cytologic evaluation should be supported by other findings and confirmed with histopathology when possible.

A veterinary bladder tumor antigen test (V-BTA test; Alidex, Inc., Redmond, WA) is commercially available and may serve as a quick screening test for TCC. The V-BTA test can be performed in-house on a free-catch urine sample. It requires 0.5 ml of test urine, which should be spun before testing and evaluated within 48 hours of sample collection. The author and others assessed the V-BTA in a prospective, multi-site study in which urine samples were collected from healthy dogs, as well as dogs with TCC, non-TCC urologic disease, and non-urologic disease.[34] A total of 229 specimens were analyzed including 48 samples from dogs with confirmed (n = 45) or suspected (n = 3) TCC. Calculated sensitivities (the likelihood of getting a positive test result in an affected patient) were 88%, 87%, and 85% for all TCC cases, confirmed TCC cases, and confirmed bladder TCC cases, respectively. Calculated specificities (the likelihood of getting a negative test result in an unaffected patient) were 84%, 41%, and 86% when samples from healthy dogs, dogs with non-TCC urinary tract disease, and dogs with non-urinary disease, respectively, were tested. Hematuria and proteinuria were associated with some false-positive test results. These causes of false-positive test results have been previously reported, as has glucosuria.[35] The high sensitivity of the V-BTA

test indicates that negative test results correlate well with the absence of TCC. The clinical value of this test lies in its ability to determine which dogs do not warrant further workup for TCC, and in its potential for earlier detection of bladder cancer in high-risk dogs. As with any screening test, positive results should prompt further patient evaluation to confirm a diagnosis.

Imaging and Confirmatory Testing

Definitive diagnosis of bladder or urethral cancer is based on demonstration of a mass, along with cytologic or, preferably, histopathologic evidence of neoplastic cells. The mass may be detected with radiography and ultrasonography or directly visualized using cystoscopy or at the time of exploratory laparotomy. Contrast cystography (Figure 22-12) is reliable for detection of bladder masses in more than 95% of cases.[2] Bladder ultrasonography (cystosonography) is best performed when the bladder is distended, either with urine or infused saline. Cystosonography (Figure 22-13) permits better visualization of intra-abdominal metastasis and can guide tissue sampling via urinary catheterization. Although ultrasound guidance improves diagnostic yield, a limitation of obtaining biopsy specimens via catheterization is the small sample size that is obtained.[36] As an alternative, biopsies can be obtained via cystoscopy or laparotomy.

Histopathologic examination of biopsy tissues allows verification of a diagnosis, as well as tumor grading using a modified WHO system.[37] Tumor grade I, II, or III is

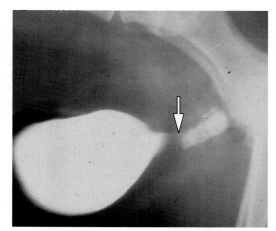

FIGURE 22-12 Contrast cystography demonstrates a filling defect *(arrow)* in the trigone and urethra of a dog with transitional cell carcinoma.

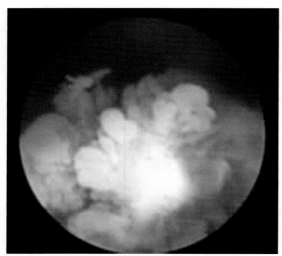

FIGURE 22-13 Cystoscopy allows visualization of a bladder mass in a 12-year-old dog. A diagnosis of TCC was confirmed with histopathologic examination of a biopsy from the visualized mass.

assigned based upon growth patterns, cell type, degree of differentiation, and depth of invasion, with grade III tumors being the most anaplastic. In a published review applying this grading system to tissues from bladder and urethral tumors of 110 dogs, the authors concluded that tumor grade and peritumoral desmoplasia were significantly associated with survival. They also found considerable variability within single tissue samples, suggesting that obtaining biopsy specimens from multiple sites is ideal for complete characterization of tumor tissue.

Tumor staging of bladder and urethral cancer requires evaluation of the primary tumor and assessment for lymph node and distant metastasis (see www.smallanimaloncology.com for tumor staging forms). Bladder tumor stage has been shown to be prognostic for survival in dogs affected with TCC.[5] Median survival times were 118 days for dogs with T3 tumors compared with 218 days for dogs with T1 or T2 tumors. Dogs lacking nodal metastasis survived a median of 234 days, compared with 70 days for dogs with nodal metastasis. Likewise, distant metastatic disease was associated with a shorter median survival time (105 days vs. 203 days for dogs without distant metastasis at the time of diagnosis). Abdominal ultrasound is useful for staging, not only to assess tumor size and degree of invasion within the bladder, but also for detecting intra-abdominal metastasis. Likewise, three-view thoracic radiographs are recommended to detect pulmonary metastasis. CT

(Figure 22-14) may aid in tumor staging and provide information vital for radiation treatment planning.

Biological Behavior/Metastasis

Distant metastases occur in approximately a third of all dogs with urethral TCC and SCC and one half of those with urinary bladder TCC.[2,8,38] There are many reported sites of metastasis, including lymph nodes, lung, and bone. The radiographic appearance of pulmonary metastatic disease from TCC can be misinterpreted if one is unfamiliar with the several distinct radiographic patterns that can occur with the disease. These include nodular interstitial opacity, diffuse unstructured interstitial opacity, cavitating pulmonary lesions, lobar interstitial/alveolar infiltrates, multiple nodules, and normal pulmonary opacity.[39,40] Thoracic radiographs should also be assessed for evidence of hilar lymph node enlargement, indicative of nodal metastasis. The lung lesions in dogs with unstructured interstitial opacity are described as a lace-like haze of semi-dense diffuse opacity. This pattern can be easily misinterpreted as age-related change, as evidenced in one report where three of eight dogs with pulmonary metastasis were incorrectly diagnosed as having normal age-related changes on thoracic radiographs.[40] The cavitating metastatic pattern that has been described for TCC is likely due to central necrosis of the metastatic lesions. This pattern has also been noted uncommonly with metastatic transitional cell carcinoma in people.[41]

Metastatic disease is apparently less common in cats with lower urinary tract tumors. In a series of 20 cats with urinary bladder TCC, only three presented with pulmonary metastasis and one had nodal metastasis.[7]

Therapy and Prognosis

Surgery

The decision of whether or not to pursue surgery for treatment of lower urinary tract tumors should be based on tumor histology, location, and invasiveness, as well as the client's goals. For benign lesions and smooth muscle malignancies that have not metastasized, surgery may be curative. In general, surgery is considered to be a palliative procedure for canine TCC because of the high metastatic rate and because even grossly normal tissue often contains neoplastic or preneoplastic tissue. Several surgical options exist including partial cystectomy, total cystectomy with urinary diversion (ureterocolonic or ureterourethral anastomosis), permanent cystostomy tube placement, or stent placement to relieve obstruction.[1,5,42,43] Clients often opt for the least invasive of these techniques, based on

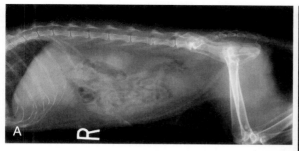

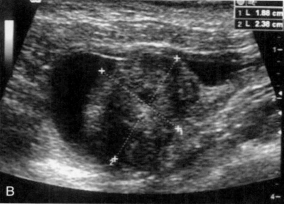

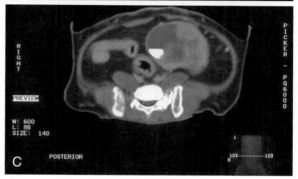

FIGURE 22-14 Radiographic (**A**), ultrasound (**B**), and computed tomography (CT) (**C**) images of a large bladder tumor identified in a 17-year-old male DSH with a history of recent hematuria. Note contrast within the bladder on CT image, demonstrating the greatly reduced lumen volume caused by infiltration of tumor mass within the bladder.

concerns regarding patient quality of life and client convenience. In one report describing partial cystectomy in 11 dogs, the 1-year survival rate exceeded 54%. Importantly, the authors reported that visual assessment at the time of cystectomy was inaccurate for determining tumor-free margins.[42] Therefore, if surgical excision of a bladder mass is attempted, wide surgical margins are imperative. Partial cystectomy may be reasonable for localized TCC and is most practical for tumors located in non-trigonal sites. However, resection does not address the problem of metastasis and is a poor treatment option for advanced TCC. Even with complete tumor excision, TCC recurrence is likely in dogs, as it is in people following partial cystectomy. Recurrence rates of 30% to nearly 50% are reported for people undergoing partial or radical cystectomy, and the recurrence usually occurs within 1 year.[44,45] This may be due to microscopic tumor at the surgical margins or due to development of *de novo* tumors. Because the underlying cause of bladder cancer is likely

related to exposure of the bladder mucosa to carcinogenic substances, *de novo* tumors may develop in the non-excised tissues as a result of the same carcinogenic mechanisms that led to initial tumor development, rather than a failure of surgical technique. In one published report that described outcome for 102 dogs undergoing surgery for TCC, only two had complete surgical excision of their disease and both later developed tumor recurrence or progression.[5] Carbon dioxide (CO_2) laser ablation of trigone or urethral TCC has been described in a case series of eight dogs. The procedure was well tolerated and resulted in rapid resolution of clinical signs.[46] The dogs in the series were subsequently treated with mitoxantrone and piroxicam, which is described below.

Finally, a palliative option for management of outflow obstruction associated with bladder cancer is the placement of a permanent cystostomy catheter. This procedure relieves stranguria and may prevent complications associated with urinary outflow obstruction.

TABLE 22-19   Published Results of Medical Therapy for Canine TCC of the Bladder

Drugs	Dosage	No. of Dogs	Prospective or Retrospective	Response Rate	MST (days)	Comments	Ref
Cisplatin alone	50 mg/m² q4wk	15	Retro	20%	NR	Increased dosage did not equate to improved response rate	48
	60 mg/m² q3wk	18	Pro	16%	130		49
Carboplatin alone	300 mg/m² IV q3wk	14	Pro	0%	132		50
Piroxicam alone	0.3 mg/kg/day PO	34	Pro	18%	181		51
Carboplatin/ Piroxicam	300 mg/m² IV q3wk 0.3 mg/kg/day PO	31*	Pro	38%	161	No nephrotoxicity noted, but GI toxicity in 74% and bone marrow toxicity in 35%	52
Doxorubicin/ Cyclophosphamide	30 mg/m² IV q21d 50–100 mg/m² PO once daily on days 3–6 after doxorubicin	11	Retro	NR	259		53
Mitoxantrone/ Piroxicam	5 mg/m² IV q3wk × 4 0.3 mg/kg/day PO	49	Pro	35%	350	75% of dogs had clinical improvement, even if tumor did not have measurable remission; GI and renal toxicity in <15%	23
Laser ablation, then Mitoxantrone/ Piroxicam	Same as above	8	Pro	100%†	299	Response rate reflects the fact that tumors were laser ablated	46
Cisplatin/Piroxicam	60 mg/m² IV q3wk 0.3 mg/kg/day PO	14	Pro	71%‡	246	Renal toxicity in 12/14 dogs	54
Cisplatin, then Piroxicam	Same as above, but not given simultaneously	8	Pro	0%, then 25%§	309	Response rate low, but survival improved over simultaneous cisplatin/piroxicam	54
Cisplatin/Piroxicam	50 or 40 mg/m² IV q3wk 0.3 mg/kg/day PO	14	Pro	7%	307	Renal and GI toxicity seen at both cisplatin dosages	55

*Of the 31 enrolled, only 29 were evaluated for response.

†100% response rate relates to the fact that all dogs underwent surgery.

‡Renal toxicity encountered in 12/14 dogs.

§No dogs responded to cisplatin alone, but 2 of 8 responded once started on piroxicam.

Because cystostomy tube placement will not relieve ureteral obstruction, excretory urography is recommended prior to the procedure in order to ensure that ureteral involvement will not negate the palliative benefit of tube placement. In one report of cystostomy tube placement in seven dogs with known or suspected TCC, six dogs had resolution of stranguria and owners reported satisfaction with the procedure.[47] MST was 106 days.

Medical Therapy/Chemotherapy for TCC

Because of the likelihood of recurrence and metastasis, treatment of lower urinary tract cancer should include systemic medical therapy from the outset or as adjuvant therapy after surgery if one hopes to achieve long-term remissions or cures. Several drugs and combination protocols have been evaluated for the treatment of canine lower urinary tract cancer, with an emphasis on TCC. The most commonly used protocols are the mitoxantrone and piroxicam combination protocol evaluated in a Veterinary Cooperative Oncology Group (VCOG) study[23] or various combinations of cisplatin and NSAIDs. Because of the potential for nephrotoxicity with cisplatin administration, care must be taken to evaluate renal function before initiation of cisplatin therapy, as well as before each treatment. NSAIDs can exacerbate nephrotoxicity and should be used with caution in dogs with any degree of renal insufficiency or in dogs undergoing platinum-based chemotherapy. Current research is focused on evaluating newer NSAIDs that are more COX-2 selective, in hopes of improving the safety profile of protocols combining platinum agents with NSAID therapy. Published results of various chemotherapy protocols for treatment of canine TCC are shown in Table 22-19.

Radiation Therapy

Radiation therapy, both intraoperative and postoperative, has been described for the treatment of canine bladder cancer.[2,56-59] Intraoperative radiation has not gained widespread popularity because of the technical difficulty of transporting patients to a radiation source intraoperatively. Likewise, complications including bladder fibrosis and ureteral stenosis and fibrosis with secondary hydroureter and hydronephrosis have dampened enthusiasm for this method. Similar complications have been reported with external beam radiation of the bladder and have led to hesitation to suggest this therapy option.[2,59] In order to minimize the likelihood of ureteral fibrosis, the radiation dose delivered to the ureters should not exceed 3000 cGy.[56,57,60] Although early reports described complications associated with

bladder irradiation, a more recent study evaluating the combination of mitoxantrone, piroxicam, and coarsely fractionated radiation for 10 dogs with TCC of the bladder suggests that this may be a reasonable treatment alternative.[59] The protocol included six weekly 575-cGy fractions of external beam radiation therapy, piroxicam (0.3 mg/kg/day orally) and mitoxantrone (5 mg/m^2 IV q21d) until evidence of disease progression was noted. Side effects were considered mild and consisted of dermatitis (n = 1), hyperpigmentation (n = 1), and mild urinary incontinence (n = 4). Although no complete or partial remissions were reported, 7 dogs had disease stabilization and clinical improvement for a median of 3 months (range = 47–320 days).

Photodynamic Therapy

Photodynamic therapy has been used to treat bladder cancer in people, with variable results. Although an effective protocol for PDT of canine bladder cancer has not been established, investigations are ongoing. More information about PDT can be found in Chapter 17.

Selected References*

Henry CJ, McCaw DL, Turnquist SE, et al: Clinical evaluation of mitoxantrone and piroxicam in a canine model of human invasive urinary bladder carcinoma, *Clin Cancer Res* 9:906, 2003.
This manuscript details a prospective clinical trial of one of the most common chemotherapy protocols used in the treatment of canine TCC.
Knapp DW, Richardson RC, Chan TC, et al: Piroxicam therapy in 34 dogs with transitional cell carcinoma of the urinary bladder, *J Vet Intern Med* 8:273, 1994.
This was the original report of piroxicam use for the treatment of canine TCC of the urinary bladder.
Norris AM, Laing EJ, Valli VEO, et al: Canine bladder and urethral tumors: a retrospective study of 115 cases (1980-1985), *J Vet Intern Med* 6(3):145, 1992.
This is the largest retrospective study of lower urinary tract tumors in dogs to date.
Wilson HM, Chun R, Larson VS, et al: Clinical signs, treatments, and outcome in cats with transitional cell carcinoma of the urinary bladder: 20 cases (1990-2004), *J Am Vet Med Assoc* 231(1):101, 2007.
This manuscript describes the clinical features, treatment options, and prognosis for cats with TCC of the urinary bladder.

---

*For a complete list of the references cited in this chapter, please go to www.smallanimaloncology.com.

SECTION J: Prostate Tumors

Jeffrey N. Bryan

KEY POINTS

- Prostate cancer is an aggressive disease that is often diagnosed in an advanced stage.
- Effective treatment of prostate cancer has not been described, but most oncologists use piroxicam, chemotherapy, and occasionally radiation therapy to manage urinary signs and control metastatic disease.
- Prostate cancer is most likely to occur in castrated, older dogs.

Incidence/Etiology and Risk Factors

Prostate cancer is uncommon in dogs in general, but breed and castration have been shown to be risk factors for developing the disease. Epidemiologic data from the Veterinary Medical Database (VMDB) revealed that castrated males are at 3.86 times the risk of developing prostate carcinoma and up to 8 times the risk of developing prostate transitional cell carcinoma (TCC) compared with intact males.[1] Other studies have found similar increased risk among castrated males.[2,3] In spite of the reported increased risk among castrated males, prostate cancer only represented 72 cases out of 7723 accessions reported for the highest incidence year from 19 academic referral institutions across the United States between 1964 and 2004.[1] Breeds including Doberman pinscher, Shetland sheepdog, Scottish terrier, beagle, and German shorthaired pointer were found to be at increased risk of developing prostate cancer.[1] Dachshunds and miniature poodles were found to be at lower risk of developing the disease.[1]

Prostate cancer in cats is extremely rare, with only a few case reports present in the literature. It is generally described as an aggressive disease in cats.[4,5] No clinical trial of therapy or necropsy series of cats with the disease has been published.

Signalment and Clinical Features

Dogs that develop prostate cancer are typically medium to large breed and average 10 years of age.[6] The most common clinical signs associated with prostate cancer are hematuria, stranguria, and urinary incontinence.[6] Many dogs will have signs of systemic illness as well. Up to a third of affected dogs have been reported to display signs of tenesmus from prostatic enlargement.[6] Up to a third of affected dogs have also been reported to appear with musculoskeletal or neurologic signs as a result of metastasis.[6]

Physical examination generally reveals an irregular, firm prostate. Disease may palpably extend into the urethra caudally or the bladder cranially. Careful attention should be paid to the sublumbar lymph nodes on rectal examination. Particular attention should also be paid to the presence of pain in distant locations, potentially signaling metastatic sites.

Diagnosis and Staging

Definitive diagnosis of prostate cancer is made by histopathologic examination of samples collected using percutaneous or transrectal needle biopsy or surgical biopsy (Figure 22-15). The most commonly recorded histologies are carcinoma, adenocarcinoma (ACA), or TCC and can include mesenchymal differentiation in mixed tumors.[1,6] ACAs have been associated most frequently with intact males and are thought to arise from the glandular portion of the prostate. Development of ACA may be preceded by the premalignant lesion "high-grade prostatic intra-epithelial neoplasia" (HGPIN), much like the androgen-dependent form of disease in men.[7] Urothelial origin tumors appear to be most common in castrated males.[1,3,6] The clinical significance of cell of origin has not been well defined. Canine prostate cancers tend to stain positive for cytokeratin 7, arginine esterase, and uroplakin III, whereas prostate-specific membrane antigen (PSMA) and prostate-specific antigen (PSA) staining is more variable.[3,8] Cytokeratin and vimentin staining suggest that the canine forms of the disease are not as well differentiated as the human forms.[9]

It is common that dogs presenting with prostate cancer have locally advanced or metastatic disease. Careful staging is necessary to clearly define the total disease burden and develop a treatment plan that will maximize quality of life. Evaluation of CBC, chemistry profile, and urinalysis to identify organ (particularly renal) dysfunction, urinary tract infection, and cytopenias is imperative prior to beginning cytotoxic chemotherapy. Thoracic (three-view) and abdominal radiographs should be evaluated carefully for metastatic disease to bone or soft tissue and displacement of the colon that might lead to obstruction (Figure 22-16). Abdominal ultrasound should be used to carefully evaluate not only the major organs, but the lymph nodes and tissues local to the

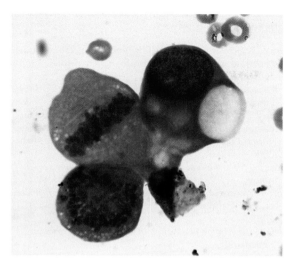

FIGURE 22-15 Photomicrograph of a cytology preparation from the peritoneal fluid of a Schnauzer that developed 7 months after chemotherapy treatment began. Local extension and intra-abdominal metastasis is common with prostate carcinoma of dogs. (Courtesy of Washington State University.)

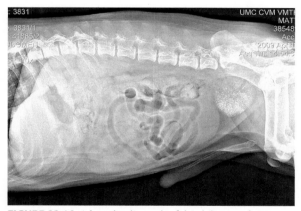

FIGURE 22-16 A lateral radiograph of the abdomen of a 9-year-old male castrated dog with prostate carcinoma. Note the large mineralized soft-tissue mass caudal to the bladder through which the urinary catheter passes. This dog presented with hematuria and ureteral obstruction leading to unilateral hydronephrosis. (Courtesy of the University of Missouri.)

prostate for evidence of metastasis and local extension of the prostate tumor. Ultrasound can be used to guide collection of cytology samples of the prostate and suspected metastatic lesions. Cytologic evidence of epithelial cells displaying characteristics of malignancy from primary prostate and metastatic location is sufficient grounds for a presumptive diagnosis of prostate carcinoma.

Biological Behavior/Metastasis

Unlike hormone-responsive early prostate cancer in men, prostate carcinomas in dogs are generally aggressive tumors. One study reported a metastatic rate of 80% at necropsy.[6] Metastatic sites included lymph nodes, lung, and bone most commonly, with rarer spread to the liver, colon, kidney, heart, adrenal gland, brain, and spleen.[6] When skeletal metastasis was observed, the bones most commonly affected were the lumbar vertebrae, pelvis, and femur, often with multiple bones involved.[6] Radiographically, these lesions were both osteoproductive and osteodestructive with a mixed pattern predominating.[6] Skeletal metastasis has been associated with younger age of onset of disease.[6] Castration after diagnosis will generally not slow progression of the disease but may shrink concurrent benign prostatic hypertrophy and improve quality of life.

Therapy and Prognosis

Because of the highly metastatic nature of prostate cancer, chemotherapy is indicated in definitive treatment. However, no therapy trials have been published for the disease, so no optimal agent has been identified. Piroxicam has been found to be beneficial in urinary tract carcinomas and may offer at least palliative benefit as a single agent to dogs with prostate cancer.[10] Because of demonstrated efficacy in urinary bladder TCC, the author recommends piroxicam and mitoxantrone for prostate carcinoma (see Table 22-19).[11] Doxorubicin or carboplatin may be expected to have efficacy in a proportion of cases as well. Carboplatin and piroxicam in combination were observed to be associated with significant gastrointestinal toxicity when used to treat urinary bladder TCC.[12] In the same study, no renal toxicity was observed, but the combination could be toxic for patients with preexisting renal impairment.[12] Regular monitoring of renal function, including BUN, creatinine, and urine specific gravity, during piroxicam therapy is warranted.

Radiation therapy has been used to treat prostate cancer in dogs. Intraoperative radiation therapy resulted in some response in a study of 10 dogs.[13] More recently, Proulx reported external beam therapy in 10 dogs with prostate cancer, but considered the response insignificant (Proulx, personal communication, 2002 Veterinary Cancer Society Annual Conference Proceedings). In the author's practice, clinicians perform radiotherapy as part of a complete protocol, including chemotherapy and piroxicam. Radiation, both external beam and brachytherapy, is a mainstay of therapy for men with prostate cancer and may become more standard in veterinary medicine when appropriate protocols are devised for dogs in the future.

Prostatectomy and partial prostatectomy have been performed to manage prostate tumors without metastasis.[14] Transurethral partial prostatectomy was used to alleviate stranguria in one study and was effective at rapidly relieving urinary obstruction signs.[15] Prostatectomy requires detailed understanding of nerve and vascular supply to the prostate to avoid hemorrhage, necrosis, and irreversible incontinence. In most cases, partial resection does not prevent localized disease progression, and metastasis should be anticipated, even with complete prostatectomy.[14,15] Laser partial prostatectomy has been reported in dogs, as has photodynamic therapy.[16,17] Experimentally, laser ablation, ultrasound ablation, and novel agent photodynamic therapy have been performed in dogs. These techniques may be clinically available one day.[18,19]

Recently, proteins unique to prostate cancer among urinary tract tissues were identified that may form the basis of future, targeted therapy.[20] Researchers expect such tumor markers to result in earlier diagnosis and more effective therapy.

Selected References[*]

Bryan JN, Keeler MR, Henry CJ, et al: A population study of neutering status as a risk factor for canine prostate cancer, *Prostate* 67:1174, 2007.
Large-population study of dogs in the VMDB that definitively associates castration with the development of prostate cancer.
Cornell KK, Bostwick DG, Cooley DM, et al: Clinical and pathologic aspects of spontaneous canine prostate carcinoma: a retrospective analysis of 76 cases, *Prostate* 45:173, 2000.
Describes the forms and metastatic behavior of canine prostate cancer.
Turrel JM: Intraoperative radiotherapy of carcinoma of the prostate gland in ten dogs, *J Am Vet Med Assoc* 190:48, 1987.
The only description of a radiation protocol to treat prostate cancer in dogs.

Tumors of the Skin, Subcutis, and Other Soft Tissues

SECTION A: Skin Tumors

Nicole Northrup and Tracy Gieger

KEY POINTS

- Most tumors of the skin and subcutis can be cured if diagnosed early.
- Owners should be instructed to perform monthly examinations of their pets to look for skin masses.
- All cutaneous and subcutaneous masses should be aspirated for cytologic evaluation.
- If cytology of a skin mass does not yield a diagnosis, biopsy is indicated.

This section discusses management of skin and subcutaneous tumors of cats and dogs. The reader is directed to discussions on mast cell tumors (MCTs) (see Section D), soft-tissue sarcomas (STSs; see Section E), and lymphoma (Chapter 25, Section A) for information about these tumors.

Incidence

Tumors of the skin and subcutaneous tissues are common in veterinary patients.[1-5] They are classified as epithelial, mesenchymal, melanocytic, or round cell (discrete cell) in origin. Most are primary tumors, but metastases and cutaneous paraneoplastic conditions are possible. In cats, skin tumors are more likely to be malignant.[4,5] The most common cutaneous tumors of cats and dogs are listed in Tables 23-1 and 23-2.

Diagnosis and Staging

Cutaneous tumors are readily identified by inspection and palpation of the skin. In patients with thick haircoats, effort should be made to palpate the skin and part the hair to identify any masses. It is important to examine areas less visible to owners, including lips, ears, ventrum, paws, and the axillary, ventral cervical, inguinal, perianal, and genital regions. Clinicians should look for preneoplastic lesions including non-healing scabs, discolorations, and skin texture changes in lightly pigmented, thin-haired areas susceptible to solar damage. Skin lesions should be documented in the medical record on a body map (included on the website, www.smallanimaloncology.com) or with a digital photograph. Masses should be measured with calipers, and fine-needle aspirates should be obtained for cytology. Biopsy and histology are indicated for masses that are growing, changing in appearance, or irritating the patient and when cytology does not provide a definitive diagnosis.

The decision of whether incisional or excisional biopsy is appropriate (see Chapter 6) is based on the size, location, and suspected diagnosis of the mass. Histology provides important information including diagnosis, assessment of completeness of excision with margin measurements, mitotic index, histologic grade, and identification of vascular/lymphatic invasion. For some tumors, immunohistochemistry or special stains may be required to determine the diagnosis. In addition, assessment of proliferation indices is a valuable prognostic indicator for some tumors.

Therapy

For most skin tumors, surgical excision is the treatment of choice. The extent of surgery required depends on the tumor type (see Chapter 14). Tissues shrink and shift in formalin,[6] so small samples should be placed in cassettes; for larger excisions, the subcutaneous tissue should be sutured to the skin. A complete history and description of the mass should be provided for the pathologist. Any resected tissues should be submitted in entirety for histology, even if a benign diagnosis is expected, and the surgical margins should be marked with India ink or the multi-colored Davidson Marking

TABLE 23-1   FREQUENCY OF SKIN TUMORS IN CATS*

Tumor	Frequency (Miller)	Frequency (Goldschmidt)
Basal cell tumor*	26%	15%
Mast cell tumor	21%	13%
Squamous cell carcinoma	15%	10%
Fibrosarcoma	15%	17%
Sebaceous adenoma	4%	2%
Fibroma	3%	Not reported
Apocrine adenocarcinoma	3%	3%
Apocrine adenoma	3%	5%
Malignant fibrous histiocytoma	3%	1%
Hemangiosarcoma	2%	3%
Hemangioma	1%	2%
Melanocytic tumors	<1%	1%
Lymphoma	<1%	3%
Trichoepithelioma	<1%	<1%
Fibropapilloma	<1%	Not reported
Lipoma	<1%	6%
Undifferentiated carcinoma	<1%	Not reported
Undifferentiated sarcoma	<1%	Not reported
Basal cell carcinoma	Not reported	1%

*Based on biopsy and necropsy specimens from 340 cats submitted to the University of Missouri Veterinary Medical Diagnostic Laboratory[4] and 3260 surgical biopsy specimens from skin lesions of cats submitted to the Laboratory of Pathology at the University of Pennsylvania, School of Veterinary Medicine.[5]

TABLE 23-2   FREQUENCY OF SKIN TUMORS IN DOGS

Tumor Type	Frequency (Goldschmidt)
Histiocytoma	12%
Perianal adenoma	12%
Mast cell tumor	10%
Lipoma	8%
Hemangiopericytoma	7%
Sebaceous adenoma	4%
Trichoepithelioma	4%
Hemangioma	4%
Melanocytic tumor	4%
Basal cell tumor*	4%
Fibroma	2%
Fibrosarcoma	2%
Squamous cell carcinoma	2%
Intracutaneous cornifying epithelioma	2%
Plasmacytoma	1%
Pilomatricoma	1%
Lymphoma	1%
Hemangiosarcoma	1%
Papilloma	<1%
Basal cell carcinoma	<1%
Apocrine gland carcinoma	<1%

Based on 29,510 surgical biopsy specimens from skin lesions of dogs submitted to the Laboratory of Pathology at the University of Pennsylvania, School of Veterinary Medicine.[5]

EPITHELIAL TUMORS

Epidermal Tumors

Squamous Cell Carcinoma (SCC), Multi-Centric Squamous Cell Carcinoma *in situ* (MSCCIS; Bowenoid *in situ* Carcinoma)

Incidence/Etiology and Risk Factors

Cutaneous SCC is common in cats and dogs[4,5] and accounts for 25% to 52% of digital tumors in dogs.[10,11] SCC is most commonly seen in sparsely haired, poorly pigmented areas of the epidermis.[12-15] In these cases, it is considered to be solar induced and is often preceded by evidence of solar-induced inflammation (actinic keratosis). SCC may develop consequent to chronic inflammation as a result of immune-mediated, infectious (e.g., viral papillomatosis in dogs[16,17]) causes, and burns. Multi-centric SCC *in situ* of cats is not solar induced; rather, a viral etiology is suspected.[18,19]

Nail bed SCC occurs most commonly in older (median age, 10 years) male dogs > 30 kg and is seen

System (Davidson Marking System, Bradley Products, Inc., Bloomington, MN).

Primary re-excision of the scar or radiation therapy should be considered for incompletely excised skin tumors. Re-excision is indicated when a relatively conservative surgery was performed to remove a malignant tumor in an area where there is adequate tissue to allow resection of the scar with 2- to 3-cm lateral margins and an intact tissue plane at the deep margin. For tumors not amenable to complete excision, radiation therapy is appropriate for local control. Chemotherapy is indicated for some malignant skin tumors based on diagnosis, grade, and the presence of vascular/lymphatic invasion on histology or nodal metastasis. Treatment protocols depend on the patient's overall health and diagnosis. Consultation with an oncologist is recommended.

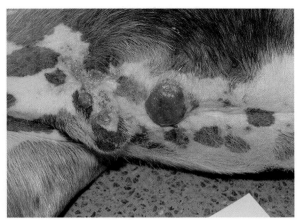

FIGURE 23-1 Solar-induced squamous cell carcinomas are frequently seen on the ventral abdomen in non-pigmented skin of dogs with sparse haircoats and a history of sunbathing.

most commonly on the forelimbs.[10,11] Giant schnauzers and standard poodles are breeds at risk for development of multiple digital SCC.[20,21]

Clinical Features

SCC appears as solitary or multiple erosive, proliferative, or nodular dermal lesions that may be accompanied by erythema, scale, and concurrent solar-induced tumors (e.g., dermal hemangioma and hemangiosarcoma [HSA]; Figure 23-1). In cats, SCC is most commonly seen in white cats on poorly haired areas of the ear tips, preauricular areas, nasal planum, and periocular regions.[12,13,15] Early lesions are often mistaken for scratches but do not heal.

Multi-centric SCC *in situ* (MSCCIS) is seen in cats of all colors. Lesions appear as multiple, alopecic, non-healing scabs on the trunk, limbs, and head.[22] Histologically, MSCCIS does not invade the epidermal basement membrane, but in some cases, focal areas of invasive SCC are present. These areas are firm, crusted, crateriforme masses.[22]

Nail bed SCCs are frequently incidental but may be accompanied by lameness, split toenails, and bleeding.[10] Eighty percent of dogs with digital SCC have radiographic evidence of bone lysis.[10,11] Multiple digital SCCs are occasionally seen in dogs.[10,11,20,21] In cats, nail bed carcinomas may represent metastasis from a primary lung carcinoma; most commonly, these cats are evaluated because of lameness, not respiratory signs.[23]

Diagnosis and Staging

The diagnosis of SCC should be histologically confirmed, since inflammation may confound cytologic diagnosis. Three-view thoracic radiographs and a regional lymph node aspirate should be performed. Biopsy of superficial facial lesions may be accomplished by shaving the lesion with a scalpel blade. Since the resulting biopsy samples are thin and fragile, placement into a tissue cassette prior to submerging in formalin is indicated.

In dogs and cats with nail bed SCC, radiographs of the affected digit(s), three-view thoracic radiographs, and a regional lymph node aspirate are indicated to evaluate the patient for bony lysis of the digit and pulmonary metastasis or a primary bronchogenic carcinoma (cats).[10,11,23]

Biological Behavior/Metastasis

Cutaneous SCC is locally invasive. Metastasis to regional lymph nodes is uncommon and pulmonary metastasis is rare. In a study of cats with planum SCC, 6 of 15 (40%) of necropsied cats had regional lymph node metastasis, and 1 (6%) had pulmonary metastasis.[13] Only 3% to 13% of dogs with nail bed SCC have radiographic evidence of pulmonary metastasis at the time of diagnosis,[10,11] and, in one study, 29% eventually developed metastasis.[10]

Therapy and Prognosis

For dogs with solitary or multiple dermal SCC, surgical excision and behavioral modification to avoid sun exposure are recommended. When multiple lesions are present, topical imiquimod cream (Aldara, 3M Pharmaceuticals, St. Paul, MN) may slow the progression of dermal SCC and other skin lesions.[24] Although the extent of disease in most patients limits its use, electron beam radiation therapy could be considered for localized SCC. Anecdotally, laser removal[25] and oral COX-2 inhibitors have been used to control SCC lesions. Oral and topical retinoids are uncommonly used for multiple SCC in dogs because of cost, potential for serious side effects, and questionable efficacy.[26]

For cats with SCC lesions on the face, treatment options are limited by the size and invasiveness of the tumor, so early treatment is best. Untreated SCC invades normal tissues, resulting in disfigurement and loss of function.[15] Pinnectomy and nosectomy can be effective in controlling the disease.[15] Tumor control is better for cats with tumors amenable to surgical excision when compared with external beam radiation therapy, and cryotherapy is associated with shorter control times when compared with either of these modalities.[15]

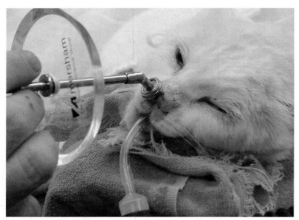

FIGURE 23-2 Strontium-90 (^{90}Sr) beta irradiation is an effective treatment for superficial squamous cell carcinoma in cats. Here the ^{90}Sr probe is applied to a lesion on the nasal planum.

Strontium-90 beta radiation (^{90}Sr) is effective for lesions < 2 mm in depth and incompletely excised small lesions (Figure 23-2).[27,28] ^{90}Sr is effective for superficial SCC, with nearly 90% of cats tumor free at 1 year and 80% tumor free at 2 years after therapy.[27] In a study of 90 cats with nasal planum SCC treated with external beam radiation therapy, 1- and 5-year progression-free rates were 60% and 10%, respectively. Cats with tumors < 2 cm had a better prognosis than those with tumors > 3 cm in diameter.[13] For more advanced local disease, external beam radiation therapy may provide long-term tumor control.[13,15] Intratumoral administration of carboplatin (Paraplatin, Bristol-Myers Squibb Co., Princeton, NJ),[29] photodynamic therapy,[30,31] and cryotherapy[15] have also been used for superficial lesions but are associated with shorter control times. SCC is poorly responsive to systemic chemotherapy.[15] In one study, none of the feline cutaneous SCC tested expressed COX-2, suggesting that COX-2 inhibition is unlikely to be useful in this species.[32]

Client education about SCC prevention is essential. Techniques to minimize sun exposure in dogs and cats include limiting access to the outdoors and windows during peak sun hours and the use of topical sunscreen or protective clothing.

Surgical excision can provide local control of MSCCIS lesions; however, cats frequently develop lesions at other sites.[22] In a recent report of 12 cats with MSCCIS treated with imiquimod, all cats showed improvement in lesions.[33] Observed toxicities included local erythema, gastrointestinal signs, elevated liver enzymes, and neutropenia. ^{90}Sr may also be useful for lesions < 2 mm in depth.[34] In cats with MSCCIS, local recurrence following surgical excision is rare; however, long-term monitoring is required because of the multifocal nature of the disease.[22] Long survival times are observed.[33]

For dogs with nail bed SCC, wide amputation with disarticulation of the first phalanx or metacarpal/metatarsal bone is the treatment of choice. Radiation therapy and chemotherapy may be indicated for incompletely excised or metastatic tumors.[10] In one study of dogs with nail bed SCC, the 1- and 2-year survival rates were 95% and 74%, respectively, for subungual SCC, and 60% and 44% for SCC from other parts of the digit.[11] A more recent study showed a 1-year survival rate of 50% and a 2-year survival rate of 18%.[10] Only 15% had metastasis at the time of death or last follow-up, and dogs treated with surgery survived longer than those not treated.

For cats with nail bed tumors resulting from metastasis of primary bronchogenic carcinomas, surgical resection of the digit is rarely palliative because of the poor prognosis associated with this syndrome.[23] In one study, the mean survival time for these cats was 58 days from diagnosis, regardless of treatment.[23]

Papilloma (Table 23-3)

FOLLICULAR TUMORS

Multiple tumor types are associated with the hair follicle.[4,35] Most are solitary benign lesions that are diagnosed and cured with surgical excision and histologic examination. Benign follicular tumors are described in Table 23-3. Their malignant counterparts (malignant trichoepithelioma and pilomatricoma) are rare and reported only in dogs. The exception is basal cell carcinoma (BCC), which is discussed subsequently.

Basal Cell Tumors

The term *basal cell tumor* describes epithelial tumors without epidermal or adnexal differentiation and has historically included a group of diverse epidermal, follicular, and adnexal tumors. In recent years, these tumors have been reclassified based on morphologic and immunohistologic features.[36,37] The majority are suspected to be trichoblastomas; however, to date, the term *basal cell tumor* remains in common use in veterinary histopathology. Basal cell tumors are common in cats and dogs[4,35-38,42] (Figure 23-3). See Table 23-3 for further information.

TABLE 23-3	BENIGN EPITHELIAL TUMORS OF THE SKIN OF DOGS AND CATS[42]					
	Papilloma	Basal Cell Tumor (Trichoblastoma; Epithelial Tumor Without Epidermal or Adnexal Differentiation)	Trichoepithelioma	Pilomatricoma	Trichilemmoma	Infundibular Keratinizing Acanthoma (Ika; Formerly Intracutaneous Cornifying Epithelioma)
Tissue of origin	Benign proliferation of the epidermis	Benign tumor of hair germ; recently, immunohistochemistry has resulted in reclassification of basal cell tumors as the follicular tumors trichoblastoma and trichoepithelioma or as ductular sweat gland tumors[36,37]	Benign tumor of the hair follicle that differentiates into all three segments of the hair follicle; incomplete trichogenesis may be present[39]	Benign tumor of the hair bulb showing matrical differentiation ± dystrophic mineralization and bone formation[39,40]	Benign tumor of the outer root sheath of the hair follicle; a bulb type and an isthmus type have been described[35,38-40]	Benign tumor of squamous cells of the follicular isthmus with a central accumulation of keratin[40]
Incidence	Uncommon in dogs; rare in cats[7,8]	Most common pigmented tumor of cats; common in dogs[4,35-38]	Common in dogs; rare in cats[4,35,38-40]	Relatively common in dogs; rare in cats[4,35,38-40]	Uncommon, mainly in dogs[35,38-40]	Common in dogs[40,41]
Risk factors/ etiology	Caused by species-specific papillomaviruses in young animals; may also be non-viral (squamous papilloma)[7,8]	No breed predilection in cats[4]; predisposed canine breeds include Kerry blue terrier, soft coated Wheaton terrier, bichon frise, cock-a-poo, Shetland sheepdog, husky, cocker spaniel, poodle, Airedale terrier, English springer spaniel, collie, Yorkshire terrier, and mixed breed[36,37]; most common in middle-aged animals	Predisposed breeds include Basset hound, bull mastiff, English springer spaniel, golden retriever, Gordon Setter, Irish Setter, German shepherd, and standard poodle[35,39,40]; most common in middle-aged to older dogs	Kerry blue terriers markedly predisposed; other predisposed breeds include soft-coated Wheaton terrier, standard poodle, Old English sheepdog, bichon frise, Airedale terrier, basset hound, miniature poodle, Lhasa apso, and miniature schnauzer[35,39,40]; most common in middle-aged dogs	None known	Norwegian elkhounds are markedly predisposed and often develop multiple lesions; other predisposed breeds include Yorkshire terrier, Lhasa apso, bichon frise, German shepherd, standard poodle, keeshond, Samoyed, and Shetland sheepdog[39,40], most commonly seen in middle-aged dogs

(Continued)

TABLE 23-3	BENIGN EPITHELIAL TUMORS OF THE SKIN OF DOGS AND CATS[42]—cont'd					
	Papilloma	Basal Cell Tumor (Trichoblastoma; Epithelial Tumor Without Epidermal or Adnexal Differentiation)	Trichoepithelioma	Pilomatricoma	Trichilemmoma	Infundibular Keratinizing Acanthoma (Ika; Formerly Intracutaneous Cornifying Epithelioma
Clinical features	Small, slow-growing, cauliflower-like, proliferations of squamous epithelium; single or multiple lesions possible; most commonly located on the head or paws[7-9]	Solitary, pigmented, well-circumscribed, cystic or solid masses[36-38] (Figure 23-3)	Slow-growing solitary or multiple masses; most commonly found on the dorsum, neck, thorax, or tail[39,40]	Masses most common on the dorsum, neck, thorax, and tail[39,40]	Alopecic, well-circumscribed dermal or subcutaneous mass(es)[40]	Multiple variably sized masses; most commonly on the dorsum, tail, and neck; masses have a central pore filled with grayish-white inspissated keratinous material that is pasty[40]; release of keratinous material results in inflammation and secondary infection is possible
Diagnosis and staging	Clinical presentation suggestive, but definitive diagnosis requires biopsy; intranuclear inclusion bodies are seen in viral-induced papillomas[7,8]	Cytology is suggestive, definitive diagnosis with biopsy	Cytology is suggestive, definitive diagnosis with biopsy	Cytology is suggestive, definitive diagnosis with biopsy	Cytology is suggestive, definitive diagnosis with biopsy	Cytology is suggestive, definitive diagnosis with biopsy
Therapy and prognosis	Generally, no treatment is required as most regress spontaneously within 1 year with associated infiltration of T cells[7,8]; surgical excision indicated for inverted papilloma (endophytic variant) or squamous papillomas that are irritating or bleeding	Most cured with excision	Most cured with excision; some breeds (especially Bassett hounds) develop multicentric lesions	Most cured with excision	Most cured with excision	Surgical resection for solitary lesions; dogs with multiple tumors are prone to developing more lesions and may benefit from long-term retinoid therapy[41]

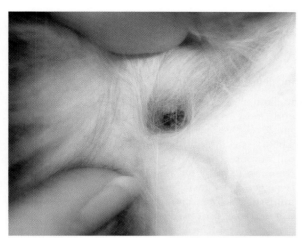

FIGURE 23-3 Trichoblastomas (previously termed *basal cell tumors*) are the most common pigmented tumor of the skin in cats.

Basal Cell Carcinoma

Incidence/Etiology and Risk Factors

Basal cell carcinomas (BCCs) are uncommon, although their true incidence is unknown since many of these tumors were previously classified as basal cell tumors or have been confused with ductular adenomas or carcinomas.[43]

Clinical Features

BCCs often appear as plaques or nodules, and may have a blue or black pigment caused by the presence of melanin. The overlying epidermis may be ulcerated. Multicentric lesions are common in cats, usually occurring on the nose, face, and ears. In dogs, BCCs are usually truncal.[43]

Diagnosis and Staging

The diagnosis may be obtained by cytology or biopsy. Regional lymph node aspiration and three-view thoracic radiographs are indicated, although the incidence of metastasis is low.[43]

Therapy and Prognosis

The treatment of choice for BCC is wide surgical excision. Adjuvant radiation therapy may be indicated if excision is incomplete. The role of chemotherapy is unknown but may be considered if BCCs are metastatic.[44,45] Long-term survival is expected for completely excised lesions. Pulmonary and regional lymph node metastases have been reported in BCC.[45] The prognosis for metastatic BCC is unknown.

SEBACEOUS GLAND TUMORS

Sebaceous glands produce sebum, an oily white fluid. In addition to cutaneous sebaceous tumors, dogs and cats develop tumors of modified sebaceous glands including hepatoid gland tumors of the perianal region (see Section G) and meibomian gland tumors (Chapter 20, Section C).

Incidence/Etiology and Risk Factors

Sebaceous adenoma, ductal adenoma, and epithelioma are benign tumors that are common in dogs and rare in cats. Sebaceous carcinoma is uncommon.[46,47] Sebaceous tumors are most common in middle-aged to older dogs and cats. Predisposed breeds include English cocker spaniel, cocker spaniel, Samoyed, Siberian husky, cock-a-poo, Alaskan malamute, West Highland white terrier, cairn terrier, dachshund, miniature poodle, toy poodle, shih tzu, and Persian cats.[46]

Clinical Features

Sebaceous tumors may be solitary or multiple. Common sites are the head and dorsum. Sebaceous tumors present as elevated alopecic nodules that may contain keratin or may have a wart-like appearance. Sebaceous epitheliomas may be pigmented.[46-48]

Diagnosis and Staging

Cytology may be suggestive of the diagnosis, and biopsy is needed for definitive diagnosis. Regional lymph node aspiration and three-view thoracic radiographs are indicated for sebaceous carcinomas.

Biological Behavior/Metastasis

Sebaceous carcinomas are locally invasive. Rarely, sebaceous carcinomas and epitheliomas metastasize to local lymph nodes or other sites.[46-48]

Therapy and Prognosis

Wide surgical resection is curative for most sebaceous tumors. Rarely, sebaceous carcinomas and epitheliomas metastasize.[46-48]

APOCRINE GLAND TUMORS

Apocrine glands are sweat glands typically associated with hair follicles. In addition to tumors of cutaneous apocrine glands, dogs and cats commonly develop tumors of modified apocrine glands including adenoma or adenocarcinoma of the apocrine gland of the anal sac (see Section G), ceruminous gland adenoma or adeno-carcinoma (see Chapter 20, Section D), and mammary adenomas and adenocarcinomas (see Chapter 22, Section F).

Incidence/Etiology and Risk Factors

Benign apocrine tumors, including apocrine cyst, cystadenoma, ductular adenoma, and secretory adenoma, are common in the dog and uncommon in the cat. Cutaneous apocrine gland carcinomas are uncommon.[49,50] Apocrine tumors are most common in middle-aged to older dogs. Predisposed breeds for adenomas include Lhasa apso, Old English sheepdog, collie, shih tzu, great Pyrenees, chow chow, malamute, and Irish setter; for carcinomas, they include the Old English Sheepdog, shih tzu, German shepherd, cocker spaniel, Coonhound, Norwegian Elkhound, and Siamese cats.[49,50]

Clinical Features

Apocrine tumors usually present as solitary masses on the head (cats and dogs) and legs (dogs).[49,50] Multiple masses are also possible.[51] Tumors may be freely movable or invasive.

Diagnosis and Staging

Cytology may be suggestive of the diagnosis, and biopsy is needed for definitive diagnosis. Regional lymph node aspiration and three-view thoracic radiographs are indicated for apocrine carcinomas.

Biological Behavior/Metastasis

The growth rate of apocrine carcinomas is variable and metastasis is uncommon, usually to lymph nodes and lungs. Inflammatory carcinomas are associated with rapid growth and metastasis.[49]

Therapy and Prognosis

Surgical resection is curative for most apocrine tumors.[51,52] In a study of 25 dogs with apocrine gland carcinomas treated with surgery, only 1 dog was euthanized for tumor-related causes and the median survival time (MST) was 30 months (17 dogs still alive).[51] Occasionally, lymphatic and distant metastasis may be seen. Metastasis is predicted by vascular invasion and tumor grade.[50,51] For incompletely excised carcinomas or those with vascular/lymphatic invasion or regional lymph node metastasis, adjunctive therapy with radiation or chemotherapy is indicated. Protocols for these tumors are not well described, but protocols effective for anal sac gland adenocarcinoma (see Section G) or mammary

adenocarcinomas (Chapter 22, Section F) would be logical choices.

MELANOCYTIC TUMORS

Incidence/Etiology and Risk Factors

Melanoma is common in dogs[4,53,54] and the second most common tumor of the digit in this species.[10,11,53,55,56] Melanoma is rare in cats.[4,5,53,56] The most common pigmented tumor in cats is basal cell tumor (trichoblastoma). Melanomas are more common in purebred dogs.[57] Genetic predisposition is suggested by increased prevalence in standard and miniature schnauzers, Doberman pinschers, Scottish terriers, Boston terriers, boxers, Airedale terriers, Irish and Gordon setters, cocker and Springer spaniels, and Golden retrievers.[58] More recently, for melanoma of the haired skin, Labrador retrievers, miniature schnauzers, and Rottweilers were overrepresented and for melanoma of the digit, Labrador retrievers, Golden retrievers, and Rottweilers were overrepresented.[59]

Clinical Features

Although melanomas are typically pigmented dermal masses, some are amelanotic.

Diagnosis and Staging

Cytology may be suggestive of the diagnosis, but melanoma is diagnosed with biopsy and histology. Immunohistochemical stains (S100 and MelanA) for proteins expressed by melanomas may be required for diagnosing anaplastic tumors.[60] For dogs with negative prognostic indicators (i.e., digital or mucocutaneous junction location, malignant histologic appearance, high mitotic index, or vascular/lymphatic invasion), cytology of regional lymph nodes, and three-view thoracic radiographs are indicated. Abdominal ultrasound should also be considered. Because the behavior of cutaneous melanomas in cats is less predictable, these tests are recommended routinely.

Biological Behavior/Metastasis

Cutaneous melanoma is typically behaviorally benign in dogs.[61,62] Malignant melanoma metastasizes via lymphatics to lymph nodes, lungs, and other sites. The behavior of cutaneous melanomas in cats is less predictable. In cats, melanomas are often slow growing and some are cured with surgical excision, but others recur locally or spread to lymph nodes, lungs, and other sites, including viscera or bone.[63,64]

Therapy and Prognosis

Most dogs with cutaneous melanomas are cured with complete surgical excision.[61,62] The histologic tumor grade is an important predictor of survival; in one study of 59 dogs treated with surgery for cutaneous melanoma, 10% of dogs with a mitotic index ≤ 2/10 HPF and 73% of dogs with a mitotic index ≥ 3/10 HPF died of melanoma within 2 years of surgery.[62] In a more recent study, only 12% of 227 cutaneous melanomas exhibited recurrence or metastasis, and it was difficult to predict which tumors would be more aggressive using histologic features.[61] Nuclear atypia was thought to be most reliable. For malignant melanomas of the canine digit, digital amputation is often required. This location is associated with more aggressive behavior, including local invasion and metastasis to lymph nodes, lungs, and other sites. For dogs with digital melanomas, reported 1- and 2-year survival rates are 42% to 44% and 11% to 13%, respectively.[10,11]

Adjunctive therapies may be indicated for patients with malignant melanoma. Radiation therapy is effective for malignant oral melanomas in dogs (Chapter 20, Section A) and may be useful for control of incompletely excised malignant cutaneous melanomas and involved regional lymph nodes. Chemotherapy with carboplatin may be helpful for slowing local progression and metastasis. One study demonstrated a 28% response rate of measurable malignant melanomas to this drug.[65] In addition, because melanomas are highly immunogenic, there has been great interest in developing immunotherapy as a treatment for these tumors.[57,66,67] A xenogenic DNA canine melanoma vaccine is currently commercially available (Canine Melanoma Vaccine, Merial Limited, Duluth, GA). Plasmid DNA encoding human tyrosinase (a melanocytic protein) is injected into the muscles of the medial thigh. Canine myocytes express the DNA, and the resultant human tyrosinase induces an immune response. Human and canine tyrosinase are similar enough that the immune response can cross over to be directed at canine melanocytic cells.[66,68] This vaccine has been demonstrated to be safe and active in phase 1 and 2 clinical trials in dogs and survival times > 1 year have been described. It is recommended that this vaccine be used as adjunctive therapy once locoregional tumor control has been achieved. Currently, the canine melanoma vaccine is licensed for use by veterinary oncologists only.

The behavior of cutaneous melanomas in cats is much less predictable, and even histologic diagnosis as benign or malignant may not predict behavior.[63] In one study of cats with cutaneous melanoma treated with surgery with or without adjuvant therapies, survival times ranged from 0 to 1003 days, with 5 of 19 cats dying of melanoma.[63] Another study described 45 cats with cutaneous melanoma treated with surgery[64]; 22 of 37 cats that died during the study had local recurrence. Sixteen of these 37 cats were necropsied and all had metastasis.

MESENCHYMAL TUMORS

Cutaneous mesenchymal tumors are usually STSs (see Section E), a group of tumors with similar histologic and clinical features. Although they are mesenchymal tumors of soft tissue, cutaneous hemangiosarcomas (HSAs) are considered separate from STS because of their distinct etiology and behavior.

Hemangioma/Hemangiosarcoma

Incidence/Etiology and Risk Factors

HSAs and hemangiomas are tumors of vascular endothelium. They occur more frequently in dogs than any other species but are uncommon in the skin of dogs and less common in cats.[69,70] In dogs, cutaneous hemangioma is more common than HSA. Cutaneous HSA is more common in older animals. Predisposed breeds include the Italian greyhound, greyhound, whippet, Dalmatian, pit bull, boxer, and Basset hound.[69-71] Solar radiation induces dermal hemangiomas and HSA in dogs with short hair and lightly pigmented skin.[71] Subcutaneous HSA is not solar induced. The identification of pairs of affected sibling Italian greyhounds and whippets suggests a possible genetic predisposition.[70,71]

Clinical Features

Dermal hemangiomas and HSAs appear as red or purple discolorations or raised masses, and lesions may be solitary or multiple. Dermal HSA frequently occurs in lightly haired and unpigmented areas, including the ventral abdomen, limbs, neck, dorsum, and head.[69-72] Subcutaneous lesions are firm or soft masses that often appear bruised and have no site predilection.

Diagnosis and Staging

Diagnosis of HSA is accomplished with biopsy and histology. For anaplastic tumors, immunohistochemical staining for Factor VIII–related antigen (von Willebrand factor), and CD31 can be used to confirm the diagnosis.[73,74] Solar-induced changes such as dermal elastosis and actinic keratosis may be observed in the skin surrounding dermal HSA. Because HSA of the skin can metastasize or may represent metastasis from visceral HSA, further staging tests are indicated. A CBC, serum chemistry profile, urinalysis, thoracic and abdominal radiographs, abdominal ultrasound, cytology of local lymph node, and echocardiogram are recommended, particularly for subcutaneous lesions, multiple lesions, or lesions not consistent with solar etiology. A staging scheme has been described for canine cutaneous HSA: stage I is a primary tumor confined to the dermis, stage II is a primary tumor involving the hypodermis, and stage III is a primary tumor with underlying muscular involvement.[69]

Biological Behavior/Metastasis

Patients with solar-induced hemangioma and HSA can have multiple lesions and are at risk of developing future lesions. HSA is locally invasive and metastasis is uncommon with dermal HSA, but common with subcutaneous HSA.[69] Common sites are skin, lymph node, and lung.

Therapy and Prognosis

Most hemangiomas and dermal HSAs are cured with complete surgical excision, but additional lesions may develop and avoidance of sun exposure is important. Subcutaneous lesions require wide surgical excision. Completeness of excision is prognostic for survival of dogs and cats with cutaneous HSA treated with surgery alone or in combination with doxorubicin (Adriamycin, Ben Venue Laboratories, Inc., Bedford, OH).[70,75,76] In dogs with HSA, subcutaneous tumors have been associated with a poorer prognosis than dermal tumors; in one study, the median survival of dogs with stage I disease was 780 days compared with 172 and 307 days for stage II and III dogs.[69] However, with aggressive therapy and complete excision, good prognoses may be achieved for some dogs with subcutaneous HSA.[70] This is supported by a recent study that showed a median disease-free interval of > 4 years for dogs with subcutaneous HSA treated with surgery and doxorubicin with or without radiation therapy.[77] In the same study, four dogs with intramuscular HSA had a median DFI of 265 days.

Radiation therapy may improve local control of incompletely excised cutaneous HSA in dogs and cats, and patients with non-resectable tumors may benefit from palliative radiation therapy. Fourteen of 17 dogs with evidence of soft tissue involvement with HSA (including SC and IM tumors) had tumor reduction (including four complete responses) following a palliative course of radiation therapy with or without doxorubicin chemotherapy.[78] The MST was approximately 3 months.

For subcutaneous tumors or those with vascular/lymphatic invasion or metastasis, adjunctive chemotherapy may improve survival time. Treatment protocols are those used for splenic HSA (Chapter 22, Section D) and should include doxorubicin. In a study evaluating vincristine (Vincasar, SICOR Pharmaceuticals, Irvine, CA), doxorubicin, and cyclophosphamide (Cytoxan, Mead Johnson Oncology Products, Princeton, NJ) chemotherapy for dogs with HSA, an MST of 425 days was reported for 6 dogs with subcutaneous HSA,[79] and in a study evaluating doxorubicin and cyclophosphamide for dogs with HSA, survival times ranged from 183 to 704 days for four dogs with subcutaneous HSA.[80] In one study of 17 dogs with subcutaneous HSA treated with doxorubicin chemotherapy with or without radiation therapy, the median survival was 1189 days.[77] The role of continuous low-dose oral chemotherapy for subcutaneous HSA has not been defined, but a preliminary study of cyclophosphamide, etoposide (Etoposide, Gensia Sicor Pharmaceuticals, Irvine, CA), and piroxicam (Feldene, Pfizer Incorporated, New York, NY) administered in this fashion after splenectomy to dogs with splenic HSA demonstrated a similar MST (6 months) to dogs treated with doxorubicin.[81] There is much interest in immunotherapy and antiangiogenic therapy for HSA,[82,83] but these therapies are not readily available at this time.

In cats, subcutaneous HSA is more likely to recur or metastasize than cutaneous HSA, but complete excision can be associated with long survival.[72,76] In one study, 10 cats treated with surgery for subcutaneous HSA lived 13 to >112 weeks.[84] In another study of 18 cats with cutaneous HSA, the MST was 912 days (range, 4–1460; 5 cats still alive at 120–1186 days), and cats treated with surgery lived significantly longer than those not treated with surgery.[72] For incompletely excised HSA, radiation therapy should be considered. There is little information regarding adjuvant chemotherapy for HSA in cats, but doxorubicin (as a single agent or in combination with vincristine and cyclophosphamide), carboplatin, and a combination of mitoxantrone (Novantrone, Immunex Corp, Seattle, WA) and cyclophosphamide have been used.[72,76,85]

ROUND/DISCRETE CELL TUMORS

Round/discrete cell tumors exfoliate as individual round cells and have distinguishing cytologic features that frequently allow diagnosis. Tumors included in this group are MCT (see Section D), lymphoma (see Chapter 25, Section A), plasmacytoma (PCT), histiocytoma, and canine transmissible venereal tumor (CTVT; see Chapter 22, Sections F and G). Any of these tumors can occur in the skin.

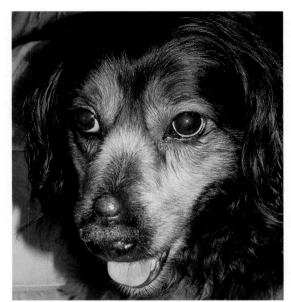

FIGURE 23-4 Cutaneous plasma cell tumors frequently appear as pink, alopecic lesions on the face, ears, or feet. This dog was treated with chemotherapy for multiple cutaneous plasmacytomas and lived > 3 years, before dying of unrelated causes.

Plasmacytoma

Incidence/Etiology and Risk Factors

Plasma cell tumors are uncommon in the skin of dogs and are very rare in cats. They are more common in older animals, and cocker spaniels may be overrepresented.[86,87]

Clinical Features

Plasmacytomas appear as raised, hairless, pink dermal nodules and are typically found on the face, ears, or feet (Figure 23-4).[86,87] In dogs, they are usually solitary, but multiple PCTs are possible.

Diagnosis and Staging

Cytology is often diagnostic and histology provides a definitive diagnosis. For more anaplastic tumors, immunohistochemical staining may be required to definitively differentiate PCT from lymphoma or MCT. For most dogs, a CBC, serum biochemical profile, urinalysis, and regional lymph node aspirate provide complete staging information. For dogs with multiple tumors, lymph node metastasis, or hyperglobulinemia, serum and urine protein electrophoresis or immunoelectrophoresis, thoracic

and abdominal radiographs (including axial skeleton), abdominal ultrasound, and bone marrow aspirate are indicated. Because of the systemic nature of PCT in cats, all of the staging tests listed are recommended.

Biological Behavior/Metastasis

Most cutaneous PCTs in dogs are primary tumors.[86,87] Rarely, canine cutaneous PCT may be associated with multiple myeloma and/or paraneoplastic syndromes (including hyperglobulinemia and hypercalcemia).[86,87] In contrast, in cats PCT may be more commonly associated with metastasis or multiple myeloma.[88,89]

Therapy and Prognosis

Most cutaneous PCTs in dogs are benign and are cured with surgical excision.[86,87] In one study of 57 dogs with cutaneous PCT, 46 had no recurrence at 1 to 62 months after surgery, and 4 were euthanized for systemic disease related to the tumor.[87] Histologic grading of canine PCT does not predict behavior.[90] Rarely, dogs develop multiple cutaneous PCTs or lymph node metastasis. These dogs may enjoy long survival times with chemotherapy. A chemotherapy protocol for multiple myeloma (combination of melphalan [Alkeran, Cardinal Health for GlaxoSmithKline, Albuquerque, NM] and prednisone; see Chapter 25, Section C) is indicated for cats and for dogs with metastatic disease or multiple PCTs. Radiation therapy can provide long-term control for tumors in locations not amenable to surgery. There is little information describing the prognosis for PCT in cats, but association with systemic disease would suggest a poorer prognosis.[88]

Histiocytoma

Incidence/Etiology and Risk Factors

Histiocytic proliferative disorders (HPDs) of dogs include cutaneous histiocytoma, reactive histiocytosis (cutaneous and systemic histiocytosis [believed to be an immunoregulatory disorder]), and malignant histiocytosis (localized and disseminated histiocytic sarcoma [HS] [Section F]). These diseases are distinguished by histologic appearance, immunophenotype, and varying clinical presentations/courses.[91-94] Histiocytomas are benign tumors of Langerhans' cells (antigen-presenting cells of the epidermis). They are most common in young, purebred dogs but can be seen in any dog.[95] Breeds at risk include Scottish terriers, boxers, Doberman pinschers, Labrador retrievers, cocker spaniels, Rottweilers, and miniature schnauzers.[95] They are extremely rare in cats.

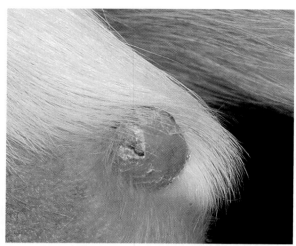

FIGURE 23-5 Histiocytomas frequently appear as pink alopecic lesions on the limbs of young dogs and spontaneously regress within a few months.

Clinical Features

Histiocytomas are hairless, raised, and white, pink, or red dermal nodules that can become inflamed and ulcerated, especially when regressing (Figure 23-5). Most commonly they occur on the head or limbs.

Diagnosis and Staging

Cytology is usually diagnostic for histiocytoma. Because of the possibility of misdiagnosis of cutaneous lymphoma or another round cell tumor, in cases with an atypical presentation (old dog, multiple lesions, not regressing), biopsy and histologic confirmation of diagnosis are indicated. Rarely, immunophenotyping[91-93] may be necessary to rule out other diagnoses and confirm that a mass is a histiocytoma.

Biological Behavior/Metastasis

Histiocytomas are usually solitary and do not metastasize; however, multiple regressing cutaneous histiocytomas have been reported. Langerhans cell histiocytosis (LCH) is a syndrome of multiple cutaneous histiocytomas that may be slow to regress, wax and wane for a period, or progress to organ involvement.[96,97] LCH is seen in children and has been reported in young dogs.

Therapy and Prognosis

Most canine histiocytomas regress spontaneously within 2 to 4 months, and recurrence or development of additional lesions is rare. If a histiocytoma does not resolve, is

irritating to the patient, or has an atypical presentation, surgical resection and histology are indicated.

Selected References*

Bergman JP, Camps-Palau MA, McKnight JA, et al: Development of a xenogeneic DNA vaccine program for canine malignant melanoma at the Animal Medical Center, *Vaccine* 24:4582, 2006.
This article presents details of the development, efficacy, and safety of the first tumor vaccine licensed for treatment of cancer in veterinary patients, the canine melanoma vaccine.
Bulakowski EJ, Philibert JC, Siegel S, et al: Evaluation of outcome associated with subcutaneous and intramuscular hemangiosarcoma treated with adjuvant doxorubicin in dogs: 21 cases (2001-06), *J Am Vet Med Assoc* 233(1):122, 2008.
This study describes a good prognosis for dogs with subcutaneous hemangiosarcoma if treated aggressively.
Gross TL, Ihrke PJ, Walder EJ, et al: *Skin diseases of the dog and cat: clinical and histopathologic diagnosis,* ed 2, Oxford, England, 2005, Blackwell Science.
This is a useful text providing detailed information regarding cutaneous neoplasia and is particularly useful for benign and rare skin tumors, topics for which little literature is available.
Hammond GM, Gordon IK, Theon AP, et al: Evaluation of strontium Sr 90 for the treatment of superficial squamous cell carcinoma of the nasal planum in cats: 49 cases (1990-2006), *J Am Vet Med Assoc* 231(5):736, 2007.
This study demonstrates that strontium-90 is a safe and effective treatment for superficial squamous cell lesions in cats.
Johannes CM, Henry CJ, Turnquist SE: Hemangiosarcoma in cats: 53 cases (1992-2002), *J Am Vet Med Assoc* 231:1851, 2007.
This is the largest study to date describing the behavior of hemangiosarcoma in cats.
Spangler WL, Kass PH: The histologic and epidemiologic bases for prognostic considerations in canine melanocytic neoplasia, *Vet Pathol* 43:136, 2006.
This study examines prognostic indicators for predicting the behavior of melanocytic tumors.

SECTION B: Nail Bed Tumors

Kim D. Johnson

KEY POINTS

- Approximately one half to one third of subungual (nail bed) tumors in dogs are squamous cell carcinomas.
- Surveillance for digital masses should be part of routine wellness examinations for all dogs, but especially Rottweilers, black Labrador Retrievers and black Standard Poodles.
- Tumors of the digits are rare in cats and more often are metastases from a primary lung tumor, rather than truly a primary digital tumor.

Clinical Behavior

Tumors comprise approximately 12% of all disorders of the nail and nail bed and should be included in any differential list for disease of this anatomical site.[1] Primary subungual tumors are common in the dog and rare in the cat, with approximately one third to one half of these tumors being squamous cell carcinoma (SCC) in the dog and the vast majority reported to be SCC in cats.[1,2] However, the latter has been disputed by a 2007 report in *Veterinary Pathology* suggesting that most primary feline digital tumors are mesenchymal.[3] Other reported tumor types include malignant melanoma, osteosarcoma, fibrosarcoma, and mast cell tumor (MCT).[4-6] These tumors are often secondarily infected and initially misdiagnosed as chronic paronychia or osteomyelitis.

Etiology/Risk Factors

In most reports of dogs with nail bed tumors, large breed dogs with black hair coats appear to be predisposed. SCC is overrepresented in Labrador Retrievers and Standard Poodles and other breeds with darkly pigmented skin such as Giant Schnauzers, Rottweilers, Flat-Coated Retrievers, and Dachshunds.[2,6-9] It has been postulated that because the forelimbs bear more weight and are exposed to more carcinogens during digging than the hind limbs, they are a predisposed site.[6,7]

Clinical Features

Clinical manifestations of digital lesions are similar regardless of whether the lesion is a malignant neoplastic, benign, or inflammatory process (Box 23-1).[4,6] A visible digital mass and/or lameness are the most common presenting complaints for dogs with digit tumors. Ulceration of the toe and a breaking or splitting of the toenail of the involved digit have also been reported.[1,7,8] In a study of 64 dogs,

---

BOX 23-1 DIFFERENTIAL DIAGNOSES FOR LESIONS AFFECTING THE CANINE DIGIT

Malignant Neoplasm
- Squamous cell carcinoma
- Melanoma
- Soft-tissue sarcoma
- Mast cell tumor
- Osteosarcoma
- Round cell sarcoma
- Adenocarcinoma
- Chondrosarcoma
- Giant cell tumor of bone
- Hemangiosarcoma
- Plasmacytoma
- Undifferentiated sarcoma

Benign Neoplasm
- Keratoacanthoma
- Sebaceous adenoma
- Histiocytoma
- Keratoma
- Hamartoma
- Infundibular keratinizing acanthoma
- Plasmacytoma
- Trichoblastoma
- Basal cell epithelioma
- Fibroma
- Hemangioma
- Inverted papilloma

Non-inflammatory, Non-neoplastic
- Epithelial inclusion cyst
- Adnexal dysplasia
- Follicular cyst
- Apocrine gland cyst
- Calcinosis circumscripta
- Sebaceous hyperplasia inflammation

---

almost 60% had lesions affecting the forelimbs, and the majority of these tumors were > 5 cm and invaded fascia or bone.[7] In a large study of 428 dogs undergoing digital amputation as a result of neoplastic disease, 7.9% had multiple digits affected.[6] Cats also present with a primary complaint of lameness, but swelling, ulcerated skin with or without purulent discharge, deviation or loss of the nail, and multiple digit involvement have also been reported; lysis of the phalangeal bone may be observed.[3,10-12]

CANINE TUMORS

Squamous cell carcinoma and malignant melanoma are the most commonly reported digital tumors.[4,7] Subungual SCC in the dog arises from the subungual epithelium and is locally invasive, has a low metastatic rate, and almost always results in bony lysis of the third phalanx. It occurs in older dogs (mean age, 9 years) and no gender predilection is known. Approximately 75% of cases involve large breed dogs, and more than two thirds of these lesions occur in dogs with primarily black hair coats such as black Labrador Retrievers, Standard Poodles, and Rottweilers.[1,7] The lesions are usually ulcerative, solitary, and occasionally hemorrhagic and expansile. The associated nail may be fractured or absent.

Subungual melanomas are potentially malignant in the dog.[13] Approximately one third to one half of melanomas that originate in the nail bed develop distant metastasis to the lymph nodes and lungs, and approximately half of dogs die as a result of distant metastasis.[7,14,15] One report suggests that Scottish terriers are predisposed to digital melanoma development.[6] Soft-tissue sarcomas involving the nail bed appear to behave similarly to their counterparts at other cutaneous locations. They are locally aggressive, but uncommonly metastatic. Mast cell tumors of the nail bed are typically high-grade, poorly differentiated tumors that carry a poor prognosis.[7]

FELINE TUMORS

Primary nail bed tumors are rare in the cat, with most studies reporting that SCC predominates. However, in one large study of 85 amputated feline digits, primary digital tumor types similar to those found in the dog were also reported, with over 55% of primary malignant lesions being mesenchymal tumors.[3] Of the 63 digital lesions that were neoplastic, tumor types included fibrosarcoma, adenocarcinoma, osteosarcoma, hemangiosarcoma, MCTs, and giant cell tumor of bone. A complete differential list can be found in Box 23-2.

Metastatic nail bed tumors are far more common in cats than are primary digital tumors. Metastatic lesions are generally carcinomas and originate from primary tumors including bronchiolar adenocarcinoma and pulmonary SCC (also referred to as "lung-digit syndrome") and cutaneous SCC and apocrine sweat gland carcinoma.[1,10-12] In one study of 36 cats with bronchogenic carcinoma metastatic to the digit, 19 had records available for review. In all 19 cases, the presenting complaint was lameness and none of the cats had respiratory signs.[10]

BOX 23-2 DIFFERENTIAL DIAGNOSES FOR LESIONS AFFECTING THE FELINE DIGIT

Malignant Neoplasm
 Squamous cell carcinoma
 Sweat gland carcinoma
 Fibrosarcoma
 Malignant fibrous histiocytoma
 Soft-tissue sarcoma
 Mast cell tumor
 Osteosarcoma
 Basal cell tumor
 Adenocarcinoma
 Giant cell tumor of bone
 Hemangiosarcoma
 Undifferentiated sarcoma
Benign Neoplasm
 Hemangioma
 Inflammation

Thus, a diagnosis of metastatic lung cancer cannot be excluded in cats with digital lesions simply based on a lack of respiratory signs.[10-12]

As a general rule, primary SCC affects a single digit, whereas multiple digits are involved with metastases from pulmonary carcinomas.[12]

Diagnosis and Staging

Clinical staging is desirable in cases of canine and feline digital tumors in order to establish the extent of disease, most appropriate treatment, and parameters by which to evaluate response to treatment. Complete clinical staging includes a minimum database (complete blood count, chemistry panel, urinalysis), three-view thoracic radiographs, radiographs of the affected limb, with or without fine-needle aspiration, and cytology of the primary site and any palpable regional lymph nodes.

Treatment Modalities

Numerous treatment modalities can be used in an attempt to control local disease. These options can be initiated alone or in combination and include amputation of the digit, amputation of the limb, cryosurgery, radiation therapy, and chemotherapy.[7] Amputation is commonly performed to both treat and diagnose conditions affecting the digit.[5,15]

Treatment for subungual tumors in the dog should include a disarticulation amputation at the metacarpophalangeal, metatarsophalangeal, or proximal interphalangeal level.[1,2] Partial foot amputation, whereby two adjacent digits are amputated, has also proven successful.[5] Adjuvant therapy does not appear to be required for most SCC or soft-tissue sarcomas but is recommended for malignant melanoma, MCTs, and osteosarcoma. A xenogeneic DNA vaccine (Canine Melanoma Vaccine, Merial, Ltd., Duluth, GA) has been developed for treatment of canine malignant melanoma and may be used as adjuvant therapy for dogs with digital melanoma. The vaccine must be administered by a board-certified oncologist, and the protocol involves one injection every 2 weeks for four treatments, with a booster given every 6 months (see Chapter 16 for more details).[17]

Digital malignancy is rarely a surgical disease in cats. Amputation may help establish the diagnosis but will not necessarily achieve palliation of symptoms and is contraindicated when the digital mass is known to represent metastasis from another site.[3,10-12]

Prognosis and Survival

Subungual SCC is potentially less malignant than SCC that originates in other parts of the digit, with reported 1- and 2-year survival rates of 95% and 75%, respectively, and the metastatic rate ranges from 4.7% to 24.1%.[4,6,7]

The reported metastatic rate for digital melanomas in dogs is higher than that of melanoma at other cutaneous sites, with a reported metastatic rate of 38% to 58% and a 1-year survival rate of 42% to 70%.[4,6,7,9] Local recurrence rates of 30% can be expected in malignant melanoma; thus, the prognosis is fair to guarded.

Long-term survival with local control can be achieved after surgical excision of subungual soft-tissue sarcomas. Amputation with adequate margins alone represents an effective method of treatment.[6,7] The survival rate for dogs with nail bed MCT is lower than that reported for dogs with MCT elsewhere on the extremities. Digital MCTs warrant a poor prognosis, similar to that of MCTs at other mucocutaneous sites. A recent publication of 20 dogs reported 1- and 2-year survival rates of 75% and 62.5%, respectively.[6]

The 2-year survival rate for digital melanomas was only 56%, compared with 83.8% for non-oral melanomas at other cutaneous sites.[16] Histologic malignancy, mitotic index > 3, and Ki-67 proliferative index (percentage of positive cells of 500 neoplastic cells counted) > 15% have been identified as negative prognostic factors for cutaneous melanoma, including those of the canine digit.[16]

Primary SCC of the feline digit warrants a guarded prognosis, with median survival time of approximately 3 months. The prognosis is very poor for cats with metastatic lesions in the digits, with reported median survival time of approximately 1.5 months.[1,3,10-12]

Selected References*

Gottfried SD, Popovitch CA, Goldschmidt MH, et al: Metastatic digital carcinoma in the cat: a retrospective study of 36 cats (1992-1998), *J Am Anim Hosp Assoc* 36:501, 2000.
This retrospective study evaluated metastasis of primary pulmonary neoplasia to the digit and reported that metastasis to and primary neoplasia of the digit is rare in the cat.

Henry CJ, Brewer WG Jr, Whitley EM, et al: Canine digital tumors: a veterinary cooperative oncology group retrospective study of 64 dogs, *J Vet Intern Med* 19:720, 2005.
This relatively large retrospective study compared the clinical characteristics and outcomes for canine digital tumors.

Marino DJ, Matthiesen DT, Stefanacci JD, et al: Evaluation of dogs with digit masses: 117 cases (1981-1991), *J Am Vet Med Assoc* 207:726, 1995.
This is the initial retrospective study evaluating digit masses in a large number of dogs, providing a description of the most common neoplasms and associated survival times.

van der Linde-Sipman JS, van den Ingh TS: Primary and metastatic carcinomas in the digits of cats, *Vet Q* 22:141, 2000.
This relatively large retrospective study of primary and metastatic carcinomas in the digits of cats found that most of these tumors represent metastases from primary pulmonary carcinomas.

Wobeser BK, Kidney BA, Powers BE, et al: Diagnoses and clinical outcomes associated with surgically amputated canine digits submitted to multiple veterinary diagnostic laboratories, *Vet Pathol* 44:355, 2007.
This large retrospective study evaluated the prevalence, prognosis, and survival times of neoplasms of the canine digit.

Wobeser BK, Kidney BA, Powers BE, et al: Diagnoses and clinical outcomes associated with surgically amputated feline digits submitted to multiple veterinary diagnostic laboratories, *Vet Pathol* 44:362, 2007.
This large retrospective study evaluated the prevalence, prognosis, and survival times of neoplasms of the feline digit.

*For a complete list of the references cited in this chapter, please go to www.smallanimaloncology.com.

SECTION C: Foot Pad Tumors

Kim D. Johnson

KEY POINTS

- Tumors of the foot pad are rare in dogs and cats, with forelimb lesions predominating.
- Malignant melanoma, squamous cell carcinoma, sarcoma, mastocytoma, liposarcoma, eccrine sweat gland tumor, lymphangioma and lymphangiosarcoma have been reported to occur in the canine foot pad, with a few studies reporting undifferentiated sarcoma, hemangiosarcoma, and squamous cell carcinoma in the foot pad of cats.
- Treatment involving digit or limb amputation, along with chemotherapy and radiation can prolong survival.

Clinical Behavior

The heavily pigmented foot pad is the toughest area of canine and feline skin. The surface of the pads is smooth in cats and rough in dogs. The thick pads insulate the feet and serve as the "housing" for retracted claws. This specialized part of the body absorbs the shock and pressure from standing, running, and jump landings. The thick epidermis protects against mechanical trauma, and the large fat deposits, also referred to as the *digital cushion*, provide shock absorbing elasticity.[1-4] The pad areas on the digits are referred to as the *digital pads*, and the larger pads located more proximally are referred to as the *metacarpal pad* on the forelimb and the *metatarsal pad* on the hind limb. A small non-weight-bearing carpal pad also exists on the forelimb[2] (Figure 23-6). Squamous cell carcinoma, sarcoma, mastocytoma, liposarcoma, eccrine

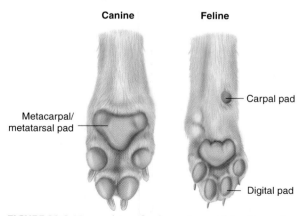

FIGURE 23-6 Nomenclature for the canine and feline foot pad.

BOX 23-3 PATHOLOGY ASSOCIATED WITH THE FOOT PADS IN DOGS

Non-neoplastic
Trauma
  Physical
  Chemical
  Thermal
Foreign body
Infection
  Bacterial
  Mycotic
  Viral
Autoimmune disorder
Vasculitis

Neoplastic
Benign
  Histiocytoma
  Basal cell tumor
  Lymphangioma
  Fibroma
Malignant
  Malignant melanoma
  Mastocytoma/mast cell tumor
  Squamous cell carcinoma
  Sarcoma
  Hemangiosarcoma
  Plasmacytoma
  Fibrosarcoma
  Liposarcoma
  Eccrine sweat gland adenocarcinoma
  Mixed carcinoma of the sweat gland
  Lymphangiosarcoma
  Atrichial sweat gland adenocarcinoma
  Angioleiomyosarcoma
  Myxosarcoma

sweat gland tumor, melanocytic tumors, atrichial sweat gland adenocarcinoma, lymphangioma, lymphangiosarcoma, and others have been reported to occur in the canine foot pad, with a few studies reporting undifferentiated sarcoma, hemangiosarcoma, and squamous cell carcinoma in the foot pad of cats (Boxes 23-3 and 23-4). In a retrospective review of 16 cases of canine foot pad tumors by the author and others, malignant

BOX 23-4 PATHOLOGY ASSOCIATED WITH THE FOOT PADS IN CATS

Non-neoplastic
Eosinophilic granuloma complex
Plasma cell pododermatitis
Trauma
   Physical
   Chemical
   Thermal
Multiple cutaneous horns
Foreign body
Infection
   Bacterial
   Mycotic
Neoplastic
Benign
   Histiocytoma
   Basal cell tumor
Malignant
   Malignant melanoma
   Squamous cell carcinoma
   Undifferentiated sarcoma
   Apocrine gland adenocarcinoma
   Hemangiosarcoma

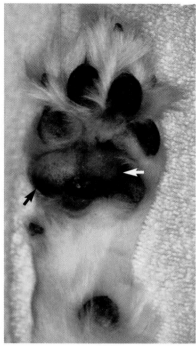

FIGURE 23-7 Myxosarcoma *(arrows)* was diagnosed in this dog that presented for soft tissue swelling of the metacarpal pad.

melanoma was the most common tumor type diagnosed (unpublished data). The prevalence of foot pad tumors in dogs and cats has not been reported but this appears to be a very rare condition in both species.

Etiology/Risk Factors

The cause of footpad tumors is unknown; however, the location of the pad tissue increases the likelihood of exposure to environmental carcinogens and trauma. In addition, genetic susceptibility may play a role. The vertical force that dogs exert on the front foot pads is approximately 1.1 times the body weight compared with the 0.8 times the body weight exerted on the back foot pads. This may help explain the predominance of pad tumors in the forelimbs.[5-7] In a case report of a cat with undifferentiated sarcoma affecting several foot pads, exposure to beryllium from old broken fluorescent tubes was postulated to be the cause.[8]

Clinical Features

Foot pad tumors occur in relatively old dogs and cats with a possible predilection for the metacarpal pad. Affected animals show signs such as swelling, bleeding,

non-healing wounds, lameness or lack of weight bearing, pain on palpation of the pad, excessive licking, discoloration of the pad, or a visible tumor on the footpad (Figures 23-7 and 23-8).[4,6,7,9-12]

Metastasis

The metastatic rate for foot pad tumors is dependent upon tumor histology. Of 16 dogs with footpad tumors in a study conducted by the author, none had evidence of pulmonary metastatic disease at the time of diagnosis, but three had lymph node metastasis (unpublished data).

Diagnosis and Staging

Complete clinical staging includes a minimum database (complete blood count, chemistry panel, urinalysis), three-view thoracic radiographs and radiographs of the affected limb. Fine-needle aspiration and cytology or surgical biopsies are the most commonly used methods to determine the type of tumor affecting a pad. Regional lymph node evaluation by fine-needle aspiration should be attempted to assess for metastasis. Advanced diagnostic imaging such as CT may be necessary for radiation therapy planning.

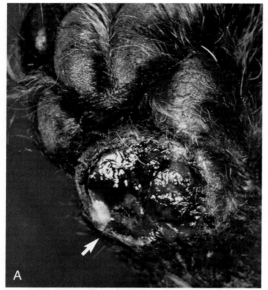

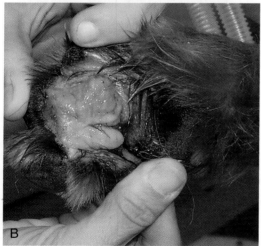

FIGURE 23-8 These ulcerative lesions of the canine footpad were diagnosed as a melanoma (**A**) and a mast cell tumor (**B**).

Treatment Modalities

Neoplasia involving the pad may require complete resection of the epidermal surface and underlying adipose tissue. Because of the constant pressure and use of the foot, wound healing may be complicated when major resections are performed. Several surgical techniques are reported to eradicate pad disease, including digital pad transposition, digit or limb amputation, with the type of reconstruction dictated by the extent and position of the surgical defect.[1,2,4,6,12] Results of chemotherapy and radiation therapy are limited to case reports; thus, efficacy of these treatment modalities for primary therapy is unclear. Adjuvant chemotherapy or radiation therapy may be indicated for lesions that cannot be completely excised or when histology suggests a high likelihood of metastasis.

Prognosis and Survival

Surgical excision may include digital or limb amputation and carries the potential for cure. In one case report, surgery eliminated local disease and resulted in normal weight-bearing within 1 to 2 months following surgery.[12] Outcomes after radiation or chemotherapy for pad tumors have not previously been summarized in the veterinary literature. In the author's review of 16 cases of canine pad tumors, diagnoses included soft-tissue sarcomas, malignant melanomas, histiocytoma, basal cell tumors, and squamous cell carcinoma. Treatment data are available for 13 of 16 cases, and treatment response data are available for 11 of the 13 cases. Various treatments were pursued, including digit and limb amputations, radiation therapy, chemotherapy, and a DNA vaccine. Complete responses were reported for 9 of the 11 cases, whereas 2 of the 11 had partial responses. Patients diagnosed with malignant melanoma had shorter survival times than other tumor types.

Selected References*

Hutton WC, Freeman MAR, Swanson SAV: The forces exerted on the pads of the walking dog, *J Small Anim Pract* 10:71, 1969.
Provides the first description of forelimb versus hind limb weight distribution during ambulation.
Olsen D, Straw RC, Withrow SJ, et al: Digital pad transposition for replacement of the metacarpal or metatarsal pad in dogs, *J Am Anim Hosp Assoc* 33:337, 1997.
Describes a unique surgical option for tumors of the canine foot pad.
Swaim SF, Garret PD: Foot salvage techniques in dogs and cats: options, "do's" and "don'ts," *J Am Anim Hosp Assoc* 21:511, 1985.
Describes foot pad pathology and various treatment modalities available.

■ *For a complete list of the references cited in this chapter, please go to www.smallanimaloncology.com.

SECTION D: Mast Cell Tumors

Dudley L. McCaw

KEY POINTS

- Surgery is the best treatment for mast cell tumors.
- Surgery should include tissue for 2 cm laterally from the tumor and to the next fascial plane deep.
- Canine mast cell tumors should be histopathologically graded and mitotic index determined.
- Feline mast cell tumors are usually less aggressive than canine.
- The grading criteria used for dogs are not reliable for feline mast cell tumors.

Mast cell tumors (MCTs) can occur in any location but are commonly described as cutaneous or visceral. In dogs, cutaneous MCTs are the more common form and perhaps the most frustrating tumors because their clinical course ranges from a benign tumor that clinically never affects the dog to an aggressive tumor that causes the dog's demise within a few weeks. The clinical course of visceral (occurring in spleen, liver, intestines) MCTs in dogs (Box 23-5) is more predictable but generally fatal. Both cutaneous and visceral MCTs are less aggressive in cats.

CANINE MAST CELL TUMORS

Cutaneous Mast Cell Tumors

Appearance of MCTs is variable; therefore, all skin masses should be cytologically examined. Studies from Australia, Canada, Greece, United Kingdom, United

---

BOX 23-5 CANINE VISCERAL MAST CELL TUMORS

- Involvement of visceral organs (spleen, liver, intestines, stomach, abdominal lymph nodes)
  - Uncommon in dogs without history of a cutaneous mast cell tumor.[31]
  - Most often in the gastrointestinal tract, especially the small intestine.
    - Common signs are vomiting, diarrhea, and melena.
    - Survival is short—usually fewer than 30 days.[31]
    - Most reported cases have been Maltese and other small dogs.[32]

States, and Zimbabwe suggest that MCTs are the most common canine skin tumor, accounting for 13% to 20% of skin tumors.[1-9] Most cases of cutaneous MCT involve single lesions; however, about 9% present with multiple tumors.[10]

Causes

As with most canine tumors, the cause of MCTs is largely unknown. A report of an MCT occurring in a surgical scar 16 months after a bite wound would suggest inflammation as a cause.[11] Certain breeds have been historically reported to be predisposed to MCTs, including the boxer and Boston terrier.[12] More recent reports suggest that Labrador and Golden retrievers may be overrepresented.[13,14] Injection of moxidectin for heartworm prevention has been associated with an increased risk of MCT development.[15] Genetic changes are responsible for some mast cell tumors, with abnormalities of the c-kit oncogene present in 33% of tumors.[16] Contrary to the case for some other skin tumors, sunlight exposure appears not to be a cause.[2,7,9]

Clinical Course

Mast cell tumors can occur in any tissue of the body but are most common in the skin. The presentation is varied, and the physical appearance is unpredictable and can be mistaken for other tumors, especially lipomas. Some tumors can be present for long periods and not grow, whereas others grow very rapidly. The history may also include a mass that has been present for a long time but is now growing rapidly. This would suggest a change in degree of malignancy. Metastasis is most often to the regional lymph nodes, then to liver and spleen, but can go directly to liver or spleen. As time passes, MCTs can spread to any organ.

Mast cell tumors are known to secrete histamine, which promotes hydrochloric acid release from the parietal cells of the stomach and can lead to gastric ulceration. Thus, patients may present with clinical signs referable to gastric ulceration, rather than for an identified cutaneous mass. Local release of histamine from malignant mast cells may initially cause lesions that are misdiagnosed as insect bites, based on appearance and acute swelling. A waxing and waning course of tumor swelling and regression is suggestive of MCT.

Prognosis

Historically, 46% of dogs with cutaneous MCTs died as a result of the tumor.[17] Fortunately, improved therapy has reduced the percentage of dogs that die of their disease. As clinicians, we would like to be able to provide an accurate prognosis to our clients, and there are certain factors that can aid us in arriving at a prognosis, including those discussed below.

Clinical Staging

Staging of tumors is based upon the extent of disease in the body, with higher stage disease generally warranting a worse prognosis. The process of staging involves assessing the number and size of the tumors (T), local and distant lymph nodes (N), and sites of potential distant metastasis (M).

Tumor. Complete excision of a MCT leads to a better prognosis; thus, smaller tumors have a better prognosis than large tumors that cannot be completely excised.[18] Most dogs have single MCTs; however, multiple tumors occur in 7% to 14% of cases.[10,19] The prognosis is the same in cases with single or multiple tumors, provided that all the tumors are completely excised.[10,14,20] Although the traditional staging system for canine cutaneous MCT has automatically placed dogs with multiple cutaneous lesions into Stage III, there is interest amongst the veterinary oncology community in redefining the staging categories such that Stage III designation is a reflection of more advanced disease, rather than just multiple primary MCTs that may not have aggressive clinical behavior.[14,20]

Node. Since cutaneous MCT likes to spread to the regional lymph node, it should be evaluated. Even if the node is normal size, it should be aspirated because malignant cells can be present without the node being enlarged. A problem with mast cells is that the mast cells in the node may be inflammatory. Normal lymph nodes can contain an average of 5 mast cells in the typical cytology slide and up to 16 per slide.[21] Spread of a MCT to a lymph node indicates the malignant nature of that tumor; therefore, the prognosis worsens.

Metastasis. Mast cell tumors spread to the spleen and liver more commonly if the regional lymph node is involved, but can spread without local node involvement; therefore, abdominal ultrasound should be performed with aspiration of the spleen and/or liver if suspicious lesions are present.[22] Thoracic radiographs, which should be taken to check for metastasis of most tumors, are typically unrewarding for MCTs because most MCTs that spread to lungs do so in a diffuse pattern that will not be apparent radiographically. However,

nodal metastasis may be detected in some cases, so thoracic radiographs are indicated when the primary tumor is located in an area that would have lymphatic drainage to nodes within the thoracic cavity.

Grading

In an effort to predict their behavior after surgical removal, MCTs are graded I, II, or III. The grading is based upon degree of cellular differentiation, degree of cellular pleomorphism, characteristics of the cytoplasmic granules, frequency of mitotic figures, and depth of invasion.[17] Higher grade indicates a worse prognosis, and this is most pronounced in a grade III tumor, which is usually very malignant and likely to metastasize.

Treatment and Outcome

Effective treatment options are surgery, radiation therapy, and chemotherapy (Box 23-6).

Surgery

Surgical removal is the primary treatment and should be performed in all cases if possible. Surgical margins should be at least 2 cm laterally and include the next fascial plane deep.[23] The removed tissue must be examined histopathologically to determine tumor grade and completeness of excision. In addition, use of immunohistochemical markers for Ki67 and c-kit mutations (using CD117), as well as indicators of proliferation including AgNOR staining and mitotic index, are recommended to help determine if adjuvant therapy is needed.[24] Mitotic index is especially helpful in determining MCT behavior and is readily available because it is determined by the pathologist during routine histopathology. If the mitotic index (number of mitotic figures per ten 400× fields) is ≤ 5, the reported median survival is 70 months; if > 5, the median survival is 2 months regardless of tumor grade.[25]

Radiation Therapy

Mast cell tumors are sensitive to radiation, which is used as a primary treatment when surgery is not an option or as adjuvant therapy when the excision has been incomplete.[26] When excision is incomplete, irradiation of a 3-cm margin around the surgical scar as a minimum, and 5 cm if anatomically possible, decreases tumor recurrence.[27]

Chemotherapy

Chemotherapy is a less effective treatment than surgery and radiation. The role of chemotherapy in treating MCTs is for treating cases in which systemic spread exists. The most effective chemotherapy is prednisone and vinblastine. Overall response rate is about 50%, with the complete resolution of tumors in about one

---

BOX 23-6   CLINICAL MANAGEMENT OF CANINE MAST CELL TUMORS

- Complete evaluation for multiple tumors and metastasis (lymph node, spleen, liver, bone marrow).
- Surgical removal is the recommended procedure.
  - ° Spread of tumor to visceral organs necessitates chemotherapy.
- Regional lymph node involvement requires removing the tumor and lymph node.
  - ° Excision with margins of at least 2 cm laterally and the next fascial plane deep.
- Submitted for histopathological examination for grading and checking for complete excision. Panel of proliferation markers (Ki67, AgNOR, CD117, and mitotic index) is useful for predicting prognosis and informing therapy decisions.
- If surgical excision is complete:
  - ° Fewer than 10% of grade I, fewer than 20% of grade II, and more than 80% of grade III tumor will recur locally and/or metastasize.
    - ▪ Monitor grade I or II tumors for recurrence.
    - ▪ Grade III tumors: chemotherapy for metastasis and radiation to lessen chance of local recurrence.
- If the excision is not complete:
  - ° Grade I or II: Surgery to remove the surgical scar and surrounding tissue to obtain clean margins. Check margins with histopathology. Complete margins, no further treatment. Monitor for recurrence.
    - ▪ If the margins are still involved, then radiation therapy. If not available, then chemotherapy with vinblastine/prednisone.
  - ° Grade III: Radiation and chemotherapy
- Multiple tumors: surgically remove all and check all histopathologically for grade and margins. Further treatment should be based on each individual tumor.
- Recurrence of tumor, whether local or distant, should be treated as new tumor.
- Tumors too large to be surgically removed:
  - ° Radiation therapy. If not available, chemotherapy.
- Any dog that has a grossly detectable tumor:
  - ° Give H_1 (diphenhydramine) and H_2 (ranitidine, famotidine) blockers or a proton pump inhibitor (omeprazole).

---

third of the dogs.[13] Duration of response is reported to be from 28 to >645 days.[13] The same chemotherapy protocol was used in dogs with incomplete surgical margins when radiation therapy was not available and only 5% of tumors recurred locally.[28] Lomustine given orally every 3 weeks is a good choice when tumors do not respond to vinblastine/prednisone. About half the dogs will have some reduction in tumor size, but very few will completely resolve.[29] A potentially effective chemotherapy involves the use of receptor tyrosine kinase inhibitors. As mentioned in the causes of cancer, mutations in the c-kit gene allow for the constitutive activation of the tyrosine kinase signaling pathways, resulting in overstimulation for cell growth. The recently approved compound Palladia (Pfizer Animal Health, New York) has the ability to block the tyrosine kinase signaling, thus reversing some of the cell growth stimulation. Fifty percent of dogs with MCTs that were given Palladia in clinical trials had tumor shrinkage.[16] An investigational drug that shows promise as adjuvant immunotherapy against canine MCT is LDI-100 (Milkhaus Veterinary Products, Delanson, NY). This compound, which is a combination of BCG and hCG, was administered subcutaneously to 46 dogs with Grade II or III cutaneous MCT and provided responses in 28.6% of dogs compared with 11.7% in the control group of 49 dogs receiving single-agent vinblastine.[30]

FELINE MAST CELL TUMORS

Mast cell tumors in cats can be cutaneous or visceral. The cutaneous tumors are classified as mast cell or histiocytic type. Visceral mast cell tumors occur in the spleen, liver, intestines, and stomach.

Cutaneous Mast Cell Tumors

See Box 23-7.

Visceral Mast Cell Tumors

See Box 23-8.

BOX 23-7   FELINE CUTANEOUS MAST CELL TUMORS

Mast Cell Type
- Account for about 20% of skin tumors in cats, making them the second most common skin tumor after basal cell carcinomas.[33]
- The average age of occurrence is 10 years.
- Siamese are predisposed.[33]
- The usual appearance is a 0.5- to 2-cm mass that is usually hairless and often ulcerated.[33,34] The most common location is the head, especially the base of the pinna.[33]
- Diagnosis of feline mast cells can be made by fine-needle aspiration. Their cytologic appearance is individual round cell containing metachromatic granules that are smaller than other species.[35]
- The grading system used in dogs does not predict outcome in cats.[36]

Clinical Course
- Solitary tumors are most common, with about 12% having multiple tumors.[36]
- Usually do not metastasize; however, spread to other skin locations or to spleen has been recognized.[35,37]
- Sometimes multiple skin mast cell tumors may be the result of cutaneous metastasis of a visceral mast cell tumor.[37]

Treatment
- Surgical removal with wide excision to remove the complete tumor.
   ° Recurrence following surgery occurs in about 15% of cases.
      ▪ No difference in recurrence based upon completeness of the surgical excision.
      ▪ Most recurrences are at distant cutaneous sites.[36]
   ° Radiation therapy appears to be effective.[38]
   ° Corticosteroids are not effective.[35]

Histiocytic Type
- Occurs in young cats.
- With microscopy, no granules can be seen.
   ° Electron microscopy reveals granules that resemble those of mast cells.[39]
- Appear as flat lesions commonly on the head of cats < 4 years of age.
   ° Originally described as a disease of Siamese[39]
   ° Larger study disputes this.[33]
- Lesions will spontaneously regress.

BOX 23-8   FELINE VISCERAL MAST CELL TUMORS

- Occur in the spleen, liver, intestines, or stomach.
- Splenic mast cell tumors occur frequently.
   ° Are the most common splenic disease in cats.[40]

Diagnosis
   ° Palpation of enlarged spleen, liver, or intestinal mass
   ° Mass detected on ultrasound
   ° Cytologic examination of aspirates taken from the affected organs will be indicative of mast cell disease
   ° Circulating mast cells are commonly found

Treatment and Prognosis
   ° In spite of what appears to be a severe disease, many cats with splenic mast cell tumor will benefit from removal of the spleen.
   ° Splenectomy is beneficial even if circulating mast cells or mast cell infiltration in the liver is present.
   ° Cats are likely to survive at least 8 months after splenectomy.
   ° Tumors involving the gastrointestinal tract carry a poor prognosis.[41]

Selected References*

Miller MA, Nelson SL, Turk JR, et al: Cutaneous neoplasia in 340 cats, *Vet Pathol* 28:389, 1991.
Report of a large number of feline skin tumors and describes frequency and description of mast cell tumors.

Mullins MN, Dernell WS, Withrow SJ, et al: Evaluation of prognostic factors associated with outcome in dogs with multiple cutaneous mast cell tumors treated with surgery with and without adjuvant treatment: 54 cases (1998-2004), *J Am Vet Med Assoc* 228:91, 2000.
Describes large number of cases of multiple mast cell tumors in dogs and shows that multiple tumors do not have a worse prognosis than single tumors. Previously multiple tumors were thought to be associated with a poor prognosis.

Murphy S, Sparkes AH, Blunden AS, et al: Effects of stage and number of tumors on prognosis of dogs with cutaneous mast cell tumours, *Vet Rec* 158:287, 2006.
This paper proposes changing the grading scheme for cutaneous MCT as it applies to dogs with multiple cutaneous lesions.

Patniak AK, Ehler WJ, MacEwen EG: Canine cutaneous mast cell tumor: morphologic grading and survival time in 83 dogs, *Vet Pathol* 21:469, 1984.
Description of the most commonly used grading system for canine mast cell tumors.

Scase TJ, Edwards D, Miller J, et al: Canine mast cell tumors: correlation of apoptosis and proliferation markers with prognosis, *J Vet Intern Med* 20:151, 2006.
Discusses the use of proliferation markers applied to biopsy samples to determine prognosis for dogs with MCT.

Thamm DH, Mauldin EA, Vail DM: Prednisone and vinblastine chemotherapy for canine mast cell tumor – 41 cases (1992-1997), *J Vet Intern Med* 13:491, 1999.
Provides the chemotherapy protocol that is most effective against canine mast cell tumors.

■ *For a complete list of the references cited in this chapter, please go to www.smallanimaloncology.com.

SECTION E: Soft-Tissue Sarcomas

Kim A. Selting

KEY POINTS

- Soft-tissue sarcomas are mesenchymal tumors characterized by locally aggressive behavior and high recurrence rates.
- Excellent long-term control of these tumors can be achieved by combining surgery and radiation therapy in dogs and cats.
- The role of chemotherapy is not clearly defined but is often recommended for non-resectable or high-grade tumors. The benefit of chemotherapy in terms of improving local control is more compelling than for systemic control.

Clinical Behavior

The term *sarcoma* is applied to malignant neoplasms of mesenchymal origin (mesoderm and some neuroectoderm). This includes tissues that provide structural support to the body. Soft-tissue sarcomas (STSs) are tumors derived from nonepithelial extraskeletal tissue and include tumors of fat, muscle, and connective tissue.[1] There are a wide variety of tumors in this category (Box 23-9). Hemangiopericytomas are theoretically derived from pericytes surrounding blood vessels and tend to be low-grade sarcomas[2]; however, the true origin of these tumors has been questioned. Hemangiosarcoma and extraskeletal osteosarcoma are more systemically aggressive than other STS. Hemangiosarcoma of the skin and subcutis will be presented here, and visceral hemangiosarcoma and extraskeletal osteosarcoma are presented elsewhere. Similarly, visceral tumors such as

---

BOX 23-9 COMMON SOFT-TISSUE SARCOMAS

Histologic Subtypes of Soft-Tissue Sarcoma
Fibrosarcoma
Liposarcoma
Myxosarcoma
Malignant fibrous histiocytoma
Peripheral nerve sheath tumor (PNST)—also called neurofibrosarcoma or schwannoma
Leiomyosarcoma
Rhabdomyosarcoma
Hemangiopericytoma (see text)

*This group of tumors behaves similarly based upon histologic criteria of grade such as mitotic index, regardless of histologic subtype. Exact cell lineage can sometimes be difficult to determine based on routine histopathology and morphology, although immunohistochemistry can better define cell type. Tumors without distinguishing features may be reported as sarcomas or spindle cell tumors.

gastrointestinal and reproductive smooth muscle tumors are discussed elsewhere.

Behavior of STS is strongly linked to histologic characteristics, and a grading scheme has been established for veterinary medicine, similar to that used in human medicine. Although in human medicine the final grade based upon percent necrosis, degree of differentiation, and mitotic index is independently associated with outcome, in veterinary medicine mitotic index has been most helpful.[1,3,4]

STS can occur anywhere in the body, and these tumors are locally aggressive (Figure 23-9). Although metastasis can occur in 40% to 50% of dogs with high-grade STS (grade 3), the metastatic rate for low- to moderate-grade tumors (grades 1 and 2) is generally < 20%.[4-6] Treatment approach typically parallels tumor behavior, and local modalities such as surgery and radiation therapy are the mainstay of treatment. STS occur most commonly in large-breed dogs, with Rhodesian ridgebacks and mixed-breed dogs overrepresented in one study.[6] Flat-coated retrievers seem to be at risk for developing STS (more than half the reported malignancies in one survey), specifically malignant fibrous histiocytoma (more than half the reported STS).[7-9]

Skin and subcutis are common locations for hemangiosarcoma, but behavior differs from their visceral counterpart (see Section A for additional information). In general, the deeper within the body a hemangiosarcoma is located, the more systemically aggressive it will behave. Lesions truly limited to the skin can often be treated with local therapy only, whereas subcuticular

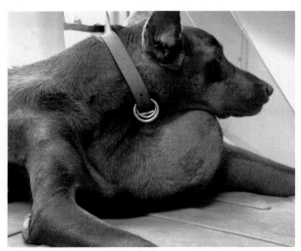

FIGURE 23-9 Because of their locally aggressive behavior, soft-tissue sarcomas can grow to be quite large without causing death of the animal.

involvement would warrant both surgery and chemotherapy. Tumors that invade muscle are as aggressive as visceral hemangiosarcoma.

Etiology

The most widely publicized cause of soft-tissue sarcoma is the association of vaccination and sarcoma development in cats. Although feline leukemia virus and rabies vaccination have been most commonly implicated, long-acting injectable medications such as penicillin and methylprednisolone acetate are also of concern.[10,11] Risk factors include multiple vaccinations at one site, although no individual vaccine manufacturer or brand has been implicated.[10] Vaccine practices such as reused syringes, vaccination at time of viral infection, history of trauma at the tumor site, mixing vaccines within the same syringe, needle gauge, massaging the vaccination site, or residence of the cat did not affect risk in one multi-center study, although vaccine temperature before injection (cold vaccinations associated with odds ratio of approximately 2) may be related to sarcoma formation.[10] Interestingly, reports of dogs with sarcomas at injection sites are rare, suggesting variation across species in response to vaccines and their components. Limited information suggests similar histopathologic characteristics for these tumors in dogs compared with cats.[12]

In addition to breed predilections in dogs, alterations in genetic content such as loss of chromosomes, mutation of p53 tumor suppressor gene or amplification of the p53 regulatory molecule mdm2, and point mutations in the *neu* oncogene, have been investigated.[13-15] Cutaneous hemangiosarcoma has been linked to ultraviolet light exposure in non-haired skin such as the ventral abdomen.

Clinical and Laboratory Abnormalities

Dogs and cats with STS typically are presented for the mass itself. Depending upon location, clinical signs referable to the mass may be seen, such as difficulty eating with oral tumors or neurologic deficits with tumors located near the spine or nerve roots. Schwannomas have been reported in association with the trigeminal nerve.[16,17] Rhabdomyosarcomas have been found often in the bladder, tongue, heart, and larynx, and can be seen in young dogs.[18-23] An interesting subtype of oral fibrosarcoma has been described in which histologically low-grade, biologically high-grade tumors may appear benign on histopathology, but behave in an aggressive, fast-growing manner. These tumors are often seen in Golden retrievers and are more common on the maxilla.[24]

There are no findings specific to, nor pathognomonic for, STS on hematology or blood chemistry in cats and dogs. Isolated case reports of schwannoma and leiomyosarcoma describe paraneoplastic erythrocytosis, possibly caused by erythropoietin production by the tumor cells.[25-27]

Histopathologically, vaccine-induced STSs are characterized by a transition zone with inflammation, cystic areas, aluminum-containing macrophages, and the presence of myofibroblasts. In addition, these tumors are often positive by immunohistochemistry for platelet-derived growth factor receptor, as well as other growth factors and expression of p53.[28-30] Also noted in vaccine-associated STS, multi-nucleated giant cells correspond to high-grade tumors when present.[31] Tissue of origin for STS in general ascertained is often by a combination of morphologic and immunohistochemical findings.[32] For example, schwannomas exhibit a characteristic Antoni A and B pattern.[15] Hemangiopericytomas similarly have a characteristic perivascular whorled pattern in most cases, or identifiable storiform or epithelioid patterns in some cases.[33]

Diagnosis and Staging

Mesenchymal tumors often have low yield on fine-needle aspiration, and neoplastic fibroblasts can sometimes be difficult to differentiate from reactive fibroplasia.[6] However, fine-needle aspiration is still an appropriate first step in diagnosis since it can help to rule out round cell and epithelial tumors, and the cells may be abnormal enough to suggest sarcoma, especially in the absence of inflammation. Reports cite up to 93% accuracy with high specificity for diagnosis of malignant mesenchymal tumor with cytology, although determination of histologic subtype is unreliable.[34,35]

As with other tumor types, staging is very important to success of treatment. If a patient has metastatic disease at the time of diagnosis, local therapy will only be palliative. Sarcomas most commonly spread hematogenously, rather than by lymphatics, which means that the lungs are the most common site of metastasis. Therefore, three-view thoracic radiographs are very important (right lateral, left lateral, and ventrodorsal) since it is possible to miss approximately 20% of metastasis with only one lateral view. Visceral sarcomas will often metastasize to the liver. Therefore, abdominal ultrasound is important for complete staging for patients with tumors located in the abdomen or caudal half of the body. Lastly, although lymph nodes are a less common route of spread, the regional lymph node should be checked by palpation and, if possible, aspiration or biopsy.

Ultimately the definitive diagnosis lies in the biopsy. An incisional biopsy should be performed in many cases to improve planning of the definitive surgery. Sarcomas are often locally invasive and require wide excision; therefore, careful surgical planning is critical to treatment success. In addition, advanced imaging of the tumor (CT, MRI, ultrasound) can help determine the likelihood of surgical success and the possible use of radiation therapy in the adjuvant (after surgery) or neoadjuvant (before surgery) setting.

Treatment Options

Surgery is the first treatment of choice when possible, and excision should involve gross tumor margins of at least 3 cm laterally and one fascial plane deep of normal tissue. Fascial planes appear to act as biologic barriers for sarcomas. Histologic margins of at least 5 mm laterally and at least one fascial plane deep will offer excellent local control.[36] Sarcomas can develop a characteristic "pseudocapsule," which is a non-adherent layer between the bulk of the tumor and the underlying tissue. Tumor cells invade tissue beyond the pseudocapsule, which means that a tumor that "shells out" easily has certainly left microscopic tumor behind and recurrence is highly likely. When surgery is incomplete, or if resection of a mass is not possible, radiation therapy or scar re-excision can be used to improve local tumor control, with median survival times exceeding 3 years, and reported up to 5 years.[37-39] In both human and veterinary medicine, surgery followed by radiation therapy for STS of the extremities has been found to be equivalent to amputation for low-grade tumors.[37,40]

As with dogs, standard-of-care treatment for cats with vaccine-associated STS includes surgery and radiation therapy. Because of the very locally aggressive behavior of this tumor in cats, and the prevalence at vaccine injection sites including the interscapular space, which makes complete excision challenging, radiation therapy is routinely recommended following surgery. Median survival times often exceed 2 years, and chemotherapy does not seem to improve outcome when added to surgery and radiation therapy, although it may prolong disease-free interval if given concurrently.[41-43]

The role of chemotherapy is much less clearly defined. While high-grade sarcomas have up to a 40% to 50% risk of systemic metastasis, the benefit of chemotherapy has not been proven.[5] In large meta-analyses of STS in people, there is a marginal, if any, benefit to long-term survival, although there does appear to be a modest improvement in local control with adjuvant chemotherapy.[44] Doxorubicin is considered the single most effective agent in this setting and has been used alone and in combination with alkylating agents such as cyclophosphamide, ifosfamide, and dacarbazine in dogs, cats, and people.[45,46] Interestingly, combination chemotherapy in people offers little advantage over single-agent doxorubicin regimens.[47,48]

TABLE 23-4   PROGNOSTIC FACTORS AND OUTCOME FOR CANINE SOFT-TISSUE SARCOMAS*

Prognostic Factor	Measure	Outcome	Statistical Significance	Reference
Margins	Complete	Median tumor-free interval not reached[4]	Prognostic on multivariate analysis[4]	4,6,36,61
	Incomplete	10.5 times more likely to develop recurrence[4] Median tumor-free interval 1850 days[4]		
Grade	Grade 1	13% metastasis	Significant on univariate but not multivariate for both development of metastasis and overall survival	4
	Grade 2	7% metastasis		
	Grade 3	41% metastasis		
Mitotic index[†]	≥9	Median ST 49 wks	Significant $P < .01$	2
	<9	Median ST 118 wks		
	>19	Median ST 236 days	Significant on univariate analysis	4
	10-19	Median ST 532 days		
	<10	Median ST 1444 days		
	≥20	5 times more likely to develop metastasis, and 2.5 times more likely to die of tumor-related causes	Significant on multivariate analysis	4
Percent necrosis	≥10%	2.78 times more likely to die of tumor-related causes		
Location	Oral	Median ST = 540 days	$P = .0167$	38
	Non-oral	Median ST = 2270 days		
	Spinal tumors	32% euthanized at surgery, median ST for PNST = 180 days	No control group	62
	Distal to stifle or elbow	No dogs developed metastasis	n/a	4
Prior surgery	Yes	More likely to develop local recurrence, OR = 1.6, but less likely to develop metastasis, OR = 0.2	$P = .43$ for local, $P = .0029$ for distant recurrence/ metastasis	61
Hyperthermia	Yes	More likely to develop local recurrence, OR = 2.4, and metastasis, OR = 8.1	$P = .22$ for local, $P = .0002$ for distant recurrence/ metastasis	61
Neuter status	Intact	More likely to develop metastasis, OR = 5.2, no bearing on local recurrence	Significant on univariate and multivariate (for metastasis)	61
Total radiation dose	57 Gy in 3 Gy fractions	More likely to have local tumor control than other radiation protocols	$P = .007$	61
Adjuvant chemo-therapy	Doxorubicin for resected high-grade tumors	n = 21 with and 18 without doxorubicin Overall DFI = 724 days, median ST = 856 days	No difference between groups	5

*From selected references

[†]*Mitotic index* = number of mitotic figures per ten 400× high-powered fields; *DFI*, disease-free interval; *OR*, odds ratio; *ST*, survival time.

In cats, doxorubicin may offer improved local control following excision of vaccine-associated sarcoma. Whereas surgical resection alone often results in early recurrence within the first 3 to 6 months, the addition of postoperative doxorubicin yielded a median survival time of 1 year.[49,50] Liposome-encapsulated doxorubicin is equally effective but does not allow dose escalation without nephrotoxicity.[50] Chemotherapy may be useful in nonresectable sarcomas in both dogs and cats. Approximately 40% to 50% of cats with vaccine-associated STS will have a clinical response to doxorubicin-based chemotherapy, although responses are short lived and response rates are much lower for dogs.[46,50,51] Novel treatments include electrochemotherapy in which electrical currents applied in biphasic pulses open pores in cell membranes to increase drug delivery. This approach has been tried with bleomycin in cats and dogs with STS with some success.[52-54]

Prognosis

Prognosis for soft-tissue sarcomas is often good if complete excision can be achieved and if the tumor is low grade (Table 23-4). Complete excision can be difficult because of the locally aggressive nature of STS, and recurrence rates with incomplete excision following surgery alone can be high.[55-57] Wide excision, however, can offer surgical cure.[6] More axially located nerve sheath tumors may have a less favorable outcome than those that are peripherally located.[4,38,58] Fixation of the mass to surrounding tissues has been listed as a negative prognostic factor for STS but has not been evaluated prospectively.[59] Additional prognostic factors and outcome following treatment are summarized in Table 23-4. Unfortunately, there are no tests currently available to better determine which STS is likely to metastasize and which dogs may respond to chemotherapy. Proliferative indices including Ki67 and AgNORs are becoming commercially available and may offer better definition of grade and behavior of these tumors.

The metastatic rate for cats with vaccine-associated sarcomas is low (15%–22%). Median survival with surgery followed by radiation therapy is approximately 2 years. Although chemotherapy does not seem to improve outcome following surgery and radiation therapy, adjuvant doxorubicin may benefit cats with soft-tissue sarcomas compared with surgery alone. Median time to recurrence was 3 months with surgery alone in one study, and 1 year with surgery followed by doxorubicin chemotherapy in another.[49,50]

Cutaneous hemangiosarcoma often has a favorable prognosis with surgical excision alone. Median survival times approach 2 years.[60]

In conclusion, STSs in dogs, cats, and people include a diverse group of histologic subtypes often considered as a group, the behavior of which depends largely on the histologic characteristics of grade and mitotic index. These tumors are highly locally invasive and often recur with inadequate surgical excision. Metastatic rates are typically low, and the addition of radiation therapy in select cases can markedly improve case outcome.

Selected References*

Clark MA, Fisher C, Judson I, et al: Soft-tissue sarcomas in adults, *N Engl J Med* 353:701, 2005.
Recent, complete review of soft-tissue sarcoma diagnosis and treatment in people. Aspects of treatment closely parallel recommendations for dogs and cats.

Ehrhart NE: Soft-tissue sarcomas in dogs: a review, *J Am Anim Hosp Assoc* 41:241, 2005.
Recent manuscript reviewing diagnostic, therapeutic, and prognostic aspects of case management for dogs with soft-tissue sarcoma.

Hendrick MJ, Brooks JJ: Postvaccinal sarcomas in the cat: histology and immunohistochemistry, *Vet Pathol* 31:126, 1994.
One of the original manuscripts describing the association between vaccination sites and sarcoma formation, this study was published by the pathologist who recognized and popularized the syndrome. This paper focuses on the histologic appearance of these tumors and discusses the epidemiology.

Kuntz CA, Dernell WS, Powers BE, et al: Prognostic factors for surgical treatment of soft-tissue sarcomas in dogs: 75 cases (1986-1996), *J Am Vet Med Assoc* 211:1147, 1997.
This is the initial study in which the grading system used in people is applied to non-visceral soft-tissue sarcomas in dogs and examines a variety of prognostic factors.

McKnight JA, Mauldin GN, McEntee MC, et al: Radiation treatment for incompletely resected soft-tissue sarcomas in dogs, *J Am Vet Med Assoc* 217:205, 2000.
Dogs in this study had excellent control of their tumors with surgery and radiation therapy, illustrating the fact that amputation is not necessary when soft-tissue sarcomas occur on limbs, similar to human medicine.

Selting KA, Powers BE, Thompson LJ, et al: Outcome of dogs with high-grade soft tissue sarcomas treated with and without adjuvant doxorubicin chemotherapy: 39 cases (1996-2004), *J Am Vet Med Assoc* 227:1442, 2005.
This retrospective study includes a relatively large group of dogs with high-grade soft-tissue sarcoma, and evaluates the lack of benefit of doxorubicin chemotherapy in the truly adjuvant setting.

■ *For a complete list of the references cited in this chapter, please go to www.smallanimaloncology.com.*

SECTION F: Histiocytic Diseases

Craig A. Clifford, Katherine A. Skorupski

KEY POINTS

- The canine histiocytic proliferative disorders (HPDs) include cutaneous histiocytoma, the reactive histiocytoses, histiocytic sarcoma, and hemophagocytic histiocytic sarcoma.
- Cutaneous histiocytoma is most common in young dogs and usually regresses spontaneously.
- The reactive histiocytoses (cutaneous and systemic histiocytosis) are usually responsive to treatment with systemic immunosuppressive therapy.
- Histiocytic sarcoma is associated with a poor prognosis except in cases of localized disease when multi-modality therapy can be effective.
- Hemophagocytic histiocytic sarcoma is most common in the spleen, and no effective treatment has been reported.

The canine histiocytic proliferative disorders (HPDs) encompass a wide spectrum of diseases characterized by a variety of biologic behaviors. These are an extremely frustrating group of diseases because the clinical presentation and behavior and responsiveness to therapy vary tremendously. At the present time, four well-defined HPDs have been considered as recognized in the canine. These include cutaneous histiocytoma, the reactive histiocytoses (cutaneous and systemic histiocytosis), histiocytic sarcoma (localized and disseminated [i.e., malignant histiocytosis]), and hemophagocytic histiocytic sarcoma. Overall, the neoplastic HPDs represent < 1% of all tumors affecting the lymphoreticular system.

CUTANEOUS HISTIOCYTOMA

Histiocytomas are benign dermal tumors of Langerhans' cells that often occur as a single lesion in young dogs typically younger than 3 years of age.[1,2-4] The most commonly affected breeds include Boxers, Dachshunds, cocker spaniels, Great Danes, Shetland Sheepdogs, and Bull Terriers, although any breed may be affected.[5-10] These tumors usually appear as "button-like" raised, hairless lesions that appear suddenly and grow quickly within the first 1 to 4 weeks.[5-10] The extremities, head, ears, and neck are the most common anatomic sites of involvement.

Diagnosis

Histiocytomas are usually easily diagnosed through fine-needle aspiration. Classified as round cell tumors, these tumors usually exfoliate high numbers of pleomorphic round cells with abundant pale grey cytoplasm, centrally located round to slightly indented nuclei, and inconspicuous nucleoli. Inflammatory cell infiltrate may be present and usually precedes spontaneous lesion regression.[5-10] Histopathology demonstrates sheets and cords of pleomorphic histiocytes infiltrating the dermis and subcutis. The presence of CD8+ (cytotoxic) T cells is common in regressing lesions.

Treatment and Prognosis

The majority of histiocytomas will spontaneously regress within 3 months.[5-9] For rare, non-regressing tumors, surgical excision, cryosurgery, or electrosurgery are expected to be curative.[10-12] Cases with multiple histiocytomas may have a more protracted clinical course, but spontaneous resolution of all nodules is still likely.[13]

CUTANEOUS HISTIOCYTOSIS

Cutaneous histiocytosis (CH) represents a benign, diffuse aggregation of histiocytes within the skin and subcutaneous tissue.[13-18] This disease is limited to the skin and subcutis but can be multifocal. Dogs present with multiple cutaneous nodules, crusts, and/or areas of depigmentation located on the face, ears, nose, neck, trunk, extremities (including foot pads), perineum, and scrotum.[13-19] Lesions will often wax and wane.[13-18] Middle-aged to older dogs are commonly affected with no sex predilection; however, Collies and Shetland Sheepdogs may be predisposed.[13-18]

Diagnosis

Cytologic samples from affected areas of skin often resemble granulomatous inflammation because of the presence of large numbers of benign histiocytes possessing abundant cytoplasm, round to indented nuclei, and inconspicuous nucleoli.[8,16,20] Skin biopsy is usually necessary for definitive diagnosis, and findings consist of a pleocellular histiocytic perivascular infiltrate within the dermis and subcutaneous tissue. Infiltrative histiocytes lack criteria of malignancy. Lymphoid infiltrates are also common, and vascular invasion by histiocytes may be present.

Treatment and Prognosis

Cutaneous histiocytosis has a benign clinical course and is often responsive to immunosuppressive therapy.[5,14,15] Prednisone, tetracycline and niacinamide, cyclosporine A, and azathioprine are some of the more commonly used therapies for CH (Table 23-5). In a recent retrospective study evaluating outcome in 32 dogs with CH, all dogs achieved resolution of dermatological lesions, and 9 dogs had one or more relapses.[16] As with other immune-mediated disorders, maintenance therapy may be required to prevent recurrence; however, affected dogs usually enjoy prolonged survival. Spontaneous regressions of CH have also occasionally been reported.

SYSTEMIC HISTIOCYTOSIS

Systemic histiocytosis (SH) represents a disseminated form of CH; together, CH and SH are referred to as the "reactive histiocytoses." SH is characterized by diffuse aggregation of benign histiocytes within the skin (with a high prevalence at mucocutaneous junctions) and ocular and nasal mucosa but can also affect lymph nodes, lung, spleen, liver, and bone marrow.[15,19-24] SH is common in Bernese Mountain Dogs, Rottweilers, Irish Wolfhounds, and Golden and Labrador retrievers.[15,20,22] The age of onset of SH is usually between 3 and 9 years. The exact etiology is unknown but dysregulation of the proliferation, activation, and function of dendritic cells and T cells or their direct interactions following antigenic stimulation is hypothesized.[15,20,22] Superficial lesions may appear erythematous to ulcerated, and they may be asymptomatic or painful. SH can be distinguished from CH by the presence of peripheral lymphadenopathy and/or multi-organ involvement.[15,20-24]

Diagnosis

Dogs with SH may have abnormal laboratory findings including anemia, monocytosis and lymphopenia.[22-25] Similar to CH, cytologic evaluation of involved organs appears much like granulomatous inflammation with large numbers of benign histiocytes with occasional multi-nucleated giant cells.[8,21] Histiocytic cells are large, contain voluminous cytoplasm, and have indented nuclei with variable nucleoli.[8,21] Lymphocytes, eosinophils, and neutrophils may be interspersed with the histiocytic population of cells. Histologically, SH is characterized by multi-centric, nodular, angiocentric histiocytic infiltrates within the deep dermis, panniculus, and other affected organs.[13,21] Variable populations of lymphocytes, neutrophils, and eosinophils may also be present.[22] The histiocytes involved in the pathology of both CH and SH are activated interstitial dendritic cells.[1,4,15,25]

Treatment and Prognosis

SH lesions may wax and wane but generally do not spontaneously resolve. Glucocorticoids and cytotoxic drugs are generally ineffective long term.[12-23] Azathioprine, cyclosporine A, or leflunomide have yielded long-term control in some cases, and a response to doxorubicin has been reported (see Table 23-5).[12-23] Ocular lesions may require the application of cyclosporine-containing ophthalmic drops. The clinical course of this disease is often prolonged but rarely results in death. Episodic periods of response followed by recrudescence are common, with some dogs being euthanized because of repeated relapses or failure to respond to therapy.[15]

TABLE 23-5   DRUGS USED IN THE TREATMENT OF CANINE HISTIOCYTIC DISEASES

Drug	Dosage	Indication	Reference	Comments
Prednisone	1–3 mg/kg/day	Cutaneous or systemic histiocytosis	16, 47	
Tetracycline and niacinamide	250–500 mg each PO q 8 hr	Cutaneous or systemic histiocytosis	16, 47	Dose based on weight Caution with seizure history
Cyclosporine A	2.5–5.0 mg/kg PO q 12 hr	Refractory cutaneous or systemic histiocytosis	11, 46, 47	Adjust to trough level of 500 ng/ml
Leflunomide	4 mg/kg PO q 24 hr	Refractory cutaneous or systemic histiocytosis	11, 46, 47	Adjust to trough level of 20 μg/ml
Azathioprine	1–2 mg/kg PO q 24–48 hr	Refractory cutaneous or systemic histiocytosis	11, 46, 47	Monitor for myelosuppression
Lomustine (CCNU)	70–80 mg/m^2 PO q 3 wk	Histiocytic sarcoma	33	Monitor for myelosuppression and hepatotoxicity
Liposomal Doxorubicin	1 mg/kg IV q 3 wk	Refractory histiocytic sarcoma	37	Administer pyridoxine concurrently

HISTIOCYTIC SARCOMA

Canine histiocytic sarcoma (HS) is a rare neoplasm representing < 1% of canine cancers of the lymphoreticular system.[24] HS occurs most commonly in Bernese Mountain Dogs, Rottweilers, and Retrievers but may be seen in any breed and at any age. Dogs may present with either localized organ involvement or disseminated, multi-organ involvement. Reported sites of involvement include lung, lymph node, liver, spleen, stomach, pancreas, mediastinum, skin, skeletal muscle, central nervous system, nasal passages, eye, bone, and bone marrow.[26-34] Localized histiocytic sarcoma occurs most commonly in the joints, skin, and subcutaneous tissues, but metastasis to lungs, lymph nodes, and abdominal viscera is frequent.[3,32-34]

Immunohistochemical evidence indicates that most cases of localized HS and many cases of disseminated HS arise from malignant transformation of interstitial dendritic cells.[3] Hemophagocytic HS arising from malignant macrophages has recently been described and has a different clinical presentation and behavior than HS of dendritic cell origin.[35] Splenic involvement and anemia from hemophagocytosis by tumor cells are the hallmarks of hemophagocytic HS. Table 23-6 summarizes the differences between these types of HS.

Diagnosis

A diagnosis of HS can be obtained via cytologic or histologic examination of tumor tissue (Figure 23-10); however, definitive diagnosis can be challenging in pleomorphic tumors. Confirmation and subtyping may be performed through immunocytochemistry or immunohistochemistry using antibodies to CD18 (the β_2 subunit of the major adhesion molecule family of leukocytes), CD1, and the CD11 subunits.[3,35]

Clinical signs of HS vary depending on the type of HS and locations of tumor involvement. Table 23-7 summarizes presenting signs in a cohort of 59 dogs with

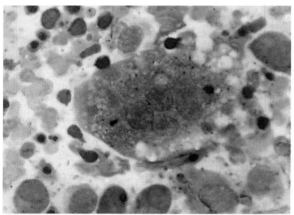

FIGURE 23-10 Cytology of histiocytic sarcoma: A single giant multi-nucleated neoplastic cell contains variably sized nucleoli surrounded by a large volume of pale-staining cytoplasm containing small clear vacuoles. Erythrophagocytosis is also present in this sample.

TABLE 23-6   COMPARISON OF LOCALIZED, DISSEMINATED, AND HEMOPHAGOCYTIC HISTIOCYTIC SARCOMA

Disease	Cell Type	Anatomic Predilections	Clinicopathologic Features	Outcome
Localized histiocytic sarcoma	Interstitial dendritic cell	Skin and subcutaneous tissue Joint space Others less common	Often normal	70%–91% metastatic rate to lymph node, lung, spleen 3–4 months untreated 6–12+ months with local and systemic therapy
Disseminated histiocytic sarcoma	Interstitial dendritic cell	Multi-organ involvement Lymph nodes, liver, lung, spleen most common	Variable	MST 1–2 months untreated MST 6 months if responds to chemotherapy
Hemophago-cytic histiocytic sarcoma	Macrophage	Spleen with or without liver involved Bone marrow Lung and lymph node less common	Anemia (regenerative) Thrombocytopenia Hypoalbuminemia Hypocholesterolemia	Poor response to chemotherapy MST 1–2 months

MST, Median survival time.

TABLE 23-7   CLINICAL SIGNS OF HISTIOCYTIC SARCOMA[38]

Presenting Sign	Dogs (%)
Lethargy	39
Presence of a mass	36
Cough or dyspnea	32
Inappetence	31
Lameness	25
Weight loss	12
Vomiting	10
Fever	8
Diarrhea	7
Lymphadenopathy	7
Polyuria/polydipsia	5
Epistaxis	2
Ocular signs	2

advanced HS. Because most dogs have metastasis or disseminated disease at diagnosis, complete staging is recommended. Complete blood count and biochemical screens are often abnormal in dogs with disseminated or hemophagocytic HS. Anemia is common and usually regenerative when caused by erythrophagocytosis from neoplastic cells. Leukocytosis, thrombocytopenia, increased liver enzymes, and hypoalbuminemia are frequent findings, and hypercalcemia or hypocholesterolemia may also be noted.[26-28,33,35] On thoracic radiography, pulmonary involvement may appear as a diffuse interstitial infiltrate, patchy consolidated areas, or focal or multi-focal mass lesions. Radiographic evidence of sternal, cranial mediastinal or tracheobronchial lymphadenopathy may also be noted. Hepatosplenomegaly, splenic or hepatic mottling, or masses in these organs are the most common abdominal ultrasonographic abnormalities.[36] Bone marrow aspiration cytology may reveal tumor infiltrate, especially in patients with cytopenias.

Treatment and Prognosis

Information regarding effective treatment of HS in dogs is scarce, but response and survival appear to vary depending on the type of HS. Localized HS is the most responsive to therapy, and outcomes are best in dogs without regional or distant metastasis. In a series of 18 dogs with localized HS of the joint, the overall median survival time (MST) was 3.6 months, the MST for dogs undergoing amputation was 6 months, and the metastatic rate was 91%.[32] In another series of 37 flat-coated retrievers, the MST for dogs without distant metastasis at diagnosis was 6 months and the metastatic rate was 70%.[34] Outcomes appear to be better with combination

therapy for localized HS and, in a pending publication by the authors, 16 dogs treated with combined local therapy and adjuvant chemotherapy consisting of single agent CCNU had an MST of over 18 months.

The clinical course of hemophagocytic HS is rapid and uniformly fatal. In a cohort of 17 dogs with immunohistochemically confirmed hemophagocytic HS, the MST was 4 weeks.[35] Likewise, another study showed that dogs with anemia, splenic involvement, thrombocytopenia, or hypoalbuminemia were less likely to respond to chemotherapy and/or had shorter survival times.[33] All of these factors are significantly more common in hemophagocytic HS than disseminated HS.[35] The clinical course of disseminated HS is variable and depends on the presence of prognostic factors listed above and response to chemotherapy. Surgery is often not an option because of multi-organ involvement, but radiation and chemotherapy can be used palliatively. MST for dogs responding to chemotherapy was 6 months versus 2 months for non-responders in one study.[33]

Few chemotherapeutics have been studied for HS. CCNU was recently reported to have a 46% response rate in 56 dogs with advanced HS.[33] Median remission duration was 84 days and overall MST was 106 days. In this group, thrombocytopenia ($< 100,000/\mu l$) and hypoalbuminemia were associated with a grave prognosis. Anecdotal reports exist describing dogs with HS responding to liposomal doxorubicin and paclitaxel chemotherapy.[37,38] In addition, a case report of a dog with cutaneous disseminated HS documented temporary remissions resulting from multiple protocols including cyclophosphamide, vincristine, prednisone, mitoxantrone, dacarbazine, and etoposide.[39]

Radiation therapy for HS has not been adequately reported; however, anecdotal reports of excellent responses exist. A recent study reported a 7-month MST in dogs receiving palliative radiation combined with CCNU chemotherapy.[34] Further investigation into the efficacy of radiation and use of multi-modality therapy to treat HS is necessary.

FELINE HISTIOCYTIC SARCOMA

Histiocytic neoplasms are more rare in cats than dogs. Most cats present with multi-focal or disseminated HS, and reported organs of involvement include CNS, spleen, liver, lymph nodes, lung, trachea, mediastinum, kidney, bladder, and bone marrow.[40-44] Severe regenerative or non-regenerative anemia and thrombocytopenia are common findings, and bone marrow involvement appears more commonly in cats, with 3 of 3 cats in a case series having positive bone marrow on post-mortem evaluation.[42] An aggressive clinical course is typical of HS in cats, and results of treatment have not been documented. Localized HS has also been reported in the tarsus of a cat, and lymph node metastasis was present at diagnosis.[45] To date, it has not been determined whether hemophagocytic HS of macrophage origin occurs in cats.

Selected References*

Craig LE, Julian ME, Ferracone JD: The diagnosis and prognosis of synovial tumors in dogs: 35 cases, *Vet Pathol* 39:66, 2002.
Describes cases of localized histiocytic sarcoma of the joint that can be confused with less aggressive synovial tumors.
Moore PF, Affolter VK, Vernau W: Canine hemophagocytic histiocytic sarcoma: a proliferative disorder of CD11d+ macrophages, *Vet Pathol* 43:632, 2006.

Documents the macrophage origin of a highly aggressive histiocytic sarcoma subtype.
Palmiero BS, Morris DO, Goldschmidt MH, et al: Cutaneous reactive histiocytosis in dogs: a retrospective evaluation of 32 cases, *Vet Dermatol* 18(5):332, 2007.
Provides a good summary clinical presentation and treatment outcome in dogs with cutaneous reactive histiocytosis.
Skorupski KA, Clifford CA, Paoloni MC, et al: CCNU for the treatment of dogs with histiocytic sarcoma, *J Vet Intern Med* 21:121, 2007.
Documents the efficacy of CCNU chemotherapy against advanced histiocytic sarcoma.

*For a complete list of the references cited in this chapter, please go to www.smallanimaloncology.com.

SECTION G: Perianal and Anal Sac Tumors

Mary Lynn Higginbotham

KEY POINTS

- Perianal adenomas are most common in the intact male dog and are usually cured by castration and surgical removal of the mass.
- Apocrine gland adenocarcinoma of the anal sac occurs in both male and female dogs and is characterized by aggressive, malignant behavior.
- Surgical excision of the primary tumor and lymph node metastases significantly improves survival for dogs with metastatic anal sac adenocarcinoma.

Incidence—Morbidity and Mortality

Most tumors of the perianal region are of sebaceous or apocrine origin. Those of sebaceous origin most often arise in the perianal glands, also referred to as *circumanal glands*. Most perianal gland tumors are benign. Perianal adenomas have been reported as the third most common canine tumor[1] and account for approximately 80% of tumors[2] of the intact male dog. Because they are androgen dependent, perianal adenomas are seldom seen in female dogs.[1-3] Perianal gland adenocarcinoma (ACA) is less common, accounting for 10% to 20% of all canine perianal tumors.[1,4,5] This tumor occurs in both sexes regardless of neutering status,[1,2,4-6] but appears to be more common in males than females.[5] Cats do not have sebaceous perianal glands and, therefore, do not develop tumors analogous to canine perianal gland tumors.[1,8,16]

Apocrine gland ACA of the anal sac is a perianal tumor of apocrine gland origin and is reported to account for 2% of canine skin tumors[9] and approximately 17% of canine perianal tumors.[10] Rare apocrine gland ACAs have been reported in the cat.[14,15]

Etiology and Risk Factors

The perianal glands are modified sebaceous glands located in the tail base, prepuce, hind limb, trunk and perianal regions of dogs.[1,8] These glands are described as "aborted sebaceous glands,"[1] and, although their function is not well understood, they enlarge during an animal's lifetime under the influence of androgens.[1,4] Because of their microscopic similarity to hepatocytes, perianal gland tumors are also referred to as "hepatoid" tumors.[1,8] When stimulated by androgens, the perianal glands undergo hypertrophy, whereas estrogen causes involution. Because of their androgen dependency, perianal adenomas occur primarily in intact male dogs but have been reported in intact and spayed females,[1,4,6] notably in an ovariohysterectomized female with hyperadrenocorticism and subsequent hypertestosteronism.[3] Perianal ACA also occurs primarily in male dogs.[1,4,5] In females, perianal ACAs are more common than perianal adenomas.[1,2] Perianal ACAs do not respond to castration, and the role of androgens in this disease is unclear. A recent study evaluated androgen expression in benign and malignant perianal gland tumors and found similar expression in both.[7] As suggested by Vail et al.,[5] androgens may be a promoter for the proliferation of the glands, acting with initiation events in a multi-stage model of carcinogenesis.

Breeds at risk for the development of perianal adenomas include the cocker spaniel, beagle, English bulldog, and Samoyed.[6] German shepherds and Arctic Circle breeds (including Samoyed, Siberian husky, Alaskan malamute, and Norwegian elkhound) were found to have increased incidence of perianal ACA compared with the hospital population in one study,[5] and Siberian husky, shih tzu, and mixed-breed dogs were at increased risk in another report.[8,10] German shepherds have been overrepresented in multiple studies of anal sac adenocarcinomas.[9,17,18] Perianal tumors most frequently occur in middle- to older-aged dogs.

Other tumor types that can affect the perianal region include lymphoma, STS, melanoma, leiomyoma, mast cell tumor,[2] SCC,[2,22] melanoma,[13,23] papillary cystadenoma,[13] transmissible venereal tumor,[24] and rhabdomyosarcoma.[25]

Clinical Features

Perianal gland adenomas are typically small, raised, hairless, non-painful masses. Lesions are most often solitary but may be multi-focal or diffuse in nature.[2] Benign masses may have been present for months to years, but malignant tumors typically grow more rapidly and are often ulcerated and fixed to underlying tissue. Any perianal mass in a neutered male should be considered potentially malignant.[2] Dogs may also present for tenesmus, obstipation, and constipation, as a result of physical obstruction from the mass or from lymphadenopathy caused by regional metastasis. Because of the aggressive nature of anal sac ACA, the primary tumor may be small at presentation, yet still have detectable lumbar or iliac lymphadenopathy. Bilateral anal sac ACAs occur in approximately 10% of cases.[13,18] Perianal gland tumors may be incidental findings on physical examination, with no clinical signs of disease. In two studies of anal sac ACAs, 34% and 39% of tumors were incidental findings on rectal palpation.[12,18]

Paraneoplastic hypercalcemia (see Chapter 11) is frequently associated with anal sac ACA, with an incidence ranging from 25% to 51%.[11,12,18] The hypercalcemia is due to parathyroid hormone related-peptide (PTHrp) produced by the tumor cells.[19-21] Polyuria, polydipsia (PU/PD), and anorexia are presenting complaints associated with hypercalcemia.[11,12,18] Paraneoplastic hypercalcemia may be a negative prognostic indicator for survival of dogs with anal sac ACA[12,18] but this has not been found in all studies.[11,13] Post-treatment recurrence

of hypercalcemia is an indication of disease recurrence or metastasis.

Diagnosis and Staging

Lesion aspiration and cytology may be used to rule out non-neoplastic etiologies and to exclude other tumor types such as mast cell tumor from the differential diagnosis list. However, the distinction between benign and malignant perianal gland tumors is difficult with cytology alone and, in most instances, histopathology is necessary to differentiate and evaluate for invasion into surrounding structures.

Thorough staging is recommended if a perianal malignancy is suspected. Staging should include a physical examination with rectal examination (evaluating all perianal tissues and the lumbar lymph node region), CBC, biochemical profile and urinalysis, ionized calcium, thoracic radiographs, abdominal radiographs, and/or abdominal ultrasound. An abdominal CT scan may be indicated to evaluate resectability of abdominal lymph nodes. However, many surgeons feel that the only way to assess resectability is to surgically explore the region.[2] For perianal adenoma, complete staging is less important, since this tumor type does not metastasize. However, a rectal examination should be performed to evaluate for occult masses in the region.

Metastasis

The most frequently reported site of metastasis for perianal gland carcinomas is the lumbar lymph nodes. Approximately 15% of dogs with perianal gland carcinomas have metastasis at the time of diagnosis.[5] Other reported metastatic sites include the liver and lungs.[8,9] Apocrine gland adenocarcinomas of the anal sac are highly metastatic, with metastasis present in up to 80% of cases at the time of diagnosis.[11] The lumbar lymph nodes are the most common sites of metastasis. Other reported sites include liver, spleen, vertebrae, femur, lungs, heart, mediastinum, and pancreas.[11] Dogs with anal sac ACA have also been reported to present for acute paralysis associated with lumbar vertebral metastasis.[26]

Treatment Modalities

The primary treatment for intact male dogs with perianal adenoma is mass excision and castration.[1,4,27] Should the mass be too extensive for removal, castration may cause sufficient involution of the tumor to facilitate excision at a later time. Estrogen causes involution of the perianal glands[1] but is not recommended as a primary treatment because of the significant potential for toxicity. Cryosurgery and radiation therapy have also been described as treatment for this tumor type. Although effective, because of the potential for late radiation effects,[28,29] the author would reserve radiation therapy for invasive tumors with malignant potential.

Treatment for perianal gland carcinoma includes aggressive surgical removal and, in the case of intact males, castration. One study found no difference in survival between dogs whose masses were completely excised and those who had a debulking surgery followed by cryotherapy to the surgical bed or surgery followed by radiation therapy.[5] Because surrounding tissue is often involved, fecal incontinence is of concern. However, up to one half of the anal sphincter may be removed with preservation of continence.[2]

Because of the malignant nature and tendency for early metastasis of anal sac ACA, multi-modality treatment is recommended. A combination of surgery, radiation therapy, and chemotherapy is considered ideal. Extirpation of lumbar nodes in addition to primary tumor excision has been advocated, regardless of whether or not metastatic disease is diagnosed. A recent study showed prolonged survival (median survival = 20.6 months) for dogs with lymph node metastasis that had surgical removal of the metastatic disease.[30] Adjuvant radiation therapy to the sites of both the primary tumor and the lumbar lymph nodes may help reduce the likelihood of recurrence, as well as control metastatic disease. Chemotherapy has also been recommended for control and prevention of metastatic disease. Various agents including melphalan,[11-13] cisplatin,[12,13] carboplatin,[12,13,31] doxorubicin with or without cyclophophamide,[11,12,17] mitoxantrone,[11,12] actinomycin D,[11,12] piroxicam,[11,12] epirubicin,[11,12] 5-fluorouracil,[11] mithramycin,[11] vincristine and cyclophosphamide,[11] piroxicam,[12] and chlorambucil have been tried.[12] However, comparative efficacy of these has not been clearly established. Carboplatin has been shown to significantly improve survival in dogs with unresectable lymph node metastasis[31] and generally, the platinum agents or anthracyclines (doxorubicin/mitoxantrone) are advocated for this tumor.

Prognosis and Survival

Prognosis for dogs with perianal adenoma treated with surgery and castration is good. Because androgen exposure can affect all the glandular tissue, rectal examination is prudent with routine evaluations. The prognosis for perianal ACA appears to be dependent upon stage of the disease. Dogs treated with surgical resection (with or without adjuvant cryosurgery or radiation therapy) whose tumors were < 5 cm in diameter with minimal or no invasion of the surrounding tissues had an MST of

24 months, which was significantly longer than that of dogs with larger or more invasive tumors.[5] Several studies have reported prognosis and treatment options for dogs with anal sac ACA; however, most studies contain too few similarly treated animals to evaluate for differences between treatment groups. A published study by Polton and Brearley[31] proposes an updated staging scheme for dogs presenting with anal sac ACA. Significant differences in survival were demonstrated when this modified staging scheme was applied. Negative prognostic factors included lack of therapy, presence of distant metastases, presence of lymph node metastases, and large size of the primary tumor (> 2.5 cm). Two studies have shown that dogs presenting with hypercalcemia have shorter survival (6–8.5 months MST) than do normocalcemic dogs (11.5–19.5 months MST). This has not been corroborated in other studies, but case numbers may have been too small to elucidate a difference.[11,13] Treatment options for dogs with anal sac ACA range from palliative therapy with piroxicam to multi-modal therapy with surgery, radiation and chemotherapy and reported MST range from 8.3 to 24.7 months.[11-13,17,31] Surgical excision appears to be important in the management of anal sac ACA, as evidenced by the MST of 18.2 months for dogs undergoing surgery (with or without other treatment) versus 13.4 months for those that do not.[12] Dogs with nodal metastases may have a surprisingly prolonged survival (MST = 20.6 months in one report) after surgical excision.[30] Dogs treated with surgery, radiation therapy, and chemotherapy had a 24.7-month MST.

Selected References*

Polton GA, Brearley MJ: Clinical stage, therapy and prognosis in canine anal sac gland carcinoma, *Vet Intern Med* 21:274, 2007.
A new staging scheme is proposed for anal sac ACA and evaluated for its relationship to treatment, prognosis, and survival in affected dogs.
Vail DM, Withrow SJ, Schwarz PD, Powers BE: Perianal adenocarcinoma in the canine male: a retrospective study of 41 cases, *J Am Anim Hosp Assoc* 26:329, 1990.
Discusses canine perianal ACA in male dogs and factors associated with survival.
Williams LE, Gliatto JM, Dodge RK, et al: Carcinoma of the apocrine glands of the anal sac in dogs: 113 cases (1985-1995), *J Am Vet Med Assoc* 223:825, 2003.
Large retrospective study of anal sac ACA in dogs.

█ *For a complete list of the references cited in this chapter, please go to www.smallanimaloncology.com.

24 Tumors of the Musculoskeletal System

David Ruslander

KEY POINTS

- In dogs and cats, osteosarcoma and chondrosarcoma are the most common primary tumors of the musculoskeletal system.
- Most dogs with appendicular osteosarcoma have no evidence of metastatic disease at diagnosis, but most will eventually develop metastasis. The metastatic rate is lower for chondrosarcoma.
- Osteosarcoma and chondrosarcoma metastatic rates are lower in cats than in dogs.
- Aggressive surgical resection including amputation is the mainstay of local therapy, although limb-sparing surgeries and palliative radiation therapy are potential options for local control.
- Adjuvant chemotherapy with doxorubicin, carboplatin, and cisplatin, or a combination thereof, has been shown to increase the median survival time (MST) in dogs with osteosarcoma.

Tumors of the musculoskeletal system are relatively rare in dogs and cats with the exception of osteosarcoma (OSA), which accounts for the vast majority of primary skeletal tumors in dogs. This chapter covers primary and metastatic tumors, but osseous manifestations of other tumors including multiple myeloma, plasmacytoma, and lymphoma are covered in separate chapters.

PRIMARY APPENDICULAR SKELETAL TUMORS

Incidence and Etiology

Osteosarcoma is the most common primary bone tumor in dogs, accounting for approximately 5% of all neoplasia and the overwhelming majority of canine bone tumors.[1-3] Other tumors of bone include, but are not limited to, chondrosarcoma (CSA), fibrosarcoma (FSA), hemangiosarcoma (HSA), and histiocytic sarcoma.

Synovial cell sarcoma is a tumor of the joint capsule and not a classic bone tumor, but has similar clinical features to the skeletal tumors. Digital tumors such as squamous cell carcinoma (SCC) and malignant melanoma, although not classical musculoskeletal tumors, also affect the bones of the digit and need to be considered here (additional information is available in Chapter 23, Section A). The overall incidence of canine OSA is low in the general population but quite high in certain breed groups. The incidence is much lower in cats. Classically, OSA affects the long bones, but can be seen in any bone of the appendicular and axial skeleton including unusual sites such as the os penis. Appendicular OSA occurs in large breed dogs in classic locations (see later discussion), but axial OSA can be seen in any breed in any location.[4-6] The exact etiology is unknown, but it has been theorized that microfractures in the weight-bearing portion of the bone lead to malignant transformation of the osteoblasts.[7] Metallic implants, ionizing radiation (resulting from therapeutic radiation), and bone infection (osteomyelitis) have also been reported as potential risk factors for development of OSA.[8-16] Height of the dog, rather than weight, has also been shown to be a risk factor.[17] Neutering status has been implicated as a risk factor, and in one study Rottweilers that were spayed or neutered prior to 12 months of age had a 4× increased risk for the development of OSA.[18] Extraskeletal OSA has been reported in both species, can include cutaneous and non-cutaneous locations, and is associated with a poor prognosis.[19-21]

Genetic factors appear to play a role in the development of OSA, given the increased risk of OSA in specific breeds. Recently, a host of genes have been shown to be differentially expressed in dogs with OSA including the tumor suppressor genes p53, retinoblastoma (Rb) and insulin-like growth factor (IGF-1), PTEN, c-met,

Ezrin, erbB-2, and possibly c-kit.[22-33] Cyclooxygenase-2 (COX-2) expression has also been identified in OSA tissue in dogs.[34] Expression and mutation of these and other genes have varying levels of prognostic significance for OSA. Molecular aspects of feline OSA are poorly described.

Multicentric digital SCC is a recognized syndrome in which dogs appear with multiple digit involvement, without metastatic disease. Labrador retrievers, giant schnauzers, and standard poodles are breeds that appear to be overrepresented for this poorly understood disease process, suggesting a genetic predisposition.[35]

Clinical Features

Most dogs with primary bone neoplasia appear to be in pain because of bone destruction. Many are presented with swelling of the affected limb, but acute lameness may be all that is apparent, especially with proximal bone lesions. Advanced cases may be presented with an acute pathologic fracture. Axial lesions in the oral cavity, spine, and ribs may be more chronic in nature, and clinical signs more subtle. Cats generally are presented with lameness or swelling.

Diagnosis in many situations is delayed by failure to recognize the disease entity and a tendency to initially treat with non-specific pain management and forego radiographs. Ideally, all large breed dogs with significant or persistent lameness should be evaluated with multiple-view radiographs of the affected limb at presentation. Long-standing discomfort in patients can lead to systemic signs such as weight loss and anorexia, but this obviously should be differentiated from metastatic disease or concurrent disease.

Diagnosis and Staging

Patients presenting for evaluation of any suspected bone neoplasia should be properly staged before initiation of therapy. Radiographs of the affected limb are often diagnostic when the lesion is in a classic location and demonstrates the "sunburst" appearance of simultaneous proliferation and destruction of bone (Figure 24-1) that does not cross the joint. This is in contrast to synovial cell sarcoma, which will produce radiographic changes on both sides of the affected joint. Some lesions can be more proliferative, whereas others are more lytic. Differentials for such radiographic findings are limited to bone neoplasia, bacterial or fungal osteomyelitis, bone cysts, and healing bone injury. A predominance of lysis without proliferation should alert the clinician to the possibility of alternative diagnoses, including metastatic carcinoma. However, primarily lytic lesions may

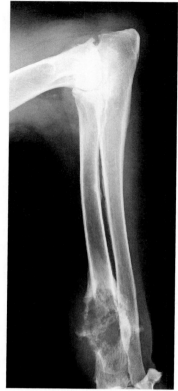

FIGURE 24-1 Lateral radiograph of a 9-year-old St. Bernard showing classic radiographic appearance of an osteosarcoma. Note the distal radius location and both osteolytic and osteoproductive lesions.

be a feature of OSA, especially in greyhounds, which are more likely to appear with a pathological fracture. Location of the lesion in the bone is often helpful, since most primary bone tumors are located in the metaphyseal region whereas metastatic lesions are often diaphyseal. The vast majority of primary OSAs are seen in the following locations: distal radius, proximal humerus, proximal tibia, and distal femur. Other sites including distal tibia, distal humerus, ulna, and proximal femur are less commonly affected. Three-view chest radiographs should be evaluated before any biopsy or surgical intervention. Non-OSA neoplasia may have a higher rate of nodal and systemic metastasis, especially histiocytic neoplasia, so lymph node aspiration should be considered in patients with suspected non-OSA (non-classic breed, location, or cytologic finding) even if the regional lymph node is not enlarged. The incidence of overtly metastatic disease is low in OSA (approximately 6%) at diagnosis, but should it exist, prognosis and treatment may be dramatically altered.[36] CT scanning may help identify early subtle lesions in the lungs. Abdominal ultrasound is indicated when bone lesions are suspected to be metastatic. Otherwise, abdominal ultrasound is not routinely used unless clinical signs or the biochemical profile is abnormal. Nuclear imaging (bone scan) can be useful in determining the extent of the bone lesions and to determine if the patient has metastasis to other bones prior to surgical intervention.[37]

Although bone biopsy facilitates histologic confirmation, diagnosis can often be made via fine needle aspiration under mild sedation. Differentiation between OSA and other bone neoplasia on cytology may be difficult short of special staining for alkaline phosphatase; however, this is often not necessary if the location and breed is consistent with OSA.[38-43] Histopathologic confirmation may be needed in situations in which the cytology is non-diagnostic or the owner wants confirmation or additional prognostic information before making therapy decisions.[44] Owners should be warned about false-negative biopsy results, which can occur in 10% to 20% of cases. Bone biopsy (described in Chapter 6) can be accomplished with an open or closed approach using either a Jamshidi needle or Michelle trephine instrument. The latter is more aggressive and more likely to cause iatrogenic pathologic fracture or other complications, although the risk of fracture is probably overstated. Care should be taken when choosing the biopsy site so that contaminated tissue can be excised at the time of limb-sparing surgery if this option is being considered.

Biological Behavior

OSA is characterized by aggressive local bone destruction and high likelihood (>90%) of eventual metastasis, although fewer than 10% of affected dogs have overt metastatic disease at presentation.[45] The concept of micrometastatic disease is difficult for owners to comprehend, but it is critical to understanding the disease process since most dogs eventually will succumb to metastatic disease even after local control of the tumor is accomplished via amputation or limb-sparing procedures. Early metastatic lesions are below the level of detection with conventional imaging such as radiographs or even CT scans, but likely will grow over the ensuing months to years following diagnosis. It has been suggested that the metastatic rate of axial OSA may be lower than appendicular disease, but this may be a manifestation of poor local disease control with tumors in the oral cavity, ribs, or vertebrae, since many of these patients succumb to local recurrence of the tumor before

the development of metastatic disease.[46-49] CSA, while seen primarily in the nasal cavity and other flat bones, can also occur in the appendicular skeleton and tends to be less metastatic than OSA, although this appears to be dependent upon grade of the tumor.[50,51] FSA of the bone is extremely rare in dogs and may be cured with surgery alone. The metastatic rate appears to be low but may be influenced by mitotic rate and grade of tumor, similar to soft tissue sarcomas. Synovial cell sarcomas are locally aggressive and have the potential to metastasize, depending on the grade of the tumor.[52,53] HSA and histiocytic sarcoma (previously known as malignant histiocytosis) of the bone may be primary or metastatic tumors and are considered highly malignant and highly metastatic even if no distant disease is noted at presentation. Multiple synchronous metastatic lesions may occur, affecting bone and other sites such as skin or internal organs.

Digital neoplasia has a moderate rate of metastasis. Accordingly, lymph node aspiration and chest radiographs are recommended.[54-57] In addition, abdominal ultrasound is advised for patients with hind limb digits affected.

Treatment Options (Table 24-1)

Surgery

Treatment of bone neoplasia is both local and systemic in nature, especially for OSA, HSA, and histiocytic sarcoma. Surgical options include amputation or limb-sparing procedures. Although effective at removing the source of pain, amputation by itself does not appear to prolong survival in OSA (other than preventing pain-related death) but may be curative for CSA or FSA. Amputation of the affected limb is well tolerated, assuming the patient does not have severe concurrent musculoskeletal or neurologic conditions. Most properly screened dogs tolerate the procedure very well, and owner satisfaction with amputation is excellent.[58] Tumors located in the scapula can be surgically removed via a partial or total scapulectomy, not necessitating limb amputation.[59,60]

Over the last decade, there have been tremendous advances in limb-sparing procedures allowing preservation of limb function. These procedures are life saving in patients who would not be able to undergo an amputation because of physical impairments or owner reluctance. Owners need to be made aware that limb-sparing procedures do not increase the median or overall survival time over that achieved with amputation, and metastatic disease is still the life-limiting factor for dogs with OSA.[61-63] Various techniques have been described for these procedures, all of which use combinations of

TABLE 24-1   SUMMARY OF OSTEOSARCOMA TREATMENT OUTCOMES

Treatment	Details	Median Survival	1-Year Survival	2-Year Survival	No. of Cases	Author
Amputation Alone						
		19.2 wks	11.5%	2.0%	162	Spodnick[45]
		175 days	21%	0%	19	Mauldin[88]
		14.5 wks	0%	0%	8	Shapiro[89]
		119 days	11%	4%	35	Straw[91]
		168 days	20%	0%	15	Thompson[93]
Amputation and Chemotherapy						
	Cisplatin × 2	~272 days	38%	17%	36	Straw[91]
	Cisplatin/doxorubicin × 2 (alt)	300 days	36%	26%	19	Mauldin[88]
	Cisplatin × 2-6	43 weeks	30%	10%	11	Shapiro[89]
	Cisplatin × 1-6 (some had limb sparing)	46.4 weeks	45.5%	20.9%	22	Berg[61]
	Cisplatin × 6	413 days	62%	19%	16	Kragel[90]
	Cisplatin × 2 before or after Sx	262/282 days	38%/43%	18%/16%	19	Straw[91]
	Cisplatin × 2	290 days	33.3%	6.6%	15	Thompson[93]
	Doxorubicin (2 or 3 pre-Sx)	52.3 weeks	50.5%	9.7%	35	Berg[94]
	Carboplatin/Doxorubicin (concurrent)	235 days	8.3%	4.1%	24	Bailey[101]
	Carboplatin × 3 (1 pre-SX)	230 days	30%	30%	21	Khanna[98]
	Cisplatin/Doxorubicin concurrent × 4	300 days	28.5%	5%	35	Chun[104]
	Lobaplatin × 4	?	31.8%	?	28	Kirpensteijn[99]
	Liposome Cisplatin	333 days	50%	40%/0%	20	Vail[100]
	Carboplatin × 4 (1 pre-Sx)	207 days	25%	20%	18	Vail[100]
	Carboplatin × 4 (1 pre-Sx)	321 days	35.4%		48	Bergman[95]
	Cisplatin/Doxorubicin concurrent (2 or 10 days post-Sx) × 3	11.5 months	47%	28%	102	Berg[96]
	Carboplatin/Doxorubicin alternating × 3	227 days	48%	18%	32	Kent[103]
Limb-Sparing Surgery						
	Misc protocols	8 months	?	?	20	Larue[62]
	No chemotherapy					Thrall[66]
	Intraarterial Cisplatin ± RT				49	Withrow[79]
	Extra Corporeal RT (70Gy) + OPLA-PT + chemo	298 days	23%	15%	13	Liptak[80]
	OPLA – PT + Carbo or Carbo/Doxorubicin	429 days	NA	NA	47	Lascelles[69]
	Humerus ± chemotherapy	172 days	?	?	17	Kuntz[68]
Radiation Therapy						
	Palliative 10 Gy × 3 (0.7.21 day)	125 days	6.6%	0%	15	McEntee[76]

(Continued)

TABLE 24-1   SUMMARY OF OSTEOSARCOMA TREATMENT OUTCOMES—Cont'd

Treatment	Details	Median Survival	1-Year Survival	2-Year Survival	No. of Cases	Author
	Axial Palliative (20–30 Gy)/ Curative (45–57 Gy)	137 day (79 Palliative vs. 265 Curative)			22	Dickerson[71]
	Curative intent (48–59.4 Gy) ± OPLA-Pt + chemotherapy	209 days	21%	7.1%	14	Walters[72]
	Stereotactic RT (20–30 Gy)	363 days	27.2%	9.0%	11	Farese[73]
	Palliative 8 Gy × 4 weekly + chemotherapy	313/162 days (appendicular/axial)	20.8%	0%	24	Green[74]
	Intra-arterial Cisplatin + RT	4.9 months	25%		12	Heidner[75]

surgical resection of the affected bone and replacement with an implant, either an allogeneic (donor) or autologous (from patient itself) bone graft implant or surgical steel endoprosthetic implant. Alternatively, the affected bone can be sterilized via extracorporeal irradiation and then replaced into position.[64-67] Bone plating and arthrodesis is necessary for stabilization of the joint and mobility of the limb. Given the location of these tumors, residual disease is likely to remain, necessitating some additional form of local control, either with radiation therapy, intra-arterial cisplatin, or more recently local chemotherapy delivered via an open cell polylactic acid impregnated with cisplatin (OPLA).[67] Not all dogs are candidates for limb-sparing procedures, especially dogs with greater than 50% bone length involvement, significant soft tissue involvement, pathologic fracture, or circumferential involvement of the limb. Distal radius or ulnar lesions are more amenable to limb-sparing surgeries than proximal humeral and proximal and distal femoral tumors.[68] Complications including local infection, recurrence, and fracture are common, and many dogs require a second or even third surgery to handle these complications. Interestingly, wound infections have been shown to improve local control and overall survival, most likely related to host immune response.[69] Cats with appendicular bone neoplasia are best treated with amputation, and it is rare for a cat to have other orthopedic issues precluding such a procedure. Primary digital lesions can be effectively treated with amputation of the affected digit. In order to achieve proximal margins for complete excision, the digital amputation should extend at least one phalanx above the affected bone, and complete excision should be confirmed with histopathology.[54-57]

Isolated metastatic OSA lesions can be managed surgically in specific clinical situations such as with lung or renal metastasis. Pulmonary metastasectomy has been described in dogs, and outcome was variable with an MST of 176 days (20–1495 days) following surgical removal. Specific criteria for surgical intervention in these situations has been adapted from human oncology and include control of the primary tumor, fewer than three metastatic lesions visible, more than 300 days from initial diagnosis, and no evidence of extrapulmonary disease.[70]

Radiation Therapy

Radiation therapy plays a role in the local management of OSA and other bone neoplasia, especially for patients who are not ideal candidates for amputation. Goals of radiation therapy may be simply palliative in nature, designed to control pain and improve quality of life with limited hospitalization time. Definitive or curative intent radiation therapy results have not been encouraging, primarily because of the significant amount of gross disease that is often present in patients at the time of presentation.[71,72] Radiation therapy has also been used effectively in prepping patients for limb-sparing procedures as described previously.[62,73,74]

No particular palliative protocol has been shown to be superior to others. The majority of dogs with appendicular or axial OSA respond favorably (75%–93%) and achieve some form of palliation, although duration is highly variable and often for only several months.[71-79] In one study of 95 dogs, those whose tumors had less bone involvement or were located in the humerus fared better in terms of local tumor control.[78] Local control is generally transient and can be durable (>1 year), but most studies have indicated median duration of control of 4 to 6 months. Dogs receiving chemotherapy before, during, or after radiation had a higher rate of control compared with radiation alone in one study.[76] Radiosurgical techniques that allow a one-time high dose of radiation to be delivered to the affected limb with minimal dose to surrounding tissues have been described. Preliminary results are encouraging, with an MST of almost 1 year.[73] Extracorporeal radiation therapy is a new technique in which the affected bone is removed from the patient either completely or with associated nerve and vessel attachments and a very large (70-Gy) dose is delivered, resulting in sterilization of the tumor cells contained in the bone but preservation of the support structure of the bone. This sterilized bone is then replaced in the patient with surgical plating and arthrodesis.[80]

The radioisotope, samarium (Sm-153-EDTMP), has been used in human and veterinary medicine and appears to be helpful in controlling bone destruction both in primary and metastatic bone tumors. The systemic delivery of this compound is especially useful in the management of multiple skeletal metastases, and side effects appear minimal but include prolonged bone marrow suppression.[81-86]

Chemotherapy

As stated previously, local therapy of OSA will control pain and recurrence of the primary tumor, but metastatic disease will develop quickly following amputation or limb-sparing surgery if adjuvant chemotherapy is not given in some fashion. Chemotherapy has improved the MST such that adjuvant chemotherapy following amputation is considered a standard of care. With amputation and no chemotherapy, the MST is approximately 4 months, with almost 90% to 100% mortality within a year. Depending on the study and specific chemotherapy protocol, OSA patients have approximately 40 to 50% chance of 1-year survival and 20% to 25% chance of 2-year survival following amputation and chemotherapy. Most studies have evaluated doxorubicin, cisplatin, and carboplatin in varying combinations and protocols, but no single protocol has been proven to be of greater benefit than another in randomized controlled studies.[87-104] The timing and number of chemotherapy cycles have varied and an ideal number of cycles has not been clearly defined, although it does appear that more than two cycles is better than less than two. Although chemotherapy is life prolonging, it is rare for dogs to be cured of OSA, and most (95%) will eventually succumb to metastatic disease. Management of metastatic disease is complex and may include surgery (if feasible; see previous discussion), additional chemotherapy, Sm-153-EDTMP and/or immunotherapy, but the prognosis is guarded to grave.[105]

Other Therapies

There has been a tremendous amount of recent literature on the use of bisphosphonates in the management of OSA in dogs. Bisphosphonates are osteoclast inhibitors used commonly in human patients with osteoporosis to inhibit bone resorption.[105a] Breast and prostate cancer patients with diffuse skeletal metastasis benefit from this therapy as well. Although inhibition of bone resorption appears to be the primary mechanism of action, direct cytotoxicity has been reported, suggesting possible interactions between bisphosphonates and chemotherapy and/or radiation therapy. Clinical trials are underway evaluating the role of bisphosphonates in canine OSA, but recent results indicate promising *in vitro* and *in vivo* activity.[106-111] Nephrotoxicity is the main toxicity, so a fluid diuresis is recommended.[112] Dosing recommendations are shown in Table 18-9, P. 182.

Immunotherapeutic approaches to OSA have been shown to have anti-tumor activity. One such approach is the use of liposome-encapsulated muramyl tripeptide phosphatidylethanolamine (L-MTP-PE), which activates alveolar macrophages and enhances cellular toxicity when combined with doxorubicin or cisplatin. In fact, the longest median survival of any OSA study was with L-MTP-PE after 4 cycles of cisplatin, resulting in a median survival of 14.5 months versus 9.7 months with cisplatin alone. Although not commercially available, human clinical trials of L-MTP-PE are ongoing.[113] Inhaled interleukin-2 (IL-2) has been shown to cause clinical regression of advanced pulmonary nodules in dogs with metastatic OSA.[114]

COX-2 inhibitors such as deracoxib, carprofen, and others have been suggested as a non-cytotoxic approach to OSA, given reports of COX-2 overexpression in canine OSA, as well as *in vitro* cytotoxicity.[34,115] Four dogs developed what appeared to be spontaneous regression of OSA in one report, although several of these dogs were receiving carprofen, leading to speculation of an anti-cancer benefit of this drug.[116] Similar approaches can be considered for digital melanoma and SCC, given responses noted with oral tumors of similar histology.

Prognosis

The MST after amputation alone for dogs with appendicular OSA is approximately 19.2 weeks, based on a large retrospective study with only 2% of dogs still alive at 2 years.[45] This study has served as an historical control for most current studies and evaluation of new chemotherapy approaches. There are several well-established prognostic factors for dogs with OSA, including adjuvant chemotherapy, low-grade histology (rare for OSA), normal total and bone-specific alkaline phosphatase, and possibly small body size.[44,117,118] Percent tumor necrosis and bone scan uptake have also been shown to predict outcome.[119] Dogs less than 5 years of age have also been reported to have shorter survival times, as do dogs with overt metastatic disease (lungs, lymph node).[36,45,120] As previously mentioned, limb-sparing patients with infection in the surgical site have a longer disease-free interval and survival.[69] Extraskeletal tumors and larger tumors are associated with shorter survival time.[19-21]

The prognosis for cats with appendicular OSA is good to excellent. Many cats are cured of the disease with amputation alone, although metastasis can occur.[121-123] Factors associated with more aggressive variants of feline OSA have not been identified.

The prognosis for CSA is good to excellent with amputation or complete surgical excision, since most are low-grade neoplasms. High-grade CSA predicts a more aggressive disease. MSTs exceed 800 days for low-grade CSA but are much shorter with higher-grade neoplasia, which, fortunately, is less common.[50,51]

Histiocytic sarcoma and HSA carry a guarded prognosis because of the likelihood of metastatic disease.[124,125] Low-grade synovial cell sarcomas may be cured with surgery alone, although high-grade tumors have a much higher risk of metastasis, with an MST of 7 months.[52,53]

Digital SCC warrants a good prognosis, although metastasis to regional lymph nodes can occur in approximately 20% to 30% of patients. Digital melanoma has a more guarded prognosis, with up to 50% eventually metastasizing. Although not considered as aggressive as oral malignant melanoma, adjuvant therapy should be considered for digital melanomas.[54-56]

PRIMARY AXIAL SKELETAL TUMORS
Incidence and Etiology

Tumors of the axial skeleton include tumors of the flat bones (i.e., skull, ribs, pelvis, and spine). Spinal, skull, and rib tumors are covered more completely in Chapters 19; 20, Section E; and 21, Section D. Although less common, tumors of the axial skeletal system are similar to appendicular tumors and include OSA, CSA, plasma cell tumors, and undifferentiated sarcomas. Etiology of axial OSA is likely similar to that of appendicular OSA in many regards. However, microtrauma on weight-bearing

bones is an unlikely etiologic factor in development of axial disease. Large breed dogs are at greater risk for the development of axial disease, reinforcing the concept of genetic predisposition.

Multilobular osteochondrosarcoma (MLO) is a unique subtype of primary bone tumor occasionally seen in dogs, primarily associated with the flat bones of the skull. This tumor appears to have a lower metastatic rate than OSA, with metastasis occurring later in the course of the disease.[126,127] See Chapter 20, Section E for additional information.

Clinical Features

Dogs and cats with axial tumors may be presented for evaluation of a noticeable and/or painful mass, or the finding may be incidental. Patients with vertebral body tumors may be presented with lameness or neurologic abnormalities. Maxillary and mandibular tumors produce clinical signs including halitosis, difficulty eating, and bleeding from the oral cavity, typical of oral tumors of other sites. Failure to thrive and weight loss are seen in advanced cases, even if metastatic disease is not present.

Diagnosis and Staging

Similar staging is recommended for axial and appendicular neoplasia. Baseline blood and urine tests and three-view chest radiographs are performed before any additional therapy. Cytology and/or biopsy should be performed to confirm the diagnosis. Given the uncommon occurrence and variable histology of axial tumors, a biopsy is recommended to rule out metastatic or nonsarcoma neoplasia because treatment and outcome is vastly different. In addition, CT scan or other advanced imaging is recommended before surgical intervention, since anatomic obstacles may preclude surgery or dictate preoperative radiation therapy rather than simple surgical removal (Figure 24-2).

Biological Behavior

Controversy exists in the literature about whether axial OSA has a lower metastatic rate, compared with appendicular disease. This may in fact be a manifestation of the aggressive local problem axial disease presents, especially in areas such as the rib and vertebral bodies. As such, all OSAs should be considered potentially metastatic, regardless of site. CSA, on the other hand, can be cured if complete surgical excision is accomplished. This is difficult, if not impossible, with vertebral lesions, but feasible with the rib and oral lesions. Plasmacytomas are considered to be locally aggressive, but progression to systemic disease/multiple myeloma occurs.

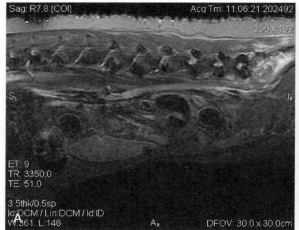
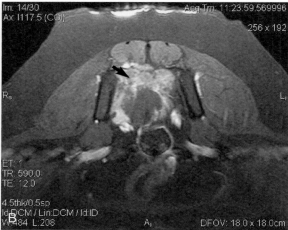

FIGURE 24-2 A, Sagittal and, **B,** transverse magnetic resonance imaging (MRI) scans from a 13-year-old male castrated Golden Retriever with a suspected sarcoma of the sacrum (*arrow*), causing pain and hind limb neurologic abnormalities because of invasion of the neural canal. Note the lack of involvement of the ilial wings on the transverse image. No primary tumor was identified.

Treatment Options

Surgery

Aggressive surgical excision remains the cornerstone of treatment and is possible even in locations such as the ribs, scapulae, and oral cavity. Significant portions of the scapula can be removed with good functional outcome. The same is true of other locations, but owners should be warned that although surgery may be locally curative, tumor cells may still be present after surgery. Should surgical margins contain tumor cells, adjuvant radiation therapy is recommended. Decompressive surgery can be attempted with vertebral body tumors and may serve to relieve clinical signs even though residual disease is likely to remain.

Radiation Therapy

For OSA and CSA, radiation therapy as a primary treatment is generally palliative and not of long-standing benefit. If there is significant pain associated with lytic bone lesions in any of these tumors, palliative radiation and bisphosphonate therapy (pamidronate) is helpful. Dogs with axial OSA treated with definitive-intent radiation therapy had longer remission times, compared with those receiving palliative-intent radiation (265 days vs. 79 days, respectively).[71] Plasmacytomas are extremely sensitive to radiation therapy and patients may benefit from radiation therapy even if surgery is not possible.

Chemotherapy

Chemotherapy is recommended for axial OSA and higher grade CSA, similar to appendicular disease. Plasmacytomas can be managed with melphalan and prednisone for both residual tumor and to help prevent or delay systemic progression, but there is little in the literature regarding this approach.

Prognosis

As discussed previously, OSA of the axial skeleton carries a guarded prognosis similar to appendicular OSA, but control of local disease is a greater concern given the anatomic sites involved. In a retrospective review of MLO, 56% of dogs developed metastatic disease. This was higher than previously reported, but not to the degree of classic OSA; it also occurred later in the course of the disease. The MST in this study was 800 days. Grade of tumor appears to be predictive of outcome for dogs with MLO.[126,127]

Rib OSA in the dog has a guarded prognosis. An MST of 3 months with surgery alone and 8 months with surgery and adjuvant chemotherapy has been reported. Many dogs will have metastatic disease at diagnosis. CSA of the rib has a much better prognosis, with MST of over 1000 days and many long-term survivors.[128-130] Accordingly, it is critically important to determine the histologic diagnosis before making definitive case management decisions for dogs with rib tumors.

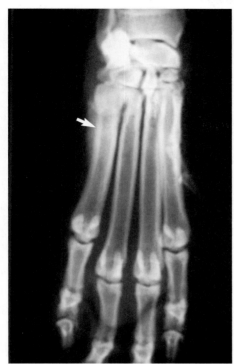

FIGURE 24-3 Carpal/metacarpal radiograph of a 3-year-old male castrated Golden Retriever with primary osteosarcoma of the rib. Complete surgical resection was accomplished followed by adjuvant chemotherapy with carboplatin, but metastasis to lungs and lateral metacarpal bone occurred 9 months following surgery. Note the subtle bone changes in the metastatic lesion *(arrow)*, which cannot be differentiated from a primary neoplasm based on location or radiographic findings.

METASTATIC SKELETAL TUMORS

Metastatic bone cancer is much less common in dogs and cats than it is in people. Any tumor can theoretically spread to bone, but epithelial neoplasias including prostatic, bladder, and mammary carcinoma are the most common tumor types.[4,131-132] Metastases can occur in any bone, but classically are reported in the diaphyseal region of the long bones as well as in the ribs, lumbar vertebrae, and pelvic bones (Figure 24-3). For patients with suspected metastatic lesions, aspiration cytology and/or biopsy will help confirm the diagnosis. Bone scans can be helpful in determining extent of disease and feasibility of treatment, but prognosis is obviously very poor. Radiation therapy (either with external beam or bone-targeting radiopharmaceuticals such as Sm-153-EDTMP) can be given for palliation of pain. Chemotherapy should be considered for control of disease outside the radiation field.

SCC of the digits affecting solitary or multiple digits is occasionally seen in cats with metastatic primary lung carcinoma. It is not clear why the tumor has a propensity to metastasize to the digits.[133,134]

MUSCLE TUMORS

Incidence, Etiology, and Risk Factors

This discussion includes tumors of the skeletal muscle, but does not include visceral disease such as gastrointestinal, splenic, or gynecologic tumors of smooth muscle origin, which are included in Chapter 22. Primary muscle tumors are extremely rare in the dog and even more so in the cat. The literature is limited to a small number of case reports. Rhabdomyosarcomas—and the benign equivalent, rhabdomyomas—are neoplasms of striated muscle with the myoblast being the tissue of origin. The two most common forms of rhabdomyosarcoma are alveolar and embryonal. Alveolar rhabdomyosarcoma is typically seen in the muscles of the extremities and head region, but any striated muscle can be affected. Embryonal or embryonal botryoid rhabdomyosarcoma is seen in the bladder of young dogs, the latter characterized by a polyploid grape-like presentation.[135-138] St. Bernards may be genetically predisposed to develop this tumor type.

Affected animals are presented with a non-painful swelling or mass. These tumors must be considered to be potentially metastatic, although overall metastatic rate is unknown.

Diagnosis and Staging

Definitive diagnosis is best made with an incisional or trucut biopsy, depending on the location. Given the potential for metastasis, chest radiographs, abdominal ultrasound, and lymph node aspiration are recommended before aggressive surgical intervention. CT scan may be indicated for surgical and radiation treatment planning.

Treatment

Aggressive surgical excision is the mainstay of therapy for skeletal muscle tumors. Amputation should be considered for highly invasive non-resectable tumors. If complete excision is not possible, radiation therapy should be considered, although there is minimal information in the literature on this mode of therapy in this instance. Adjuvant chemotherapy is of potential benefit in cases with documented metastatic disease or with high mitotic rate and aggressive histology. No grading system has been applied to this tumor in dogs or cats, given the low incidence.

Prognosis

Prognosis is widely variable. Published case reports indicate both long-term control and rapid recurrence, with outcome apparently dictated primarily by surgical margins.

Selected References*

Fan TM, de Lorimier LP, O'Dell-Anderson K, et al: Single-agent pamidronate for palliative therapy of canine appendicular osteosarcoma bone pain, *J Vet Intern Med* 21(3):431-439, 2007.
This recent paper described a new approach to managing pain in the OSA patient using a bisphosphonate (pamidronate, an osteoclast inhibitor that appears not only to prevent bone loss and improve bone deposition, but also to have anti-tumor properties as well).
Ramirez O, Dodge RK, Page RL, et al: Palliative radiotherapy of appendicular osteosarcoma in 95 dogs, *Vet Radiol Ultrasound* 40(5):517-522, 1999.
This paper is one of many investigating the use of radiation therapy with palliative intent for OSA in dogs but is distinguished with large case numbers. Seventy-five percent of dogs responded to low-dose radiation for a median of 73 days. Positive prognostic factors included concurrent use of chemotherapy, minimal bone involvement, and non-humerus locations.
Spodnick GJ, Berg J, Rand W, et al: Prognosis for dogs with appendicular osteosarcoma treated by amputation alone: 162 cases (1978-1988), *J Am Vet Med Assoc* 200:995-999, 1992.
This paper serves as a baseline from which all future papers are compared where adjuvant chemotherapy was administered. Key points included median survival of 4 months and a worse prognosis for younger dogs.
Straw RC, Withrow SJ: Limb sparing surgery vs. amputation for dogs with bone tumors, *Vet Clin North Am* 26:135-143, 1996.
This paper showed similar survival times of dogs treated with limb-sparing procedures and indicated that while local control can be achieved without amputation, metastatic disease remains the greatest obstacle.

*For a complete list of the references cited in this chapter, please go to www.smallanimaloncology.com.

25 Tumors of the Hematopoietic System

SECTION A: Lymphoma

Jeffrey N. Bryan

KEY POINTS

- Lymphoma is a systemic disease requiring chemotherapy in almost all cases.
- Approximately 80% of dogs treated with chemotherapy will experience complete remission.
- Younger cats tend to have FeLV-related mediastinal lymphoma and older cats have non-FeLV-related intestinal lymphoma.

LYMPHOMA IN DOGS

Incidence/Etiology and Risk Factors

Lymphoma is a collection of neoplasms arising from the malignant transformation of lymphocytes. Incidence in dogs increases with increasing age, leveling off somewhat after 6 years.[1] Lymphoma can appear in dogs of any age, breed, or sex, although certain breeds (Table 25-1) and intact females (relative risk of 0.7) appear to have a lower incidence of the disease.[1] The development of lymphoma has been associated with exposure to the 2,4D herbicide, although an industry re-examination of these data weakened the initial association.[2-4] Industrial living and chemical use by owners have been associated with development of lymphoma.[5] The disease has also been demonstrated to be genetically heritable in families of dogs.[6] Immunosuppressive medications such as cyclosporine increase the risk of lymphoma in humans and likely cats, suggesting that this may be true in dogs as well.[7] Genomic loss of methylation of cytosine bases in the canine chromosomes has also been associated with lymphoma.[8]

Signalment and Clinical Features

Presentation can be indolent or aggressive. Lymphoma can be solitary or multicentric, node based or associated with any organ in the body. Early, accurate diagnosis and careful staging are keys to proper clinical decision making. Dogs typically present with non-painful lymphadenomegaly. Tumor stage has been shown to be prognostic (Table 25-2), and staging tests should be performed routinely. Prognostic variables are listed (Table 25-3). Canine lymphoma is generally the non-Hodgkin's form of the disease, although Hodgkin's lymphoma has been reported.[9-11]

Diagnosis and Staging

A diagnosis of lymphoma is most commonly established using cytology or biopsy. Cytology allows rapid identification of a monomorphic, abnormal lymphocyte population, but does not give complete classification and grading information (Figure 25-1). Histopathologic examination allows complete classification and grading, as well as immunophenotyping of the disease, yielding prognostic information. Classification systems in use include the National Institutes of Health Working Formulation and the Kiel system.[9,10,12] Both systems evaluate architecture and cellular morphology; the former does not include immunophenotype, but the latter includes immunophenotype in classification. Low-grade lymphomas, including mantle-zone, marginal-zone, follicular, and T-zone origins, have been associated with a significantly better survival prognosis than intermediate- and high-grade lymphomas.[13] Recently, flow-cytometry and immunoglobulin-gene and T-cell receptor gene rearrangement have been used to diagnose and type lymphomas.[14-24] Cytogenetics have also been used to identify chromosomal abnormalities in canine lymphomas.[25] Many extranodal locations have been reported (Table 25-4). Complete staging is critical for effective therapeutic decision-making (Table 25-5). Positron emission tomography (PET) imaging may offer an extremely sensitive staging

TABLE 25-1   LYMPHOMA RISK IN DOG BREEDS

Breed	Relative Risk[1]
Increased Risk	
Boxer	4.5
Basset Hound	4.1
St. Bernard	4.0
Scottish Terrier	3.2
Airedale	2.7
Labrador Retriever	1.8
Bulldog	2.2
Lower Risk	
Dachshund	0.1
Pomeranian	0.1
Pekingese	0.3
Miniature/Toy Poodle	0.3
Chihuahua	0.2
Brittany Spaniel	0.1

TABLE 25-2   WHO LYMPHOMA STAGING SCHEME

Stage	Characteristics
I	1 lymph node affected
II	>1 lymph node affected, same side of diaphragm
III	Multiple nodes, both sides of diaphragm
IV	Liver or spleen involvement +/- I-III
V	Marrow or extranodal tissue involvement +/- I-III
Substage	
A	No clinical signs referable to lymphoma
B	Clinical signs referable to lymphoma

TABLE 25-3   PROGNOSTIC VARIABLES IN CANINE LYMPHOMA

Prognostic Variable	Critical Factor	Prognosis
WHO stage	Stage I/II	+
	Stage III–V	–
WHO substage	b	–
Histologic subtype	Low grade	Longer survival, lower chemoresponsiveness
	High grade	Higher chemoresponsiveness, shorter survival
Immunophenotype	T cell	–
Hypercalcemia	Elevated iCa	–
Sex	Female	+
P-glycoprotein expression	Present	–
Prednisone prior to chemotherapy	If prolonged exposure	–
Mediastinal location	Present	–
Extranodal location	GI, renal, or cutaneous	–
Trisomy 13	Present	+

in a single examination in the future.[26] Thorough patient evaluation allows the detection of prognostic factors that may have bearing on a client's decision to treat, and allow careful staging of induction with chemotherapy to minimize patient morbidity through toxicity.

Biological Behavior/Metastasis

Lymphoma is most commonly a systemic illness and is assumed to be metastatic at presentation. Localized lymphomas have been reported, but systemic therapy is nearly always warranted for effective management. Multicentric lymphoma is the most common presentation. This disease appears to arise in one node or group of nodes and progress to involve many nodes,

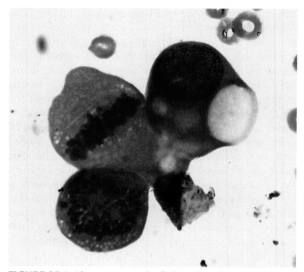

FIGURE 25-1 Photomicrograph of a lymph node aspirate cytology preparation. Note the large cellular size relative to the red blood cell. The lymphoma cells display anisokaryosis as well as large and irregular nucleoli, and at least one mitotic figure is visible.

TABLE 25-4   EXTRANODAL LOCATIONS OF LYMPHOMA AND PARANEOPLASTIC SYNDROMES

Location	Canine Reference	Feline Reference	Comments
Cardiac	27	28	
Hepatosplenic	29,30		
Ocular/orbital	31		
Conjunctiva	32,33	34	
Synovial	35		
Cutaneous	36–38	39–41	
Intestinal	42,43	44–52	
Hypercalcemia	53	54,55	T-cell lymphoma
Skeletal muscle	56,57	58	
Bone	59		
Brachial plexus		60	
Spinal cord		61,62	
Brain		63	
Tympanic bulla		64	
Hypereosino-philia	43	47	T-cell lymphoma
Intravascular	65–68	69	
Upper respira-tory	70,71	72–74	
Trachea		75	
Lung		58	
Kidney	76	77	
Urinary bladder	78		
Urethra	79		
Myasthenia gravis	80		

TABLE 25-5   STAGING TESTS APPROPRIATE TO LYMPHOMA

Staging Tests	Purpose	Stage If Positive
Lymph node aspirate	Rapid diagnosis	I–V
CBC	Detect cytopenias or anemia that complicate treatment or the presence of leukemia	V
Chemistry profile	Detect organ dysfunctions that complicate treatment/indicate organ involvement	IV or V possible
Urinalysis	Detect complicating urinary tract disease or renal compromise	V possible
Lymph node biopsy	Establish tumor grade and immunophenotype	I–V
Thoracic radiographs	Detect thoracic node or pulmonary involvement	V if pulmonary lymphoma
Abdominal ultrasound	Detect organ or abdominal node involvement	IV if liver/spleen lymphoma
Bone marrow aspirate	Detect bone marrow compromise	V if lymphoma cells present
Ophthalmic examination	Detect ocular involvement	V if lymphoma present

any lymphoid tissue, and even non-lymphoid tissue, as reflected by the World Health Organization (WHO) staging scheme. Alimentary lymphoma occurs less frequently than multicentric lymphoma. This form of lymphoma may be associated with significant hypoproteinemia, which has been identified as a negative prognostic factor for survival. Alimentary lymphoma must be differentiated from lymphocytic/plasmacytic enteritis. Chronic lymphocytic enteritis has been suggested to precede the development of alimentary lymphoma, although this has not been definitively demonstrated. A reported hallmark of lymphoma is invasion of the muscularis of the intestine, ruling out lymphocytic enteritis. Early literature suggested B-cell origin for the majority of these tumors, but recent reports suggest that T-cell origin may be frequent and associated with an eosinophilic infiltrate.[42,43,81,82] Central nervous system (CNS) lymphoma can occur as the primary presentation, or lymphoma may affect the CNS

as a secondary site. CNS infiltration may be focal or diffuse (see Chapter 19). The cutaneous form of lymphoma is most classically represented by epitheliotropic T-cell lymphoma (mycosis fungoides), although B-cell cutaneous lymphoma has been reported. This form of the disease is progressive and usually becomes systemic in its course. Renal lymphoma in dogs has been associated with a poor prognosis, but case reports exist of long-term survival.[76]

Therapy and Prognosis

Chemotherapy

The mainstay of therapy for canine lymphoma is cytotoxic chemotherapy. Numerous protocols have been evaluated in the literature (Table 25-6). Of these, the multi-drug protocols that include doxorubicin, vincristine, cyclophosphamide, and prednisone (CHOP)

TABLE 25-6   CHEMOTHERAPY PROTOCOLS FOR LYMPHOMA

Chemotherapy Protocol	CR Rate	Median Survival or Response	Reference
COP	70%–75%	7.5 mo	107,108
Madison-Wisconsin 25 wk*	94%	13.2 mo	83
Lomustine alone (cutaneous disease)	17%	3.5-mo response	97
Madison-Wisconsin 25 wk w/Actino		7 mo	94
VELCAP-S*	94%	12.5mo overall and 17 mo if CR	84
VELCAP-SC*	70%	6 mo	
VELCAP-HDC*	93%	32 mo for high-dose cyclo w/transplant	99
Madison-Wisconsin 25 wk w/Half Body RTX*	85%	19 mo if CR	109
Doxorubicin single agent	59%–79%	7.3–9 mo	
Mitoxantrone	25%	3-mo median remission	95

*CHOP-based protocol.

TABLE 25-7   A 25-WEEK CHOP CHEMOTHERAPY PROTOCOL

Week 1	L-Asparaginase/Vincristine/Prednisone	10,000 U/m² IM/0.7 mg/m² IV/2 mg/kg PO daily
Week 2	Cyclophosphamide/Prednisone	250 mg/m² PO divided over 4 days/1.5 mg/kg PO daily
Week 3	Vincristine/Prednisone	0.7 mg/m² IV/1 mg/kg PO daily
Week 4	Doxorubicin*/Prednisone	30 mg/m² IV/0.5 mg/kg PO daily
Week 6	Vincristine	0.7 mg/m² IV[†]
Week 7	Cyclophosphamide	250 mg/m² PO divided over 4 days
Week 8	Vincristine	0.7 mg/m² IV
Week 9	Doxorubicin*	30 mg/m² IV
Week 11	Vincristine	0.7 mg/m² IV
Week 13	Cyclophosphamide	250 mg/m² PO divided over 4 days
Week 15	Vincristine	0.7 mg/m² IV
Week 17	Doxorubicin	30 mg/m² IV
Week 19	Vincristine	0.7 mg/m² IV
Week 21	Cyclophosphamide	250 mg/m² PO divided over 4 days
Week 23	Vincristine	0.7 mg/m² IV
Week 25	Doxorubicin	30 mg/m² IV

*Administer (qs 30 ml in 0.9% NaCl) over 1/2 hour minimum.
[†]Doxorubicin dosage decreased to 1 mg/kg in dogs weighing < 10kg.
Perform a CBC with platelet count before and 7 days after every treatment.
Vincristine dosage range = 0.5 to 0.7 mg/m².

have met with the greatest success. Given in various combinations, these drugs typically yield greater than 80% complete response, remissions of approximately 9 months, and median survival greater than 1 year when followed by rescue therapy. The Madison-Wisconsin 25-week protocol, reported by Garrett and others,[83] led to a 94% complete response rate with 100% of those patients achieving a second remission after reinduction with the same protocol (Table 25-7). The 25-week version has no maintenance phase, which allows dogs to live for a period after chemotherapy without treatment. This may lead to greater responsiveness after loss of remission by lack of selection for resistance during the new rapid growth phase. Similarly, Moore and

others[84] found no loss of effectiveness of disease control by using a discontinuous protocol of VELCAP without a maintenance phase in the initial therapy period. It now appears that there is no survival benefit to a maintenance phase of initial chemotherapy for the average canine patient. Both protocols described include L-asparaginase. MacDonald and others[85] published a follow-up study to the original Wisconsin-Madison 25-week protocol that found no difference in response rate or survival with the omission of the L-asparaginase during induction. This suggests that reserving that drug for rescue may be most appropriate.[85,86] If used, L-asparaginase should be administered intramuscularly.[87] Drug resistance may be mediated by *p*-glycoprotein encoded by the multi-drug

TABLE 25-8   RESCUE CHEMOTHERAPY PROTOCOLS

Rescue Chemotherapy Protocol	No. of Dogs	CR Rate	PR Rate	Median Duration of Response	Notes	Reference
Actinomycin-D	9	33%	44%	1.5 mo		110
Actinomycin-D	25	0%	0%	0 mo	No response observed	111
Mitoxantrone	34	38%	26%	4 mo if CR	Not dissimilar to mitoxantrone first	95
Mitoxantrone	15	47%	47%	3 mo if CR	Much lower than doxorubicin	96
Doxorubicin	12	42%	33%	5 mo	No dog responded to second dose if failed first	112
Doxorubicin/ Dacarbazine	15	53%	33%	1 mo	All had received doxorubicin prior	113
MOPP	117	65%	31%	2 mo if CR	9/76 had longer rescue remission	114
Cisplatin/cytosine arabinoside	10	30%	10%	1.5 mo	Abstract	Ruslander
Etoposide	12	15%	7%		Cutaneous reactions to Polysorbate-80	115
CCNU (Lomustine)	43	27%	7%	3 mo overall, 4 mo if CR		116
B(Carmustine)OPP	14	29%	21%	4 mo if CR	Neutropenia, thrombocytopenia, and GI tox	117
L(Lomustine)OPP	40	27%	25%	4 mo if CR	Neutropenia, thrombocytopenia, and GI tox	117

OPP, Vincristine, procarbazine, prednisone.

resistance gene (MDR1).[88-91] *P*-glycoprotein expression has been documented in lymphomas and is likely a negative prognostic factor.[89,90,92] Mutation of this gene may be associated with increased chemotherapy toxicity.[93]

A chemotherapy protocol must be selected and tailored to meet the patient's and client's needs. The ideal protocol (1) will be within the client's budget and have a toxicity profile on par with the client's willingness to assume risk, (2) will avoid drugs with toxicity profiles that could target a particular weakness of the patient in question, and (3) will result in remission for the patient. The chronic chemotherapy toxicity of most concern in canine lymphoma patients is the cardiotoxicity associated with doxorubicin. Doxorubicin has been associated with the most durable remissions of the drugs available to treat lymphoma. The chronic cardiotoxicity associated with its administration can be a contraindication to its use. In these patients, the use of dexrazoxane, an iron-free radical scavenger, may prevent damage to an already compromised myocardium. The use of other anthracycline drugs has also been explored. Unfortunately, actinomycin-D as a replacement for doxorubicin resulted in diminished survival in an otherwise identical protocol.[94] Mitoxantrone has also been associated with a lower response rate.[95,96]

One of the greatest apparent benefits of chemotherapy protocols without a maintenance phase is the high proportion of patients who will reenter remission when the protocol is repeated following loss of remission after therapy is completed. This simplifies initial rescue therapy decisions. When patients have failed resumption of initial therapy, it is necessary to choose among a series of single drug and combination chemotherapy options, each with toxicity and efficacy differences (Table 25-8). Subsequent remissions tend to be shorter than the initial remission. The MOPP (mechlorethamine, vincristine, procarbazine, prednisone) protocol has been associated with longer second remissions in a subset of patients, however. Subsequent losses of remission portend a worsening prognosis.

Clinically ill or Stage V dogs with low neutrophil or platelet counts require cautious initiation of chemotherapy. In these patients, treatment with L-asparaginase and prednisone after complete staging may cause downstaging of the disease without causing myelosuppression. Cytotoxic therapy may be initiated 3 to 5 days later when the animal feels clinically well or the cell counts have returned to normal.

Lomustine has been evaluated for the treatment of epitheliotropic lymphoma. A dosage of 70 mg/m² administered every 3 weeks resulted in a 78% overall response rate (17% complete) for a median of 3 months in a study of 36 dogs.[97] Retinoic acid derivatives isotretinoin and etretinate may be used as well, with varying success reported.[37,98]

Stem Cell Transplantation

Recent reports from two institutions have examined the addition of hematopoietic stem cell transplant (bone marrow transplant) to chemotherapy.[99,100] These patients exhibited longer survival with median survival in optimally treated dogs up to 139 weeks.[99] The toxicity appears to be manageable, but the procedure remains quite expensive.[100]

Radiation Therapy

The addition of half-body radiation to standard chemotherapy has resulted in improved median survival times in several studies.[101] In the largest study to date, including 52 dogs, median remission duration was 486 days CHOP chemotherapy plus half-body radiation therapy.[101] The cost and toxicity has been judged by some to be excessive for the modest gains in survival.[101] Low-dose, whole body radiation was recently evaluated as a consolidation therapy, and was judged to be well tolerated.[102] The pilot study was too small to identify any survival benefit. Total skin irradiation with electrons has been described by Prescott and others (personal communication, 2004) for cutaneous lymphoma, but is not widely available.[103] Radiation therapy is effective as a palliative measure for bulky, localized disease, or to relieve neurologic signs associated with central nervous system lymphoma.[37] Treating a single area with radiation is almost never undertaken with curative intent.

Diet

Dietary n-3 fatty acid supplementation has been shown to be beneficial in canine patients. Metabolic parameters were improved in lymphoma patients eating an n-3 fatty acid–supplemented diet, and most importantly, survival times and disease-free interval were improved. Supplementing this nutrient in home-prepared diets may be of benefit to clinical patients.[104-106] (See Chapter 18, Section B, for additional details on dietary modification.)

Management Considerations

In the clinical setting, the question often arises as to whether patients should be vaccinated. Two veterinary studies addressed the question of whether a lymphoma patient can mount an appropriate antibody response while affected by an immunosuppressive disease and receiving immunosuppressive therapy. Henry et al.[118]

demonstrated that titers against canine parvovirus, canine distemper, and rabies were maintained during therapy for lymphoma in 16 dogs relative to 122 control dogs. Walter et al.[119] showed that doxorubicin therapy did not significantly affect T- and B-cell numbers, whereas combination chemotherapy caused a decrease in circulating B-cells in 12 lymphoma patients. Antibody titers were unaffected by chemotherapy, remaining stable throughout the course of treatment.[119] The same authors presented an abstract that demonstrated the ability of dogs to mount an antibody response against a novel antigen during chemotherapy for lymphoma. These data suggest that dogs can maintain adequate protective titers against vaccines for infectious disease following chemotherapy. What is less clear is whether there is a risk of vaccination contributing to relapse. To date, no study has documented this. However, stimulation of the lymphoid system could theoretically lead to recurrence of the cancer. As always, vaccination decisions should be dictated by assessment of the individual's risk.

LYMPHOMA IN CATS

Incidence/Etiology and Risk Factors

The risk of lymphoma in cats has been reported to rise until 1.5 years of age, and then becomes essentially stable throughout life thereafter.[1] Lymphoma can appear in cats of any age, breed, or sex, although Manx (RR of 4.6) and Burmese (RR of 3.1) appear to be at increased risk and intact females (RR of 0.7) appear to have lower-than-expected risk of the disease.[1] Unlike dogs, retroviral causes of feline lymphoma are well defined, with feline leukemia virus (FeLV) infection increasing risk 62 fold, feline immunodeficiency virus (FIV) infection increasing risk 6 fold, and concurrent FeLV and FIV infection increasing risk 77 fold.[120] Of cats with persistent FeLV infection undergoing necropsy, 23% died with lymphoma/leukemia complex.[121] Second-hand cigarette smoke also increases risk of lymphoma 2.5 to 3.2 fold, depending on duration of exposure.[122] Chronic inflammation has been postulated to lead to gastrointestinal lymphoma.[48] Immunosuppressive therapy for renal transplantation has also been associated with development of lymphoma.[123,124] Six cats were reported to develop lymphoma after treatment for vaccine-associated sarcoma, five of which were FeLV negative.[125]

Signalment and Clinical Features

Cats with lymphoma tend to present in two groups. The first are young cats with FeLV-associated disease. These cats often have respiratory signs associated with mediastinal lymph node enlargement and pleural effusion.[126] Older cats most commonly present with gastrointestinal lymphoma or extranodal lymphoma and are serologically negative for FeLV.[46] Siamese have been reported to be over-represented as a breed.[46,126] Lymphoma in an extranodal location can have widely variable presentations (see Table 25-4), from solitary masses in typical locations (e.g., cutaneous) to masses that destroy bone (Figure 25-2). Feline lymphoma has even presented as hypoadrenocorticism.[127] Hypercalcemia may be present, but less commonly than for dogs.[54] The presenting characteristics and clinical behavior of feline lymphoma may vary significantly with geographic location.[128-133]

Diagnosis and Staging

Staging is accomplished in cats with a similar battery of examinations as dogs (see Table 25-5). The traditional WHO stages have not been as useful to describe prognosis in cats as in dogs. Instead, cat lymphoma tends to be described in a syndromic fashion based on anatomic location of disease. These include mediastinal, gastrointestinal, multicentric, nasal, and extranodal locations. Each appears to have clinically different progression and potentially useful therapy. Each also presents a unique set of therapeutic challenges. Diagnosis of mediastinal lymphoma is made on cytological examination of pleural fluid or aspirate of the mediastinal mass. Biopsy can be complicated by location within the confines of the

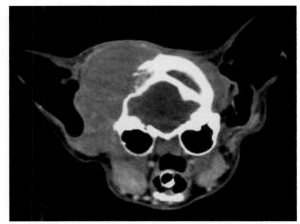

FIGURE 25-2 Presented is a single slice of a CT scan of a cat's skull that presented with a firm, immoveable mass caudal to the left ear. The scan reveals significant destruction of the bony calvarium, as well as a large soft-tissue mass overlying the area of destruction. Biopsy confirmed the diagnosis of lymphoma. Feline lymphoma can occur in atypical locations and demonstrate aggressive local invasion.

thoracic cavity, increasing risk of puncture of a lung or vascular structure. Diagnosis of gastrointestinal lymphoma is made using immunohistochemistry on histopathology of biopsy specimens of an endoscopically or surgically collected sample.[45] Nasal lymphoma most commonly requires a biopsy to confirm and has been reported to have a characteristic neoplastic appearance on skull CT examination.[73,134] Multicentric and extranodal presentations can usually be diagnosed by fine-needle aspirate or biopsy. If histopathology is inconclusive, immunoglobulin gene or T-cell receptor gene rearrangement clonality assessment can lend further support for neoplastic transformation.[135,136] After definitive diagnosis is made, complete staging is indicated to optimize therapy and minimize toxicity.

Biological Behavior/Metastasis

As in dogs, feline lymphoma tends to progress to systemic involvement. It also is generally the non-Hodgkin's form of lymphoma, although Hodgkin's lymphoma has been reported with Reed-Sternberg cells observed.[137,138] Because of the unusual anatomic presentations of feline lymphoma, the standard WHO staging scheme is less prognostic than for dogs. Immunophenotype can vary by location and etiology. Of retrovirus-induced tumors, FeLV-related lymphomas tend to be of T-cell lineage, whereas FIV-related lymphomas tend to be of B-cell origin.[46] Tumors resulting from FeLV tend to involve the mediastinum.[46] FIV-associated lymphomas tend to involve extranodal locations.[139] A study of nasal lymphomas found 17 of 18 to be of B-cell origin.[140] De Lorimier[141] presented an abstract including 16 cases of nasal lymphoma in which 8 were B-cell in origin. This form of lymphoma has been reported to be curable by radiation therapy alone; however, systemic metastasis has been reported.[142] Intestinal lymphomas have been reported to derive from large granular lymphocyte origin, which are often null cells or T-cells.[143] A study of intestinal lymphoma in Great Britain found 15 of 32 cats to have B-cell and 8 of 32 cats to have T-cell lymphoma.[45] In this series, 5 of 32 appeared to be inflammatory, contradicting the earlier diagnosis of lymphoma and emphasizing the diagnostic difficulty this disease can present.[45] Systemic spread of this disease may be less important than the consequences of local progression resulting in malassimilation. Immunophenotype does not appear to have the prognostic significance seen in dogs.[44,52] Age, weight, gender, FIV status, and stage have also been found not to be useful prognostic factors.[44,144] More than one study has found FeLV infection to be negatively prognostic, but other studies did not find this to be true.[145,146]

TABLE 25-9   COP-DOX PROTOCOL FOR FELINE LYMPHOMA AT UNIVERSITY OF MISSOURI-COLUMBIA

Drug	Dosage
First 6 Weeks	
Vincristine	0.5 mg/m^2 IV on day 1 of each treatment week for 6 weeks; VESICANT
Cyclophosphamide	150 mg/m^2 PO on same day as vincristine for 6 weeks; WEAR GLOVES
Prednisone	40 mg/m^2 PO daily for first week, then 20 mg/m^2 PO every other day thereafter
Beginning Week 7	
Doxorubicin	25 mg/m^2 IV q21d for 6 doses or until relapse Dilute to 20 ml in saline and administer IV over 20–30 min; SEVERE VESICANT

Complete blood counts are performed weekly at the time of vincristine injection and prior to each doxorubicin dose. If the total segmented neutrophil count is < 3000, cyclophosphamide is not administered until count increases above 3000. Then cyclophosphamide is restarted at three-fourths dose. Above protocol is discontinued after 6 months.

Watch for sterile hemorrhagic cystitis resulting from cyclophosphamide therapy. If it occurs, discontinue cyclophosphamide and replace with chlorambucil at 8 mg/m^2 po for first 3 days of each treatment week. Myelosuppression associated with chlorambucil occurs later than with cyclophosphamide (21 days vs. 7-10 days). Prednisone and cyclophosphamide administration in the morning are recommended.

Serum biochemistry profiles and urinalysis should be checked once monthly.

Therapy and Prognosis

The mainstay of therapy for aggressive or lymphoblastic lymphoma is combination chemotherapy. The combination of COP (cyclophosphamide, vincristine, and prednisone) may be expected to result in a complete remission for approximately 50% to 70% of cats.[133,144] Doxorubicin as a single agent has been less successful, generally resulting in complete remission rates less than 50%.[147,148] However, doxorubicin is associated with the most durable remissions.[144] For this reason, the COP-Dox protocol (Table 25-9) is used at the University of Missouri-Columbia. Achieving a complete remission appears to be the most reliable positive prognostic factor for survival with median survival approaching 1 year and long-term survival reported.[44,48,51,145] One study from Australia suggested that one quarter of cats achieving complete remission may never relapse, although this has not been the author's experience and may reflect geographic differences.[132] Failure to achieve complete remission is associated with median survivals of only a few months.[44,48,51,145] The University of Wisconsin-Madison protocol, described above for dogs, has been reported in a series of 38 cats. The complete remission rate was 47% with median duration of complete remission of 654 days.[44] This is very similar to the results achieved with COP. Lomustine has been administered to cats as a primary or rescue agent at a dosage of 45.5 to 60 mg/m^2 and appears to be well tolerated at those doses.[41,149] Cats with renal lymphoma have been shown to have the risk of CNS metastasis reduced

significantly by the addition of cytosine-arabinoside to a standard COP protocol (COAP).[77]

Radiation therapy has been reported for therapy of localized lymphoma.[72,138,141,142,150] Although it has been shown to be effective for local control, particularly for nasal lymphoma, adjunctive systemic chemotherapy is usually advisable to delay or prevent systemic progression. Survival times in cats treated with radiation therapy for nasal lymphoma often exceed 1 year.[72,141,142]

Feline alimentary lymphoma presents a therapeutic challenge. Median survival times for cats experiencing complete remission with chemotherapy can exceed 11 months.[48,151] It is clear that lymphoblastic forms of the disease should be treated with combination chemotherapy. What is less clear is the need for aggressive therapy with lymphocytic forms. One study reported a 69% complete remission rate for alimentary lymphocytic lymphoma treated with chlorambucil and prednisone.[152] It may be appropriate to treat indolent-appearing lymphomas with this combination.

Selected References*

Garrett LD, Thamm DH, Chun R, et al: Evaluation of a 6-month chemotherapy protocol with no maintenance therapy for dogs with lymphoma, *J Vet Intern Med* 16:704, 2002.
This study describes the chemotherapy most widely used currently for canine lymphoma.

Louwerens M, London CA, Pedersen NC, et al: Feline lymphoma in the post-feline leukemia virus era, *J Vet Intern Med* 19:329, 2005.
This reference is a thorough discussion of current presentations of feline lymphoma.
Rassnick KM, Mauldin GE, Al-Sarraf R, et al: MOPP chemotherapy for treatment of resistant lymphoma in dogs: a retrospective study of 117 cases (1989-2000), *J Vet Intern Med* 16:576, 2002.

This study describes the only rescue protocol published that resulted in some second remissions longer than the first.

■ *For a complete list of the references cited in this chapter, please go to www.smallanimaloncology.com.

SECTION B: Leukemia

Jeffrey N. Bryan

KEY POINTS

- Chronic lymphocytic leukemia in the dog is highly manageable.
- Leukemia in the cat is most frequently associated with FeLV infection.
- Immunohistochemical or flow cytometric typing should be performed early to identify leukemia lineage and establish therapy options and prognosis.

Incidence/Etiology and Risk Factors

Leukemias are malignancies arising in the bone marrow from leukocyte, erythrocyte, or megakaryocyte progenitor cells and are classified according to their aggressiveness and cell of origin. The incidence of true leukemias of dogs and cats is not known, but they appear to be very rare, with chronic lymphocytic leukemia (CLL) and acute lymphocytic/lymphoblastic leukemia (ALL) predominating over chronic myelogenous leukemia (CML) or acute myelogenous leukemia (AML).[1] Polycythemia vera (primary erythrocytosis) and megakaryocytic leukemias have been reported as well.[2,3] Lymphoid leukemias appear to be more frequent in dogs than in cats.[2] In dogs and cats, the best recognized and understood etiology of leukemia is FeLV, which can cause myelogenous, erythroid, or lymphoid leukemias in cats.[2] In a study of 16 cats with myelodysplastic syndrome, of which four transformed to AML, 15 were seropositive for FeLV.[4] Infectious retroviral particles were isolated from a large granular lymphocytic leukemia in a dog, but this finding has not been replicated.[5] Exposure to radiation and prior chemotherapy, particularly with alkylating agents, has been associated with the development of leukemias in dogs.[6-8] No specific risk factors of breed or gender have been identified.[9]

Signalment and Clinical Features

Cats affected by FeLV tend to be young.[2] Dogs with acute leukemias also appear to be affected at younger ages. In a series of 30 dogs with ALL, a median age of 5.5 years was reported (range, 1–12 years).[10] Dogs affected by AML appear to be similarly young.[9] Dogs with chronic leukemias tend to be older, with reported median age for CLL of approximately 10 years[9,11] and a median age of 8 years for CML.[12] Clinical signs with acute leukemias tend to be much more prominent, but are non-specific, including lethargy, inappetence, and gastrointestinal signs of vomiting or diarrhea.[2,10] CLL tends to be clinically occult and is often an incidental discovery on routine CBC or may cause vague clinical signs of illness.[11] Physical examination findings in leukemic dogs and cats may include lymphadenomegaly or abdominal organomegaly.[9,11-13] Particularly in dogs, the differentiation between ALL and Stage V lymphoma can be difficult, with degree of disease burden in the bone marrow relative to peripheral locations being the primary deciding factor. Manifestations of concurrent and secondary complications may be apparent as well, including petechiation, ecchymosis, or frank hemorrhage.[10,13] Clinical pathology findings in acute leukemias can include total nucleated cell counts that range from subnormal (aleukemic) to extremely elevated with moderate to poor differentiation (Figure 25-3).[9,13] Affected animals may have severe anemia, neutropenia, or thrombocytopenia, which may complicate treatment.[9,13] Animals with chronic leukemias tend to uniformly have elevated white cell counts of moderately to well-differentiated cells.[9,11,13] These counts can exceed 200,000 cells/µl (Figure 25-4), and may be accompanied by thrombocytopenia.[11,12]

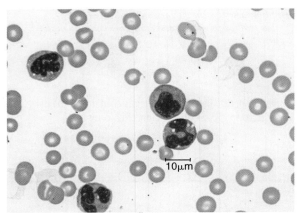

FIGURE 25-3 Peripheral blood smear from a dog with acute myelogenous leukemia. Note the lack of clear lineage differentiation of the two uppermost large cells. *(Courtesy of the University of Missouri-Columbia Oncology Service.)*

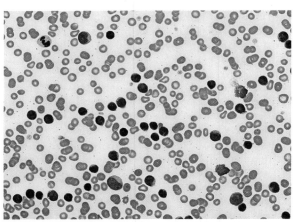

FIGURE 25-4 Peripheral blood smear from a boxer dog with chronic lymphocytic leukemia. Note the marked increase in number of primarily well-differentiated lymphocytes. *(Courtesy of the University of Missouri-Columbia Oncology Service.)*

Diagnosis and Staging

The diagnosis of leukemia is made by positively identifying neoplastic cells in circulation or the bone marrow. This is easier in chronic leukemias, since the cells are better differentiated. Acute leukemias may be comprised of cells so immature that their type is distinguishable only through cytochemistry, immunohistochemistry, or flow cytometry (Tables 25-10 and 25-11). In the case

TABLE 25-10   IMMUNOHISTOCHEMICAL STAINS USED TO DIFFERENTIATE LEUKEMIAS

Stain	Cell Type
Peroxidase	Neutrophils, eosinophils, ± monocytes
Chloracetate esterase	Neutrophils, basophils, mast cells
Leukocyte alkaline phosphatase	Eosinophils
Non-specific esterase	Monocytes, lymphocytes, megakaryocytes, ± plasma cells, granulocytes
Toluidine blue	Mast cells

TABLE 25-11   CLUSTER OF DIFFERENTIATION DESIGNATIONS ASSOCIATED WITH VARIOUS CELL TYPES

Cluster of Differentiation	Cell-Type
CD1c	Myeloid cells
CD3	T-cells
CD4	T-helper
CD8	T-cytotoxic
CD11	Leukocytes
CD14	Monocytes, granulocytes
CD18	Leukocytes
CD21	B-cells
CD25	T-regs
CD34	Immature leukocytes
CD45	All leukocytes
CD56	Natural killer, some T
CD57	Natural killer, some T
CD79a	B-cells
CD90 (Thy-1)	Leukocytes

of lymphocytic leukemias, immunoglobulin and T-cell receptor gene rearrangement PCR assays may also be used to identify a clonal expansion of lymphocytes, supporting neoplastic expansion over inflammatory response in most cases.[9] Leukemias are typed according to cell of origin, degree of bone marrow infiltration, and degree of differentiation by the French-American-British (FAB) classification system (Table 25-12). Complete blood cell count, serum chemistry profile, FeLV serology in cats, thoracic radiographs, and abdominal ultrasound are recommended. Particular attention should be paid to cytopenias or organ dysfunction that might complicate chemotherapy. Often, neutropenia and thrombocytopenia will limit the frequency and dosage of cytotoxic

TABLE 25-12   FEATURES OF VARIOUS TYPES OF LEUKEMIA

Type Of Leukemia	FAB AML Classification	Features
Acute undifferentiated	AUL	All BM cells UD blasts
ML without differentiation	M0	All BM cells are myeloblasts
ML with minimal maturation	M1	< 10% maturing granulocytes
ML with maturation	M2	>10% maturing granulocytes
Promyelocytic leukemia	M3	Predominantly promonocytes
Myelomonocytic leukemia	M4	Mix of granulocytes and monocytes
Monoblastic leukemia	M5a	>80% BM cells are monoblasts
Monocytic leukemia	M5b	>30% and <80% BM cells are monoblasts
Erythroleukemia	M6	>50% BM cells are nucleated erythroid
Erythroleukemia	M6Er	Erythroblasts predominate
Megakaryocytic leukemia	M7	>30% BM cells are megakaryoblasts

BM, Bone marrow; *ML*, myelogenous leukemia; *UD*, undifferentiated.

agents that can be delivered.[9-13] Well-differentiated leukemias must be distinguished from inflammatory responses, leukemoid reactions, and paraneoplastic elevations in white blood cell lines. Polycythemia vera must be distinguished from secondary polycythemias (see Chapters 11 and 22, Section H).

Biological Behavior/Metastasis

Acute leukemias are extremely aggressive neoplasms that severely impair the function of the normal bone marrow elements. Identification of neoplastic cells in the lymph nodes, liver, and spleen is not uncommon in dogs and cats with these leukemias,[9,13] but probably does not represent metastasis of the primary reproducing elements of the disease. These diseases are systemic at the time of diagnosis and require systemic chemotherapy. The expected survival in most cases of acute leukemia is extremely short, usually less than 1 week after diagnosis.[9,13]

Chronic leukemias are much more indolent in their clinical course.[11,12] Mean survival times in dogs with CLL and CML have been reported to be 452 days (range, 30–1000) and 108 days (range 41–>690), respectively. Blast crisis, in which chronic disease transforms to a fulminant acute form, appears to occur in CML and is usually a terminal event.[12] Dogs with CLL have been reported to lapse terminally into generalized lymphoma,[11] which would be expected to be drug resistant. The majority of cases of CLL in one study were of T-cell origin.[9]

Dogs or cats with leukemia have impaired immune response to pathogens.[2,11,12] The majority of dogs with CLL and CML may be expected to ultimately succumb to infectious causes of death.[11,12] For this reason, patients should be evaluated carefully for sources of septicemia.

Therapy and Prognosis

Therapy for acute leukemias is generally unrewarding. For AML, cytosine arabinoside, 6-thioguanine, doxorubicin, and mitoxantrone have been suggested, but there are no reports of successful treatment.[15] Therapy for ALL is similar to that for Stage V lymphoma, with the addition of cytosine arabinoside during induction.[10] With the success of CHOP-based protocols (see Section A) for treating advanced lymphoma, these should be considered for primary therapy of ALL. Bone marrow transplant may become routine for treating this, as well as lymphoma, but is of limited availability.[16] One dog with ALL experienced a remission after treatment with plasma and whole blood transfusion, presumably because of the immunologic effect of the engrafted immune components.[17]

Therapy for chronic leukemias has been reported to be more successful. For CLL, induction with a COP protocol and maintenance with chlorambucil and prednisone can result in complete remissions, even in patients with extremely high cell counts at diagnosis (Table 25-13).[11] Long-term survival has been reported with no therapy as well.[18] For CML, hydroxyurea has been recommended at a dosage of 50 mg/kg orally once daily, with remission typically occurring within 1 month.[12] Polycythemia vera may be treated with hydroxyurea or with serial phlebotomy.[19] Polycythemia vera and chronic megakaryocytic leukemia have been reported to respond to radioactive phosphorus-32.[3]

TABLE 25-13   INDUCTION PROTOCOL FOR CLL

Week	Drug	Dosage
1	Cytosine Arabinoside	50 mg/m^2 subcutaneously bid × 4 days
1	Prednisone	40 mg/m^2 PO daily
1–8	Vincristine	0.5 mg/m^2 IV once on Day 1 of each week
1–8	Cyclophosphamide	50 mg/m^2 PO daily × on Days 1-4 of each week
2–8	Prednisone	20 mg/m^2 PO daily
After week 8	Chlorambucil	8 mg/m^2 PO daily for the first 4 days out of 14
After week 8	Prednisone	20 mg/m^2 PO daily

CBC performed weekly at the time of vincristine injection. If the total segmented neutrophil count is < 3000, cyclophosphamide is not administered until count increases > 3000. Then cyclophosphamide is restarted at three-fourths dose. Daily temperature monitoring is recommended for first 3 weeks of therapy.

Every-other-week maintenance therapy is performed for four treatments (8 weeks). If dog is in remission and doing well after 8 weeks of twice-monthly maintenance therapy, treatments are decreased to every third week for four additional treatments (12 weeks) and prednisone is continued as before. If dog is doing well after completion of every-3-week regimen, chemotherapy is discontinued. Relapses are treated with induction protocol, then maintenance.

Selected References*

Hardy WD: Hematopoietic tumors of cats, *J Am Anim Hosp Assoc* 17:921, 1981.
This paper provides a complete review of hematopoietic tumors of cats associated with FeLV and those that arise spontaneously.
Leifer CE, Matus RE: Chronic lymphocytic leukemia in the dog: 22 cases (1974-1984), *J Am Vet Med Assoc* 189:214, 1986.
This manuscript provides a good overview of CLL and its expected outcomes in dogs.

Vernau W, Moore PF: An immunophenotypic study of canine leukemias and preliminary assessment of clonality by polymerase chain reaction, *Vet Immunol Immunopathol* 69:145, 1999.
This is an excellent review paper on the topic of canine leukemias and includes information related to flow cytometry and PCR evaluation.

█ *For a complete list of the references cited in this chapter, please go to www.smallanimaloncology.com.

SECTION C: Multiple Myeloma

Chelsea Tripp and Jeffrey N. Bryan

KEY POINTS

- Multiple myeloma is a systemic disease requiring chemotherapy in almost all cases.
- Approximately 80% of dogs treated with chemotherapy will experience complete remission.
- Clinical presentation for cats with multiple myeloma is quite variable.

Incidence/Etiology and Risk Factors

Multiple myeloma is a neoplasm of clonal proliferation of malignant plasma cells that most often produce an immunoglobulin. In most instances, the population of neoplastic plasma cells is monoclonal, although biclonal and polyclonal plasma cell neoplasms

have been reported.[1,2] The secreted protein produces a narrow peak on serum and urine electrophoresis, most commonly in the gamma globulin region, although beta peaks are reported.[3,4] A variety of plasma cell neoplastic syndromes exist, including multiple myeloma, immunoglobulin M (IgM) (Waldenström's) macroglobulinemia, immunoglobulin-secreting lymphoma, and solitary osseous or soft-tissue plasmacytomas. Multiple myeloma is most frequently reported in older dogs (average 8–9 years). German shepherds are reported to be overrepresented in one study.[5] Genetic predisposition, viral infection, chronic antigenic stimulation, and exposure to carcinogens have all been implicated in the development of multiple myeloma in humans.[6] Reports of two cases among siblings suggest that genetic predisposition may exist in cats.[7] Solitary osseous plasma cell tumors have been reported to progress to multiple myeloma in both dogs and cats.[8]

Signalment and Clinical Features

Clinical signs of multiple myeloma are non-specific, including depression, chronic infections, bleeding diathesis, bone pain, paresis, or polyuria/polydipsia. Associated pathologic syndromes include osteolytic lesions or pathologic fracture, cytopenias, coagulopathies, hyperviscosity syndrome, hypercalcemia, renal disease, and cardiac failure. Signs may be quite variable and present for long periods prior to diagnosis in cats.[9] Electrophoresis consistent with a monoclonal gammopathy of unknown significance has been reported in both dogs and cats, similar to humans.

Osteolytic lesions can be solitary or appear as diffuse osteopenias. Bones of active hematopoiesis are more frequently affected, including ribs, pelvis, vertebrae and proximal and distal long bones.[10]

Normocytic, normochromic, non-regenerative anemia can result from marrow infiltration, increased destruction caused by hyperviscosity syndrome, blood loss from coagulation defects, or low iron stores from anemia of chronic disease. Similar factors may lead to thrombocytopenia or leukopenias. Approximately half of cats will have anemia and thrombocytopenia at presentation, and one third will be neutropenic.[11]

Hypercalcemia of malignancy associated with multiple myeloma has been reported for dogs and cats.[12] Proposed mechanisms of hypercalcemia include increased production of an osteoclast-activating factor by neoplastic cells and direct bony osteolysis.[9,12,13] Binding of calcium to myeloma proteins with resultant normal serum-ionized calcium has been documented in a dog, as it is in humans.[4] Polyuria and polydipsia may be present from renal failure or as a result of hypercalcemia. Renal dysfunction is often associated with multiple myeloma and may be the result of tumor infiltrate, hypercalcemia, amyloidosis, decreased perfusion, or Bence-Jones proteins.[14] Hyperviscosity syndrome may be present in patients with extremely elevated globulin levels. This may manifest as hypertension, epistaxis, retinal detachment, cardiac failure, or seizures.

Diagnosis and Staging

A diagnosis of multiple myeloma requires identification of a combination of factors. A minimum database should include a complete blood count, serum biochemistry profile, urinalysis, and protein electrophoresis to detect a monoclonal gammopathy and characterize the immunoglobulin present. Diagnosis of multiple myeloma in both humans and dogs has traditionally required the demonstration of at least two of the following criteria: (1) monoclonal gammopathy (M component), (2) lytic bone lesions (Figure 25-5), (3) atypical plasma cell proliferation within the bone marrow, and (4) Bence-Jones proteinuria.[14-16] Newer guidelines for diagnosing multiple myeloma in humans require inclusion of one major criteria and one minor criteria. The major criteria are as follows: (1) tissue evidence of plasmacytoma, (2) bone marrow plasmacytosis of > 30% plasma cells, or (3) a monoclonal globulin spike on serum electrophoresis > 3.5 g/dL for IgG or 2.0 g/dL for IgA. The minor criteria are (1) bone marrow plasmacytosis between 10% and 30%, (2) lytic bone lesions, or (3) a monoclonal globulin spike below the previous threshold. Cytology of the spleen or bone marrow identifying clustering of monomorphic plasma cells is suggestive of plasma cell tumor. Normal bone marrow should contain < 5% plasma cells. Current standards suggest that plasma cells in excess of 20% indicate myeloma. However, a cutoff of 10% with cellular atypia may also be considered.[11] Aspiration of lytic bony lesions may yield a diagnosis of plasma cell infiltrate.

Biological Behavior/Metastasis

Multiple myeloma is a systemic illness and by definition considered metastatic at presentation. Extramedullary plasmacytoma (EMP) has been reported in conjunction with multiple myeloma; thus a diagnosis of EMP warrants patient evaluation for metastatic lesions suggesting the presence of multiple myeloma. EMP is defined as a neoplastic plasma cell infiltrate in soft tissue without evidence of bone marrow involvement.[17] In dogs, this condition appears to arise from mucosal

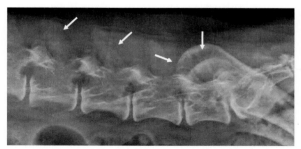

FIGURE 25-5 This lateral radiograph of the lumbar spine and pelvis demonstrates the punctate lysis *(arrows)* typical of aggressive, bone-based multiple myeloma.

or cutaneous tissues, most commonly in the oral cavity and skin of the head and digits.[18,19] The oral form of plasmacytoma may also be associated with periodontal disease. Special stains for amyloid and cyclin D1 may be positive on histopathology, but do not predict biological behavior.[18,20] Although both conditions appear to derive from functional B-cell lymphocytes, studies have not shown cutaneous EMP to progress to multiple myeloma.[8,21] In cats, EMP typically results in the production of a monoclonal gammopathy, which may lead to hyperviscosity syndrome, whereas a secreted paraprotein is rare in dogs with EMP.[20,22] A literature report exists of 1 of 4 vertebral solitary osseous plasmacytoma progressing to multiple myeloma.[23]

Therapy and Prognosis

Recommended therapy for multiple myeloma is chemotherapy, pain management, and reduction of serum levels of immunoglobulins. The chemotherapeutic drug of choice for the treatment of multiple myeloma is melphalan. In the dog, the starting dose of 0.1 mg/kg is given orally once daily for 7 to 10 days and then reduced to 0.05 mg/kg given orally once daily thereafter.[14] The addition of prednisone appears to improve response to therapy. Melphalan is continued daily for the duration of remission or until a dose reduction is necessary because of myelosuppression. The most common clinically significant toxicity associated with long-term administration of melphalan is thrombocytopenia. Patients should be monitored with bi-weekly CBCs for the first 2 months of therapy and monthly thereafter. An alternative pulse-dosing schedule (7 mg/m^2 given orally daily for 5 consecutive days every 3 weeks) has been described for patients experiencing hematopoietic toxicity.[24]

Other alkylating agents such as cyclophosphamide have been used alone or in combination with melphalan in multiple myeloma.[5,14] Induction therapy with vincristine has been advocated in patients with widespread tumor burden, hyperviscosity syndrome, or systemic hypercalcemia.

When patients have failed initial therapy, rescue therapy may be attempted. Successes with standard-dose doxorubicin, vincristine, and cyclophosphamide are anecdotally discussed, but not published.

For patients with localized plasma cell tumors causing pain or neurologic dysfunction, radiation therapy appears to be effective in relieving the clinical signs and resolving the local disease.[23] Radiation therapy is generally not appropriate for systemically affected patients unless it is used primarily for palliation of pain. Chemotherapy is necessary to manage systemic manifestations of the disease.

Management Considerations

Multiple myeloma patients are immunologically compromised. Careful evaluation for concurrent infections during chemotherapy is important for these patients.

Selected References*

Matus RE, Leifer CE, MacEwen EG, et al: Prognostic factors for multiple myeloma in the dog, *J Am Vet Med Assoc* 188:1288, 1986.
This manuscript provides the most comprehensive description of prognostic factors for canine multiple myeloma currently published.
Mellor PJ, Haugland S, Murphy S, et al: Myeloma-related disorders in cats commonly present as extramedullary neoplasms in contrast to myeloma in human patients: 24 cases with clinical follow-up, *J Vet Intern Med* 20:1376, 2006.
This manuscript provides a good overview of the presentation of myeloma diseases in cats.
Wright ZM, Rogers KS, Mansell J: Survival data for canine oral extramedullary plasmacytomas: a retrospective analysis (1996-2006), *J Am Anim Hosp Assoc* 44:75, 2008.
This retrospective study provides information about oral extramedullary plasmacytomas and their clinical behavior in dogs.

■ *For a complete list of the references cited in this chapter, please go to www.smallanimaloncology.com

26 Tumors of the Endocrine System

SECTION A: Adrenal and Pituitary Tumors in Dogs and Cats

Amy E. DeClue and Jeffrey N. Bryan

KEY POINTS

- Adrenal tumors may produce a variety of different hormones, and a thorough endocrinologic evaluation should be performed on any animal with an adrenal tumor.
- Dogs with adrenal tumors treated with surgery have an excellent long-term prognosis.
- Because of the episodic nature of clinical signs, pheochromocytomas are difficult to recognize. Surgery is the treatment of choice, and careful pre-operative management is essential.
- The majority of cats with adrenal cortical or pituitary tumors present for diabetes mellitus.
- An aldosterone-secreting adrenal cortical tumor should be suspected in any cat with acute blindness, polymyopathy, hypertension, hypokalemia, and/or metabolic alkalosis and an adrenal mass. Both medical and surgical therapies result in a good to excellent prognosis.
- Care should be taken to rule out a pituitary macroadenoma in any dog with pituitary-dependent hyperadrenocorticism.

Tumors involving the adrenal gland may arise from the adrenal cortex or medulla or may be due to metastatic disease. It is important to note that metastatic lesions represent 26.7% of canine and 60% of feline adrenal neoplasms.[1] Metastatic disease should be considered in any patient with an adrenal mass.

ADRENAL CORTICAL TUMORS IN DOGS

Incidence/Etiology and Risk Factors

Tumors of the adrenal cortex may be adenomas or carcinomas. Although some adrenal cortical tumors are hormonally silent, a myriad of hormones either singly or in combination can be produced, with cortisol being the most common (Table 26-1).

Signalment and Clinical Features

Adrenal tumors are most commonly recognized in middle-aged to older (median age, 11–12 years), large breed (median weight, 20 kg), female dogs.[2,3] Clinical signs and clinicopathologic abnormalities are related to the type of hormone produced (see Table 26-1).

Diagnosis and Staging

Definitive diagnosis of an adrenal tumor requires histopathologic evaluation, although a presumptive diagnosis can be made based on clinical signs, endocrinologic testing, and the presence of an adrenal mass. Radiographic evidence of adrenal calcification is present in about half of cases but fails to differentiate benign from malignant lesions.[4,5] Ultrasound or CT are the most commonly used imaging modalities for the detection of adrenal tumors and abdominal metastases. Atrophy of the contralateral adrenal gland is inconsistent and, therefore, a lack of atrophy does not rule out a functional cortical tumor.[4] Any animal with a suspected adrenal tumor should undergo thorough endocrinologic evaluation to determine functionality (Table 26-2).

Biological Behavior/Metastasis

Tumors of the adrenal glands occur with equal frequency in the left and right gland with 14 to 30% of dogs having bilateral tumors.[2,4] Approximately 56% to 83% of adrenal cortical tumors are carcinomas.[2,6] Tumor size > 2 cm in diameter is associated with adrenal cortical carcinomas.[7] Metastatic lesions are recognized in 14% to 28% of dogs with adrenal neoplasia, with the lungs, liver, and lymph nodes being the most common sites.[2,8]

TABLE 26-1   CLINICAL FINDINGS AND CLINICOPATHOLOGIC ABNORMALITIES IN DOGS AND CATS WITH ADRENAL TUMORS

Tumor Type	Hormone Produced	Clinical Findings		Clinicopathologic Abnormalities	
		Dogs[*]	Cats[†]	Dogs[*]	Cats[†]
Adrenal cortical adenoma/ carcinoma	Cortisol Progesterone 17-OH progesterone Corticosterone Testosterone Estradiol Androstenedione	Polyuria/ polydipsia[‡] Polyphagia[‡] Panting[‡] Pendulous abdomen[‡] Alopecia Hyperpigmenta- tion Calcinosis cutis	Polydipsia[‡] Polyuria[‡] Polyphagia[‡] Weight loss[‡] Increased skin fragil- ity[‡] Hepatomegaly Alopecia Uncontrolled diabetes mellitus[‡]	Stress leukogram[‡] Mildly to severely ↑ ALP[‡] Hypercholesterolemia Mildly ↑ALT Proteinuria	Hyperglycemia[‡] Hypercholester- olemia Glucosuria[‡]
	Aldosterone	Rare, similar to cats	Sudden blindness[‡] Hypokalemic polymyopathy[‡] Cervical ventroflexion Polyuria/polydipsia Hyporexia Weight loss Nocturia Abdominal distension Mydriasis	Rare, similar to cats	Hypokalemia[‡] Mild hypernatremia Metabolic alkalosis Hypophospha- temia Hypomagnesemia Azotemia Increased CK
Pheochromo- cytoma	Norepinephrine Epinephrine	Asymptomatic[‡] Syncope, weakness Anxiety, panting Hypertension Seizure Cardiac arrhythmia Polyuria/ polydipsia	Rare, similar to dogs	Mild thrombocytopenia Mild anemia Increased ALT Hypoalbuminemia Hypercholesterolemia Azotemia Proteinuria	Unknown

ALP, Alkaline phosphatase; *ALT,* alanine transaminase; *CK,* creatine kinase.
[*]References 2,5,9,11,14,16,64-68.
[†]References 29,33,36,37,69-72.
[‡]Most common findings.

Therapy and Prognosis

Adrenalectomy is the treatment of choice for any hormonally functional adrenal cortical tumor or any adrenal cortical tumor > 2 cm. Although reported post-operative mortality is high (19%–30%), patients that survive 2 weeks after adrenalectomy have a good long-term prognosis (mean survival, 778 days).[2,6,9] It is important to note that tumor size, patient age, histopathologic diagnosis, and presence of tumor thrombi of the vena cava are not prognostic.[2,9] For patients that are poor surgical candidates, medical management is possible (Table 26-3).[10-13] Since it is adrenolytic, mitotane is the

preferred medical treatment for adrenocortical tumors with a median survival of 11.5 months.[10] In addition, mitotane may be administered to control cortisol- or androgen-related clinical signs associated with metastatic disease.

PHEOCHROMOCYTOMA IN DOGS

Incidence/Etiology and Risk Factors

Pheochromocytomas arise from the chromaffin cells of the adrenal medulla and produce the catecholamines epinephrine and norepinephrine.

TABLE 26-2   ENDOCRINE EVALUATION OF ADRENAL CORTICAL TUMORS IN DOGS AND CATS[29,36,37,65,67,70,73-75]

Diagnostic Test	Sensitivity	Specificity	Interpretation	Comments
LDDST	Excellent	Good	Failure to suppress at 8 hr is consistent with HAC; suppression at 4 hr is consistent with PDH, not AT	Diagnostic test of choice to diagnose HAC because of the high sensitivity in dogs and cats
ACTH stimulation test: Cortisol	Poor	Good	Hyperstimulation is consistent with HAC	Poor sensitivity makes this test less desirable; cannot differentiate PDH from AT. This test is not recommended in cats.
ACTH stimulation test: Androgens*	Unknown	Unknown	Hyperstimulation is consistent with an androgen-secreting AT	Consider in patients with adrenal tumors and negative LDDST
UCC	~100%	Poor	UCC ≤ the reference range is inconsistent with HAC	Because of poor specificity, this test cannot be used to diagnose HAC
Aldosterone	Unknown	Unknown	Elevation may be consistent with an aldosterone secreting tumor	Evaluate prior to starting antihypertensive medications, potassium supplementation, or fluid therapy

ACTH, Adrenocorticotropic hormone; *AT,* adrenal tumor; *HAC,* hyperadrenocorticism; *LDDST,* low-dose dexamethasone suppression test; *PDH,* pituitary dependent hyperadrenocorticism; UCC, urine cortisol:creatinine.

*Androgens include androstenedione, estradiol, progesterone, testosterone, and 17-hydroxyprogesterone.

TABLE 26-3   MEDICAL MANAGEMENT OF ADRENAL CORTICAL TUMORS SECRETING CORTISOL OR ANDROGENS IN DOGS[10-13,21,48,67]

Drug	Mechanism of Action	Side Effects	Efficacy	Comments
Mitotane	Adrenal cortical lysis, enzyme inhibitor	Hypoadrenocorticism Gastrointestinal	Good	Dogs with AT typically require higher doses than dogs with PDH
Trilostane	Enzyme inhibitor	Hypoadrenocorticism	Good	FDA approved for the treatment of hypoadrenocorticism secondary to AT; no effect on tumor growth or metastasis
Ketoconazole	Enzyme inhibitor	Gastrointestinal Hepatic toxicity Hypoadrenocorticism Thrombocytopenia Lightening of haircoat	Fair	Typically used for pre-operative rather than long-term management; no effect on tumor growth or metastasis

AT, Adrenal tumor; *PDH,* pituitary-dependent hyperadrenocorticism.

*Androgens: androstenedione, estradiol, progesterone, testosterone, and 17-hydroxyprogesterone.

Signalment/Clinical Features

Pheochromocytomas are most commonly found in middle-aged to older dogs.[14,15] Clinical findings are variable (see Table 26-1) and 60% of dogs are asymptomatic.[14-16] Aortic thromboembolism and retroperitoneal hemorrhage are unique sequelae.[17,18]

Diagnosis and Staging

A presumptive diagnosis of pheochromocytoma can be made on the bases of appropriate clinical signs and the presence of an adrenal mass. Diagnostic assessment should include blood pressure, ophthalmic examination, and ECG. Because changes occur intermittently (when catecholamines are secreted), repeated evaluations may be necessary. Abdominal ultrasound is more sensitive than radiographs for detection of pheochromocytoma, and CT is ideal for detecting local invasion.[14,19] Because of the episodic nature of catecholamine release and lack of commercial assays, blood or urine catecholamine evaluation is rarely performed. Provocative endocrine testing is not recommended due to the risk of hypertensive crisis, and suppression testing has not been validated in dogs.

Biological Behavior/Metastasis

Pheochromocytomas may be benign, malignant, unilateral, or bilateral. Metastatic disease or local invasion is reported in approximately 13% to 24% or 39% to 52% of dogs with pheochromocytoma, respectively.[14,15] The most common sites for metastases include regional lymph nodes, liver, lung, spleen, kidney, and bone.[14]

Therapy and Prognosis

Because of the potentially aggressive biologic behavior and life-threatening sequelae, surgical removal should be recommended for any dog with a pheochromocytoma. Median survival is 15 months for dogs undergoing adrenalectomy for pheochromocytoma.[20] The patient should be stabilized before surgical therapy with medications such as phenoxybenzamine, an α-adrenergic blocker.[21-23] For patients with tachycardia or cardiac arrhythmias, β-blocking agents such as propranolol are indicated.[21,23,24] It is imperative that β-adrenergic blockade is not attempted without prior α-adrenergic blockade to avoid life-threatening hypertension.[21,25] Ideally, anesthesia and surgery should only be performed by individuals with great familiarity and experience with the management of pheochromocytoma.

ADRENAL TUMORS IN CATS

Incidence/Etiology/Risk Factors

Adrenal tumors are infrequent, with cortisol and aldosterone being the most commonly produced hormones.[26] Pheochromocytomas are extremely rare.[27,28]

Signalment and Clinical Features

Middle-aged to older, female cats are most commonly affected. Clinical signs vary based on hormone production (see Table 26-1).[29]

Diagnosis and Staging

Diagnosis of an adrenal tumor is based on histopathology and imaging.[30] A thorough endocrinologic evaluation is indicated (see Table 26-2) in any cat with an adrenal mass. Low-dose dexamethasone (LDDS) test is the diagnostic test of choice to detect cortisol excess in cats.

Biological Behavior/Metastasis

Approximately 50% of adrenal cortical tumors in cats are carcinomas.[26,29] Reports of metastasis are infrequent.[31]

Therapy and Prognosis

Adrenalectomy is the recommended treatment for adrenal tumors in cats.[32] There are reports of successful alleviation of clinical signs using trilostane in cats with cortisol-secreting adrenal tumors.[33-35] Prognosis is guarded to grave for cats with functional adrenal tumors producing cortisol or androgens.[29,32]

For cats with aldosterone-secreting adrenal tumors, hypertension and/or hypokalemia should be corrected prior to invasive therapy. Spironolactone (an aldosterone antagonist) and potassium supplementation can be used to stabilize the patient pre-operatively or as long-term medical management, with reported survival times of 1- to 3 years.[26,36] Adrenalectomy is definitive therapy, and for cats surviving the immediate post-operative period, survival times of 1 to 8 years have been reported.[26,37]

PITUITARY TUMORS IN DOGS

Pituitary tumors include growth hormone–producing somatotroph adenomas and adrenocorticotropic hormone (ACTH)–producing corticotroph adenomas. Carcinomas are rare. Pituitary adenomas in dogs are classified based on diameter as microadenomas (< 1 cm) or macroadenomas (> 1 cm).

Incidence/Etiology and Risk Factors

Corticotroph adenomas are by far the most common type of pituitary tumor in dogs. Corticotroph carcinomas and somatotroph adenomas are rare.[38-40]

Signalment and Clinical Features

Pituitary tumors are more common in middle-aged to older dogs, with females being slightly overrepresented. Clinical findings related to pituitary dependent HAC are similar to those seen with cortisol-secreting adrenal cortical tumors (see Table 26-1). Dogs with pituitary macroadenomas may present with neurologic signs including disorientation, ataxia, inappetence, circling, pacing, seizures, facial nerve deficits, stupor, head pressing, and adipsia.[41,42]

Diagnosis and Staging

Diagnosis of a pituitary tumor has been reviewed elsewhere.[43] Identification of a macroadenoma alters management and prognosis, so early detection is imperative. Both CT and MRI have been used to evaluate pituitary adenoma size.[41,42,44-46] Elevated plasma pro-opiomelanocortin and pro-adrenocorticotropin concentrations may be used to detect macroadenomas as well.[47]

Biological Behavior/Metastasis

Local tumor growth has the greatest effect on morbidity and mortality. Macroadenomas are identified in 50% of dogs with pituitary-dependent HAC.[45]

Therapy and Prognosis

Medical management for pituitary corticotroph microadenomas focuses on controlling excessive hormone secretion and has been reviewed elsewhere.[48] Because of a lack of efficacy, L-deprenyl (Anipryl) is not recommended.[48,49] Hypophysectomy is a successful treatment for dogs with pituitary microadenomas, but operative mortality can be high.[42,50,51]

Treatment for pituitary corticotroph macroadenomas relies on radiation therapy.[52] Although radiation therapy is successful at decreasing pituitary size, medical management of HAC is still necessary to control the hormonal effects in most dogs.

PITUITARY CORTICOTROPH TUMORS IN CATS

Incidence/Etiology and Risk Factors

Pituitary corticotroph tumors autonomously secrete ACTH and are most commonly adenomas, although carcinomas have been reported.[29,53-55] Excessive secretion of ACTH leads to stimulation of the adrenal glands and the development of HAC.[29,56]

Signalment and Clinical Features

Pituitary corticotroph tumors typically affect middle-aged to older female cats. Clinical signs (see Table 26-1) are typically associated with excessive ACTH production, although some cats will develop neurologic signs associated with tumor enlargement.

Diagnosis and Staging

A presumptive diagnosis of a pituitary tumor can be made based on appropriate clinical signs, endocrinologic testing (see Table 26-2), and imaging of the pituitary gland (CT or MRI).[53,54,57] The low-dose dexamethasone suppression test is the endocrine test of choice.

Biological Behavior/Metastasis

About 30% of cats develop a macroadenoma (defined by diameter >0.5 cm).[54]

Therapy and Prognosis

Treatment focuses on managing the hormonal consequences of pituitary corticotroph tumors. Mitotane is not efficacious.[29] There are a few reports of the use of trilostane for the successful management of pituitary-dependent HAC in cats.[58] Hypophysectomy or radiation therapy are definitive therapies.[53,54] Survival time with radiation therapy ranges from 5.5 to 20.5 months.[53] Seventy percent of cats undergoing hypophysectomy have long-term survival.[54]

PITUITARY SOMATOTROPH TUMORS IN CATS

Incidence/Etiology and Risk Factors

Pituitary somatotroph adenomas producing growth hormone most commonly affect neutered male cats over 8 years of age.[59] Acromegaly, which is excessive production of growth hormone, is associated with insulin resistance and growth stimulation.

Signalment and Clinical Features

All patients will present for uncontrolled diabetes mellitus but are rarely ketotic and often gain weight despite poor diabetic regulation.[57,59,60] Secondary hypertrophic cardiomyopathy and arthropathies are common.[59,60] Occasionally, cats will present for neurologic signs caused by tumor expansion.[59]

Diagnosis and Staging

Diagnosis is made based on clinical signs, serum IGF-1 or GH concentration, and imaging.[57,59,61]

Biological Behavior/Metastasis

Growth rate appears to be variable and metastasis rare.

Therapy and Prognosis

Radiation therapy or hypophysectomy are the best treatment modalities for cats with acromegaly.[53,61-63] Survival time ranges from 4 to 20 months (median, 20.5 months).[59]

Selected References*

Feldman EC, Nelson RW: *Canine and feline endocrinology and reproduction*, ed 3, St Louis, 2004, Elsevier.
This book contains a concise and complete review of canine and feline pituitary and adrenal gland disorders including information pertaining to diagnosis and treatment.

▌ *For a complete list of the references cited in this chapter, please go to www.smallanimaloncology.com

SECTION B: Thyroid Tumors

Jeffrey N. Bryan, Amy E. DeClue

KEY POINTS

- Thyroid carcinomas in dogs respond well to therapy with long survival times possible after appropriate surgery, radiation, and radioiodine therapy.
- Fixed, irregular thyroid masses in cats are likely to be malignant carcinomas, rather than benign adenomas.
- Metastatic thyroid carcinoma may be treated with radioiodine (^{131}I) if the lesions accumulate pertechnetate on a thyroid nuclear medicine scan.

Incidence/Etiology and Risk Factors

Thyroid neoplasia occurs more commonly in cats than dogs. In cats, tumors are most commonly benign adenomas, with carcinomas occurring much less frequently. In dogs, the tumors are most commonly follicular carcinomas, with medullary c-cell carcinomas occurring less frequently.[1,2] Carcinosarcoma, a poorly differentiated form of neoplasia with both epithelial and mesenchymal characteristics, is reported in dogs.[3] Thyroid neoplasia has been associated with experimental radiation exposure in beagle dogs.[4,5] A family of dogs of Alaskan malamute descent was observed to have a familial form of medullary carcinoma.[6] In cats, the consumption of a high proportion of canned food, exposure to pesticides, and presence of dental disease have been epidemiologically associated with the development of hyperthyroidism.[7,8] A causative agent has not been identified. A somatic mutation that is associated with hyperthyroidism has been identified in cats, and trisomy 18 has been identified in thyroid carcinomas of dogs.[9,10]

Signalment and Clinical Features

Adenomas have been reported to occur in dogs and cats at a mean age of 10.7 and 12.4 years, respectively.[11] Follicular carcinomas tend to occur in younger dogs (9 years) and older cats (15.8 years).[11] Beagles, boxers, and Golden retrievers are at greater-than-average risk for follicular carcinomas, whereas miniature and toy poodles appear to be at less-than-average risk.[12] Tumors in dogs commonly appear as cervical masses but can be located from the base of the tongue to the base of the heart.[13-15] These masses can be mobile or fixed in nature. Dogs with hyperthyroidism may exhibit tachycardia or tachypnea, behavioral changes, and weight loss despite an increased appetite.[16] Intrathoracic hemorrhage, leading to thrombocytopenia, has been reported in a dog with thyroid carcinoma.[17] In cats, thyroid masses are typically movable and well demarcated. Fixed or irregular masses are often malignant in nature.

Diagnosis and Staging

An algorithm outlining diagnosis and therapy options for canine thyroid carcinoma is provided in Figure 26-1. Diagnosis of thyroid neoplasia in dogs or cats can be facilitated by identifying a hyperthyroid condition.[16] The presence of a cervical mass along with elevated serum T3 or T4 concentration is reasonably diagnostic for thyroid neoplasia in either species. Elevated serum thyroid hormone concentration is far more common in cats than in dogs.[1] The diagnosis may be supported by further imaging, either anatomical by CT or ultrasound, or functional by pertechnetate scan.[18-20] Cytology may be diagnostic for thyroid carcinoma, but blood contamination often prevents accurate diagnosis. Biopsy from surgical excision is the ideal diagnostic test. Histopathological examination can determine follicular or medullary origin of the mass and identify evidence of vascular or lymphatic invasion.

Key Fact

Contrast agents used in CT imaging will interfere with nuclear medicine scans and radioiodine therapy for thyroid carcinoma. Accordingly, timing of diagnostic procedures must be planned in advance, and nuclear scintigraphy should be performed first if ^{131}I therapy is being considered.

Staging of thyroid carcinoma should be accomplished by careful cervical palpation, thoracic radiography, complete blood count, chemistry profile, urinalysis, serum thyroid hormone (total T4, free T4, or T3) measurement, and, for dogs, thyroid-stimulating hormone (TSH) assay. Abdominal ultrasound or radiography may be performed if signs referable to the abdomen are present, if serum chemistry profile suggests that abdominal organs are diseased, or if there is a palpable mass in the

Palpable Thyroid Mass

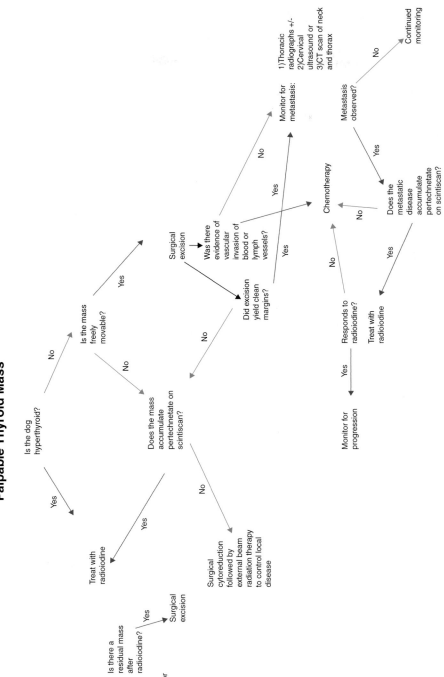

FIGURE 26-1 Algorithm for case management of dogs with thyroid carcinoma.

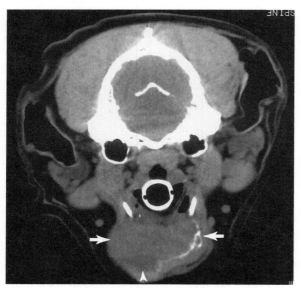

FIGURE 26-2 Computed tomography (CT) images show extent *(white arrows)* of a thyroid carcinoma in a dog. A cavitary portion of the mass *(arrowhead)* can be appreciated with the aid of these CT images.

abdomen. Complete evaluation of the cervical mass should include CT (Figure 26-2) or MRI of the affected region to determine which, if any, cervical structures are involved and whether the mass is resectable. Use of iodinated contrast agents may saturate thyroid iodine receptors, preventing adequate functional scan or successful treatment with radioiodine. Because the contrast agent for CT is iodine based, MRI using gadolinium as the contrast agent may be preferable. Therapy with radioiodine should follow iodinated contrast administration by at least 3 weeks to be most effective. Pertechnetate scintigraphy is recommended to evaluate the functional nature of the tumor, and to screen for metastases or ectopic foci. This is accomplished by injecting $^{99m}TcO_4$- intravenously at a licensed facility with a gamma camera for imaging. This radiopharmaceutical mimics iodine and undergoes trapping by the thyroid cells. Unlike iodine, however, it cannot be organified into thyroid hormone, so it does not evaluate that portion of iodine metabolism. Its accumulation in tumor cells models the distribution of iodine. Although helpful for identifying metastatic masses, at least one study did not find scintigraphy to be more sensitive than thoracic radiography for detecting pulmonary metastasis.[18]

Biological Behavior/Metastasis

Medullary thyroid carcinomas may behave less aggressively than follicular carcinomas but still can have metastatic potential.[21,22] Follicular thyroid carcinoma can be widely metastatic. Metastases have been reported in the lungs, bone, draining lymph nodes, and brain, but skin or internal organs may be affected as well.[23] The histopathological description should include mention of vascular and lymphatic invasion if present. Pulmonary metastasis is not necessarily associated with a poor prognosis, and should not automatically result in a grave prognosis.[24,25]

Therapy and Prognosis

Dogs with freely movable thyroid carcinomas treated with surgery alone have been reported to have a median survival of greater than 36 months.[26] Surgery may be beneficial, even with fixed or ectopic masses, and should be attempted by an experienced surgeon, if possible.[14] Potential complications associated with surgery include hemorrhage, damage to the vagosympathetic trunk, damage to the recurrent laryngeal nerve, and incomplete resection of the mass. If surgery results in incomplete resection it should be followed by radiation therapy. For dogs with negative pertechnetate scans, external beam irradiation should be chosen over radioiodine therapy. Dogs with invasive thyroid carcinoma treated with external beam irradiation have been reported to experience a median survival of 24.5 months with surgery, and progression-free survival rates as high as 72% at 3 years, even without surgery.[27,28] Coarse-fractionated radiation therapy has been reported as well, with a median survival of 96 weeks. In this series, presence of thoracic metastatic disease was not prognostic for survival.[24]

For dogs with positive pertechnetate scans, radioiodine may be considered. Radioiodine has been used as a sole therapy for non-resectable thyroid carcinoma, resulting in a median survival of 366 days for dogs with metastasis, and 839 days for dogs without metastasis.[29] These results were similar to an Australian study that reported 30-month median survival time for dogs receiving only ^{131}I, compared with only 3 months for dogs receiving no treatment at all.[30] Dogs should have a positive pertechnetate scan to be considered candidates for ^{131}I therapy, but need not be clinically hyperthyroid, and may even be hypothyroid (Figure 26-3).[29] Radioiodine therapy is generally well tolerated, but severe, even fatal, myelosuppression may occur, suggesting that any adjuvant chemotherapy should be delayed

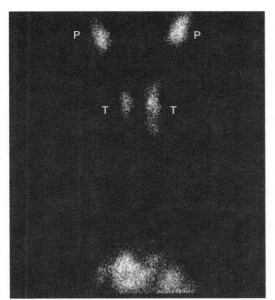

FIGURE 26-3 Ventral cervical view of pertechnetate scan of a Golden retriever with metastatic thyroid carcinoma. Uptake is present in the parotid salivary glands *(P)* at a similar intensity to the thyroid glands *(T)*. The activity visible at the bottom of the image is thoracic metastatic disease. (Courtesy of the University of Missouri Oncology Service.)

until full marrow recovery after ^{131}I administration. For metastatic thyroid carcinoma, ^{131}I may effect long-term control of the disease. A pertechnetate scan should be performed before therapy (Figure 26-4). In cases in which pertechnetate accumulation is present, ^{131}I is the treatment of choice.

Cats with thyroid carcinoma may be treated with surgery, radioiodine, external beam irradiation, or a combination of these modalities. Radioiodine therapy for thyroid carcinoma requires much higher doses than standard hyperthyroidism treatment, limiting availability to only those centers with appropriate approval (see Table 10-1 for information regarding sites for canine and feline radioiodine therapy). This option offers the hope of survival greater than 1 year in most cases.[31,32] Radioiodine therapy is most appropriate for cats with documented hyperthyroidism with positive pertechnetate scintigraphy.[32] Surgical reduction of palpable masses may improve the clinical status of hyperthyroid cats before radioiodine administration.[31] A cat with thyroid carcinoma without a positive pertechnetate scan was reported to have been managed effectively with surgery and external beam irradiation.[32]

Chemotherapy has been used to treat unresectable or metastatic canine thyroid carcinoma. Doxorubicin, cisplatin, and actinomycin D have been reported to

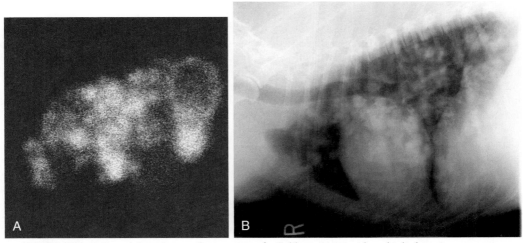

FIGURE 26-4 A, Lateral thoracic pertechnetate scan of a Golden retriever with multiple thoracic metastases. This dog was considered a suitable candidate for ^{131}I therapy. The largest mass on the image at the right edge is the stomach. **B,** The lateral thoracic radiograph is provided for comparison. (Courtesy of the University of Missouri Oncology Service.)

cause an objective response in measurable disease.[33-36] However, no study has shown a survival benefit to chemotherapy treatment. The author's current recommendation is to reserve chemotherapy for those cases of unresectable primary or metastatic disease that do not show uptake on pertechnetate scan, and for those completely or partially resected cases that demonstrate vascular or lymphatic invasion on histopathology. Optimal protocols have not been published. The author uses either doxorubicin or cisplatin as single agents at the standard dosage and frequency of administration for other malignancies.

Management Considerations

Following surgery and radiation therapy, the authors recommend maintaining dogs on thyroid supplementation indefinitely to suppress TSH secretion, a potential trophic hormone for follicular carcinoma. Measured plasma T4 levels should be maintained in the normal range, and measured TSH levels should be low. Patients receiving external beam radiation therapy may experience laryngeal, tracheal, or esophageal irritation. Clients should be advised before therapy about potential long-term complications that might affect voice or swallowing, although these are generally uncommon.[27,28] Hypothyroidism should be anticipated, but signs will be avoided with appropriate thyroid supplementation after radiation therapy.

Selected References*

Guptill L, Scott-Moncrieff CR, Janovitz EB, et al: Response to high-dose radioactive iodine administration in cats with thyroid carcinoma that had previously undergone surgery, *J Am Vet Med Assoc* 207:1055, 1995.
This paper demonstrated the benefit of radioiodine therapy and surgery, in combination, for cats with thyroid carcinomas causing hyperthyroidism.
Pack L, Roberts RE, Dawson SD, et al: Definitive radiation therapy for infiltrative thyroid carcinoma in dogs, *Vet Radiol Ultrasound* 42:471, 2001.
This paper describes the treatment of invasive thyroid carcinoma in dogs by external beam irradiation, resulting in a 2-year median survival.
Turrel JM, McEntee MC, Burke BP, et al: Sodium iodide I 131 treatment of dogs with nonresectable thyroid tumors: 39 cases (1990-2003), *J Am Vet Med Assoc* 229:542, 2006.
This study evaluated radioiodine for treating unresectable thyroid carcinomas in dogs, resulting in good control and prolonged survival.

■ *For a complete list of the references cited in this chapter, please go to www.smallanimaloncology.com

---

SECTION C: Parathyroid Tumors

Jeffrey N. Bryan and Amy E. DeClue

KEY POINTS

- The most common presenting complaints associated with parathyroid tumors are polyuria/polydipsia caused by hypercalcemia and pollakiuria or stranguria resulting from oxalate urolithiasis.
- The prognosis for patients with parathyroid tumors treated by surgery or ablation before the development of renal compromise is good, although post-treatment hypocalcemia must be managed carefully.
- Extremely elevated total calcium has been associated with increased risk of renal failure.

Incidence/Morbidity and Mortality

The development of primary hyperparathyroidism is uncommon in veterinary patients. The primary forms of neoplasia responsible for this are parathyroid adenomas and parathyroid carcinomas. The benign form may be difficult to distinguish from hyperplasia and appears to be more common than malignant forms.

Etiology/Risk Factors

Keeshond dogs are at increased risk for hyperparathyroidism.[1] Parathyroid hyperplasia is a feature of Type 2a multiple endocrine neoplasia of humans. A similar syndrome has been reported in dogs; however, the genetic etiology associated with the human syndrome has not been identified in canines.[2]

Clinical Features

Dogs and cats with parathyroid neoplasia generally present for signs referable to hypercalcemia. Polyuria/polydipsia may be seen, as well as stranguria or pollakiuria, often associated with oxalate urolithiasis.[1,3] It is rare that clients notice a cervical mass. The average age of 211 dogs with primary hyperparathyroidism was 11.2 years.[1] In cats, hyperparathyroidism has been observed in association with concurrent hyperthyroidism.[4] Primary hyperparathyroidism must be differentiated from other causes of hypercalcemia (Table 26-4).

TABLE 26-4 DIFFERENTIAL DIAGNOSES FOR HYPERCALCEMIA

	Disease	Dogs	Cats
Endocrine	Hypoadrenocorticism	X	X
Idiopathic			X
Infectious	Feline infectious peritonitis		X
	Toxoplasmosis		X
	Actinomyces		X
	Cryptococcosis		X
	Schistosomiasis	X	
	Blastomycosis	X	
Neoplasia	Lymphoma	X	X
	Thymoma	X	
	Multiple myeloma	X	X
	Leukemia	X	
	Squamous cell carcinoma	X	X
	Mammary carcinoma	X	
	Nasal carcinoma	X	
	Bronchogenic carcinoma		X
	Apocrine gland anal sac adenocarcinoma	X	
	Melanoma	X	
	Osteosarcoma	X	X
	Fibrosarcoma		X
	Parathyroid tumor	X	X
Toxic	Vitamin D toxicity	X	X
	Vitamin A toxicity	X	X
	Calcium supplementation	X	X

Diagnosis and Staging

Primary hyperparathyroidism should be suspected when hypercalcemia is present in conjunction with hypophosphatemia.[1] A hyperparathyroid state can be confirmed by detection of a normal or elevated PTH level in the face of elevated ionized calcium.[1] Development of renal insufficiency as a result of the hypercalcemia of primary hyperparathyroidism appears to be uncommon but occurs more frequently with increasing levels of total calcium.[1,5] Parathyroid tumors are most commonly diagnosed by ultrasound of the cervical region, and may be multiple.[6-8] In a study of 33 dogs, Wisner and others[6] concluded that detectable nodules > 4 mm in diameter were highly suspicious for adenoma or carcinoma, whereas nodules < 4 mm were more likely to be hyperplastic lesions. Double-phase scintigraphy has been used to identify a parathyroid adenoma in a dog.[9] However, this imaging modality has been demonstrated to be insensitive with an overall accuracy of only 27%, and ultrasound is the preferred method of diagnosis.[10]

Metastasis

No case of metastatic parathyroid neoplasia has been recorded in the literature that the authors can find.

TABLE 26-5 MANAGEMENT OF POST-TREATMENT HYPOCALCEMIA

Recommended laboratory monitoring: Measure total calcium daily for 1 week after therapy, then twice weekly for 2 weeks, then weekly until stable. If mild hypocalcemia develops, initiate oral calcium and vitamin D supplementation. If moderate or severe (symptomatic) hypocalcemia develops, initiate intravenous calcium and oral vitamin D supplementation.

CALCIUM SUPPLEMENTATION			
Drug	Initial Dose	Comments	Reference
Calcium gluconate 10%	0.5–1.5 mL/kg to effect slowly, then 5–15 mL/kg/hr as a constant rate infusion	Use IV supplementation only for severe or symptomatic hypocalcemia. Monitor calcium 2–3 times daily while on infusion.	13
Calcium gluconate	25–50 mg/kg/day	Oral supplement	13
Calcium carbonate	25–50 mg/kg/day	Common in antacids	13
Calcium lactate	25–50 mg/kg/day	Oral supplement	13

VITAMIN D ANALOGUE SUPPLEMENTS				
Drug	Initial Dose	Maintenance Dose	Onset of Action	Reference
Calcitriol	20–30 ng/kg/day PO divided BID	5–15 ng/kg/day divided BID	As short as 1 day	13
Dihydrotachysterol	30 ng/kg daily PO once daily for 2 days, then 20 ng/kg daily PO for 2 days	10 ng/kg daily PO	Within the first week	14

Treatment Modalities

Surgery to remove the abnormal parathyroid tissue is effective in managing patients with parathyroid adenomas and carcinomas.[5] In a trial of 11 dogs, 8 were successfully treated with ultrasound-guided radiofrequency ablation.[11] Out of these 8 dogs, 2 required a second treatment, and 3 were not effectively treated using this approach. Ultrasound-guided chemical ablation has also been reported with mixed results. A trial in eight dogs treated with chemical ablation resulted in resolution of clinical disease in all dogs.[12] In another study including five dogs treated similarly, resolution of disease occurred in only two dogs.[5] This suggests that the technique may be operator dependent and require appropriate case selection.

Post-therapy hypocalcemia has been reported with every modality of tumor control. Treatment with vitamin D and calcium may be necessary, particularly for those patients with presurgical total calcium > 14 mg/dL (Table 26-5).[13]

Prognosis and Survival

The prognosis associated with parathyroid neoplasia is generally favorable. Survival times as long as 3.5 years have been reported in case series.[5] The development of renal failure associated with extremely elevated total calcium is a significant life-limiting factor in these diseases; thus, early clinical detection and treatment is critical. Malignant tumors that invade locally would also be expected to be life limiting if not amenable to surgical resection or control by radiation therapy.

Selected References*

Chew D, Nagode L: Treatment of hypoparathyroidism, In Bonagura J: *Kirk's current veterinary therapy: XIII small animal practice*, Philadelphia, 2000, WB Saunders.
This chapter provides useful information regarding clinical management of post-operative hypocalcemic complications.
Feldman EC, Hoar B, Pollard R, et al: Pretreatment clinical and laboratory findings in dogs with primary hyperparathyroidism: 210 cases (1987-2004), *J Am Vet Med Assoc* 227:756, 2005.
This is the largest retrospective study of canine primary hyperthyroidism published in the literature.
Gear RNA, Neiger R, Skelly BJS, et al: Primary hyperparathyroidism in 29 dogs: diagnosis, treatment, outcome, and associated renal failure, *J Small Anim Pract* 46:10, 2005.
This case series of dogs with primary hyperthyroidism includes treatment and outcome data.

*For a complete list of the references cited in this chapter, please go to www.smallanimaloncology.com.

SECTION D: Endocrine Pancreatic Tumors

Jeffrey N. Bryan, Amy E. DeClue

KEY POINTS

- Insulinoma and gastrinoma, although uncommon, are the most commonly observed exocrine pancreatic neoplasias in dogs and cats.
- Hypoglycemia is the most life-threatening complication of insulinoma, more so than metastatic disease.
- Zollinger-Ellison syndrome manifests as vomiting and gastrointestinal ulceration as a result of hypergastrinemia from gastrinoma.

Incidence/Morbidity and Mortality

Tumors arising from the endocrine pancreas are rare, with insulinoma and gastrinoma occurring with greatest frequency.[3,4] Other reported tumors are listed in Table 26-6.

Etiology/Risk Factors

Insulinoma and gastrinoma can occur in any breed, generally in dogs 8 to 12 years old. They are extremely rare in cats.

Clinical Features

Insulinoma is associated with profound hypoglycemia, usually causing clinical signs. Common clinical signs of insulinoma include weakness, ataxia, collapse, and seizures.[8,12] Glucose may be too low to accurately measure with cageside instruments. The hypoglycemia may be severe enough to cause structural damage to the brain.[23] Insulinoma has been associated with peripheral neuropathy in a dog.[28] Insulinoma was reported in a cat associated with an aldosterone-secreting adrenal tumor and a hyperplastic nodule in the parathyroid, similar to multiple endocrine neoplasia type I in humans.[20] Gastrinomas are classically associated with Zollinger-Ellison syndrome where elevated gastrin levels lead to gastroduodenal ulcers.[7] Gastrinomas are most commonly reported in the pancreas, but one was reported to arise from the duodenum, leading to common bile duct obstruction.[30]

Diagnosis and Staging

Insulinoma is diagnosed clinically by demonstrating hypoglycemia in the face of normal or increased plasma insulin concentration. Although more sensitive, the amended insulin/glucose ratio is less specific and not recommended.[13] One case report used decreased fructosamine levels to demonstrate the presence of chronic hypoglycemia.[25] Low fructosamine was used to detect an insulinoma in a normoglycemic dog.[16] Ultrasound, CT, and single photon emission tomography (SPECT) using radiolabeled somatostatin analogues were evaluated for imaging insulinomas in the pancreas.[21] Ultrasound and SPECT were found to be equivalent, with CT demonstrating greater sensitivity, but also yielding false-positive results for lymph node metastasis.[21] The authors deemed intraoperative inspection and palpation to be the most useful tools for definitive detection in cases with a high index of suspicion.[21] Planar scintigraphy has also been reported using radiolabeled somatostatin analogue to detect insulinoma.[6,14] In a comparison of radiography and ultrasonography, the sensitivity of ultrasound was 75% for detection of pancreatic masses, compared with only 19% for radiography.[12] Ultrasound was able to detect masses as small as 0.4 cm in cats with pancreatic neoplasia, although none had endocrine neoplasia.[9] Since clinical signs of gastrinoma are often severe with a relatively small tumor burden, elevated gastrin levels in the face of normal renal function should prompt exploratory laparotomy.[7]

Pancreatic islet cell tumors and their metastases have been shown to stain positively for chromogranin A with immunohistochemistry.[18] This same study demonstrated positive levels of chromogranin A in the plasma of two dogs with insulinoma.[18] This test is not currently commercially available.

Metastasis

Insulinomas commonly metastasize to the liver and local lymph nodes.[21]

Treatment Modalities

Therapy for insulinoma has two aims: first, manage the hypoglycemia; second, control the tumor. See Table 26-7 for medications used to manage hypoglycemia.

TABLE 26-6   UNCOMMON TUMOR TYPES THAT MAY BE PRESENT IN THE PANCREAS

Tumor Type	Secreted Product	Clinical Syndrome	Reference
Neuroendocrine (type not specified)	ACTH	Cushing's disease in a dog	5
Pancreatic pseudocyst	None	Biliary obstruction; reported in dogs and cats	15,24,29
Endocrine carcinoma	Pancreatic lipase	Elevated lipase in 2 dogs with endocrine carcinoma	19
Glucagonoma	Glucagon	Necrolytic dermatitis in a dog	1,26,27
Endocrine carcinoma	Multihormonally secreting	European Lynx	11

*ACTH, Adrenocorticotropic hormone.

TABLE 26-7   DRUGS USED TO MANAGE HYPOGLYCEMIA IN PATIENTS WITH INSULINOMA

Drug	Dosage	Indication
50% Dextrose in water	1–2 mL/kg IV	Profound hypoglycemia or seizures. Must support plasma glucose after administration with D_5W.
Prednisone	0.25 mg/kg PO BID	Counter-regulatory hormone results in increased blood glucose concentration. May increase as body becomes acclimatized.
Diazoxide	5 mg/kg PO BID	Decreases insulin secretion, promotes gluconeogenesis and glycogenolysis, and antagonizes insulin at tissues. May increase dose slowly to 30 mg/kg PO BID as necessary.
Hydrochlorothiazide	1–4 mg/kg PO once daily	Use in combination with diazoxide to stabilize blood glucose.
Octreotide	1 to 2 µg/kg SC BID to TID	Somatostatin analogue. May help stabilize glucose. May cause diabetes mellitus rarely.
Diet	Feed 3–4 times daily	Feed multiple small meals high in protein and fat, and low in carbohydrates.

BOX 26-1   STREPTOZOTOCIN PROTOCOL

Seven-Hour Streptozotocin Protocol
21-day cycle for two to eight treatments
Indication: insulinoma in dogs
Pretreatment evaluation = CBC/chemistry panel/UA
Contraindications = renal failure, neutropenia,
    thrombocytopenia, diabetes mellitus
1. Fluid diuresis (3 hours) rate = 18.3 mL/kg/hr
Fluid = 0.9% NaCl_____mL/hr pre-
    treatment diuresis volume =_____mL total
2. Streptozotocin 500 mg/m^2 infused over 2 hr
Saline volume for streptozotocin dilution =
    18.3.mL/kg × 2_____mL 0.9%
    saline
Total dose streptozotocin =_____mg
3. Immediate post-treatment antiemetic:
    Butorphanol 0.4 mg/kg IM
Post-treatment diuresis (2 hr) rate = 18.3 ml/kg/hr
    fluid = 0.9% NaCl_____ml/hr
4. CBC and platelet count should be checked in
    7 to 10 days. Protocol is repeated every 21 days
    for up to 8 treatments provided the dog does
    not develop diabetes mellitus, renal failure, or
    worsening of clinical signs.

The primary tumor should be removed surgically, if possible. Streptozotocin is the primary chemotherapy for insulinoma (Box 26-1).[17] Somatostatin analogues have been used to treat both insulinomas and gastrinomas. In one study, the somatostatin analogue octreotide was able to suppress insulin levels and increase glucose levels in dogs with insulinoma.[22] Therapy of gastrinoma is primarily surgical, with medical therapy to manage the potential ulceration.

Prognosis and Survival

Prognosis for both insulinoma and gastrinoma depends on the severity and management of clinical signs. The median duration of normoglycemia in insulinoma treated with streptozotocin was 163 days.[17] Omeprazole, sucralfate, and famotidine should be used to control clinical signs of gastritis with gastrinoma.[10] Octreotide, in combination with these drugs, resulted in a 14-month survival of one dog with gastrinoma.[2] Overall, however, average survival tends to be less than 5 months.[10] Early stage tumors of both types will likely have longer survival.

Selected References*

Hughes SM: Canine gastrinoma: a case study and literature review of therapeutic options, *N Z Vet J* 54:242, 2006.
This is a case report and review of canine gastrinoma.
Meleo KA, Caplan ER: Treatment of insulinoma in the dog, cat, ferret. In Bonagura J: *Kirk's current veterinary therapy: XIII small animal practice*, Philadelphia, 2000, WB Saunders.
This chapter provides useful information regarding clinical management of insulinoma and its associated hypoglycemia.
Moore AS, Nelson RW, Henry CJ, et al: Streptozocin for treatment of pancreatic islet cell tumors in dogs: 17 cases (1989-1999), *J Am Vet Med Assoc* 221:811, 2002.
This retrospective study established the safety of streptozotocin for treatment of canine insulinoma.

INDEX

Page numbers followed by f indicate figures; t, tables; b, boxes.